ECHOCARDIOGRAPHIC DIAGNOSIS

ECHOCARDIOGRAPHIC DIAGNOSIS

Differential Diagnosis of M-Mode and Two-Dimensional Echographic Appearances

Ivan A. D'Cruz
M.D., F.A.C.C.
F.R.C.P. (Edin)
M.R.C.P. (Lond)

Director, Echocardiography Section and Attending Physician, Michael Reese Hospital and Medical Center, Chicago, Illinois; Associate Professor of Medicine, University of Chicago, Pritzker School of Medicine

Macmillan Publishing Company
NEW YORK

Collier Macmillan Canada, Inc.
TORONTO

Collier Macmillan Publishers
LONDON

Macmillan Publishing Company
866 Third Avenue, New York, New York 10022

Collier Macmillan Canada, Inc.
Collier Macmillan Publishers · London

Library of Congress Cataloging in Publication Data
D'Cruz, Ivan A.
   Echocardiographic diagnosis.

   Includes index.
   1. Ultrasonic cardiography.   2. Heart—Diseases—
Diagnosis.   I. Title. [DNLM: 1. Echocardiography.
2. Diagnosis, Differential. WG 141.5.E2 D277e]
RC683.5.U5D38   1983   616.1'207544   83–860
ISBN 0–02–326120–X

Printing: 1 2 3 4 5 6 7 8   Year: 3 4 5 6 7 8 9 0 1

Dedicated

to my

WIFE, SON, and DAUGHTER

Foreword

ECHOCARDIOGRAPHY during the past fifteen years has become established as one of the indispensable noninvasive techniques for the functional, anatomic, and diagnostic evaluation of the normal and diseased heart. Consequently, cardiac ultrasound equipment has proliferated rapidly into virtually every community hospital and cardiologist's office, as well as into medical centers. Unfortunately, accurate recording and interpretation of echocardiograms are not as simple as they are often represented, and the number of outstanding, in-depth training programs that can confer such expertise has not yet caught up with demand. As a result, aspiring echocardiographers have relied heavily on one or more of the available textbooks on the subject as the major source of self-education in this field. The format of most of these texts consists of a systematic description of the echocardiographic findings of each of the cardiac disease entities. Unfortunately, such information is not readily incorporable by the clinician into a differential diagnosis and a subsequent diagnostically reliable verdict.

Dr. D'Cruz, who has practical expertise and has made many original contributions in this field, has written a textbook that elegantly bridges the gap between the great mass of existing echocardiographic knowledge and practical diagnostic expertise. His method of presentation enables the clinician to become thoroughly familiar with a wide variety of M-mode and 2-D echocardiographic patterns—common and uncommon, typical and atypical—in terms of their broad clinicopathologic implications and, from this point, then to distinguish echographic patterns that are superficially similar but etiologically diverse. Mastery of this approach enables the physician to proceed readily from observation of an abnormal echocardiographic pattern to a cardiac diagnosis.

The text is clearly written, and original, idealized drawings render explicit the abnormalities presented in the many reproductions of actual echocardiograms. Invaluable features of the book are the innumerable helpful hints regarding technique that will enable the inexperienced echocardiographer to avoid pitfalls and facilitate obtaining reliable and accurate tracings. These are largely drawn from Dr. D'Cruz's own experience and not to be found in most other textbooks. In particular, the pitfalls and limitations of indices of ventricular function are presented with remarkable clarity. Finally, the thorough discussion of the differential diagnosis of abnormalities is also not readily available in other texts or reviews.

I am privileged to have been one of many who badgered Dr. D'Cruz to undertake this volume, and I could not put the manuscript down until I had read it from beginning to end. Dr. D'Cruz is to be congratulated for what I believe will become a classic contribution to mastering the art of echocardiography.

EARL N. SILBER, M.D.

Preface

SEVERAL EXCELLENT TEXTBOOKS on echocardiography are available that systematically describe the echographic findings of various cardiac entities, each in a separate chapter or subsection of a chapter, thus reviewing all previously published work topic by topic. However, in the everyday interpretation and reporting of echocardiograms, one has to form opinions promptly and make decisions, often far reaching, on the tracing at hand: Is it normal or abnormal? If abnormal, what is the diagnosis or differential diagnosis indicated by the graphic abnormalities? If two or more possibilities are suggested, are there any clues in the echographic appearances to favor one diagnosis over another?

The recognition of a specific clinical diagnosis by the identification of specific echographic patterns is not as simple and easy as it may seem to those whose acquaintance with cardiac ultrasound has been limited to the perusal of books or attendance at short courses, however intensive. In echocardiography, as in electrocardiography, there are few graphic patterns that are absolutely pathognomonic of a particular clinical diagnosis. Textbook descriptions, or textbook illustrations of "classic" cases, are not easily translated into the decision-making process that results in a confident and reliable diagnosis. To the contrary, most cardiac lesions are each capable of producing a wide variety of echographic manifestations. Although classic examples of the various abnormalities can be recognized at a glance, even by beginners, all of these entities can present as one of a broad spectrum of possible echocardiographic appearances. Thus, proficiency in the interpretation of echocardiograms requires that one become conversant with common and uncommon echocardiographic variations of every form of heart disease, and be aware of all the fallacies, pitfalls, normal variants, and technical artefacts that lurk in ambush along the echocardiographer's path. This is yet another reason why a comparison between echographic patterns that are superficially similar, but etiologically diverse, is important. The illustration of an extensive gamut of different patterns, grouped according to some common presenting feature but demonstrating also certain other distinguishing characteristics, will, it is hoped, strengthen the practical skills of physicians responsible for performing and reading echocardiograms.

When the echographic tracing reveals an abnormal finding, the question arises as to which disease state or states can cause it. If several possible diagnoses come to mind, it is important to know whether there is evidence in the echocardiogram pointing at one or another of them as being more likely. It often happens that initial echocardiographic scanning indicates a cardiac pathology very different from that originally suspected. Thus, every practitioner of cardiac ultrasound has encountered instances of important cardiac pathology in which the diagnosis had never been considered until the moment of truth in the echo laboratory. Therefore, echocardiographers have to base their diagnostic approach not only on the referring physician's suspicions but also on the echocardiographer's preliminary survey of the patient's cardiac anatomy as it unfolds during the course of the echographic procedure. That is another reason why one needs to be thoroughly familiar with a wide variety of ultrasound appearances and their clinical implications. The cardiologist should be able to think as readily from an abnormal echocardiographic pattern to a cardiac diagnosis as he can from a clinical diagnosis to its confirmation or exclusion by echocardiography.

This book is written with the aim of bridging the gap between textbook knowledge and practical diagnostic expertise. A thorough training and extensive experience are indispensable for achieving proficiency in clinical echocardiography, but it is hoped that an approach such as that developed in this work will expedite and encourage the process.

Because of limitations of space, it is not possible to present examples of every known echocardiographic abnormality; these are now so numerous that even doubling the number of illustrations in this book would not suffice. For readers who might fault the author for the omission of specific illustrations, references, or detailed discussions of instrumentation, technology, and pathophysiology, the exigency of restricted space must again be pleaded. However, important clinical implications of certain echographic findings—for example, left atrial enlargement and left ventricular hypertrophy—are amply discussed.

The echographic differential diagnosis of complex congenital heart anomalies in infancy is not dealt with in this book. However, the echocardiographic manifestations of cardiac defects that commonly present in older children and adults are included, because otherwise the differential diagnosis of certain echographic findings (such as right ventricular dilatation) would remain incomplete.

Over 95 per cent of the echocardiograms illustrated here were recorded personally by me. Most of the remainder were done by my associate in the Echocardiography Laboratory of Michael Reese Hospital and Medical Center, Leroy J. Hirsch, Ph.D., whose valuable support I have enjoyed over several years. I take this opportunity to thank Dr. W. Jacobs and Dr. G. Lalmalani, each of whom provided me with a couple of illustrations used in this book.

Without the encouragement so generously extended to me by Dr. Earl N. Silber, Acting Director of the Cardiovascular Institute, Michael Reese Hospital and Medical Center, this book would never have been written. I am indebted to Ms. Sibyl Waring for her expertise and unfailing patience with the diagrammatic illustrations. I must acknowledge the efficient running of the Echocardiography Laboratory by technicians Ms. Lola Buffkin and Ms. Frankie Mason, the typing skills of Ms. Marceine Lamb and Ms. Ora Benton, and the cooperation over the last several years of Mr. Don Macmillan of Picker International. Mr. Bruce Lesser, of Merck, Sharp & Dohme, provided valuable help in computerized retrieval of references, and my son, Paul, assisted in organization of illustrations and compilation of the Index. I take this opportunity to thank my colleagues and former fellows at Michael Reese, and also my fellow echocardiologists of the Chicago Society of Echocardiography, too numerous to mention individually, for their stimulating association over the years.

Ivan A. D'Cruz, M.D.

Contents

ECHOCARDIOGRAPHIC DIAGNOSIS

Abbreviations in Illustrations

AAR:	Anterior Aortic Root
AML:	Anterior Mitral Leaflet
AP:	Apex (of LV)
AR:	Aortic Root
AV or AoV:	Aortic Valve
CT:	Chordae Tendineae
DA:	Descending Aorta
ECG:	Electrocardiogram
EV:	Eustachian Valve
IVC:	Inferior Vena Cava
LA:	Left Atrium
LAA:	Left Atrial Appendage
LAPW:	Left Atrial Posterior Wall
LV:	Left Ventricle
LVPW:	Left Ventricular Posterior Wall
MAC:	Mitral Annulus Calcification
MV:	Mitral Valve
PAR:	Posterior Aortic Root
PCG:	Phonocardiogram
PER or P:	Pericardium
PER EFF:	Pericardial Effusion
PLEU EFF:	Pleural Effusion
PM:	Papillary Muscle
PML:	Posterior Mitral Leaflet
PV:	Pulmonic Valve
RA:	Right Atrium
RV:	Right Ventricle
RVAW:	Right Ventricular Anterior Wall
THR:	Thrombus
TUM:	Tumor
TV:	Tricuspid Valve
VS:	Ventricular Septum

A

Practical Aspects of Echocardiographic Recording

The following brief remarks pertain to various practical considerations in the performance of M-mode and two-dimensional (2-D) echocardiograms. For a detailed discussion of the physical principles underlying cardiac ultrasound, its instrumentation, and technique, the reader is referred to other works, notably to that of Feigenbaum (1981) and of Weyman (1982).

TRANSDUCERS

1. For routine M-mode echography in adults, a focused transducer 0.5 inch in diameter and 2.25 megahertz (MHz) is used.

2. In very large, obese, or emphysematous patients, a 1.6 MHz transducer may be more suitable because it has greater ultrasound penetration; the little that one sacrifices in fine resolution is usually acceptable.

3. In children between approximately two and eight years, a 3.5 MHz transducer is suitable; in infants, a 5 MHz one is best. These higher frequencies have better resolution capability, yet sufficient penetration for pediatric purposes. Occasionally one encounters a very thin, small adult in whom the 3.5 MHz transducer is effective. Another application of the 3.5 MHz transducer in adults is to obtain optimal resolution of right ventricular (RV) structures as, for example, in measuring RV anterior wall thickness.

4. For routine 2-D echography with mechanical oscillating scanners, ultrasound crystals of the same frequency (2.25 MHz) as those for M-mode echography are used. However, a popular mechanical scanner of rotating type contains 3 crystals of 3.0 MHz frequency.

5. Early oscillating mechanical 2-D probes had a sector cycle of 30° only. These are still available, but the mechanical 2-D probes now in most use either are adjustable from 0 to 60°, or are of the rotating type with fixed wide sector cycles of 80 to 90°.

6. Technical improvements in transducer capability have continued to develop. Thus, "quarter wave" and "double quarter wave" transducers, which became commercially available recently, have definitely upgraded image quality and ultrasound penetration.

7. The main advantages of phased-array 2-D equipment are (a) small size of the scanning head, (b) no moving parts, (c) wide angle, (d) ability to record simultaneous 2-D and M-mode echograms, using cursors to select the M-mode site, (e) better electronic focusing.

Disadvantages are (a) higher cost, (b) larger, heavier, less portable, (c) greater incidence of certain artefacts (side-lobes), (d) inability to replace older transducers with better new transducers in the scan head. (Buying a whole new scan head is rather expensive.)

8. The main advantages of mechanical 2-D scanning equipment are (a) less cost, (b) small, lighter, more portable machines that facilitate transport, (c) easily changed ultrasound crystal component of the scan head. Thus, the same 2-D oscillating probe can be used for adults, children, and infants by removing the 2.25 MHz crystal and replacing it with the 3.5 or 5 MHz one, an easy maneuver taking only a couple of minutes.

Disadvantages of mechanical scanners are (a) noise and vibration in oscillating (but not rotating) equipment, (b) narrow angle in oscillating (but not rotating) scan heads, (c) unfeasibility of simultaneous M-mode and 2-D recordings, (d) artefactual echoes produced by the plastic casing of the scan head, (d) bubble formation in the oil surrounding the rotating element, (f) fatigue with continued use of the wiring or other moving parts of oscillating or vibrating scanners.

POSITION OF PATIENT

1. Some years ago it was customary to place the patient supine, but better visualization of cardiac structures is obtained consistently with the patient partly turned to the left. Consequently, it is now routine in most centers to turn the patient so that his upper back makes a 30° angle with the horizontal, a pillow supporting the right shoulder. Very often good visualization of the ventricular septum and of the left ventricular chamber can be achieved only with a greater degree (60 to 90°) of left lateral rotation.

Caution: In the left lateral position the ultrasound beam tends to traverse the right ventricle very obliquely so that this chamber erroneously may appear large. The patient should be completely supine for proper right ventricular dimension recording.

2. Occasionally the echocardiographic examination is done with the patient sitting up, not from choice but because of orthopnea. The sitting position is also useful in patients with posterior pericardial effusions, to ascertain whether fluid moves into the anterior pericardial space, thus demonstrating that it is not loculated.

3. Care should be taken to see that the patient is comfortable and relaxed. This ensures a smooth ECG baseline without artefacts due to skeletal muscle contraction.

SITES FOR SCANNING (ECHOCARDIOGRAPHIC "WINDOWS") (Fig. A-1)

1. The window used for routine scanning is the left *parasternal,* corresponding to the anterior "bare area" of the heart. The remainder of the heart is separated from the chest wall by intervening lung tissue, through which ultrasound cannot pass. The ultrasound transducer is positioned over one of the left intercostal spaces, near the left sternal border. In normal children and young adults, cardiac echoes can usually be obtained from the second to fifth left intercostal spaces, but in elderly persons and those with some degree of pulmonary emphysema (chronic bronchitis, asthmatics, heavy smokers, and so forth), the echocardiographic window shrinks in size so that only the lower intercostal spaces are usable. In some cases, the best left parasternal window is found not at the left sternal border but near the left midclavicular line, presumably because the heart comes closest to the chest wall at this site. If no cardiac echoes can be seen from the left parasternal region, the following possibilities may be considered (Fig. A-2): (a) the left lung covers the heart completely, (b) there is gross shift of the mediastinum to the right, (c) the patient has congenital dextrocardia, (d) previous thoracic surgery or radiation therapy has produced dense fibrosis and perhaps grossly distorted normal anatomy, (e) extreme obesity, (f) the alignment of the left ventricle (LV) with the anterior chest wall is unfavorable for echographic viewing, i.e., the LV long axis tends to be perpendicular rather than parallel to the

ECHOCARDIOGRAPHIC "WINDOWS"

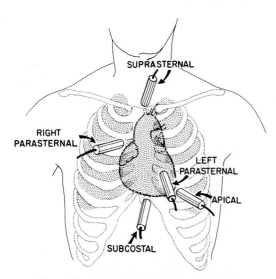

Fig. A-1. Diagram showing the various "windows" used in clinical echocardiography to scan the heart, in M-mode as well as 2-D techniques. The left parasternal is the standard site; the other sites are employed in special circumstances or for specific purposes.

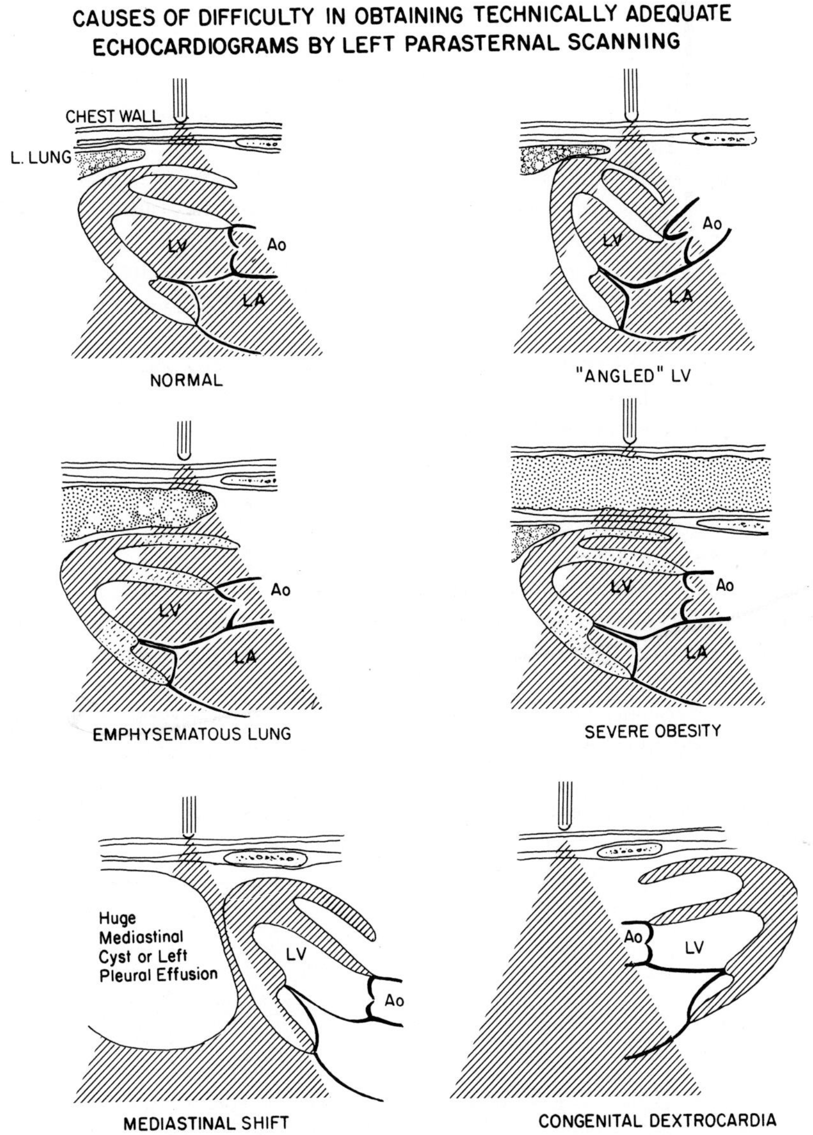

CAUSES OF DIFFICULTY IN OBTAINING TECHNICALLY ADEQUATE
ECHOCARDIOGRAMS BY LEFT PARASTERNAL SCANNING

Fig. A-2. Diagram illustrating causes of difficulty in obtaining adequate visualization of the heart from the standard left parasternal site. The normal situation is shown at top left, abnormal alignment of the heart with the chest wall at top right. Lung intervenes between transducer and heart (*center left*) in emphysema; fat can do so in obese subjects (*center right*). Displacement of the heart toward the right hemithorax can be due to mediastinal shift (*bottom left*) or to congenital anomaly (*bottom right*).

chest wall. This variant recently has been described as "angled septum."

Further attempts to visualize cardiac structures should be made (a) with the patient turned to a fully left lateral position, or (b) by the subcostal approach, or (c) if the echographic information desired is crucial and someone with equipment and experience in esophageal echocardiography is available, this technique may be considered, provided the discomfort of this approach is acceptable to the patient.

When satisfactory echoes cannot be obtained from the left parasternal region, or in certain specific situations, other echocardiographic windows are worth trying:

2. The *subcostal* (also called subxiphoid) approach is best done with the patient supine and the abdominal muscles relaxed. The transducer is placed in the upper epigastrium, pressed firmly back, and directed upward toward the patient's head with a little posterior and leftward tilt. The most suitable patient for this approach is a thin one with a scaphoid abdomen and lax abdominal wall. Obese patients with tense protuberant abdomens are least suitable. Pulmonary emphysema may actually facilitate subcostal echography by lowering the diaphragm and thereby bringing the heart closer to the transducer.

3. In *suprasternal echography,* it is convenient to place a pillow under the patient's shoulders and upper back so that his neck is extended. This facilitates manipulation of the transducer in the groove just above the manubrium, sternum, and clavicles. The transducer is positioned in the suprasternal notch and pressed firmly back so that the mediastinal structures posterior to the sternum can be explored. Suprasternal echography is appropriate for viewing the aortic arch and right pulmonary artery. It can also depict the left atrium in its superoinferior axis. Two-D echography by this approach often can provide good visualization of all upper mediastinal structures: aorta, right

pulmonary artery, superior vena cava, and brachiocephalic veins. Of particular interest to pediatric cardiologists are the possible diagnoses of a patent ductus and anomalous pulmonary venous channels.

4. The *right supraclavicular* approach provides a view very much like the suprasternal one. However, it is used only for visualizing the motion of prosthetic aortic valves, particularly the Starr-Edwards ball valve, which is not well perceived by left parasternal scanning. The transducer is pressed firmly back in the groove between the sternal and clavicular leads of the right sternomastoid muscle, i.e., above and behind the medial end of the right clavicle.

5. *Right parasternal* scanning normally is not possible because the right lung intervenes between heart and chest wall. Exceptions to this rule include marked dilatation of the ascending aorta, normal infants, marked dilatation of the heart (especially of its right chambers), large pericardial effusions, and mediastinal shift to the right. It has been used with advantage to visualize aortic root aneurysms, also to explore the atria and atrial septum.

6. M-mode echography from the cardiac

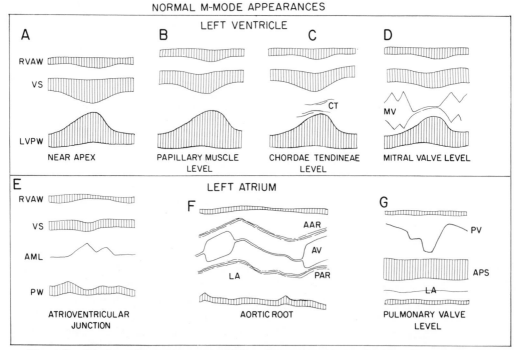

Fig. A-3. Diagrams illustrating normal M-mode appearances, progressing from the apex to the base of the left ventricle (*upper*), then to the atrioventricular junction (*lower left*), and finally to the aortic root (*lower center*) and pulmonary artery (*lower right*). Note that the posterior chamber in all 3 lower diagrams is the left atrium.

apex has been employed to record motion of prosthetic aortic valves, as for instance the Starr-Edwards ball valve. The transducer is placed at the point where the apical cardiac impulse is best felt and directed toward the base of the heart. Two-D echography from the cardiac apex (Silverman and Schiller, 1978) has become established as an extremely important part of the routine echographic examination.

The precise sequence in which the different cardiac structures are visualized need not follow a fixed protocol or ritual. The echocardiographer should first note the salient clinical features and diagnostic impression of the referring clinician. The echographer's attention and efforts then can be tailored to the specific questions that arise in that patient.

Most echocardiographers seek the mitral valve first, record motion of its anterior and posterior leaflets, then scan medially and upward toward the aortic root and left atrium as well as leftward and inferiorly to visualize the left ventricle below the mitral valve level.

The pulmonic valve is sought by tilting the transducer upward toward the left clavicle or shoulder. The tricuspid valve is found by angulating the transducer as acutely as possible rightward and somewhat inferiorly toward the patient's liver.

Normal patterns on M-mode and 2-D echography are depicted diagrammatically in Figures A-3 and A-4, respectively. Two-D echographic terminology is based on the Report of the American Society of Echocardiography (Henry *et al.*, 1980).

M-mode measurements are made as shown in Figure A-5, based on the standards adopted by the American Society of Echocardiography (Sahn *et al.*, 1978). In these diagrams, ARD = aortic root dimension; LAD = left atrial dimension; PEP = preejection period; EP = ejection period (of left ventricle); RVID = right ventricular internal dimension; LVID = left ventricular internal dimension; ST = septal thickness; LVWT = left ventricular wall thickness. The latter three measurements are made

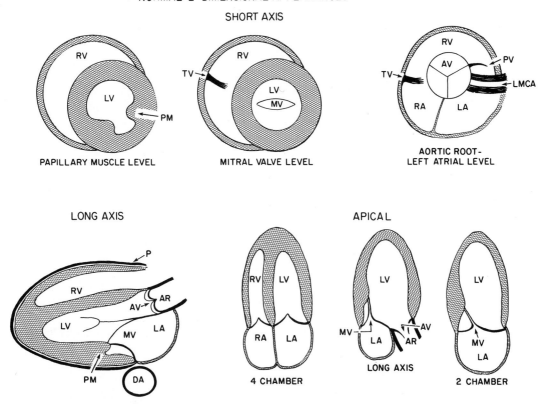

NORMAL 2-DIMENSIONAL APPEARANCES

Fig. A-4. Diagram depicting normal 2-D echographic appearances in the short-axis view (*upper*), the long-axis view (*lower left*), and apical views (*lower right*).

M-MODE ECHOGRAPHIC MEASUREMENTS

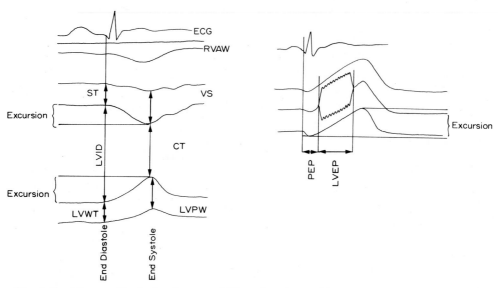

Fig. A-5.   Diagram illustrating how some M-mode echographic measurements are made: ventricular dimensions and wall thickness on the left, aortic root excursions and systolic time intervals on the right.

at end-diastole (onset of QRS on the ECG) as well as at end-systole (smallest LV dimension).

ADJUSTMENT OF OSCILLOSCOPE AND RECORDER CONTROLS

There is no substitute for "hands-on" experience and learning how to use the controls of any one machine to best advantage. A talent for obtaining echocardiographic recordings of scientific and esthetic merit has to be cultivated by long practice and meticulous attention to detail.

The following are merely some useful practical hints:

1. The near gain should be properly suppressed so as to obtain a well-defined right ventricular anterior wall and right ventricular chamber. Beginners tend to leave the right ventricle (RV) cluttered with unnecessary obscuring echoes, or to suppress all near echoes so much that the RV wall and even perhaps the right side of the ventricular septum are not seen at all.

2. Likewise, the region of the left ventricular posterior wall and pericardium may be so overfilled by dense echoes reflected from the pericardial-lung interface that it is impossible to ascertain whether pericardial effusion or pericardial thickening is present or not. Proper adjustment of the damping control will promptly clarify the situation.

3. At some stage of the echographic examination, the scale should be reduced so as to view the space behind the heart and not miss a pericardial effusion, pleural effusion, or pseudoaneurysm, any of which can present as a retrocardiac echo-free space (Fig. A-6). On the other hand, the scale may have to be expanded to demonstrate details of fine vibratory motion, such as diastolic flutter of the mitral valve or ventricular septum, that might have been equivocal or overlooked on an attenuated scale.

4. A paper speed of 25 mm/sec is usually adequate for most of the echographic tracing; 50 mm/sec may be needed if the heart rate is very fast. Faster paper speeds (50, 75, or 100 mm/sec) are necessary when time intervals are being measured as, for example, the preejection and ejection periods on the aortic valve echogram. Abnormal septal motion is also better demonstrated at fast paper speed which permits easier perception of the correlation of septal motion with simultaneous contour of the ECG, mitral valve, and left ventricular posterior wall. A slow paper speed (10 mm/sec) is suitable for recording scans from apex to base of the left ventricle, or left atrium to ventricle, such

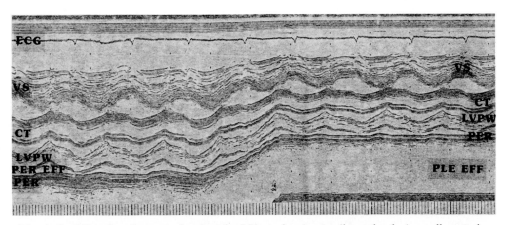

Fig. A-6. M-mode echogram showing the LV at chordae tendineae level. A small posterior pericardial effusion appears as a small echo-free space between LV posterior wall and pericardium. The unusual distortion of the echographic image in the center of the figure is due to the reduced scale. A large echo-free space is revealed posterior to the pericardium. The space represents a pleural effusion and was not evident until the scale was appropriately attenuated.

that the entire scan can be depicted within a small space, suitable for illustration or teaching purposes.

5. M-mode scans constitute an essential part of the echographic examination. Transducer direction is deliberately altered to record, in succession, different parts of the same cardiac chamber, or the transition from one chamber to another, while the recording paper is running at a constant speed. Left ventricle–left atrial scans are probably the most common. The object is to depict echographic continuity or contiguity of various cardiac valves, chambers, or walls, which in turn demonstrates or elucidates the anatomic nature of various echoes or echo-free spaces recorded. Some examples of such scans are shown here (Figs. A-8 to A-11, A-13, A-15, A-25), and numerous others appear in subsequent chapters.

In wide-angle 2-D echocardiography, the anatomic relationship of various cardiac chambers and structures visualized is usually obvious since they appear as parts of the same picture. However, deliberate scanning in a definite direction, during continuous videotape recording, does have a place in 2-D echographic technique, especially when the sector angle is 30 to 60°.

NORMAL ECHOGRAPHIC ANATOMY

Examples of normal M-mode appearances are shown in Figures A-7 to A-15, and of normal 2-D appearances in Figures A-16 to A-26.

CONTRAST ECHOCARDIOGRAPHY

When fluids are injected rapidly into a forearm vein, microbubbles are formed in the blood stream; this renders the blood "opaque" to ultrasound and so opacifies the right heart chambers (Fig. A-27). To obtain satisfactory opacification the fluid injected should be freshly drawn up in the syringe and rapidly injected as a bolus. Some claim that better results are contained with indocyanine green (1 ml in 10 ml saline); others claim saline or glucose is equally effective. At least 10 ml is needed in an adult. Although contrast echography was introduced before the era of 2-D echography, better anatomic and functional information is obtained with contrast 2-D echography than with contrast M-mode echography alone.

Contrast echography has many diagnostic uses (Nanda and Rothbard, 1981; Meltzer and Roelandt, 1982). It is used to demonstrate shunts from the right to left chambers of the heart in cyanotic heart disease. When the right atrial and ventricular chambers are densely opacified, left-to-right shunts may be detected as a stream of unopacified blood emerging through the septal defect.

PITFALLS

The interpretation of echocardiograms is beset with more potential pitfalls than most other graphic recordings. There is a real danger of overreading and of mistaking artefacts or vari-

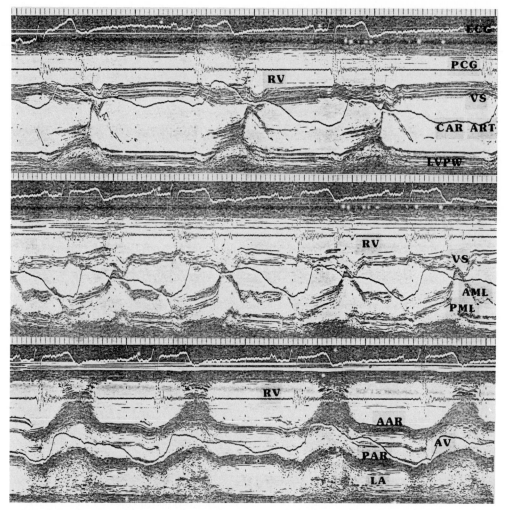

Fig. A-7. Segments from the M-mode echogram of a normal young woman with simultaneous ECG, phonocardiogram, and external carotid pulse tracing. Paper speed 100 mm/sec.

Upper. LV at chordae tendineae level.

Center. LV at mitral valve level.

Lower. Aortic root. The temporal relationship of the first, second, and third heart sounds to the motion of various cardiac structures is demonstrated.

ants of normal anatomy for evidence of cardiac pathology. *Artefacts* result from aberrant or unexpected behavior of reflected ultrasound or of the electrical signals which the ultrasound impulses have activated.

The different varieties of artefact include:

Reverberations. Echoes recorded on the echocardiographic tracing are produced by ultrasound waves reflected back from cardiac structures. It is possible for ultrasound to get reflected *again*—from the transducer face, from the chest wall, or other cardiac structures, in which case they appear on the echographic tracing as an "abnormal" echo. This reverberatory

echo would appear some distance behind the "true" echo representing that structure because it has taken longer to register eventually on the transducer. Thus echoes of the mitral valve or LV posterior wall appear posterior to the heart on the screen and tracing (Fig. A-28). These reverberations can perplex the beginner or even be mistaken for the "true" echoes if the latter have been hidden by unduly high near-gain suppression.

More important pitfalls are produced by reverberations of anterior cardiac structures—chest wall, RV anterior wall, or RV catheter (or pacemaker wire). These artefacts appear

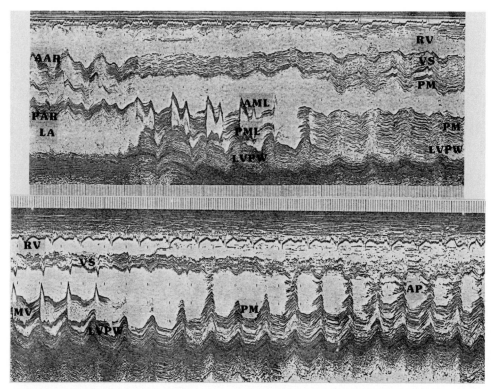

Fig. A-8. *Upper.* M-mode echographic scan, in a normal individual, from aortic root to LV at mitral valve level and then to papillary muscle level. Note that the anterior aortic root is continuous with the ventricular septum, while the posterior aortic root is continuous with the anterior mitral leaflet. As the papillary muscle comes into view, it merges with the LV posterior wall, appearing as an abrupt and striking increase in the thickness of the latter. At the same level, the anterior papillary muscle is partly visible, adjacent to the ventricular septum.

Lower. M-mode echographic scan, in a normal person, of the LV from its base (mitral valve level) toward its apex. Note that the LV internal dimension gradually diminishes from mid-LV level toward the apex. The papillary muscles produce intracavity LV echoes that tend to be more conspicuous in systole than in diastole. These echoes should not be mistaken for mural thrombi.

within the cardiac image, simulating the right or left border of the ventricular septum or even mural thrombi. They can be recognized by the fact that they run parallel to the chest wall (flat linear echo) or to the RV anterior wall echo, and so forth.

On the 2-D echogram, reverberations can resemble mural thrombi (Fig. A-29). Ultrasound reflected from the plastic casing of the scan head tends to appear within the LV image near its apex, thus mimicking mural thrombi which also have a predilection for the apex in patients with cardiomyopathy or anteroapical infarcts. A small, dense, flickering artefact, dubbed "Herbie," is peculiar to a popular rotating type 2-D scanner; it could be mistaken easily for a thrombus or vegetation unless one is aware of its artefactual nature. Side-lobe artefacts occur

mainly with phased-array equipment. They arise from extraneous beams of ultrasound generated from edges of the individual transducer elements. Abnormal echoes, often dense, appear within the 2-D image as a curved band, simulating an abnormal structure (mass, thrombus, membrane, and so forth) within the left atrium or ventricle or pericardial space.

Television persistence artefacts produce "ghosts" of echoes which had appeared on the screen a moment before and not quite faded away. Thus a faint image of the closed aortic valve may be superimposed, in systole, on the image of the open aortic valve, where possibly it could be mistaken for a vegetation.

Artefact Due to Problems of Lateral Resolution. Because ultrasound energy cannot be

[*Text continued on page 26.*]

A.

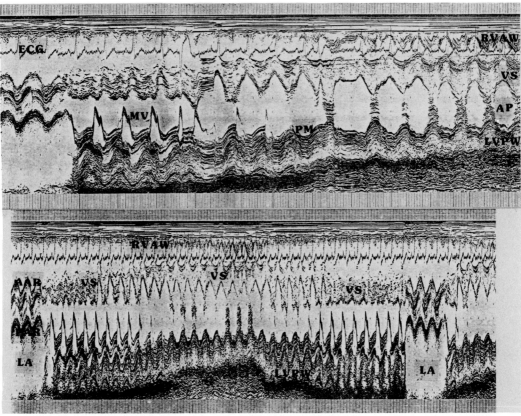

B.

Fig. A-9. *A.* M-mode echographic scan, at paper speed 25 mm/sec, from aortic root to LV at mitral valve level, and then on to papillary muscle and finally near-apical LV level. The base of the papillary muscle (PM) merges with the LV posterior wall, producing an apparent doubling of LV wall thickness at this level. The ventricular septum is continuous with the anterior aortic root; the anterior mitral leaflet, with the posterior aortic root.

Fig. A-9. *B.* M-mode echogram at slower paper speed (10 mm/sec) from aortic root to LV at mitral, papillary muscle, and near-apical levels. Note normal tapering of LV shape toward its apex (*center of figure*). The scan was then retraced, to encounter the same LV levels in reverse, back to the aortic root.

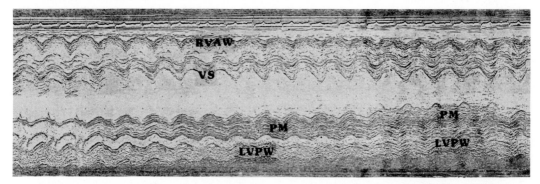

Fig. A-10. M-mode echographic scan of the LV shows continuity of mitral chordae tendineae with papillary muscle. The echo mass just anterior and parallel to the LVPW is a papillary muscle and not a mural thrombus.

A.

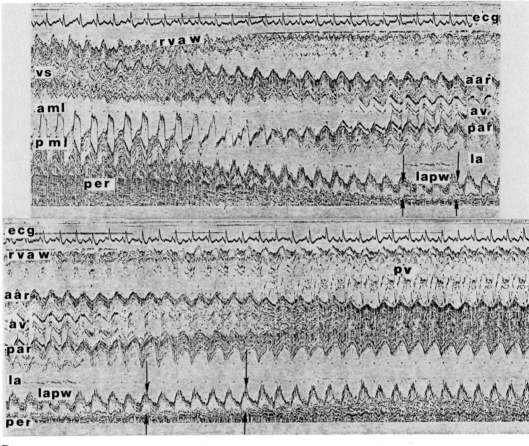

B.

Fig. A-11. M-mode echographic scans, from the parasternal area, in a patient with a pericardial effusion (*arrows*), which facilitates visualization of the RV anterior wall and LA and RA posterior wall.

Fig. A-11. *A.* Scan from LV to LA and aortic root. The ventricular septum is continuous with the anterior aortic root, the anterior mitral leaflet with the posterior aortic root, and the LV posterior wall with the LA posterior wall.

Fig. A-11. *B.* Scan from aortic root to pulmonary artery. The RV outflow tract (between RV anterior wall and anterior aortic root) is continuous with the pulmonary artery containing the pulmonic valve. The anterior and posterior aortic root echoes merge into a thick band of echoes (the atriopulmonary sulcus) posterior to the pulmonic valve. The LA appears as a wide echo-free space posterior to the aorta and pulmonary artery.

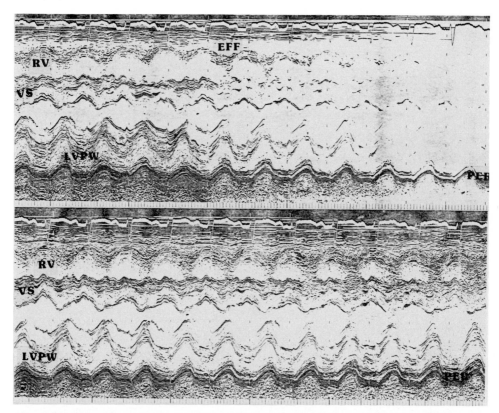

Fig. A-12. M-mode echogram showing the LV at chordae tendineae level. In the upper panel, the damping (reject) was progressively increased, suppressing echoes of the RV anterior wall, ventricular septum, and LV endocardium. The only echoes that persist (*right*) are the epicardial and pericardial ones, which are thin linear parallel echoes close to each other. In the lower panel, the demarcation between epicardium and pericardium was obtained (*right*) by slight alteration of transducer angulation.

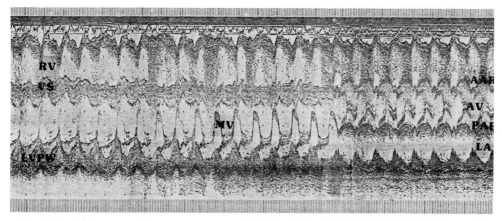

Fig. A-13. M-mode echographic scan from LV to LA. Note the gradual change in endocardial contour as the scan moves from the LV posterior wall to the atrioventricular junction and then to the LA posterior wall.

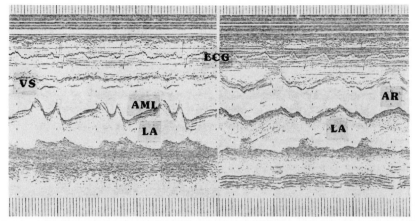

Fig. A-14. M-mode echogram showing the pattern of LA posterior wall motion at different levels. In the left panel, near the atrioventricular junction, the LV posterior wall moves anteriorly during atrial systole and posteriorly during ventricular systole. At this level the anterior mitral leaflet lies anterior to the LA posterior wall. In the right panel, the aortic root lies anterior to the LA posterior wall, which exhibits a prominent anterior excursion during atrial contraction. The echo-free space posterior to the LA posterior wall is the descending aorta.

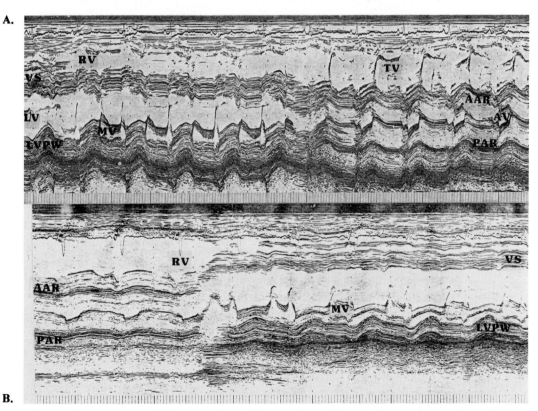

Fig. A-15. *A.* Subcostal M-mode echographic scan from LV to aortic root in a patient with chronic bronchitis and emphysema. The mitral and aortic valves are clearly visible, and their motion patterns are very similar to those commonly obtained by the conventional parasternal approach. The tricuspid valve can be partly visualized anterior to the aortic root. Note that the LV posterior wall echo tends to merge with the posterior aortic root echo, and very little of the left atrium can be seen. Left atrial dimension cannot be measured.

Fig. A-15. *B.* Subcostal M-mode echographic scan from aortic root to LV in an elderly man with chronic pulmonary disease and anteroseptal infarction. Note that the posterior aortic root appears to be continuous with the LV posterior wall, not with the anterior mitral leaflet, as is usual in the parasternal approach.

15

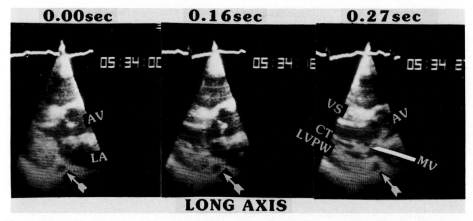

Fig. A-16. 2-D echogram of a patient with concentric LV hypertrophy. The first frame is at early diastole, the second at late diastole, and the third at eary systole. A small round echo-free space (*arrows*) at the junction of the LV posterior wall and LA posterior wall represents the coronary sinus.

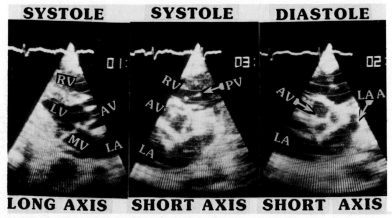

Fig. A-17. 2-D echogram demonstrating normal anatomy of left heart structures in the long-axis view (*left*) and short-axis view (*right*). The aortic valve is open in the systolic frames (*left and center*), closed in the diastolic frame (*right*). The anatomic relationship of the left atrium and its appendage to the aortic root is clear. Note also the RV outflow tract and pulmonic valve (PV) anterior to the aortic root.

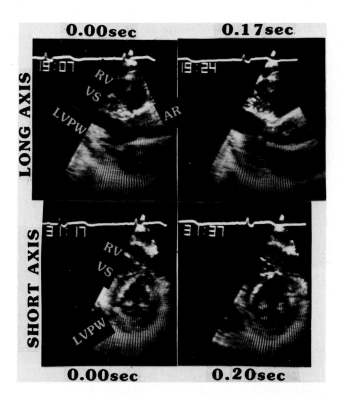

Fig. A-18. 2-D echogram of a normal young man. The two upper frames are in the long-axis view from the same cardiac cycle. The left is in systole; the right, in diastole. The two lower frames are in the short-axis view, at papillary muscle level. The left is in systole; the right, in the ensuing diastole.

Fig. A-19. 2-D echogram showing a prominent posterior papillary muscle. The two upper frames are in a near-apical long-axis view; the papillary muscle appears much thicker and shorter (*left upper frame*) in systole than in diastole (*right upper frame*). The left lower frame, in the parasternal long-axis view, shows chordae connecting the papillary muscle to the mitral valve. The right lower frame, in the short-axis view, also shows a conspicuous papillary muscle.

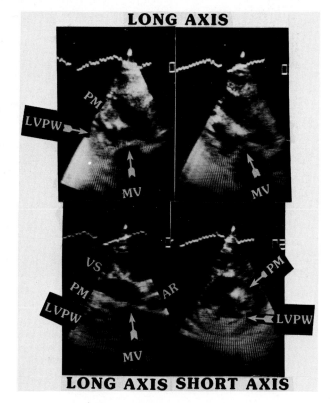

17

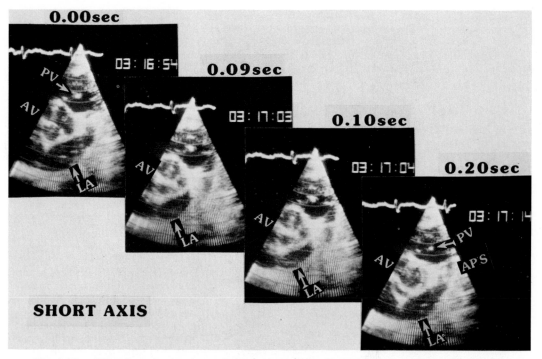

Fig. A-20. 2-D echogram showing serial frames in the short-axis view. The aortic root appears with the individual aortic valve cusps visible within it; the pulmonic valve is anterior to the aortic root. The left atrium is well visualized posterior to the aortic root. During atrial contraction (*second and third frames*) the LA size decreases considerably, but it increases during the subsequent ventricular systole (*fourth frame*).

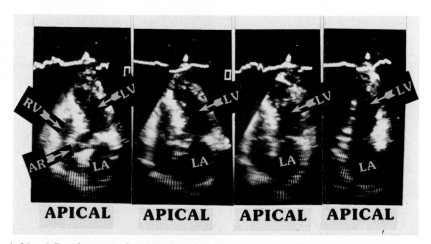

Fig. A-21. 2-D echogram of a patient with mild concentric LV hypertrophy. All four frames were recorded from the apex. The one on the extreme left shows an apical 4-chamber view with the aortic root arising from the LV. The two center frames show apical 4-chamber views in a slightly different plane, revealing the mitral valve as well as aortic root. The valve is open in diastole (*left*) and closed in systole (*right*). The frame on the extreme right shows the 2-chamber (LV-LA) view.

18

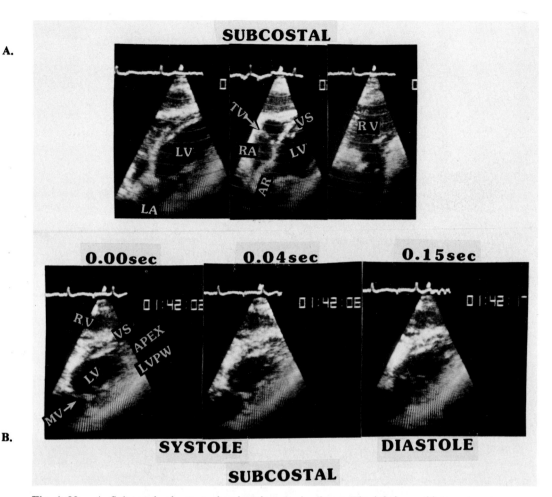

Fig. A-22. *A.* Subcostal echogram showing three basic planes. The left frame (the most posterior) shows the left atrium and left ventricle; the center frame shows the aortic root emerging from the LV; the right frame (the most anterior) shows the RV, including its outflow tract.

Fig. A-22. *B.* Three serial frames in the subcostal view showing the LA and LV. The first frame is in midsystole, the second near end-systole, the third in early diastole. The mitral valve is closed in the first two frames, open in the third. The LV wall thickens in the center frame, and the LV becomes smaller.

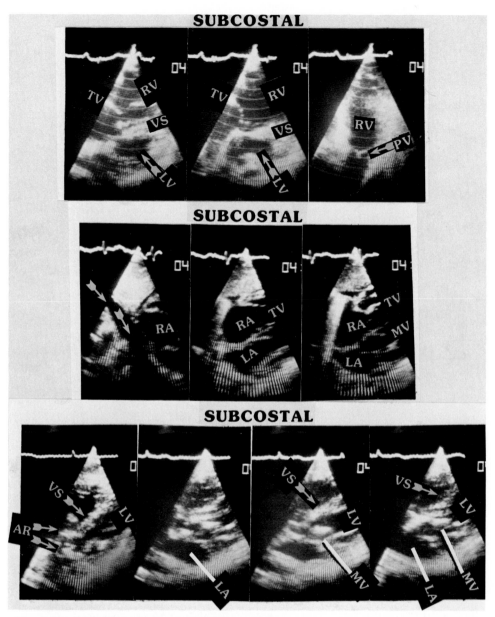

Fig. A-23. 2-D subcostal scans in 3 different patients.

Upper. Subcostal 2-D echogram of a patient with RV dilatation due to chronic cor pulmonale. The left frame shows the RA and RV anteriorly and the LA and LV posteriorly. The center frame, in a more anterior plane, shows the RA and RV anteriorly with the aortic root emerging from the LV outflow tract posteriorly. The right frame, even more anterior, shows the RV outflow tract and pulmonic valve.

Center. 2-D echographic scan in the subcostal view. The left frame, in a parasagittal plane, shows the inferior vena cava (*arrows*) entering the right atrium. The sweep is then directed to visualize the RA and LA (*center*) and then the tricuspid and mitral valves (*right*).

Lower. Subcostal 2-D echogram demonstrating a scan from the aortic root to a more posterior (mitral valve) plane. The first frame shows the aortic root arising from the LV; the last frame depicts the LA opening into the LV. The center frames are intermediate. In this patient the mitral leaflets and chordae were sclerotic and therefore more conspicuous than usual.

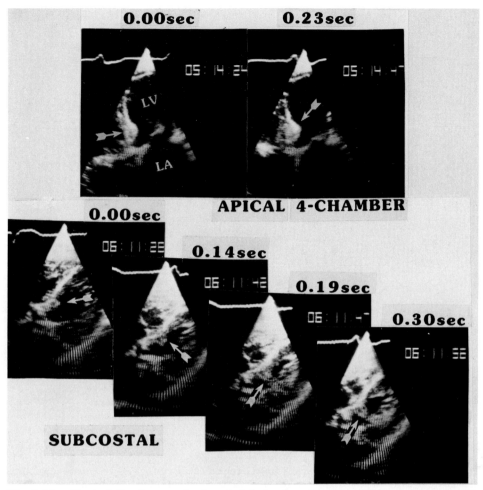

0.00sec **0.23sec**

APICAL 4-CHAMBER

0.00sec **0.14sec** **0.19sec** **0.30sec**

SUBCOSTAL

Fig. A-24. *Upper.* 2-D echogram, in the apical 4-chamber view, of a middle-aged woman with an interesting anatomic variant. The ventricular septum (*arrow*) exhibits a protuberance that bulges into the LV outflow tract. It is visible in diastole (*left*) but is more conspicuous (*arrow*) in the ensuing systole (*right*). This should not be mistaken for a mural thrombus; unlike a thrombus, it thickens visibly in systole.

Lower. Subcostal 2-D echogram of the same patient. The four serial frames are from the same cardiac cycle. The protuberance (*arrow*) on the left aspect of the ventricular septum becomes progressively more prominent in systole. The significance of this anatomic variant is uncertain. Some consider it innocuous, whereas others have called it a variety of hypertrophic cardiomyopathy.

A.

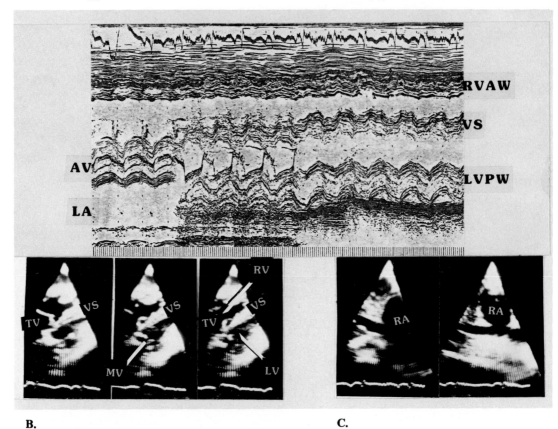

B.

C.

Fig. A-25. *A.* Subcostal M-mode echogram of an elderly man with chronic lung disease, showing a scan from aortic root to LV. The dense stratified echoes between the transducer and the heart arise from the left lobe of the liver.

Fig. A-25. *B.* Subcostal 2-D echogram of the same patient. The first frame is in systole, the second in middiastole, and the third at end-diastole after atrial contraction. The RV, LV, mitral and tricuspid valves, and aortic root can be identified.

Fig. A-25. *C.* Subcostal 2-D echogram of the same patient in a right parasagittal plane. The left frame shows the inferior vena cava entering the RA. In the right frame, the sector angle has been widened to include more of the RA and the entrance of the superior vena cava into it.

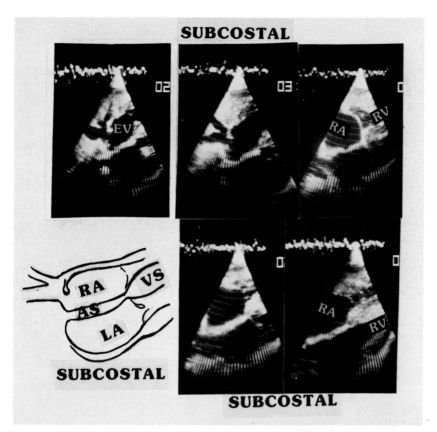

Fig. A-26. 2-D subcostal view demonstrating atrial anatomy. Note the inferior vena cava entering the right atrium in the upper left and center frames, and the eustachian valve (EV) guarding the caval orifice. The atrial septum (AS) is well visualized in all the frames.

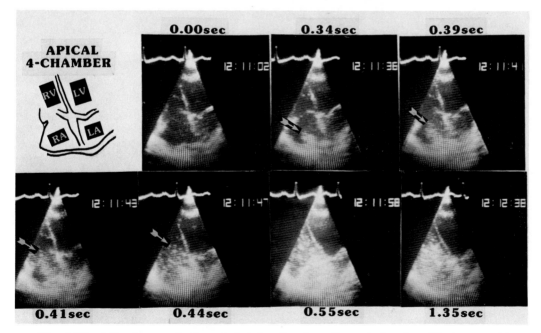

Fig. A-27. 2-D echogram in the apical 4-chamber view of a normal patient. The seven serial frames are from the same cardiac cycle. The first frame is just before entry of microbubble-bearing blood (after intravenous saline injection). The second, third, and fourth frames show the stream of opacified blood entering the RA (*arrows*). The RA and then the RV get fully opacified (*fifth, sixth, and seventh frames*).

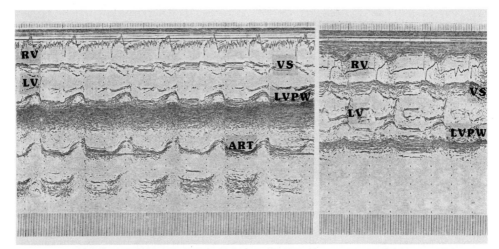

Fig. A-28. M-mode echogram of a normal person. In the left panel, the scale has been attenuated so that the heart occupies less than half the paper width, and a reverberation of the LV posterior wall echo is recorded at some distance behind the true LV posterior wall echo. The reverberatory artefact can be eliminated by an alteration of transducer direction (*right panel*); the scale is not as attenuated in this segment.

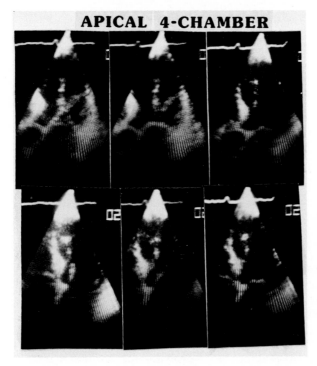

Fig. A-29. 2-D echogram of a patient with aortic regurgitation and LV dilatation. All six frames are in the apical 4-chamber view. In all there appears an "abnormal" echo within the LV, which remains in more or less a fixed position perpendicular to the chest wall. It does not bear a constant relationship to the LV (or its walls), which has been moved about by manipulation of the 2-D probe. This indicates that the abnormal echo is an ultrasonic reverberation rather than a true intraventricular mass.

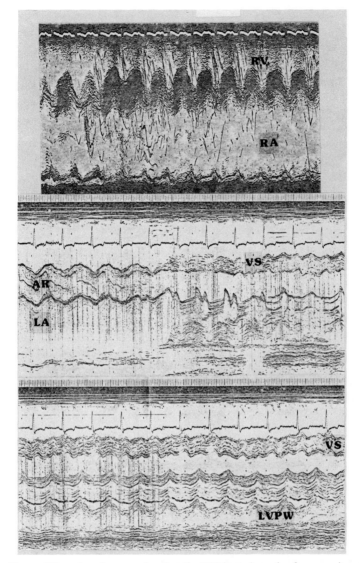

Fig. A-30. *Upper.* M-mode echogram showing the RV (anterior echo-free space) and RA (posterior echo-free space). Abnormal irregular short linear echoes appear first in the RA, and immediately thereafter in the RV. Over the next four beats these echoes persist in the RV but gradually disappear from the RA. The patient was receiving an intravenous saline drip, which spontaneously produced microbubbles in an arm vein, which were carried along to the RA and RV.

Center and Lower. M-mode echogram showing a scan from aortic root to LV (*center*) and LV at chordae and papillary muscle level (*lower*). Artefacts consisting of high-frequency fine vertical lines are superimposed on the tracing in the center panel and the first half of the lower panel. The artefacts were due to electrically operated construction equipment being used elsewhere in the building; they ceased abruptly (*middle of lower panel*) when the equipment was turned off.

25

focused over the entire depth range of the ultrasound beam, there will always be echoes generated and received from structures located away from the center of the beam (Roelandt *et al.*, 1976). Thus it is possible for two different and separate structures, side by side in the heart, to appear superimposed if both fall within the width of the same beam. This explains why structures that reflect ultrasound strongly, such as prosthetic or calcified valves, appear to extend beyond their expected site of chamber into adjoining chambers; also why, in certain circumstances, structures such as the mitral valve are represented by multiple parallel echoes rather than a single one.

Electrical interference from construction or other electrical equipment elsewhere in the building appears as irregular, fine linear markings on the tracing, with abrupt onset and cessation (Fig. A-30). They should not be mistaken for the microbubbles generated by saline or (Fig. A-30) green dye injections in contrast echography.

REFERENCES

Feigenbaum, H.: *Echocardiography,* 3rd Ed. Lea & Febiger, Philadelphia, 1981.

Henry, W. L.; DeMaria, A.; Gramiak, R., *et al.:* Report of the American Society of Echocardiography Committee on Nomenclature and Standards in Two-Dimensional Echocardiography. *Circulation,* **62:**212, 1980.

Meltzer, R. S., and Roelandt, J: *Contrast Echocardiography.* Martinus Nijhoff, The Hague, 1982.

Nanda, N. C., and Rothbard, R. L.: Contrast echocardiography. *Semin. Ultrasound,* **2:**167, 1981.

Roelandt, J.; van Dorp, W. G.; Bom, N., *et al.:* Resolution problems in echocardiography: A source of interpretation errors. *Am. J. Cardiol.,* **37:**256, 1976.

Sahn, D. J.; DeMaria, A. N.; Kisslo, J. K., *et al.:* Recommendations regarding quantitation in M-mode echocardiography: Results of a survey of echocardiographic measurements. *Circulation,* **58:**1072, 1978.

Silverman, N. H., and Schiller, N. B.: Apex echocardiography: A two-dimensional technique for evaluating congenital heart disease. *Circulation,* **57:**503, 1978.

Weyman, A. E.: *Cross-Sectional Echocardiography.* Lea & Febiger, Philadelphia, 1982.

B

The Mitral Valve

MITRAL STENOSIS

The history of echocardiography began in the 1950s with the discovery of Edler (1956) that the diastolic motion of the anterior mitral leaflet echo was distinctly abnormal in patients with stenosis of the mitral valve. Subsequently, when the posterior mitral leaflet echo was identified by echocardiographers, it soon became evident that it too moves abnormally in mitral stenosis (Duchak *et al.,* 1972). Ultrasound rapidly gained wide acceptance as the best noninvasive means of diagnosing mitral stenosis.

However, during the 1970s, an element of disillusionment crept in as evidence accumulated that a low mitral EF slope may be found in conditions other than mitral stenosis, and that anterior (paradoxic) diastolic motion of the posterior mitral leaflet, for several years considered a hallmark of the stenotic mitral valve, was occasionally absent in hemodynamically proven instances of this lesion (Levisman *et al.,* 1975). Fortunately, this provoked a reappraisal of mitral cusp motion in mitral stenosis, especially the extent of cusp separation during the various phases of diastole. New M-mode echocardiographic criteria emerged, which have partly superseded or at least amplified the original ones.

Finally, the ability to visualize the whole length and the whole width of the mitral leaflets by 2-D echocardiography led to the appreciation of abnormalities of diastolic cusp motion that were not possible with the M-mode technique. This resulted not only in new diagnostic criteria of mitral stenosis, but also in a reliable method of quantifying the area of the narrow mitral orifice.

The M-mode characteristics of mitral stenosis (Joyner *et al.,* 1963; Segal *et al.,* 1966; Edler, 1956; Effert, 1967; Winters *et al.,* 1967; Zaky *et al.,* 1968; Duchak *et al.,* 1972; Cope *et al.,* 1975); include the following:

The anterior mitral leaflet may exhibit:

1. An unusually thick and dense echo, due to sclerosis or calcification;

2. A low or flat EF slope (0 to 30 mm per sec);

3. An abnormally small amplitude of diastolic opening (DE distance, 15 mm or less);

4. A very small or absent "A" peak, in patients not in atrial fibrillation;

5. An unduly rapid AC slope (350 to 600 mm per second).

The posterior mitral leaflet may show:

1. An unusually thick and dense echo;

2. Anterior motion during diastole, or at least an absence of posterior motion.

The diastolic separation between the mitral leaflets:

1. May be abnormally small;

2. Remains constant, or almost so, throughout diastole, i.e., the anterior and posterior cusp echoes run parallel to each other on the tracing, or converge only slightly, during the whole of diastole, however long it may be.

The maximal diastolic separation between the mitral leaflets was found to correlate better with the mitral valve area (assessed hemodynamically) than did the EF slope (Fisher *et al.,* 1979).

All the above features need not be apparent in every case.

It is important to be aware of certain exceptions:

1. In patients with mild mitral stenosis, it is not uncommon to find (a) a mildly decreased EF slope, between 30 to 45 mm per sec, (b) a marginally decreased amplitude of mitral diastolic opening (DE distance, 15 to 18 mm), (c) a small "A" peak on the anterior cusp echo, (d) neither anterior nor posterior motion of the posterior leaflet in diastole, between the D and C points.

2. In patients with associated mitral regurgitation, (a) the EF slope is often in the borderline low range; it may have a concave parabolic contour, the so-called "ski-slope" appearance; (b) the two mitral leaflets tend to gradually converge in mid- to late diastole, whereas in most patients with pure stenosis, cusp separation remains constant during all of diastole.

3. In stenotic but pliable and noncalcified mitral valves, the cusp echoes may be only slightly thickened. It is not unusual for the anterior leaflet to appear heavily calcified, while the posterior leaflet, though moving abnormally, is of normal thickness. Less commonly, the reverse is true.

4. In a small minority of cases of catheterization-proven mitral stenosis, the posterior mitral leaflet can be shown to move posteriorly in diastole (Levisman et al., 1975; Flaherty et al., 1975). This finding is said to occur in about 10 per cent of patients (Levisman et al., 1975) and 17 per cent (Shiu et al., 1978). However, other echographic features of mitral stenosis such as cusp thickening, small and constant cusp separation throughout diastole, absent "A" peak (atrial wave), and small DE amplitude are usually present, so that the diagnosis of mitral stenosis need not go unsuspected.

Occasionally, it is possible to record normal as well as abnormal motion of the posterior mitral leaflet in the same patient at the same examination, at slightly different transducer angulations (Glasser and Favis, 1977). Late diastolic anterior motion of the posterior mitral leaflet (during atrial contraction) is said to be highly diagnostic of mitral stenosis, even when posterior leaflet motion is otherwise not quite typical of stenosis (Shiu et al., 1978). A variety of abnormal M-mode echographic abnormalities are shown in Figures B-1 to B-7.

The diagnostic emphasis has shifted from criteria based on a low EF slope and abnormal diastolic motion of the posterior mitral leaflet to newer criteria such as (1) abnormally small separation between anterior and posterior mitral leaflets (less than 15 mm) and (2) a fixed or constant separation (or very slight convergence) between the two mitral leaflets throughout diastole.

This important observation that the anterior and posterior mitral leaflet echoes remain parallel, or almost so, on the M-mode tracing in mitral stenosis has been expressed quantitatively by Shiu and his colleagues (1977, 1978, 1979) as the mitral valve closure index.

Shiu's index, the MCVI, correlated well with mitral valve orifice area, calculated by the Gorlin formula. The same group of authors studied the MVCI index in 54 patients one month to three years after mitral valvotomy and found it to be a sensitive index for diagnosing residual

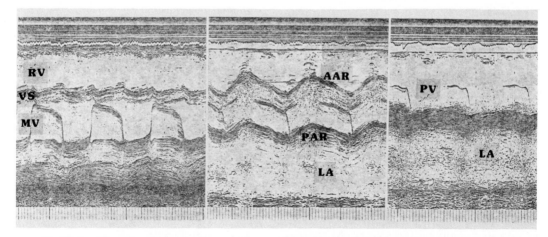

Fig. B-1. M-mode echogram of a typical case of mitral stenosis of mild to moderate severity. The left panel shows typical changes of mitral stenosis, with slightly thickened cusps, low EF slope, and abnormal posterior leaflet motion. The center panel shows mild LA dilatation. The right panel shows a small pulmonic "a" wave, suggesting mild pulmonary hypertension.

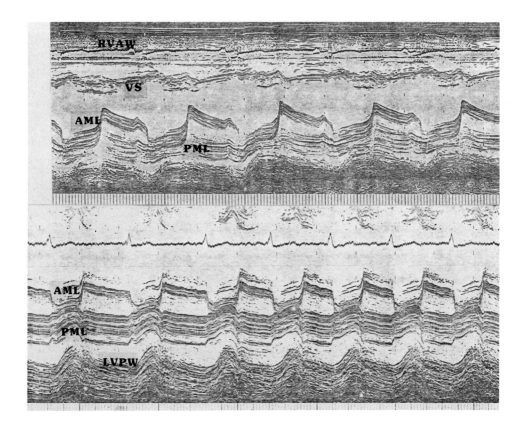

Fig. B-2. M-mode echogram of the mitral valve showing findings typical of mitral stenosis. The posterior mitral leaflet and chordae produce broad echoes posterior to the anterior mitral cusp. These are unduly prominent in some beats (first and fourth beats) and could possibly be mistaken for an LA myxoma. Unlike myxomas, these abnormal echoes are continuous with mitral cusp echoes. Mitral valve echoes appear unusually thick in systole, which supports a diagnosis of mitral sclerosis, not LA myxoma.

M-mode echogram of a patient with mitral stenosis. Diastolic separation of the mitral cusps is small and constant through all of diastole. The EF slope is low. Atypical echographic features of this case include (a) very heavy calcification of the posterior mitral leaflet, exceeding that of the anterior mitral leaflet; and (b) posterior (though small) motion of the posterior leaflet in diastole. The calcified posterior mitral leaflet can be differentiated from mitral annulus calcification by its obvious coaptation in systole with the anterior leaflet.

mitral stenosis (Shiu *et al.,* 1979). Toutouzas *et al.* (1977) devised a somewhat different index based mainly on the fact that the stenotic mitral valve remains open to its full cusp separation until the LV contracts.

MITRAL VALVE CALCIFICATION

The question often arises as to whether abnormally thick and dense echoes from a stenotic mitral valve should be reported as calcification or merely fibrous thickening. The issue is of interest to the cardiac surgeon who would like to know whether mitral valve replacement is

avoidable, i.e., whether mitral valvotomy may be feasible.

It has been assumed (Nanda *et al.,* 1975) that when diastolic mitral echoes appear:

1. Thick, conglomerate, and fuzzy, heavy calcification is present;

2. Multiple linear, layered, or tiered, the valve is lightly calcified;

3. Thin, single, or duplicate, the valve is not calcified.

Raj *et al.* (1976) correlated the echographic mitral appearances with anatomic estimation (by radiography, and calcium extraction and estimation of the excised valve) of calcification

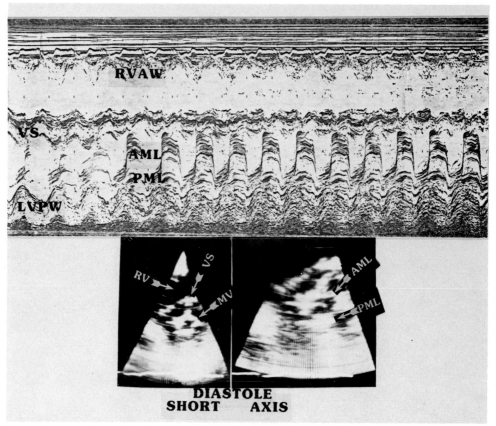

Fig. B-3. M-mode echogram (*upper*) of a patient with moderate mitral stenosis. The mitral cusps appear sclerotic or calcified, with abnormal posterior leaflet motion, small cusp separation, and a flat EF slope. In the 2-D echogram (*lower*) in the short-axis view, the calcified mitral valve is clearly visible and its orifice (about 1 cm²) is well defined. The mitral valve image has been expanded in the right frame to facilitate measurement of the mitral valve orifice area.

in 20 patients. They found that a single, thin mitral diastolic echo excludes significant calcification as well as fibrosis. On the other hand, increased thickness of the mitral valve echo in diastole could be caused by either fibrosis or calcification. However, all cases with more than 80 mg of calcium in the valve exhibited multiple dense parallel mitral leaflet echoes. Nicolosi *et al.* (1979) correlated the M-mode echocardiograms, chest x-rays, and anatomic findings (at surgery) in 87 patients with mitral stenosis. The radiographic diagnosis of mitral valve calcification was highly specific but not sensitive, whereas the echographic criteria were highly sensitive for calcification but not specific. These authors showed that the ratio of the echo representing the anterior mitral leaflet to that representing the left margin of the ventricular septum (abbreviation: MT/ST ratio) over 1.7 indicated heavy or light mitral valve calcification in all

cases. Absolute measurements of anterior mitral leaflet thickness in diastole were less reliable in predicting its calcification. Zanolla *et al.* (1982) recently correlated the 2-D echographic prediction of calcium in the mitral valve with x-ray detection of calcium in the excised valve and confirmed the very high sensitivity of ultrasound in detection of mitral calcification.

TWO-DIMENSIONAL ECHOCARDIOGRAPHY

Two-dimensional echocardiography definitely has advanced the diagnostic capabilities of ultrasound with respect to mitral stenosis (Fig. B-8). In the *long-axis view* of the left ventricle and atrium, the whole length of the anterior mitral leaflet is well seen, from its attachment to the posterior aortic root to its tip or free edge. The normal diastolic motion of the anterior mitral leaflet comprises a gentle, slow, waving motion, which corresponds to the EF slope, "A" peak, and AC slope of the M-mode echogram. In mitral stenosis, the anterior mitral cusp behaves very differently:

1. Early in diastole it assumes a curved contour, convex toward the ventricular septum, and this appearance is maintained with little change until the end of the diastole. This corresponds to the straight, flat EF segment on M-mode;

2. The separation between the tips of the anterior and posterior mitral leaflets is decreased (although the "mouth" of the mitral valve funnel may appear wide and capacious). This abnormally small distance between the tips of the mitral cusps tends to remain constant through all of diastole;

3. With the onset of ventricular systole, the anterior mitral leaflet moves posteriorly in an abrupt "slamming" motion to appose the posterior leaflet.

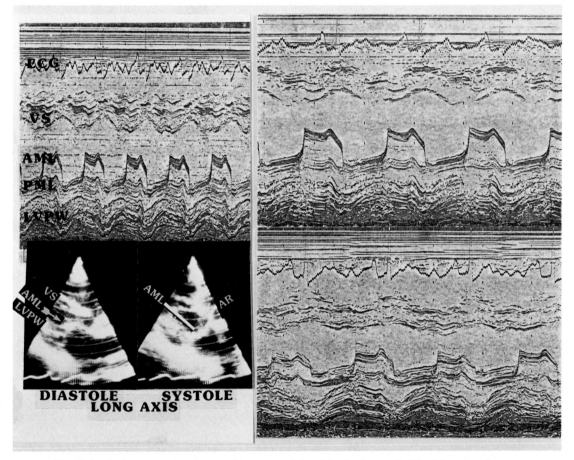

Fig. B-4. Echograms of a 40-year-old woman with mild mitral stenosis. The M-mode echogram (*left upper panel*) presents typical findings of mitral stenosis: low EF slope, small anterior diastolic excursion, constant separation of mitral cusps through all of diastole, and abnormal diastolic motion of the posterior mitral leaflet. The left lower panel shows a 2-D echogram in the long-axis view. In the left frame, the mitral valve is open in diastole: note its funnel-like shape. In the right frame, the valve is closed in systole: note that the anterior mitral leaflet is convex toward the LA, not unlike its contour in mitral prolapse. The difference in contour of the anterior mitral leaflet from diastole to systole is good evidence of good valve mobility; this rather abrupt slamming shut motion of the valve is quite distinctive and diagnostically helpful when viewed in real time.

The right upper and lower panels show the mitral valve at slightly different transducer angulations. The EF slope is abnormally low; both leaflets show an anterior motion ("A" wave) with atrial contraction. Note that cusp separation appears wider in the upper panel.

In other words, in mitral stenosis the anterior leaflet appears fixed at its attachment (base) to the aortic root and relatively fixed at its tip (narrow end of the mitral funnel), but the middle of the leaflet shows an exaggerated amplitude of motion, bulging forward early in diastole and abruptly backward as ventricular contraction begins. The presence of anterior mitral motion of this type indicates not only the diagnosis of mitral stenosis but also that the leaflet retains some pliability. In such cases the convexity of the anterior mitral leaflet in diastole has been likened to a "bent knee" (Henry et al., 1975).

The long-axis view of the mitral valve is helpful also in providing a better idea of the extent of its sclerosis and calcification than the M-mode can. Thus, the absence of gross calcific deposits, usually accompanied by good pliability, suggests to the surgeon that the stenotic valve may be amenable to valvulotomy and may not need replacement. When calcium is present in the anterior or posterior mitral leaflet, it may appear as a hunk or nodule near the free edge, the base or proximal part of the leaflet remaining partly mobile. In yet other instances, the entire leaflet produces a dense, almost immobile echo mass; in such patients mitral valve replacement is a foregone conclusion.

Nichol et al. (1977) noted that in 40 percent of their patients with mitral stenosis, the anterior leaflet bulged above the level of the mitral leaflet in systole; this may account for systolic sagging or "hammocking" sometimes seen in M-mode echograms and designated concomitant prolapse and stenosis. Not all cardiologists would agree that this constitutes true prolapse.

The short-axis view of the mitral valve, which brings into view the entire widths of the mitral leaflets, shows the following abnormalities in mitral stenosis:

1. Constant distance (separation) between the anterior and posterior mitral leaflets throughout all of diastole;

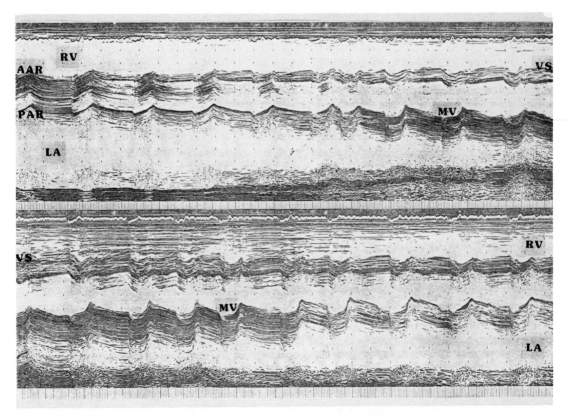

A. **Fig. B-5.** *A.* M-mode echographic scan from aortic root to LV (*upper*) and in the reverse direction (*lower*), in a man with calcific mitral stenosis. The anterior mitral leaflet is so heavily calcified that it is scarcely recognizable as such; it manifests as a large dense mass with rather restricted mobility that is continuous with the posterior aortic root.

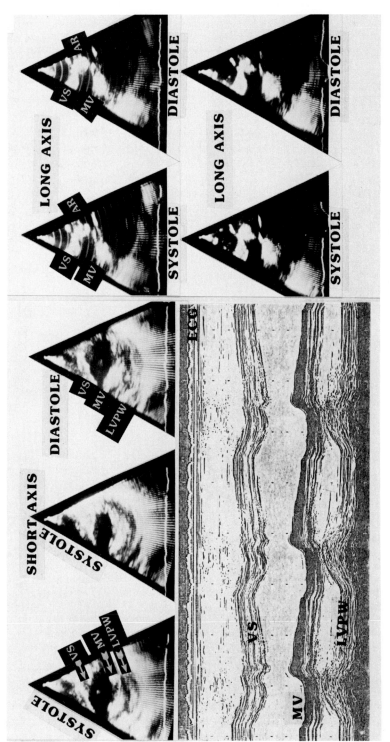

Fig. B-5. *B.* The left lower panel shows the M-mode echogram of the same patient with calcific mitral stenosis. The anterior mitral leaflet appears heavily calcified, and very little separation is visible between it and the posterior leaflet. The left upper panel shows three frames, in the short-axis view, from the same cardiac cycle. The first frame is in early systole, the second in late systole, and the third in diastole. The mitral valve is heavily calcified; no definite valve orifice is visualized, and the calcified cusps show little mobility from systole to diastole.

The four frames on the right are in the long-axis view. The two upper frames are from the same cardiac cycle; the two lower frames are from another cardiac cycle, in a slightly different plane. The anterior mitral leaflet, which shows very limited mobility from systole to diastole, consists mostly of a large mass of calcium.

B.

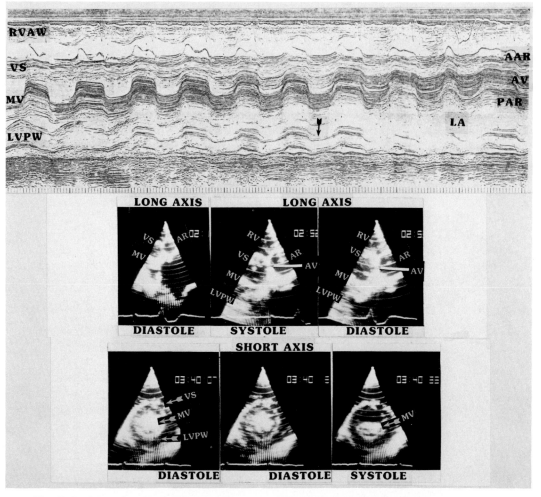

Fig. B-6. M-mode echographic scan from LV to LA in a patient with calcific mitral stenosis as well as calcific aortic stenosis. The massively calcified anterior mitral leaflet is almost continuous with the heavily calcified aortic valve. The LA posterior wall (*arrow*) is thickened to about 1 cm; at surgery this was found to be fibrous thickening.

2-D echogram of the same patient with calcific mitral stenosis and calcific aortic stenosis. The left frame shows both valves; the mitral valve is massively calcified and grotesquely deformed; the aortic valve is calcified and stenotic. Huge dilatation of the LA is clearly visible. The mitral and aortic valve image has been expanded in the center frame (systole) and the right frame (diastole). Mitral calcification appears continuous with aortic valve calcification. The aortic valve appears very immobile and stenotic.

2-D echogram in the same patient with massively calcified mitral stenosis. The three frames shown in the short-axis view are serial ones from the same cardiac cycle. The first two frames, in diastole, show the calcified valve as a large dense mass filling almost the whole LV at basal level. The right frame shows the valve closed in systole.

2. Abrupt posterior motion of the anterior leaflet at the onset of ventricular contraction;

3. The most important application of cross-sectional echocardiography to valvular heart disease is undoubtedly the ability to visualize and measure the precise cross-section area of the mitral valve orifice. The ideal patient for this purpose is one in whom the mitral cusps are thickened but not heavily calcified, the mitral orifice appearing in this view as a smooth circle or oval with sharp, regular edges. The mitral valve orifice area, thus estimated, has been shown to correlate well with the orifice area calculated by the Gorlin formula and directly measured at surgery. In some centers patients with pure mitral stenosis are sent to sur-

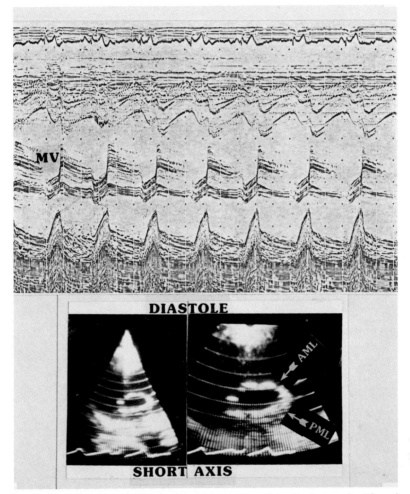

Fig. B-7. *Upper.* M-mode echogram of a patient with mild mitral stenosis. The mitral valve shows changes typical of mitral stenosis. In pure mitral stenosis, the LV is usually low normal in size. However, the LV appears to be dilated and to contract hyperdynamically, suggesting that a diastolic overload state also exists. No murmur of mitral or aortic regurgitation was heard, but hemodynamic studies revealed significant aortic regurgitation.

Lower. The mitral valve orifice is seen in short axis-view on the 2-D echogram. The parallel lines represent 1 cm calibration marks. The mitral valve orifice area, thus measured, was 3.4 cm². This patient had thickened mitral cusps that were fused at the commissures but not significantly stenotic. The LV was dilated because of associated aortic regurgitation.

gery without hemodynamic studies, on the basis of the 2-D echocardiographic demonstration of a critically narrowed mitral valve orifice.

In view of the important decision-making role of 2-D echocardiography in assessing the severity of mitral stenosis, it is worth pointing out certain difficulties and pitfalls that often arise in actual practice:

1. The mitral valve orifice area may be difficult to measure accurately if the orifice is of irregular shape, usually because of cusp scarring or calcific nodules or overlapping of one leaflet by another.

2. A calcified object appears larger than it actually is on echocardiogram, because calcium reflects ultrasound very well. Heavy calcification of the margins of the orifice will therefore tend to make the orifice appear smaller than it really is (Henry *et al.,* 1975). Too bright an image of the cusps on the Polaroid picture could also account for a falsely small orifice due to the excessive "bloom" or "glow" effect allowing the excessively augmented cusp echoes to encroach on the area of the true orifice.

3. The chordae tendineae of a stenotic mitral valve are often very thickened and matted to-

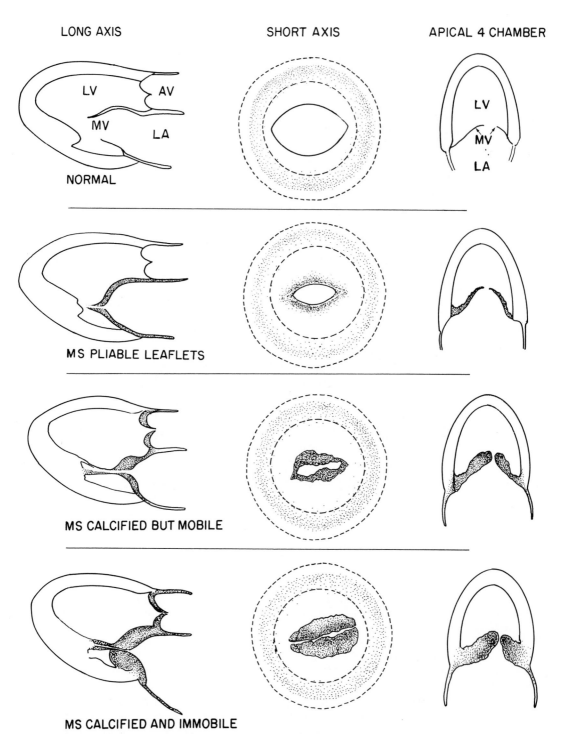

LONG AXIS   SHORT AXIS   APICAL 4 CHAMBER

NORMAL

MS PLIABLE LEAFLETS

MS CALCIFIED BUT MOBILE

MS CALCIFIED AND IMMOBILE

Fig. B-8. Diagrammatic representation of 2-D echographic appearances in mitral stenosis. The top horizontal row depicts normal echographic anatomy; the next row shows a stenotic but pliable mitral valve; the third row presents a calcified stenotic valve that has retained some mobility; the bottom row shows a very heavily calcified immobile mitral valve. The left vertical row depicts the long-axis view, the central vertical row the short-axis view, and the right vertical row the apical 4-chamber view.

gether, so that chordal structures are mistaken for one or both mitral cusps, and the area measured is not that of the true mitral valve orifice.

4. Perhaps the most dangerous pitfall is that of recording the separation or orifice between the mitral cusps near the widest level of the mitral funnel rather than at its narrowest part, which after all is the effective mitral orifice. This fallacy is most likely to occur in patients with long, pliable cusps and unlikely with very sclerotic short leaflets. The echocardiographer should attempt to avoid this pitfall by making a short-axis scan, from apex to base, of the left ventricle, i.e., sweeping slowly and carefully in an upward and medial direction so that the left ventricle is seen in short axis first at papillary muscle level, then at chordae level, and finally at the level at which both mitral cusps just come into view; it is at this level that planimetric measurement of mitral valve orifice area is made. Another possible fallacy consists in visualizing the mitral valve so that the plane imaged transects the anterior mitral leaflet twice, above and below "the bend of the knee" (Henry et al., 1975).

5. Martin et al. (1979) showed that gain settings too low led to image dropout, indicating erroneously large orifice; gain settings too high led to image saturation, indicating a falsely small valve orifice. These authors found that the mitral valve orifice is measured best at the inner black-white margin of the 2-D image as recorded on video screen or Polaroid print, in early diastole.

In the initial description of 2-D estimation of the mitral valve orifice area by this method, Henry et al. (1975) reported that this valve was within 0.3 sq cm of the valve orifice area directly measured at operation in all 14 patients (r = 0.92) with both 2-D echographic and surgical data.

Subsequently several other groups have confirmed the good to excellent correlation between the 2-D estimate of mitral valve orifice area and the area calculated by the Gorlin formula applied to cardiac catheterization data and/or measured directly at surgery. The "r" values have varied from 0.83 to 0.95 (Nichol et al., 1977; Wann et al., 1978; Martin et al., 1979; Glover et al., 1983). Using the valve areas by the Gorlin formula or surgical inspection as the "gold standard," their correlation with the mitral EF slope on the M-mode echocardiogram was rather poor, with "r" values of 0.38 (Nichol et al., 1977) and 0.49 (Wann et al., 1978).

Wann et al. (1978) also showed that the mitral valve area could be reliably estimated in patients with combined mitral stenosis and regurgitation (r = 0.09). The same group (Heger et al., 1979) have used the 2-D estimation of mitral valve orifice area to evaluate patients who had had mitral commissurotomy 10 to 14 years earlier; they found that it could distinguish reliably between those who had suffered restenosis and those who had not.

The spectrum of abnormal 2-D echographic findings in mitral stenosis is illustrated in Figures B-3 to B-12.

In addition to the various characteristics of mitral leaflet motion and morphology enumerated above, certain other echocardiographic findings have been shown to be associated with mitral stenosis. They are all a consequence of obstruction to blood flow from left atrium:

1. Left atrial enlargement is the rule in mitral stenosis, being present in all but the mildest cases. Atrial fibrillation is common in those with left atrial dimensions greater than 5 cm. Dilatation of the left atrium is, of course, the rule also in mitral regurgitation and in chronic left ventricular failure of any cause. On the other hand, the *absence* of left atrial enlargement in a patient thought to have moderate to severe mitral stenosis would be unusual. In an occasional patient the left atrium enlarges laterally rather than in an anteroposterior direction, so that it is strikingly dilated on a PA chest film or an angiocardiogram, whereas the echocardiographic dimension is normal or only slightly increased. In such circumstances, the left atrial dilatation may be better manifested by scanning from the suprasternal notch (M-mode) or in the apical four-chamber view (2-D).

2. Prominent posterior motion of the ventricular septum in early diastole. Feigenbaum (1976) commented on the brief movement of the septum toward the left ventricular chamber immediately after the end of ventricular systole, seen in some normal persons and particularly in those with mitral stenosis. Subsequently, Feigenbaum and his group (Weyman et al., 1978) studied this in further detail with 2-D

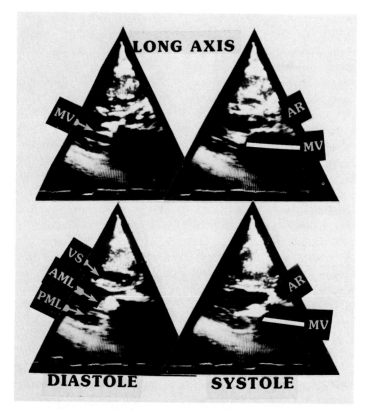

Fig. B-9. 2-D echogram of a patient with mitral stenosis, in the long-axis view. The left frames are in diastole, the right in systole. The two upper frames are in a slightly different plane than the two lower frames. Stenosis of the funnel-shaped mitral valve orifice is evident in the diastolic frames. Note that the anterior mitral leaflet is heavily calcified at its free edge but thin and mobile at its attachment.

echography and found that nearly all their patients with critical mitral stenosis exhibited a prominent early diastolic posterior septal motion. Presumably the disparity between early rapid filling of the right ventricle and slow early filling of the left ventricle (because of mitral stenosis) is so substantial as to displace the ventricular septum toward the latter chamber in early diastole. Thus, a very prominent motion of this type in a patient with mitral stenosis suggests that the stenosis is likely to be of significant severity.

3. The posterior wall of the aortic root and the anterior left atrial wall are contiguous and echocardiographically move as one structure. Strunk *et al.* (1976, 1977) studied the diastolic motion of the posterior aortic root in normals and in mitral stenosis; they found that normally 70 per cent of the posterior motion of the posterior aortic root echo takes place in the first third of the interval between the onset of dias-

tole and the onset of atrial contraction. The ratio of the amplitude of posterior aortic root motion during the first third of this interval to the total posterior excursion of the aortic root during the whole interval was designated the atrial emptying index (AEI) by Strunk *et al.* (1977). To ensure accurate measurements, paper speeds of 50 or 100 mm/sec are used and the scale expanded so as to magnify the aortic root image.

In severe mitral stenosis, Strunk *et al.* found the AEI to be 0.4 or less; in moderate mitral stenosis, 0.5 to 0.6; in mild mitral stenosis, up to 0.7. In other words, in normals the aortic root moves rapidly backward in early diastole and then remains more or less stationary in middiastole; in mitral stenosis, posterior aortic root motion is more gradual, continuing through middiastole. When pronounced, the difference between these two patterns of aortic root motion on the M-mode tracing lends itself

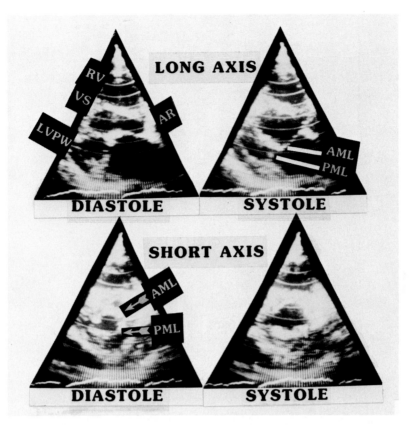

Fig. B-10. 2-D echogram of a woman who had had mitral valvotomy 12 years previously. The two upper frames are in the long-axis view, the two lower frames in the short-axis view. The left frames show the mitral valve open in diastole, the right frames show it closed in systole. The mitral cusps are thickened but mobile. In long axis the mitral valve appears funnel-shaped in diastole, and in systole loses its convexity to the LV to lie flat in approximately the plane of the mitral annulus. In short axis, the mitral orifice was well defined (*left lower frame*) and found to be 2.3 cm² in area.

to easy recognition during routine inspection of the record, apart from a quantitative assessment as expressed in the AEI.

Strunk *et al.* (1977) emphasized that the AEI is particularly useful in evaluating possible stenosis of a prosthetic mitral valve, a situation in which direct visualization and estimation of the mitral orifice area is not possible by either M-mode or 2-D echocardiography.

Naccarelli *et al.* (1979) confirmed the abnormalities of aortic root motion in mitral stenosis. They found the AEI to be 0.9 ± 0.01 in 25 normals, and only 0.47 ± 0.09 in 35 patients with mitral stenosis. A close correlation (r = 0.93) was demonstrated between the AEI and the mitral valve orifice area calculated by the Gorlin formula from catheterization data, but the AEI did not correlate well with left atrial size or with the mitral EF slope. All their patients with severe mitral stenosis had AEI of 0.42 or less, most of those with moderate stenosis had values of 0.43 to 0.51, and most with mild stenosis 0.52 or more. The predictive accuracy of the atrial emptying index in classifying the severity of mitral stenosis (mild, moderate, severe) was 86 per cent.

Whereas the AEI appears reliable in roughly grading the severity of mitral stenosis when the diagnosis of a stenotic mitral valve is made on clinical grounds or on the M-mode or 2-D appearance of the valve itself, the AEI may not be a valuable specific criterion of the *diagnosis* of mitral stenosis (Hall *et al.,* 1979). These authors confirmed that slow (less than 30 mm/sec) or prolonged (more than 240 msec) "early" diastolic posterior motion of the posterior aortic root is the rule in mitral stenosis. However, similar abnormalities were noted in patients

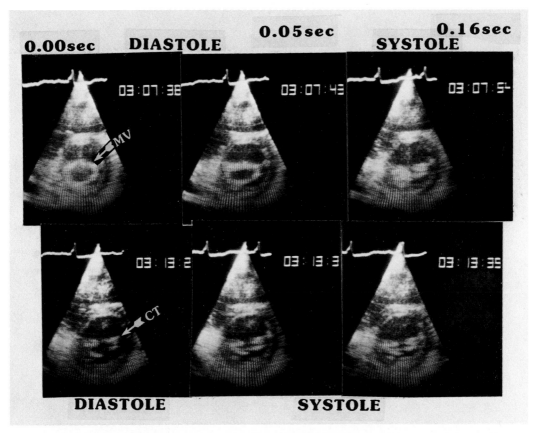

Fig. B-11. 2-D echograms from a person with a history of rheumatic fever in childhood. The 3 upper frames, from the same cardiac cycle, show that the mitral valve is thickened but not significantly stenotic. The 3 lower frames, from the same cardiac cycle, show the LV at chordae tendineae level. In the lower middle and right frames, in systole, the mitral chordae could be mistaken for a stenotic mitral valve orifice. Scanning upward to the true mitral valve level, and noting the systolic timing (from the ECG) would prevent this error.

with hypertrophic as well as congestive cardiomyopathy, aortic valve disease, aortic valve replacement, and even mitral regurgitation. Moreover, these authors found that quantitatively the parameters of aortic root diastolic motion were poor predictors of the severity of mitral stenosis.

Hall *et al.* (1979) pointed out that the amplitude and rate of diastolic posterior motion of the aortic root must depend on several factors: the relative rates of left atrial inflow and outflow of blood, the size and distensibility of the left atrium, and the mobility of the aortic root. The left atrium is frequently enlarged by mitral valve as well as LV disease, and the compliance of its walls altered by rheumatic fibrosis, mural thrombi, or scarring from previous cardiac surgery; the aortic root mobility may be affected

by scarring of previous surgery or disease of calcific degenerative type in adjacent areas of the cardiac skeleton. These theoretical considerations provide plausible reasons for lack of accord between quantitative parameters of aortic root diastolic motion and the severity of mitral stenosis.

EARLY DIASTOLIC POSTERIOR MOTION OF THE LEFT VENTRICULAR POSTERIOR WALL

Wise (1980) reported that the slope of the LV posterior wall endocardial echo in early diastole correlated well (r = 0.92) with the severity of mitral stenosis, as determined by calculation of the mitral valve orifice area by the Gorlin formula. In normals the slope of LV endocar-

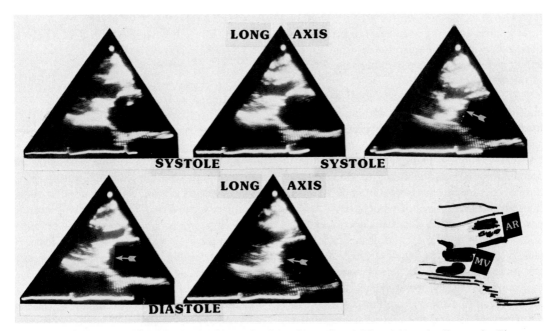

Fig. B-12. 2-D echogram in the long-axis view of a patient with calcific mitral stenosis. The five serial frames are from the same cardiac cycle. In the three upper frames, which are in systole, the dense thick mitral valve echoes (*arrow*) appear somewhat convex to the LA, suggesting mitral prolapse. However, the two lower frames, in diastole, show little change in contour, (*arrows*) suggesting that the abnormal mitral configuration is not due to prolapse but rather to deformed calcified immobile mitral cusps.

dial motion was 90 to 190 mm/sec (average, 153), whereas in mitral stenosis it was 41 to 101 mm/sec (average, 66). Wise claimed that this method predicted the mitral valve orifice area better than another indirect index of mitral stenosis, the atrial emptying index obtained by measurement of posterior aortic root motion.

CONGENITAL MITRAL STENOSIS

The patient is an infant or child, but sometimes an adolescent. Rheumatic mitral stenosis is very unusual in this age group, except in some tropical or semitropical developing countries.

The congenitally stenotic mitral valve sometimes resembles rheumatic mitral stenosis, inasmuch as the cusps are thickened and fused at the commissures. In other cases the mitral cusps are normal, but obstruction to flow from LA to LV is caused by a supravalvar ring or membrane, by cor triatriatum, or by a "parachute" mitral valve with single, large papillary muscle. It is therefore not surprising that the echographic findings have been correspondingly varied (Chung *et al.,* 1974; Goodman *et al.,* 1975;

Lundstrom, 1976; LaCorte *et al.,* 1976; Driscoll *et al.,* 1978; Snider *et al.,* 1980).

Although these anomalies causing obstruction to LV inflow are quite distinct from each other in an embryologic or developmental sense, they are very similar in hemodynamic and clinical presentation, and from the viewpoint of diagnosis it is convenient to group them together. Isolated congenital mitral stenosis is rare; more commonly it is associated with ventricular septal defects, coarctation of the aorta, or less frequently other congenital defects (Driscoll *et al.,* 1978).

The M-mode echocardiographic profile of congenital mitral stenosis may resemble that of rheumatic mitral stenosis: low EF slope, diastolic anterior motion of the posterior mitral leaflet, and absent "A" (atrial) wave (Driscoll *et al.,* 1978). Diastolic flutter of the mitral cusps occurred in 21 of 30 patients in Driscoll's series; it appears peculiar to congenital mitral stenosis since it is not seen in rheumatic mitral stenosis and has been attributed to turbulence of transmitral flow. In the hands of these authors, M-mode echography was useful in detecting the *presence* of congenital mitral stenosis, but of little value in assessing its severity or in differentiating stenosis of the mitral cusp from supravalvar membrane or the parachute valve variety of mitral stenosis.

Cor triatriatum tends to manifest with normal mitral leaflet motion but with an abnormal linear or band echo in the left atrium, in a plane posterior to the aortic root or the mitral annulus. On the other hand, supravalvar mitral membranes or rings commonly produce an abnormal linear echo closely related to or between the mitral leaflets which is associated with abnormal mitral motion (low EF slope and paradoxic diastolic motion of the posterior leaflet) (LaCorte *et al.,* 1976). However, exceptions to this general rule do occur. The presence of normal mitral leaflet motion indicates to the cardiac surgeon that the obstruction probably can be removed, leaving the mitral valve intact, whereas if the mitral leaflets move abnormally, valve replacement may be required.

Abnormal mitral valve motion, together with multiple linear diastolic valve echoes, has been reported in patients with parachute mitral valves. The echo appearances thus closely resemble those of a supravalvar membrane. In fact, the identification of an abnormal linear echo in or posterior to the mitral valve area as an abnormal stenosing membrane or diaphragm is often much more difficult than may appear from published illustrations of proven cases. Reverberations, beam-width artefacts, normal chordae tendineae echoes, or awkward transducer angulation can all be responsible for confusing echoes in this region.

Two-D echocardiography has proven diagnostically superior in dealing with congenital mitral stenosis, as it has in other congenital defects, by providing a fuller and clearer picture of cardiac anatomy (Snider *et al.,* 1980): (1) membranes or diaphragms within the left atrium can be imaged and identified as quite distinct from the mitral leaflets, which can be recognized easily by their motion characteristics, when viewed in real time; (2) mitral stenosis caused by cusp thickening and stenosis is associated with two normally placed papillary muscles in the short-axis view, whereas the parachute mitral valve is entirely attached to a large, conspicuous, central single papillary muscle.

ECHOCARDIOGRAPHIC PATTERNS RESEMBLING MITRAL STENOSIS (Fig. B-13)

MITRAL ANNULUS CALCIFICATION (Figs. B-14 to B-16)

When submitral (mitral annulus) calcification is of mild degree, it causes no significant alteration of mitral valve motion and can be identified easily as quite separate from the mitral valve. However, when submitral calcification is extensive and so located that it interferes with normal mitral cusp motion and position, one or more of the following echocardiographic features may be encountered, in spite of intrinsically normal mitral leaflets:

1. Flat or low EF slope;
2. Small DE (anterior) excursion;
3. Absence of posterior diastolic motion of the posterior mitral leaflet;
4. Posterior submitral (mitral annulus) calcification may sometimes be mistaken for a heavily calcified posterior mitral leaflet;
5. Anterior submitral calcification may be mistaken for calcification in the anterior mitral leaflet.

The differentiation between mitral stenosis and mitral annulus calcification lies in the proper visualization of the mitral leaflets, which, in the latter case, are of normal thickness and exhibit qualitatively normal diastolic motion, with "E" and "A" peaks.

Usually posterior mitral annulus calcification is easily identified as a dense bandlike echo 5 to 15 mm wide, situated between the mitral valve and left ventricular posterior wall, moving parallel to the latter. Thus, in both echographic morphology and diastolic motion, mitral annulus calcification is very different from mitral leaflets.

However, if the patient is a difficult subject because of emphysema, obesity, and so forth, or if the submitral calcification is of large extent, some skill and effort are often needed to visualize the mitral leaflets. Massive mitral annulus calcification frequently obscures the posterior mitral leaflet completely, and even to some extent the anterior mitral leaflet which may be barely visible "peeping" over the calcified mass only at a particular transducer angulation.

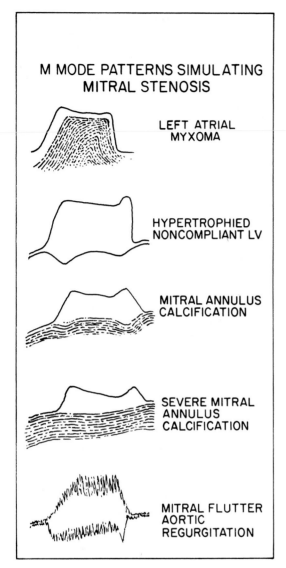

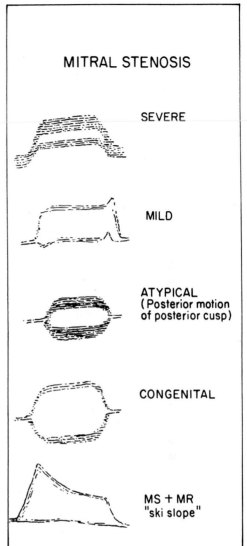

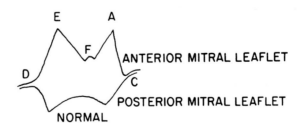

Fig. B-13. Diagram showing various M-mode patterns associated with mitral stenosis (*right*), and other M-mode patterns (*left*) that can simulate those of true mitral stenosis. The normal pattern of mitral motion is presented at bottom.

The posterior mitral leaflet, even when calcified or sclerotic, apposes the anterior mitral leaflet exactly during systole (between C and D points); this serves to distinguish it from mitral annulus calcification, which does not do so. Anterior submitral calcification, much less common than the posterior variety, may be very closely related to the anterior mitral leaflet, but scanning carefully from aortic root downward to midventricle will reveal the separation between leaflet and subjacent calcification.

The differential diagnosis between calcific stenosis of the mitral valve, on the one hand, and calcified mitral annulus with an intrinsically normal mitral valve, on the other, is important because the former is amenable to surgery while the latter is not, at least at the present day.

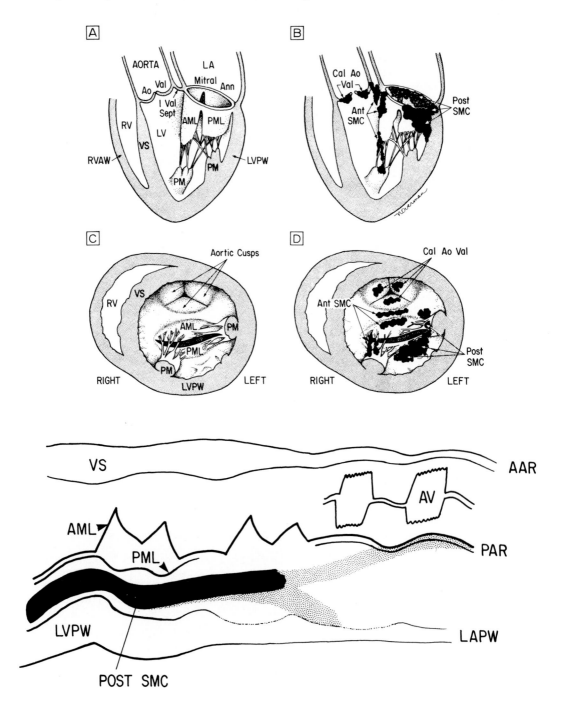

Decrease in the mitral EF slope and diminished diastolic excursions of the mitral leaflets in patients with extensive submitral calcification are attributable to restriction and modification of normal mitral leaflet motion by the mechanical interference of large calcific deposits. Not only is the amplitude of leaflet motion diminished but bulky calcification in the posterior submitral region tends to displace the mitral cusps anteriorly, toward the ventricular septum. It is also possible that massive submitral calcific accumulations could alter normal patterns of diastolic flow (vortex formation) within the left ventricle so as to reduce the EF slope of the mitral valve.

The relationship between mitral annulus calcification and mitral stenosis is complicated by the fact that, in rare instances, hemodynamically significant stenosis of the mitral orifice can occur when severe mitral annulus calcification occurs in a small-chambered, hypertrophied left ventricle (Hammer et al., 1978; Osterberger et al., 1981), even though the mitral cusps themselves are normal. This is possible because the left ventricular inflow tract is so diminished in capacity that further narrowing by encroachment of large calcific deposits in the posterior submitral region results in a significant diastolic pressure gradient between left atrium and ventricle.

Two-D echocardiography is very helpful in identifying the presence and extent of posterior mitral annulus submitral calcification, which appears as a dense conspicuous echo just anterior to the left ventricular posterior wall near its junction with the left atrial posterior wall. The calcific area appears of round or oval shape in the long-axis view, and like a bar or crescent in the short-axis view. The submitral calcification moves along with the left ventricular posterior wall and is quite independent of the brisker and larger motion of the mitral cusps anterior to it. Exceptionally, the submitral calcification is of such massive dimensions that the mitral cusp echoes are completely submerged and obscured.

Recently Come et al. (1982) have shown that calcification in the papillary muscles or chordae of the mitral valve can also present as dense echoes in the LV. This differs from "mitral annulus" calcification inasmuch as it is seen best at a level below the mitral leaflets.

Reconstructive surgery for mitral regurgitation (Fig. B-17), including plication of mitral leaflets or commissures, repair of cusp perforation, and reattachment of chordae, frequently results in echographic abnormalities of mitral motion and morphology (Snodgrass et al., 1977): mild decrease in EF slope, abnormal diastolic motion of the posterior mitral leaflet, and dense or multiple echoes in the region of the posterior leaflet or annulus; the latter were conspicuous in all three patients who had had Carpentier rings inserted in the mitral annulus.

Fig. B-14. *Upper.* Diagrams showing long-axis (*A*) and short-axis (*C*) views of the normal left ventricle in submitral (mitral annulus) calcification. In *A,* the mitral ring is shown in circumference rather than in section. In *B,* the apical left ventricle has been removed so that the aortic and mitral valves are visible from below (ventricular aspect). *B* and *D* are composite diagrams depicting the location of submitral calcification (SMC), shown as dense black areas, as observed by us in two-dimensional echocardiograms. Aortic valve calcification (Cal Ao Val) is a frequent associated finding. The intervalve septum (I Val Sept), a narrow fibrous structure bridging the space between aortic and mitral rings, may be the site of origin of some cases of anterior submitral calcification (Ant SMC). (An = annulus; Ao Val = aortic valve; PM = papillary muscles; PML = posterior mitral leaflet; Post = posterior; RVAW = right ventricular anterior wall.

Lower. Diagram depicting the different echocardiographic patterns in patients with posterior submitral calcification (POST SMC) as delineated in the scans from the left ventricle to the left atrium. This calcification is represented as a thick black bandlike echo between the posterior mitral leaflet (PML) and the left ventricular posterior wall (LVPW). As the scan continues to the left atrium, this dense band usually ends abruptly approximately midway between the posterior aortic root (PAR) and the left atrial posterior wall (LAPW). However, in some cases the calcification slopes anteriorly (upper stippled band) to merge with the posterior aortic root. In other instances the calcification inclines posteriorly (lower stippled band) to become contiguous with the posterior A-V junction.

(Reproduced from D'Cruz, I. A., *et al.:* Submitral calcification or sclerosis in elderly patients: M-mode and two-dimensional echocardiography. *Am. J. Cardiol.,* **44:**31, 1979, with permission of the publishers.)

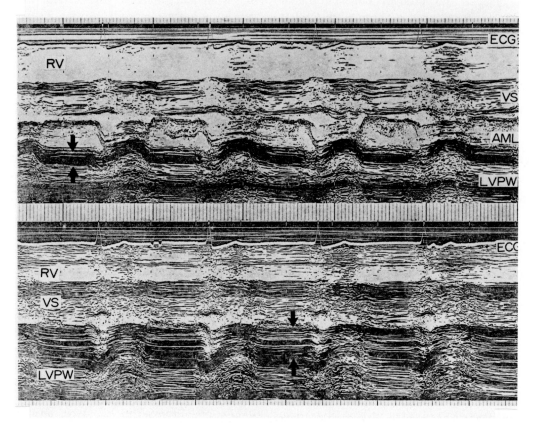

A.

Fig. B-15. *A.* Segments from an M-mode echogram with a large area of posterior submitral mitral annulus calcification, which can be seen in the upper panel as a dense echo (*arrows*) between the mitral valve and LV posterior wall. In the lower panel, at a slightly different transducer direction, the submitral calcification (*arrows*) appears much larger, almost obscuring the mitral valve. This appearance could possibly be mistaken for a mural thrombus or other LV mass.

Fig. B-15. *B.* M-mode echograms of two patients with posterior submitral "mitral annulus" calcification. The one shown in the upper panel is from a young woman with chronic renal failure on hemodialysis, with elevated parathyroid hormone levels. The one shown in the lower panel is from an elderly woman with the usual senile variety of calcification. In both cases the submitral annulus calcification appears as a dense echo between mitral valve and LV posterior wall.

Fig. B-15. *C.* M-mode echogram of an 88-year-old woman with (senile degenerative) sclerosis or calcification of the anterior mitral chordae. This can simulate the flat EF slope of mitral stenosis (*arrows at left*). However, the diagnosis of mitral stenosis is excluded by the normal motion of the posterior mitral leaflet (PML), and also the normal motion of the thickened anterior mitral leaflet (*right of figure*) as a scan is made to the aortic root.

Such abnormal, dense, bandlike echoes just posterior to the mitral valve could be easily mistaken for submitral (mitral annulus) calcification commonly seen in elderly patients, or sclerotic-calcific changes in chordae tendineae resulting from old rheumatic inflammation.

In another postoperative M-mode echographic study of mitral motion in 32 patients

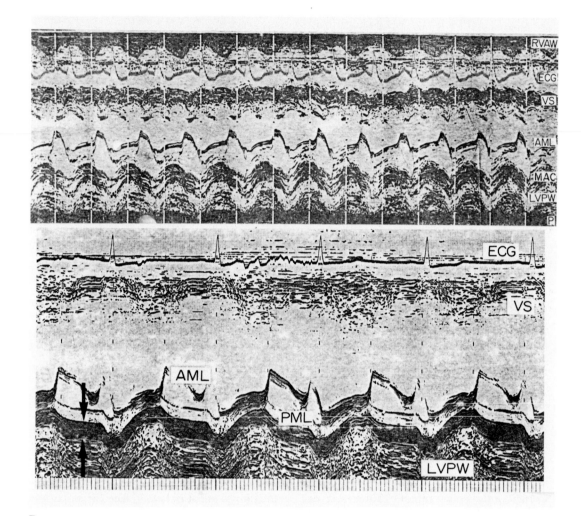

B.

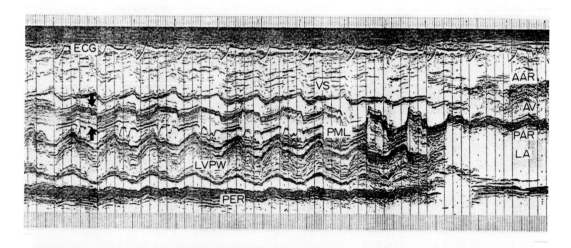

C.

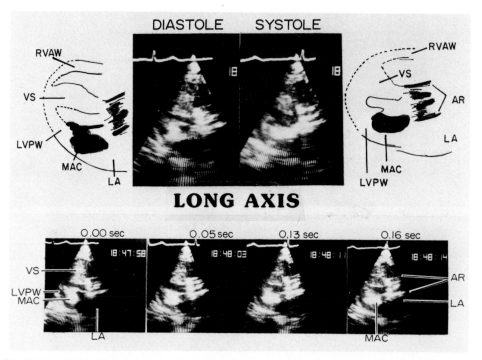

Fig. B-16. 2-D echogram, in the long-axis view, in an elderly woman with massive posterior submitral mitral annulus calcification. In the upper panel, the left frame is diastolic, the right frame systolic. The lower panel shows 4 serial frames from the same cardiac cycle. The first is near end-diastole; the second, third, and fourth are at early, mid-, and late systole. The submitral calcification appears as a large dense mass protruding into the rather small LV chamber. It also encroaches on the LV inflow from the LA. In fact, a small diastolic gradient was recorded across the mitral orifice. The aortic valve is also calcified and mildly stenotic.

who underwent mitral annuloplasty, mostly for rheumatic mitral regurgitation, Thomas *et al.* (1979) made the interesting observation that diastolic anterior motion of the posterior mitral leaflet was associated with extensive disease (fibrosis, thickening, and rigidity) of this leaflet, whereas thin, pliable posterior mitral leaflets usually showed normal posterior motion. No relation was found between the type of posterior leaflet motion and size of mitral valve orifice.

SMALL LEFT VENTRICLE WITH LOW COMPLIANCE (Fig. B-18)

Patients with thick-wall-chamber left ventricles, secondary to hypertension, aortic stenosis, or hypertrophic cardiomyopathy, may exhibit an abnormally low EF slope. Similar low EF slopes with perhaps some decrease in anterior diastolic mitral excursion also occur in patients with RV overload states (Kelley *et al.*, 1971; Goodman *et al.*, 1973; McLaurin *et al.*, 1973). During the early days of cardiac ultrasound, when only

the anterior mitral leaflet was identified by investigators, and the low or flat EF slope was hailed as a hallmark of mitral stenosis, the realization that various other cardiac conditions could be associated with a low EF slope was disconcerting. With the ability to record posterior mitral leaflet motion, and better quality strip-chart recordings, it became evident that mitral stenosis could be excluded in these cases because:

1. The mitral leaflets show no thickening or calcification;

2. The posterior mitral leaflet shows normal posterior motion in diastole (Duchak *et al.,* 1972);

3. A normal "A" peak is seen in patients with sinus rhythm; in fact the atrial contribution to ventricular filling, and consequently the "A" wave, may be unduly prominent.

LEFT ATRIAL MYXOMA

A low or flat EF mitral slope is commonly seen in patients with left atrial myxomas, but numer-

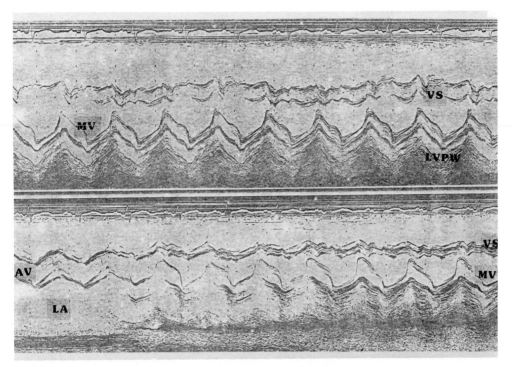

Fig. B-17. M-mode echogram of a 15-year-old girl who had had mitral annuloplasty for severe mitral regurgitation. In the upper panel, the mitral valve appearances are typical of mitral stenosis: the mitral cusp separation is small and constant through all of diastole, the "A" wave is absent, and the posterior mitral leaflet appears thickened and moves abnormally (anteriorly) in diastole. The LA is mildly dilated. On cardiac catheterization, no mitral diastolic gradient was found.

ous other echographic features of the latter serve to identify them:

1. A large stippled or layered mass of echoes which appears within the concavity of the anterior mitral valve echo in diastole;

2. A slight delay between anterior motion of the anterior mitral leaflet and that of the myxoma in early diastole produces a narrow, clear space between the two echoes (Fig. H-7);

3. The anterior mitral leaflet is of normal thickness, it is not sclerotic or calcified as in most instances of mitral stenosis;

4. During systole, the myxoma disappears from view in left ventricular scans, but may appear in the left atrium in aorta–left atrial scans. The mitral valve appears normal in systole.

On 2-D echocardiography, a left atrial myxoma is visualized as a mobile mass of variable size and density which plops abruptly into the left ventricle in diastole and moves back into the left atrium at the onset of ventricular systole with equal swiftness.

The mitral leaflets appear normal, although deprived of their normal free diastolic motion by the bulk of myxoma lying between them.

On the other hand, in mitral stenosis, the mitral leaflets are thickened or calcified and exhibit a very distinctive pattern of diastolic motion as described above (page 31).

Although the echocardiographic distinction between mitral stenosis and left atrial myxoma is usually easy and straightforward, on occasion the ultrasound appearances can be confusing. Such unusual instances are worthy of mention, since overlooking the diagnosis of an atrial myxoma on echocardiography, for technical reasons, is a catastrophe of the first order.

1. If, in a patient with mitral stenosis, the anterior mitral leaflet is heavily calcified and so aligned with the ultrasound beam in diastole as to produce multiple, dense, layered echoes, it can be mistaken for a myxoma. The true

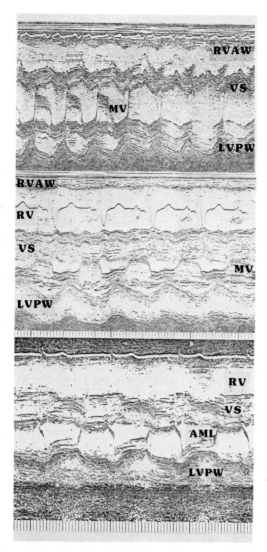

Fig. B-18. M-mode echograms of a patient with true mitral stenosis (*upper*) and two patients with "pseudomitral stenosis" due to concentric LV hypertrophy (*center and lower*). In all instances the mitral EF slope is flat. However, the posterior mitral leaflet appears abnormal and moves abnormally in true mitral stenosis (*upper*) but in pseudomitral stenosis (*center and lower*) it is normal. A flat mitral EF slope in the latter type of stenosis is attributable to low LV compliance and a small LV chamber, which interfere with those vortex flow patterns in the LV that are responsible for the normal EF slope. The mitral valve opens to the full width of the small LV chamber. Mild mitral annulus calcification (*lower*) may be an additional factor causing the flat EF slope.

diagnosis can be made by demonstrating that the narrow space (interval) between anterior leaflet and "myxomas" in early diastole is absent, and by identifying the posterior mitral leaflet which shows abnormal anterior diastolic motion typical of mitral stenosis.

2. Sometimes the physical properties of the myxomatous tumor tissue or the tumor-blood interface are such that ultrasound is not reflected adequately, so that echoes representing the tumor are weak or nebulous. These echoes may then be dismissed erroneously by the echocardiographer as artefact (reverberatory clutter), or overlooked completely if the gain is set too low or the reject set too high.

3. Whereas the vast majority of cardiac myxomas are pedunculated and attached only to a small area of atrial endocardium, in rare instances the neoplasm arising in the left atrium or mitral valve is of an invasive sarcomatous nature. In such cases the typical "plopping" of a mobile tumor mass back and forth between left atrium and ventricle is absent, and infiltration of cusp tissue by the malignant growth may resemble the sclerotic leaflets of mitral stenosis. It may also happen that as the tumor grows, it protrudes into the mitral orifice, producing a bizarre but diagnostic appearance.

AORTIC REGURGITATION

In patients with rheumatic heart disease, the association of aortic regurgitation with a stenotic mitral valve is not uncommon. On the other hand, diastolic murmurs are often heard at the apex in patients with aortic regurgitation who do not have mitral stenosis (Austin-Flint murmur). The simulation of some echocardiographic features of mitral stenosis in patients with aortic regurgitation (but normal mitral valves) is therefore of some importance, and the question "Does this patient with aortic regurgitation have mitral valve stenosis or not?" is encountered fairly frequently in cardiologic practice.

Echocardiographic appearances of the anterior mitral leaflet may, in some cases, mimic those of mitral stenosis:

1. Fine flutter on the anterior mitral leaflet can be mistaken for thickening or sclerosis of the leaflet, especially if the gain is set too high or the scale too attenuated on the tracing. Enlargement of the mitral valve echo by expansion of the scale, faster speeds, and deliberate gradual increase of the reject will clearly demonstrate the vibratory nature of fine diastolic flutter and differentiate it from sclerotic cusp thickening.

2. Low or flat mitral EF slope.

3. Decrease in or even absence of the mitral anterior excursion (opening) of the abnormalities is caused by the regurgitant jet from the leaking aortic valve impinging on the anterior mitral leaflet during diastole, particularly early diastole, so that the leaflet is held down and prevented from moving anteriorly as the mitral valve opens.

The following characteristics of mitral valve motion in patients with aortic regurgitation help in excluding mitral stenosis:

1. The posterior mitral leaflet moves normally (posteriorly) during diastole.

2. A normal "A" peak usually is seen in patients with sinus rhythm. In fact, the "A" wave may be quite prominent in cases where the regurgitant aortic jet holds the mitral valve almost closed in early to middiastole; in this situation the atrial "kick" may be the only phase of diastole during which the mitral valve opens fully.

3. If the aortic regurgitation is chronic and moderate to severe in degree, the left ventricle is dilated. In pure mitral stenosis, unassociated with mitral regurgitation, aortic regurgitation, or myocardial disease, the left ventricle is usually low normal in size.

CHRONIC LEFT VENTRICULAR FAILURE (Fig. B-19)

In patients with left ventricular dilatation and chronic decompensation, with low stroke vol-

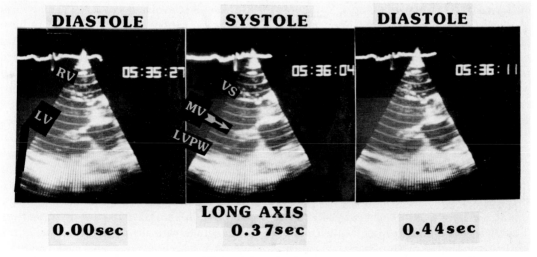

Fig. B-19.   2-D echogram, in the long-axis view, of a patient with severe congestive cardiomyopathy and refractory chronic heart failure. The three frames are serial ones from the same cardiac cycle. The first is in late diastole, the second in systole, the third in early diastole. The LV is dilated and contracts poorly. The mitral valve leaflet separation is abnormally small in diastole, due to the low stroke output. Note that the diastolic configuration of the mitral valve, in this view, is different from the funnel-shaped outline of noncalcific mitral stenosis.

ume and cardiac output, the amplitude of diastolic opening of the mitral valve is often subnormal. The underlying left ventricular failure may be secondary to congestive (dilated) cardiomyopathy, ischemic heart disease, or advanced valvular heart disease (aortic or mitral) with poor myocardial contractility. The mitral cusps in such patients may show mild nonspecific thickening. Thus, one notes thickened mitral leaflets that do not open fully, and it is not surprising that the possibility of mitral stenosis is sometimes raised. True mitral diastolic opening accompanying low-output states is identified by the following features:

1. The latter situation is usually associated with a dilated ventricle. In pure mitral stenosis the left ventricle is normal to small in size, unless a significant degree of aortic or mitral regurgitation is also present, or the left ventricular myocardium is diffusely diseased.

2. Although the diastolic excursions of the mitral leaflets are abnormally small in amplitude, they are *qualitatively normal.* The normal morphology of contour, including the "E" peak, is preserved on the anterior mitral leaflet echo; this applies also to corresponding deflections of the posterior mitral leaflet.

3. Patients in sinus rhythm exhibit the so-called double-diamond appearance, whereas those in atrial fibrillation lack the second peak, since atrial contraction and peaks are not in evidence. In either case, the mitral leaflets are so aligned with the ultrasound beam in such hearts that it is usually impossible to record one cusp without the other. On the other hand, in true mitral stenosis, the anterior mitral leaflet and its motion are conspicuous, and can be visualized easily (without the posterior leaflet) by scanning toward the aortic root.

4. On 2-D echocardiography the diastolic motion of the mitral leaflets in mitral stenosis is of a typical and distinctive nature, whereas in low-output states the mitral cusps exhibit the brisk yet gentle diastolic motion similar to that seen in normals, albeit of somewhat smaller amplitude. The diminished range of mitral diastolic excursions is partly illusory in patients with very large ventricles; the attenuation of scale necessary for encompassing the dilated ventricles within the width of the tracing tends to make the mitral cusp motion appear diminutive.

MITRAL VALVE PROLAPSE

In many centers today, more echocardiograms are done to confirm or exclude the diagnosis of mitral prolapse than for any other purpose in clinical medicine. Before beginning the discussion of specific echocardiographic criteria, a few preliminary remarks are necessary to place the problems that the clinical echocardiographer and cardiologist face in proper perspective:

1. "Classic" examples, in which the prolapse is most pronounced, are diagnosed easily by all and pose no difficulty. It is with regard to the remainder of patients with this entity, who comprise the majority, that much controversy and confusion prevail.

2. There is no easily available "gold standard." Although generally reliable, angiocardiography has certain shortcomings (Smith *et al.,* 1977) and in any case is rarely justified.

3. It is generally accepted that echocardiographic false negatives are not rare, however skillful the echocardiographer. Thus, it has been estimated that 10 to 20 per cent of instances of genuine prolapse are not detected by echocardiography.

4. The posterior mitral leaflet consists of three scallops: a central scallop and one on either side related to each commissure: the posteromedial, middle, and anterolateral scallops. Prolapse can involve only one scallop, or two scallops (in various combinations), or all three (Aranda *et al.,* 1975). Thus, it is common for part of the posterior mitral cusp (the affected scallop or scallops) to prolapse while the rest of the cusp moves normally. This explains why, in many cases, mitral prolapse may be evident only at a particular transducer angulation, whereas at a different angulation or intercostal space mitral valve motion appears quite normal. Thus, a segment of M-mode tracing showing normal posterior cusp motion is not inconsistent with an appearance indicating prolapse elsewhere in the same tracing; it is also not incompatible with the abnormal prolapse motion having been demonstrated on some other occasion by a more experienced or diligent echocardiographer.

5. Whether mitral prolapse itself is always a disease, or merely a variant of normal that is associated with symptoms or untoward effects

only in a small minority of instances, is still not clear in the minds of most clinicians. The decision to label an individual, usually perfectly healthy in every other respect (Markiewicz *et al.,* 1976), with this diagnosis is fraught with the hazard of provoking iatrogenic symptoms, anxiety in relatives, and so forth. Another way of expressing this is to say that it is difficult to decide whether less damage is done by false-negative than by false-positive diagnosis.

The diagnostic approach I outline below attempts to define a practical framework of echocardiographic diagnosis that is workable in everyday practice, that strives to avoid over-diagnosis as well as underdiagnosis, and yet is

not too complicated. In my experience it has worked well.

Abnormal posterior motion of both mitral leaflets, or of either valvar leaflet alone, is the sole echocardiographic criterion of mitral prolapse. A variety of M-mode echographic patterns (Figs. B-20 to B-28) are considered diagnostic of mitral prolapse. (Kerber *et al.,* 1971; Dillon *et al.,* 1971; Popp *et al.,* 1974; DeMaria *et al.,* 1974; Cohen, 1976; Devereux *et al.,* 1976; DeMaria *et al.,* 1977; Sahn *et al.,* 1977; Cohen *et al.,* 1979). It is convenient to group these patterns into three main types:

1. *Mid- to late systolic prolapse.* The mitral leaflets move normally during approximately

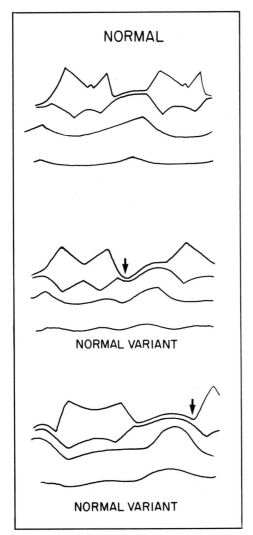
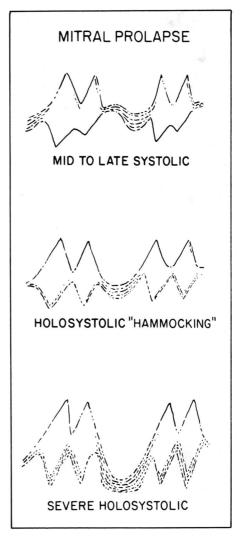

Fig. B-20. Diagram showing normal pattern of mitral motion (*top left*) and normal variants that could possibly be mistaken for mitral prolapse (*center and bottom left*). The 3 main varieties of true mitral prolapse are depicted in right half of the figure.

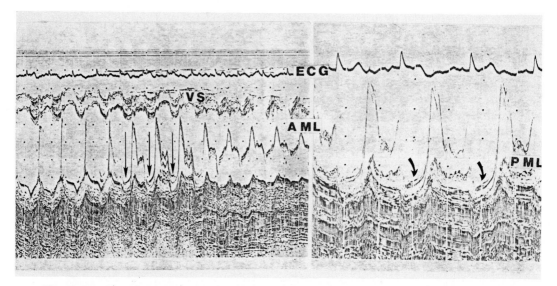

Fig. B-21. The left panel depicts an M-mode echographic scan at slow paper speed in a 20-year-old man, from mid-LV to LA. The arrows show the level at which mitral prolapse is detectable.

M-mode echogram of the same patient, obtained with a slightly different transducer angulation and faster paper speed. Mitral prolapse is evident (*arrows*). The mitral leaflet echoes are not visualized in continuity through all of systole. However, anterior mitral leaflet echoes occupy an abnormally posterior position in late systole (*arrows*), and then rapidly converge upward toward the mitral E point. This type of mitral valve pattern is frequently encountered in practice and suggests mitral prolapse, though it is not as diagnostically valuable as other patterns of prolapse, where both mitral leaflet echoes are well delineated through the whole cardiac cycle.

the first half of systole. Abruptly, in midsystole (actually, at some point during the middle third of systole) they move posteriorly for 3 mm or more and then move rapidly forward to attain the D point, when the mitral valve opens.

This pattern, if clearly recorded with good visualization of both mitral leaflets or at least the posterior leaflet through the whole cardiac cycle, is diagnostic of mitral prolapse, no matter in which intercostal space the transducer was positioned, or whether the transducer was held perpendicular to the chest wall or not. Some-

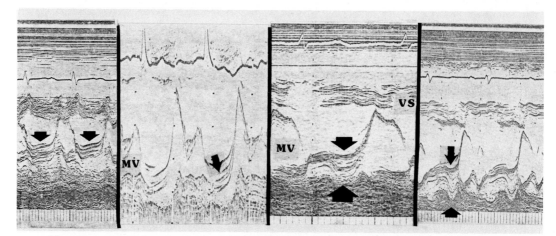

Fig. B-22. M-mode echograms of 4 different patients. All have mitral prolapse. The two on the left are called holosystolic or hammock-type, while those on the right are termed late systolic, by most observers. However, the four echograms demonstrate the range of variation in duration of systolic mitral prolapse.

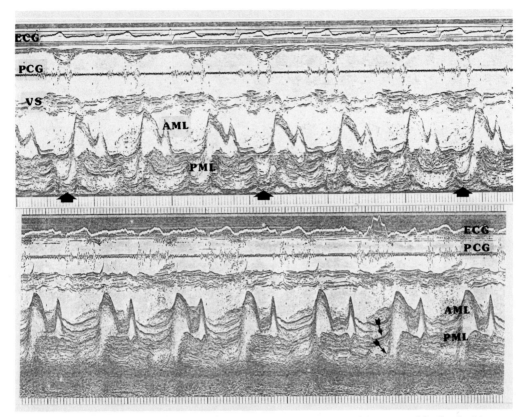

Fig. B-23. M-mode echogram and phonocardiogram of a 30-year-old woman with a loud midsystolic click. The mitral valve abruptly prolapses in midsystole (*arrows*), forming a U-shaped indentation on the endocardial contour of the LV posterior wall. The posterior mitral leaflet appears unduly thickened in diastole (simulating a vegetation) due to folding and myxomatous thickening of the redundant leaflet.

M-mode echogram of a young woman with a midsystolic click and late systolic murmur, as recorded on the phonocardiogram (PCG). During systole, multiple fine linear echoes are visible in the mitral valve area, some of which could be considered normal, while others (*arrows*) indicate late systolic prolapse. Apparent thickening and increased amplitude of motion of the mitral leaflets are associated with virtual apposition of the mitral cusps in middiastole. Such cusp thickening is partly due to redundant folds and perhaps to myxomatous change; it should not be mistaken for valvular vegetations.

times the prolapsing mitral leaflet is represented not by a single linear echo but by several thin, more or less parallel, loops, the most posterior of which may fall back almost as far as the posterior atrioventricular wall. These delicate multiple linear echoes are easily missed if the gain is set too low or the recording equipment is of suboptimal quality, but are of diagnostic value because they are highly typical of mitral prolapse.

An important variant of the late systolic type of mitral prolapse is one in which the anterior mitral leaflet moves to an anterior position in early systole, then whips abruptly backward in midsystole to occupy a posterior position of pro-

lapse until end-systole. The cause of this initial anterior mitral motion is not entirely certain; it has been attributed to "buckling" of a long, redundant anterior mitral leaflet (Gardin *et al.,* 1981) that precedes posterior motion (prolapse) of the leaflet as a whole toward the left atrial region. Such early anterior motion of small amplitude is not uncommon (Fig. B-26); occasionally it is pronounced, in which case it assumes some diagnostic significance because:

a. It could be mistaken for the systolic anterior motion (SAM) of idiopathic hypertrophic subaortic stenosis (IHSS). Close attention to the position of the mitral C point on the tracing is said to distinguish between the two: the C

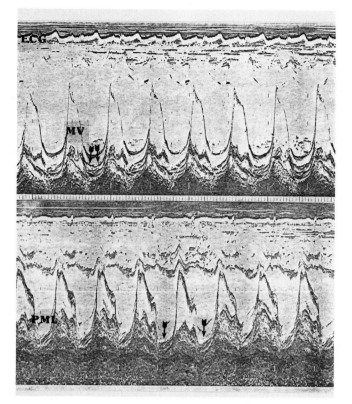

Fig. B-24. *Upper.* M-mode echogram in a young woman with mitral valve prolapse of the holosystolic or hammock type (*arrows*). As soon as the mitral leaflets close at the onset of systole, they move posteriorly to almost 1 cm behind the line joining C and D points, and remain there until they rapidly move forward at end-systole.

Lower. M-mode echogram in a young woman with severe holosystolic mitral valve prolapse. During all of systole, the mitral leaflets occupy a very posterior position (*arrows*) adjacent to the posterior atrioventricular wall. Thick multiple echoes representing the posterior mitral leaflet in diastole are attributable to redundant folds of this leaflet, commonly associated with severe instances of mitral prolapse.

point is anterior to the late systolic position of the mitral valve in mitral prolapse, but is posterior to the end-systolic mitral valve position in the SAM of IHSS (Popp *et al.,* 1974).

b. An early systolic motion of anterior mitral chordae, or tip of the anterior mitral leaflet, which does *not* continue into a posterior prolapse motion is a common normal variant. It manifests on the M-mode tracing as a fine linear echo that moves rapidly forward, anterior to the main leaflet echo, in early systole and is lost to view before midsystole. On the 2-D echocardiogram, careful observation may reveal a brisk forward flicking motion of the anterior mitral apparatus, at approximately the point of attachment of chordae tendineae to cusp. It must be emphasized that mitral prolapse is *not* diagnosed if the mitral valve does not move to an abnormally posterior position in the latter half of systole, as recorded on the M-mode and 2-D echogram. Admittedly, the echocardiographer will encounter instances where the distinction between a variant of normal and a variant of prolapse is difficult; it may be based more on a subjective opinion than on established or proven criteria.

It is worth adding that patients with late systolic prolapse (1) usually have midsystolic clicks that may or may not be followed by a late systolic murmur at the apex; (2) usually have left ventricles and left atria of normal size, because the mitral regurgitation is of mild degree; (3) in one instance, early anterior mitral motion with late systolic prolapse was thought to be associated with a partly flail anterior mitral leaflet (Zerin *et al.,* 1980).

2. *Hammock-type prolapse.* The mitral cusps sag posteriorly in systole like a suspended hammock, the C and D points representing the points of suspension. The contour of the apposed mitral cusps is that of a smooth curve, the convexity of which is directed posteriorly; however, the prolapsed leaflets usually do not abut against the posterior ventricular or atrial wall. As with the late systolic variety of prolapse, the mitral cusps may sometimes be represented not by a single linear echo or two closely apposed linear echoes, but by multiple fine parallel lines, one below the other.

It generally is accepted that prolapse can be diagnosed if the most posterior point on the hammock is 3 mm or more posterior to a line joining the C and D points, provided that the transducer is held perpendicular to the chest wall.

The latter condition, specifying the position of the ultrasound transducer, was added because it was realized (Weiss *et. al.*, 1975) that false-positive prolapse could be produced by directing the transducer caudally. When the same mitral valve is recorded from a lower intercostal space, with the transducer held perpendicular to the chest wall, this spurious prolapse is no longer apparent. Thus, a mild degree of sagging or hammocking can be artefactually produced by a downward (caudal) transducer inclination. However, a *marked* posterior sagging of the mitral cusps to the extent of 1 cm or more below the C–D level is more than can be attributed to transducer artefact and must be presumed to indicate true prolapse, even if the transducer angulation is not known.

In the hammock variety of prolapse, posterior motion of the mitral leaflets begins in early systole, whereas in late systolic prolapse it begins in the middle one third of systole. The characteristic auscultatory finding in patients with mitral hammocking is a systolic murmur occupying most of systole, but it is not uncommon for patients with the typical echographic pattern to have no murmur at all.

An "early" nonejection systolic click may be heard at or near the junction of the first one third with the middle one third of systole. In a frequent variant of the hammock type of prolapse, the mitral leaflets, or at least the posterior one, exhibit an abrupt *accentuation* of the prolapse in late systole; the resulting pattern is thus a combination of hammocking and late systolic prolapse.

3. *Severe holosystolic prolapse* is the most severe type of mitral prolapse, and is much less

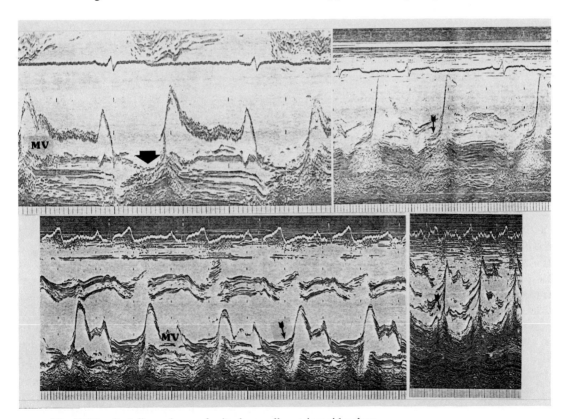

Fig. B-25. Systolic prolapse of mitral as well as tricuspid valves:

Upper. The left panel shows systolic prolapse of the mitral valve (*arrows*) and also a fine diastolic flutter of the anterior mitral leaflet, attributable to aortic regurgitation. The right panel shows late systolic prolapse of the tricuspid valve (*arrow*). It is possible that this young man had myxomatous degeneration of all three valves.

Lower. M-mode echogram of a young woman. Late systolic prolapse of the mitral valve (*arrow*) is apparent in the left panel, and of the tricuspid valve in the right panel.

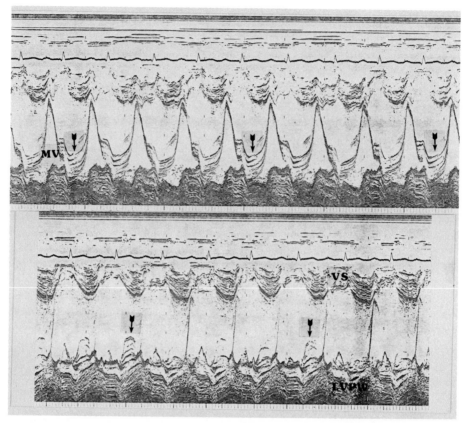

Fig. B-26. *Upper.* M-mode echogram of a 15-year-old boy with mitral prolapse of the holosystolic or hammock type (*arrows*). An unusual feature of the mitral valve pattern in this illustration is the multiple mitral echoes anterior to the main echo of the main anterior leaflet echo in late diastole.

   Lower. Echogram of the same patient with different transducer angulation. The anterior mitral leaflet is not completely visualized. Early systolic anterior motion of mitral chordae is visible (*arrows*), especially in the first two beats. Early systolic anterior chordal buckling is not rare in association with mitral prolapse.

common than the other two types. The mitral leaflets move rapidly backward at the onset of systole to lie against the left atrial posterior wall; they maintain this extreme posterior position until the end of systole, when they move rapidly forward to the mitral D point.

   Though this variety of mitral prolapse is usually lumped together with the hammock variety under the label holosystolic prolapse, there are several differences between the two, so that their separation into distinct varieties is justified. The following features associated with severe holosystolic prolapse help in distinguishing it from the hammock variety:

   1. In the M-mode echogram, the prolapsing mitral leaflets have a rectangular contour with rounded edges (Fig. B-24), whereas in the hammock type a smooth curve is inscribed, convex posteriorly.

   2. The amplitude of posterior systolic motion is greater, the mitral leaflets abutting against the left atrial wall during almost the whole of systole.

   3. The mitral leaflets tend to show a greater range of diastolic motion, which manifests as abnormally large diastolic excursions, perhaps with an element of erratic or irregular motion; such behavior of the posterior mitral leaflet is particularly characteristic.

   4. Thus severe holosystolic prolapse bears a close resemblance, on the echocardiogram, to a flail posterior mitral leaflet (rendered untethered by rupture of chordae tendineae).

   5. Mitral regurgitation is invariably present

and usually quite severe, requiring mitral valve replacement. A loud pansystolic apical murmur, well conducted posteriorly to the left scapular region, is the rule. On the other hand, lesser degrees of mitral prolapse are associated with either no murmur at all or a soft murmur localized to the area of the cardiac apex.

As Feigenbaum perspicaciously remarked (1976), echocardiographically as well as hemodynamically there is probably little difference between a regurgitant mitral valve caused by a flail posterior leaflet and one caused by very severe prolapse with intact chordae. In the former, the chordae are ruptured; in the latter, they (or the leaflets, or both) are not torn but are extremely long and redundant. In either case, the mechanical defect of the valve (regurgitation) is equally severe.

MANEUVERS TO PROVOKE OR ENHANCE MITRAL PROLAPSE

Echographic appearances of mitral prolapse can appear or be accentuated by inhalation of amyl nitrite or by sitting or standing up from the supine position. The factor common to these maneuvers is decrease in LV size, which permits the redundant mitral leaflet to fall farther into the left atrium during systole. Mathey *et al.* (1976) showed that, in susceptible persons, mitral prolapse and a systolic click occurred at a definite "critical" LV diameter, which was constant for any particular patient. It has been demonstrated (Mathey *et al.,* 1976; Winkle *et al.,* 1975) that amyl nitrite and a change in position from horizontal toward vertical result in an earlier onset of mitral prolapse on the echographic tracing and an earlier occurrence of the systolic click on the phonocardiographic tracing, i.e., the click and onset of prolapse "move" closer to the first heart sound. Such an effect sometimes can transform midsystolic prolapse to holosystolic prolapse (Winkle *et al.,* 1975). Noble *et al.* (1982) found that standing the patient up demonstrated mitral prolapse (on M-mode as well as 2-D echography) in most patients who had auscultatory signs of prolapse but whose echocardiograms were normal in the supine position. Bartall *et al.* (1978) showed that Müller's maneuver diminished the degree of mitral prolapse.

ECHOCARDIOGRAPHIC APPEARANCES SIMULATING MITRAL VALVE PROLAPSE

1. *Normal variants.* The LV posterior wall sometimes may exhibit a normal brief posterior motion, either at the very beginning or at the very end of the C–D interval, i.e., during the period of mitral cusp apposition (Fig. B-20):

a. At the onset of systole, during the isovolumic (preejection) phase (first 50 msec after onset of QRS), the LV posterior wall may show a small transient posterior motion; this has been attributed to a slight change in LV shape, characterized by slight increase in its minor axis. Being attached to the mitral annulus, the mitral valve participates in this brief posterior motion, which is immediately followed by normal anterior systolic motion of the LV posterior wall endocardium and of the apposed mitral cusps. When present, this brief posterior mitral motion is of small amplitude, not exceeding 2 or 3 mm, and limited in duration to that of the isovolumic phase. On the other hand, the posterior motion of a prolapsing mitral valve, though of variable onset with reference to the C point, always continues until the D point. Whether of early, mid-, or late systolic onset, mitral valve prolapse never ends before end-systole.

Another point of difference is that parallel motion of the apposed mitral cusps and of the LV posterior wall is "physiologic," the former passively following the latter, whereas in true prolapse the prolapsing leaflet or leaflets fall backward toward the LV posterior wall at the onset of prolapse and move forward away from it just before mitral opening.

b. The mitral valve usually opens at about the peak of anterior motion of the LV posterior wall endocardium. However, in hypertrophied hearts, especially hypertrophic cardiomyopathy, mitral opening (the D point) is somewhat delayed so that it may *follow* the peak of LV posterior wall endocardial motion. When this happens, the apposed mitral cusps show a brief posterior motion, parallel to that of LV posterior wall endocardium, just before the valve opens at the D point. It should not be mistaken for late systolic mitral prolapse, which occurs *before* the peak of LV posterior wall endocardial motion and is not characterized by parallel mitral-endocardial motion.

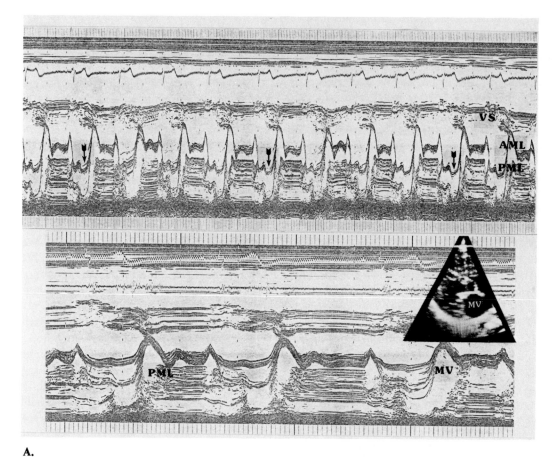

A.

Fig. B-27. *A. Upper.* M-mode echogram of a young man with conspicuous late systolic mitral valve prolapse (*arrows*). During systole the mitral valve is represented by two linear echoes, roughly parallel to each other. The posterior mitral leaflet shows exaggerated diastolic motion. At the left end of the figure the redundant folds of the posterior mitral leaflet give rise to large, multilayered echoes, simulating a left atrial myxoma.

Lower. Echogram of the same patient with late mitral prolapse at faster paper speed, showing that the mitral valve opens well in early diastole ("E" peak) and with atrial contraction ("A" peak), but during the intervening diastole the posterior mital leaflet moves forward to an abnormally anterior position. An anterior diastolic position of the posterior mitral leaflet is seen also in (1) mitral stenosis, which is excluded by large posterior motion of the posterior leaflet in early and late diastole, and normal anterior leaflet diastolic motion; (2) flail mitral leaflet due to ruptured chordae, for which there was no evidence on the 2-D echogram. The broad, multilayered echo representing the redundant posterior mitral leaflet can be seen to extend anteriorly as far as the anterior mitral leaflet in diastole. The inset, showing a long-axis 2-D echographic view of the mitral valve in diastole, demonstrates the thickened folds of the posterior mitral leaflet gathered behind the anterior mitral leaflet.

2. *Large pericardial effusions.* In large pericardial effusions the heart as a whole exhibits abnormal and exaggerated mobility. An important feature of this motion is posterior motion of the LV posterior wall during systole; the mitral valve, because of its attachment to the mitral annulus, participates in this motion. The configuration of such motion on the M-mode echocardiogram (Fig. N-10) is very similar to that recorded in the mid- to late systolic variety of mitral prolapse (Levisman and Abbasi, 1976; Owens *et al.*, 1976). It can be easily differentiated from true mitral prolapse because: (a) The posterior systolic motion of the apposed mitral leaflets is parallel to a corresponding motion of the subjacent LV posterior wall. (b) Following paracentesis or spontaneous absorption of the effusion, motion of the LV

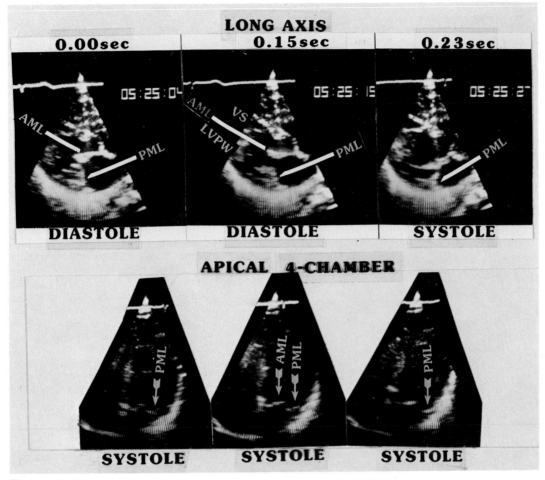

B.

Fig. B-27. *B.* 2-D echogram of same patient.

Upper. Long-axis view, showing mitral prolapse in systole (*right*); in diastole (*left and center*) the posterior leaflet forms redundant folds.

Lower. In the apical 4-chamber view in early systole (*left*), midsystole (*center*), and late systole (*right*). The prolapsing motion of the posterior mitral leaflet in mid- to late systole is evident.

posterior wall and of the mitral valve return to normal. (c) Swinging or pendulous motion of the ventricles within a large pericardial effusion is usually obvious. If the mistake is made of expanding the scale so much that the echo-free pericardial space between pericardium and ventricular wall is excluded from the tracing, the pericardial effusion could perhaps be overlooked, but, even so, abnormal systolic motion of the LV posterior wall would give the clue to "pseudoprolapse."

It has been suggested that a large pericardial effusion might provoke actual mitral prolapse by decreasing LV size, in this respect acting

in the same way as amyl nitrite inhalation or the Valsalva maneuver. This explanation is unlikely to be valid because: (a) Pseudoprolapse is seen in patients with large pericardial effusions who have no evidence of cardiac compression (tamponade). (b) When cardiac tamponade *is* present, the phasic respiratory variations in LV size are not accompanied by corresponding phasic changes in the degree of pseudoprolapse of the mitral valve.

3. Another form of pseudoprolapse can occur in *postinfarction aneurysms of the LV posterior wall;* systolic posterior motion of the mitral valve can parallel the abnormal paradoxic sys-

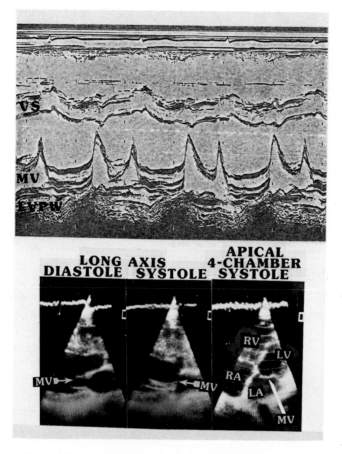

VS

MV

LVPW

LONG AXIS
DIASTOLE

SYSTOLE

APICAL
4-CHAMBER
SYSTOLE

MV→

←MV

RV
LV
RA
LA
MV

Fig. B-28. This M-mode echogram illustrates a pattern seen in everyday practice, and is included to make the point that not all patients with mitral prolapse present with the classic diagnostic features shown in most other figures in this chapter. This echogram would be read as mild late systolic prolapse by some echocardiographers, whereas others would consider it equivocal or even normal.

2-D echogram of another young woman with persistent atypical chest pain and premature ventricular beats. The appearances in the long-axis and apical views are suggestive but not absolutely indicative of mitral prolapse.

tolic motion of the LV posterior wall (Fig. K-3). Such paradoxic motion of the LV wall in this area is quite unusual, hypokinesis or akinesis being much more frequent results of infarction. The precisely congruous or parallel contours of the mitral valve and LV posterior wall endocardial echoes indicate that mitral motion is secondary to abnormal LV wall motion and also serve to distinguish it from true mitral prolapse.

4. *Patients with marked LV dilatation and decompensation,* as in congestive cardiomyopathy, often have mitral valves that show mild sagging during systole, instead of the slight anterior motion seen in normal hearts. The reason for the somewhat different mitral valve configuration in those patients with severe LV dilatation is the altered spatial plane of the mitral annulus with respect to the rest of the left ventricle and the chest wall. In addition to marked increase in the LV minor axis, the LV shape tends to be more like a sphere, as can be seen clearly in the 2-D long-axis or apical view. On the other hand, in true mitral prolapse, the LV

size is usually normal and LV contractility normal or enhanced.

5. Chandaratna *et al.* (1974) showed that individuals with a normal pattern of mitral valve motion during sinus rhythm can exhibit prolapse during *premature ventricular beats* (Fig. B-29). They speculated that this phenomenon could possibly be caused by abnormal and delayed activation of the papillary muscles and smaller ventricular volume than during normal beats. That the latter factor was an important one is suggested by the finding that prolapse was seen in early extrasystoles but not when the coupling interval was long; moreover, extrasystoles occurring in patients with very dilated ventricles did not result in prolapse.

OTHER DIAGNOSTIC CONSIDERATIONS PERTAINING TO MITRAL PROLAPSE

A detailed discussion of the auscultatory and other clinical aspects of mitral prolapse would be out of place here. However, there are certain features that the echocardiographer can easily

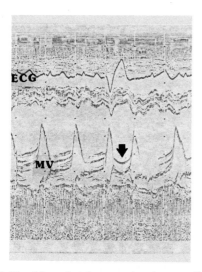

Fig. B-29. M-mode echogram showing systolic prolapse of the mitral valve during a ventricular premature beat only (*arrow*). No prolapse is seen in the other beats.

observe during the course of his examination that have a bearing on the probability that mitral prolapse is present in a given patient. Patients who have such mitral pathology are often of slender asthenic build, or sometimes of average build, but very rarely of a heavy, stocky, or obese habitus. Whereas the typical patient is usually a slim young woman, mitral prolapse is not rare in middle-aged or elderly men (Higgins *et al.*, 1976). At the other end of the gamut of age, it has been found in newborn female infants (Chandaratna *et al.*, 1979). Mitral prolapse is the rule in patients with Marfan's syndrome (Brown *et al.*, 1976), the incidence in females being 100 per cent. Mitral prolapse was reported in 31 per cent of patients with abnormal thoracic configuration, including pectus excavatum, the straight-back syndrome, and decreased anteroposterior thoracic diameter (Udoshi *et al.*, 1979). The association of mitral prolapse with prolapse (and often regurgitation) of the tricuspid and/or aortic valve is not rare (Ogawa *et al.*, 1982), myxomatous degeneration having affected multiple valves.

The association of mitral prolapse with various other cardiac conditions is reported from time to time in the literature; however, in many of them the relationship between the primary or associated entity and mitral prolapse is unexplained, uncertain, or merely coincidental. These reports are mentioned briefly here, so

that the echocardiographer, alerted to such associations, may study mitral motion with extra diligence in these patients.

It is reemphasized that mitral prolapse is extremely common in patients with Marfan's syndrome. The coexistence of mitral prolapse with asymmetric septal hypertrophy (ASH) (Chandaratna *et al.*, 1977), with rheumatic mitral stenosis (Weinrauch *et al.*, 1977), following mitral valvotomy (Gottdiener *et al.*, 1978), with coronary heart disease (Aranda *et al.*, 1975), and with hyperthyroidism (Channick *et al.*, 1981) is as intriguing as its mechanisms are obscure. The syndrome of "papillary muscle dysfunction" is often invoked when mitral prolapse is noted in patients with ECG or angiographic evidence of ischemic heart disease, the implication being that the mitral cusps and chordae are normal but impaired contraction of the papillary muscle is the primary fault.

In the area of congenital heart disease, the association of mitral prolapse with atrial septal defects (Betriu *et al.*, 1975) is now well known. Less known and less frequent is its incidence in patients with ventricular septal defect, patent ductus arteriosus, tetralogy of Fallot, congenital aortic stenosis, and Ebstein's anomaly (Rippe *et al.*, 1979).

Recently an association has been established between myotonia dystrophica and mitral prolapse (Strasberg *et al.*, 1980).

TWO-DIMENSIONAL ECHOCARDIOGRAPHY (Figs. B-30 to B-32)

Sahn *et al.* (1976) described 2-D appearances in 26 children with mitral prolapse on M-mode echography, using a linear-array system. They noted a "superior and somewhat posterior displacement of both leaflets" in prolapse, i.e., the body or central portion of each leaflet billowed toward the left atrium; both leaflets were involved in the prolapse in all their patients. Gilbert *et al.* (1976), using phased-array equipment, confirmed abnormal superior motion of the mitral leaflets, above the level of the mitral ring, as a reliable 2-D indicator of mitral prolapse (established by angiocardiography in their 34 patients). However, they found that either the anterior leaflet or the posterior leaflet, or both, could be affected in individual patients.

MITRAL PROLAPSE: 2D ECHO

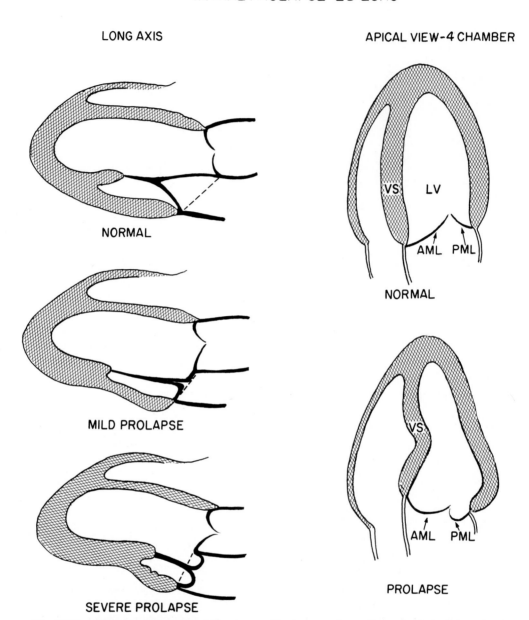

Fig. B-30. Diagram showing the 2-D echographic pattern of systolic coaptation of the mitral valve leaflets in normals and in mitral valve prolapse. In the parasternal long-axis view (*left*) the coapted mitral valve tends to form a Y outline in normals (*top left*), a T outline in mild prolapse (*top center*), and a convexity toward the LA in severe prolapse (*bottom left*). In the apical 4-chamber view (*right*), the normal pattern is shown above, whereas a pattern often seen in severe prolapses is shown below: the mitral leaflets bulge into the LA, the ventricular septum appears hypercontractile, and the posterolateral basal LV appears hypokinetic.

Gilbert *et al.* (1976) reported two additional 2-D features of mitral prolapse, as viewed in the long-axis view: (1) The anterior and posterior mitral leaflets coapt in an abnormally posterior plane (more than 8 mm posterior to the posterior aortic root). (2) "Abnormal curling of the mitral ring on the adjacent posterior LV myocardium," implying an abnormal inferior motion of the mitral annulus relative to the LV, a finding that does not lend itself to depic-

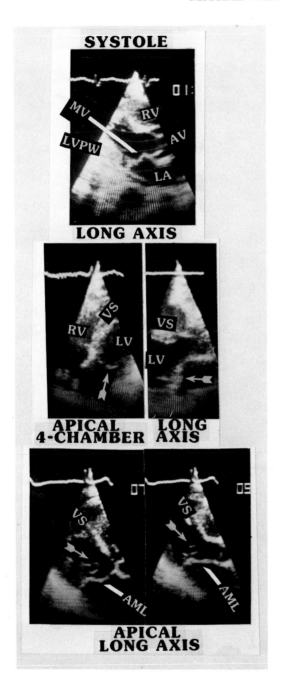

SYSTOLE

LONG AXIS

APICAL
4-CHAMBER

LONG
AXIS

APICAL
LONG AXIS

Fig. B-31. *Upper.* 2-D echogram in the long-axis view of a patient with mitral valve prolapse. The anterior mitral leaflet is mainly affected, and bulges backward toward the LA.

Center. 2-D echogram of a 58-year-old woman in the apical 4-chamber view (*left*) and long-axis view (*right*), showing mitral valve configurations suggestive of mitral prolapse (*arrows*).

Lower. 2-D echogram of a young woman with mitral valve prolapse, in the long-axis view. The 2-D probe is nearer to the LV apex in the left frame, and nearer to the left sternal border in the right frame. Mitral valve bulging toward the LA is evident in the left frame. An abnormal curved linear echo, just anterior to the anterior mitral leaflet, at about the leaflet edge, represents buckling or looping of redundant mitral anterior chordae (*arrows*).

tion on still frames but can be appreciated only on real-time viewing.

A convenient way of differentiating normal from prolapsing mitral valves, in the parasternal long-axis view, is to recognize that the coapted mitral leaflets and chordae in systole form a Y-shaped configuration in normals such that the fork of the Y is well into the LV cavity, i.e., inferior to the plane of the mitral prolapse. In most patients with mitral prolapse the Y shape alters to a T shape, so that mitral leaflets appear more or less in the same straight line, a line that meets the chordae perpendicularly and lies approximately in the plane of the mitral ring. In pronounced or severe prolapse, one or both leaflets may bulge into the left atrium so that their billowing convexities attain a position superior to a line representing the mitral ring.

It is important to note that the free edges of the mitral leaflets never project or evert into

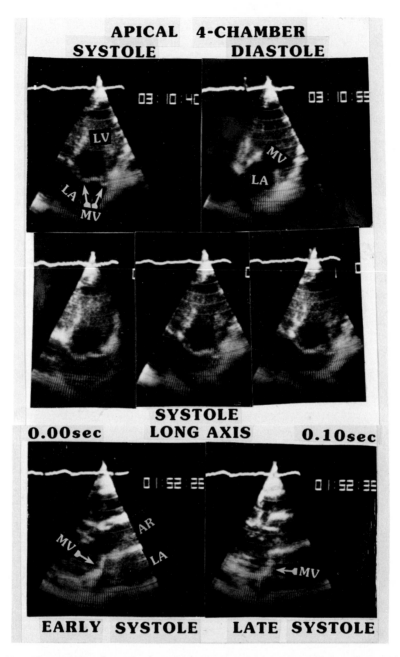

Fig. B-32. *Upper.* 2-D echogram of a young woman with definite mitral prolapse. The apical 4-chamber view shows the mitral valve closed in systole (*left upper frame and 3 lower frames*) and open in diastole (*right upper frame*). The mitral cusps bulge into the LA in systole. The systolic frames show how slightly different imaging of the anterior and posterior mitral leaflets can be obtained with slight alterations of tilt or rotation of the 2-D probe. Such maneuvering of the probe is necessary to obtain optimal visualization of both leaflets and their abnormal contours.

Lower. Parasternal long-axis view of the same patient showing abnormal bulging of the mitral valve into the LA.

the left atrium unless the leaflet has been rendered flail by chordal rupture. In other words, the redundant prolapsing cusps may bulge up into the left atrium, but their free edges always remain tethered and directed inferiorly within the LV.

Bulging of the mitral leaflets into the left atrium, beyond the plane of the mitral ring (i.e., on the atrial side of it), can also be appreciated in the apical views (Schiller and Silverman, 1978).

Morganroth et al. (1981) recently have documented the diagnostic potential of the apical four-chamber view in greater detail. They found it superior to the long-axis view, especially in detecting the milder grades of mitral prolapse. These authors found that: (1) In normal persons the mitral leaflets as well as their point of systolic coaptation were always on the ventricular side of the plane of the mitral ring. (2) In mild mitral prolapse the coaptation point was in the plane of the mitral ring, but the leaflets themselves bowed (prolapsed) on the atrial side of this plane. (3) In severe mitral prolapse both the mitral leaflets as well as their coaptation point were clearly on the atrial side of the mitral ring, i.e., within the left atrium, in systole. Morganroth's data also confirmed the general view that prolapse of both mitral leaflets is the rule and that the posterior mitral leaflet tends to prolapse more severely than the anterior one.

Caveats: (1) The posterior mitral leaflet is shorter and much less conspicuous than the anterior leaflet in the long-axis and apical views. Care therefore must be taken to angle and rotate the 2-D probe to display the posterior leaflet to the best possible advantage. (2) Abnormalities of mitral motion and leaflet position may be too rapid to appreciate in real-time viewing. It cannot be emphasized too strongly that the characteristic T configuration or superior arching of the mitral leaflets in the long-axis view easily can be overlooked unless mitral valve contour is scrutinized in slow motion over several beats, with frequent pauses to examine still frames during late systole.

An abnormal pattern of LV contraction in the apical four-chamber view recently has been described in about one third of patients with definite mitral prolapse on M-mode echography (D'Cruz et al., 1981). It is characterized by apparent hypokinesis of the LV posterolateral basal wall and a hyperdynamic systolic "bending" of the ventricular septum. It appears that this 2-D echographic pattern is specific for mitral prolapse and resembles the "ballerina-foot" and "hourglass" LV contraction patterns previously reported by angiocardiographers.

MITRAL REGURGITATION (Figs. B-33 to B-39)

It is a paradox of echocardiography, often incomprehensible to clinicians unfamiliar with the technique, that ultrasound has such an important role to play in the identification of various pathologic entities causing mitral regurgitation (Segal et al., 1967; Frankl et al., 1972; Burgess et al., 1973; Cosby et al., 1974), and yet there are few echocardiographic signs, if any, that are truly specific for the *presence* of mitral regurgitation.

There are, however, certain characteristics of mitral valve motion frequently noted in association with mitral regurgitation (Winters et al., 1969):

1. A steep EF mitral slope.

2. A large anterior excursion of the anterior mitral leaflet (DE distance).

These features are of limited diagnostic value because they are not by any means specific for mitral regurgitation. They are encountered also in mitral valve prolapse without mitral regurgitation, in hyperdynamic states such as anemia, and in some normal children and young adults. The latter often have short "functional" innocent murmurs for which cardiac consultation and echocardiography are done, and it is therefore particularly important not to make an erroneous diagnosis of mitral regurgitation.

DIASTOLIC MITRAL FLUTTER

Tremulous or coarse oscillatory behavior of a flail mitral leaflet has been well documented (see section on flail mitral valve, Fig. B-39).

Typically the diastolic flutter has an irregular or erratic quality, in contrast to the usual form of fine regular diastolic mitral flutter seen in patients with aortic regurgitation.

It is less generally known that rheumatic mitral regurgitation (with intact chordae tendineae) also can exhibit diastolic mitral flutter

VARIETIES OF MITRAL REGURGITATION

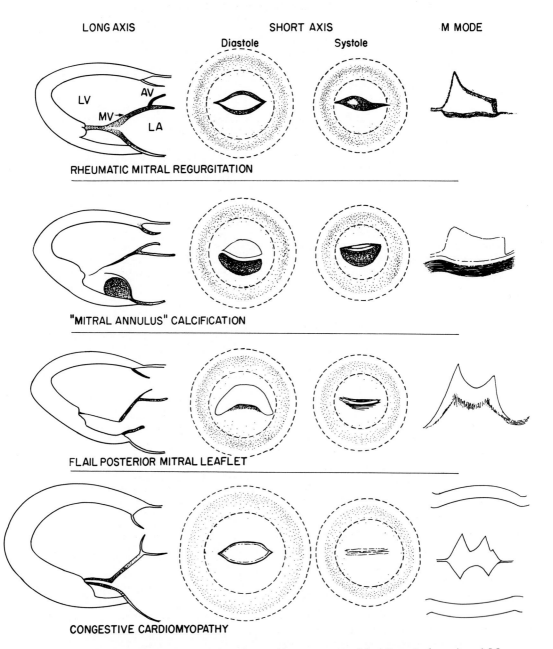

Fig. B-33.   Diagram depicting the 2-D echographic appearance (*first 3 vertical rows*) and M-mode appearances (*last vertical row*) of four common varieties of mitral regurgitation; rheumatic (*top horizontal row*); mitral annulus calcification (*second row*); flail leaflet (*third row*); and dilated cardiomyopathy (*bottom row*).

in children or young adults. Mitral valve flutter of this type differs from the better-known diastolic flutter typical of aortic regurgitation in the following respects:

1. It occurs exclusively or at least more prominently on the posterior mitral leaflet, while in aortic regurgitation diastolic flutter is always more conspicuous on the anterior mitral leaflet (D'Cruz *et al.,* 1976).

2. Flutter on the posterior mitral leaflet is

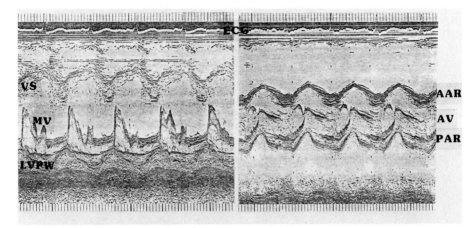

Fig. B-34. M-mode echogram of a patient with severe mitral regurgitation of recent onset due to mitral valve endocarditis. The left panel shows abnormal erratic motion of the anterior mitral leaflet and thickened cusp echoes due to vegetations. Note vigorous septal contraction. The right panel shows abnormally rapid anterior systolic motion of the posterior aortic root with rapid posterior motion in early diastole, attributable to forceful systolic expansion of the LA, which in turn was due to severe mitral regurgitation into an LA chamber of normal size.

maximal in early diastole (rapid filling phase) and wanes or ceases in mid- to late diastole.

SYSTOLIC POSTERIOR MOTION OF THE LEFT ATRIAL POSTERIOR WALL

Normally, the inferior portion of the left atrial posterior wall moves posteriorly during systole. Patton et al., (1978) studied this motion in detail in 34 normal individuals, 15 patients with mitral regurgitation, and 17 others with various cardiac lesions, including aortic valve disease and ventricular septal defect. They found that in mitral regurgitation not only the amplitude, but also the velocity, of the left atrial posterior wall posterior systolic motion was increased. Thus, in mitral regurgitation, the left atrial posterior wall abruptly attains its posterior position early in systole, whereas in normal individuals and those with other types of heart lesions the left atrial posterior wall moves gradually backward through entire systole. The mean amplitude of posterior motion in the mitral regurgitation group was 12 mm, compared to 9 mm in the normal group and in the other miscellaneous cardiac group. This disparity was not impressive, although statistically significant. A better separation was obtained as regarding the *velocity* of posterior motion of the left atrial posterior wall; the mean value for the mitral

regurgitation group was 123 mm per sec, while it was between 50 and 60 mm per sec for the others. If the product of the amplitude and the velocity of the left atrial posterior wall is multiplied by the left atrial diameter, the separation between mitral regurgitation, on the one hand, and normal hearts as well as other cardiac lesions, on the other, is even more impressive.

The limitation of left atrial posterior wall motion as an indicator of mitral regurgitation lies in the technical difficulties involved in recording sufficiently good and sharp echoes of the left atrial endocardium. It may require considerable attention to gain-setting and care in performing left ventricle–left atrial scans. Patton et al. found a 3.5 MHz ultrasound transducer better than the 2.25 MHz one for this purpose. Faster paper speeds and expansion of the scale facilitate accurate measurements of left atrial posterior wall endocardial motion. The upper part of the left atrial posterior wall shows little motion; it is the lower part, near the atrioventricular groove, that exhibits the typical patterns described above.

Posterior aortic root echo motion may also reflect left atrial volume change during the cardiac cycle, inasmuch as it reflects left atrial anterior wall motion. Thus, mitral regurgitation is associated with enhanced amplitude and velocity of anterior systolic motion of the aortic root (Akgun and Layton, 1977), as in Figure B-34.

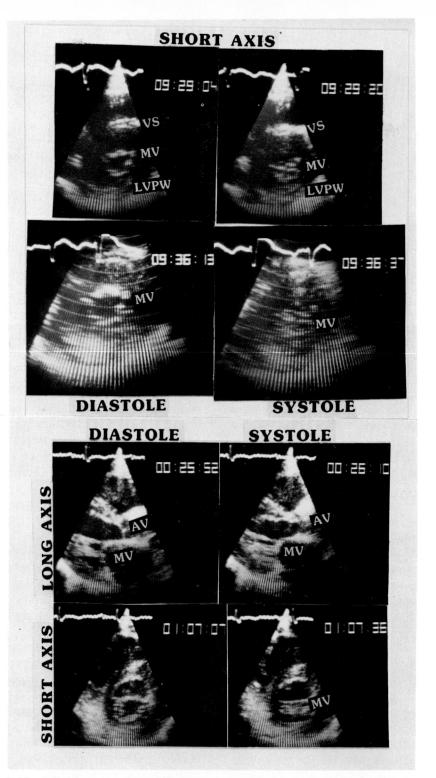

Fig. B-35. 2-D echograms of two different patients with rheumatic mitral regurgitation.

Upper. Short-axis view: the upper 2 frames are from the same cardiac cycle; the lower 2 frames, with expanded mitral image, are from another cardiac cycle. The left frames are in diastole, the right in systole. The latter show that anterior and posterior mitral leaflets do not meet in normal apposition. Normal apposition of the mitral cusps could not be visualized in spite of repeated scanning attempts from papillary muscle to mitral valve level.

Lower. The mitral valve and chordae are thickened. The two upper frames are in the long-axis view, the two lower frames in the short-axis view. The frames on the left are in diastole, those on the right are in systole.

SYSTOLIC SEPARATION BETWEEN THE MITRAL CUSPS

During systole (between C and D points) the anterior and posterior mitral leaflets are seen in apposition. Usually in normal individuals, the linear echoes of the two leaflets are identified easily; other linear echoes due to chordae tendineae may be seen anterior and posterior to the apposed leaflets. At one time it was thought by some echocardiographers that systolic separation between the anterior and posterior mitral leaflets was evidence of mitral regurgitation; it seemed plausible to view this separation as the area of nonclosure through which regurgitation occurred. However, it was soon realized that separation between the mitral leaflet echoes could occur in patients with mitral valves of proven competency, because of the ultrasound beam transecting the mitral cusps above the plane of their apposition (Fig. B-40).

A further element of confusion is added in those patients in whom multiple parallel echoes are recorded in the mitral valve area during systole; this is not uncommon in rheumatic mitral valve disease, endocardial cushion defects (ostium primum atrial septal defect with cleft mitral valve), cardiomyopathy, and mitral prolapse. In such circumstances, it may be difficult or impossible to ascertain which exactly of the several parallel echoes represent the anterior and posterior leaflets.

With the introduction of 2-D echocardiography, the visualization of systolic separation of the mitral cusps has reemerged as a sign of mitral regurgitation (Wann et al., 1978). By this technique it appears a more reliable criterion of mitral regurgitation than by the M-mode, at least in rheumatic hearts. Fortunately, the cusps of a rheumatic valve are usually thickened and reflect dense sharp echoes. In the short-axis view, therefore, the mitral valve orifice is well defined in diastole as well as systole. Normally, the two leaflets are seen to meet in complete apposition over the whole width of the orifice in systole. In mitral regurgitation, a small space may be visible between the anterior and posterior leaflets (Figs. B-5 and B-36) at either or both corners of the valve orifice or in the central area of the orifice. Failure of closure of small areas of either the medial or lateral aspect of the valve is associated with trivial or mild mitral regurgitation; failure of both sides to close or failure to close in the center of the valve indicates significant mitral regurgitation (Wann et al., 1978).

Ultrasound equipment with excellent resolution capability, careful viewing of the videotape in slow motion, and frame-by-frame scrutiny with special attention to early systole are essential. The theoretical objection that the apparent area of systolic separation may not represent the site of regurgitation but instead an area above the plane of apposition can be overcome by scanning several times in the short-axis view from papillary muscle level to mitral valve level. When this is done, one can be fairly sure that the plane of mitral leaflet apposition is well recorded.

SYSTOLIC FLUTTER OF LEFT ATRIAL WALL

A fine rapid flutter of the anterior LA wall, contiguous to the posterior aortic root echo, has been reported in a patient with a partly flail posterior mitral leaflet (Antman et al., 1978). Systolic flutter of the interatrial septum was demonstrated in four of seven patients with flail mitral valves (Tei et al., 1979). These authors visualized the atrial septum from the right parasternal area with the patient supine or in the right lateral position. Two-D scanning was done in a horizontal plane with some medial and superior tilt to display the interatrial septum separating the right atrium anteriorly from the left atrium posteriorly, and an M-mode tracing was obtained by means of a cursor passing through the midportion of the atrial septum. I have observed systolic flutter of the LA posterior wall in an elderly man with a mitral regurgitant murmur.

LEFT ATRIUM

The left atrial dimension is increased in moderate to severe mitral regurgitation. Both left atrium and left ventricle are of normal size if mitral regurgitation is trivial or slight, as for instance in most patients with the click-murmur syndrome associated with late systolic mitral prolapse. Severe acute mitral regurgitation, as for example caused by bacterial endocarditis or papillary muscle rupture or infarction, is an

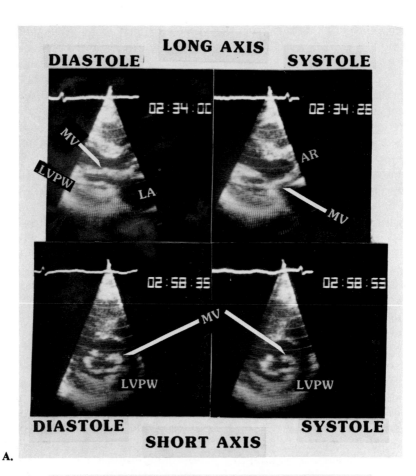

LONG AXIS

DIASTOLE SYSTOLE

02:34:00 02:34:26

MV AR

LVPW MV

LA

02:58:35 02:58:53

MV

LVPW LVPW

DIASTOLE SYSTOLE

SHORT AXIS

A.

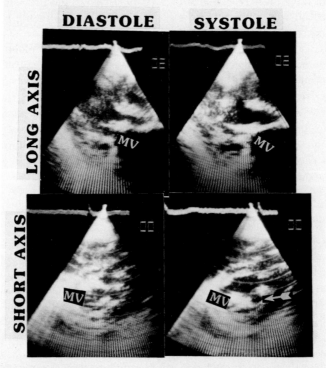

DIASTOLE SYSTOLE

LONG AXIS

MV MV

SHORT AXIS

MV MV

B.

important exception; the left atrium may be normal or only slightly dilated although the patient is in pulmonary edema.

LEFT VENTRICLE

In moderate to severe mitral regurgitation caused by rheumatic mitral involvement or mitral prolapse, the left ventricle is dilated but it contracts vigorously, as reflected in exaggerated excursions of the left ventricular posterior wall and ventricular septum. The left ventricular end-systolic dimension is thus normal or only slightly increased, and the left ventricular internal diameter shortening fraction is high normal or increased (normal, 28 to 41 per cent).

In patients with mitral regurgitation secondary to congestive cardiomyopathy or ischemic heart disease, the left ventricle is considerably dilated (values over 7 cm are common), and the indices of left ventricular performance demonstrate poor contractile function (Levisman, 1977).

On the other hand, significant mitral regurgitation can exist in association with a small left ventricular chamber in patients with concentric left ventricular hypertrophy secondary to hypertension, hypertrophic cardiomyopathy, or aortic stenosis.

Competence of the mitral valve depends on the integrity and normal motion of not only the mitral leaflets, but also of the rest of the mitral apparatus—the chordae tendineae, papillary muscles, and mitral annulus. Consequently, a wide variety of cardiac lesions can result in mitral regurgitation; often more than one component of the mitral apparatus is affected, as in fact the echocardiogram may demonstrate.

Mintz et al. (1979) recently have appraised the role of 2-D echography in the differential diagnosis of mitral regurgitation in a series of 133 unselected patients, 51 of whom had been studied hemodynamically. The etiology of mitral incompetence, in descending order of frequency, was mitral valve prolapse, rheumatic disease (either with or without associated mitral stenosis), ruptured chordae tendineae, LV dysfunction (diffuse or local), mitral annulus calcification, IHSS, cleft anterior leaflet, and atrial myxoma. The authors concluded that 2-D echocardiography could reliably separate mitral regurgitation caused by intrinsic mitral valve abnormality from that caused by myocardial (LV or papillary muscle) dysfunction. Since the former is more amenable to surgical therapy, the importance of cardiac ultrasound in the assessment of patients with mitral regurgitation is obvious.

The chief role of echocardiography in patients with mitral regurgitation is not to establish the presence of regurgitation but to detect its anatomic basis. Fortunately, most forms of mitral pathology can be identified by M-mode and 2-D techniques. Some of these abnormal echographic appearances have been described and illustrated elsewhere in this chapter; as, for example, mitral valve prolapse, bacterial endocarditis, and mitral annulus calcification. Other varieties of mitral regurgitation shown here include rheumatic mitral regurgitation (Fig. B-35), cleft mitral valve associated with ostium primum atrial septal defect (Figs. B-37 and B-38), and flail mitral valve (Fig. B-39).

Recently Smallhorn et al. (1982) described five patients with mitral regurgitation due to isolated anterior mitral leaflet cleft, unassociated with atrioventricular (endocardial cushion) defects. On 2-D echography, the defect in the anterior leaflet points toward the LV outflow tract, whereas the anterior mitral cleft associ-

Fig. B-36. *A.* 2-D echogram of a patient with chronic renal failure and mitral regurgitation. The upper frames are in the long-axis view. The right (systole) was recorded 0.2 sec after the left (diastole). The lower frames are in the short-axis view, the right (systole) 0.18 sec after the left (diastole). The mitral valve cusps and chordae appear thickened. During systole the mitral valve remains open (*lower right*), resulting in mitral regurgitation.

Fig. B-36. *B.* 2-D echogram of a young woman with an apical systolic murmur of mitral regurgitation, who had had rheumatic carditis in childhood. The two upper frames are in the long-axis view, the two lower in the short-axis view. The left frames are in diastole, the right in systole. The mitral leaflets and chordae tendineae are obviously thickened. In systole the mitral valve closes (*right frames*), but a gap or lack of apposition is seen (*arrow*) between the anterior and posterior mitral leaflets. This is presumably the site of regurgitation.

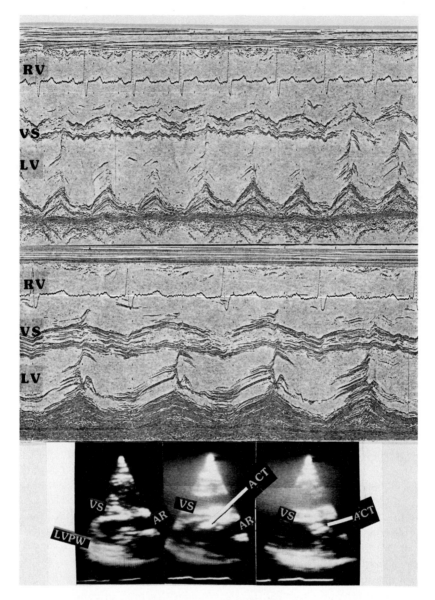

Fig. B-37. *Upper and Center.* M-mode echogram of a 53-year-old woman with an ostium primum atrial septal defect and cleft mitral valve. The RV appears dilated. At chordae level (*left*) septal systolic motion is abnormal; this is called type B septal motion. Mitral valve (*right*) echographic morphology appears abnormal; this can be seen at faster paper speed in the central panel. It was impossible to record the M-shaped contour of a normal anterior mitral leaflet.

Lower. 2-D echogram, in the long-axis view, of the same woman with an ostium primum atrial septal defect and cleft mitral valve. The left frame is in systole, with the mitral valve closed; thickened mitral chordae can be seen. In the center and right frames, which are diastolic, abnormal small dense echoes are seen in the LV outflow tract. These represent thick anomalous mitral chordae tendineae (ACT) connecting the cleft anterior mitral leaflet to the crest of the ventricular septum.

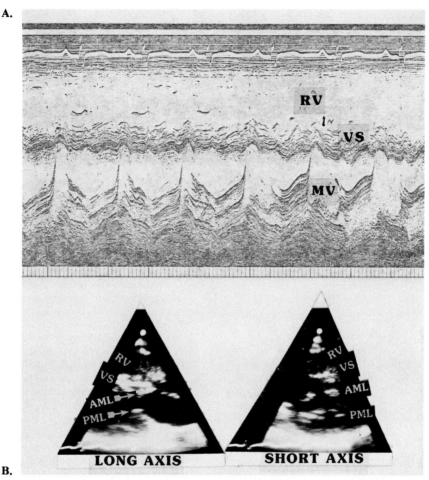

Fig. B-38. *A.* Segments from the M-mode echogram of a 15-year-old boy with Down's syndrome. Hemodynamic studies revealed an ostium primum atrial septal defect and cleft mitral valve. Note abnormalities in the echographic morphology of the mitral valve: the diastolic contour of the anterior mitral leaflet echo appears broken or discontinuous; the mitral valve in systole appears to be unduly thick and to consist of a stack of multiple parallel echoes. The RV is dilated.

Fig. B-38. *B.* 2-D echogram of the same patient with a cleft mitral valve. The long-axis view (*left*), in diastole, appears normal. However, the short-axis view, also in diastole, shows an abnormal appearance, with the anterior mitral leaflet split into two components.

ated with ostium primum atrial septal defects points toward the ventricular septum.

MITRAL VALVE ENDOCARDITIS

Mitral valve vegetations are said to be detectable by echocardiography if they are 3 mm or more in size (Wann *et al.,* 1976). The visualization of mitral vegetations is valuable in confirming the diagnosis of bacterial endocarditis suspected on clinical grounds; (Dillon *et al.,* 1973; Wann *et al.,* 1976; Roy *et al.,* 1976; Andy *et*

al., 1977); the clinician is grateful for a means of validating his diagnosis that does not entail the delay until blood cultures yield their results. Less often, echocardiography performed for some other indication uncovers a totally unsuspected diagnosis of subacute bacterial endocarditis. Even when the physician caring for a patient with bacterial endocarditis is confident of his diagnosis on the basis of clinical history, presentation, and positive blood cultures, he is anxious to know whether vegetations are recognizable by echocardiography or not because of

A.

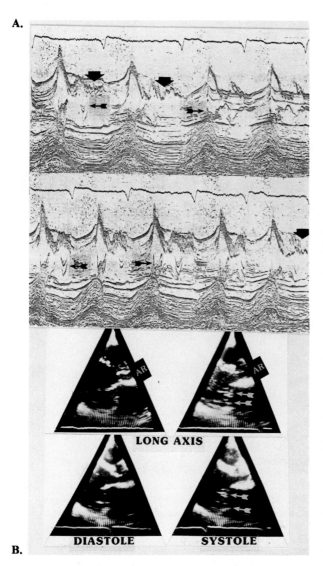

LONG AXIS

DIASTOLE   **SYSTOLE**

B.

Fig. B-39. *A.* Echogram of a 75-year-old man with severe mitral regurgitation. Hemodynamic studies and surgery were not done because of associated abdominal malignant growth. At autopsy some of the chordae tendineae of the posterior papillary muscle were ruptured and the mitral valve was partly flail. Chordal rupture was presumably spontaneous, as there was no evidence of recent or past endocarditis. M-mode echogram shows apparent thickening of the anterior mitral leaflet and an abnormal diastolic appearance of the posterior leaflet. Note irregular vibration of the anterior mitral leaflet (*broad arrows*) and also abnormal motion of the posterior leaflet (*thin arrows*).

Fig. B-39. *B.* 2-D echogram of the same patient with flail mitral valve, in the long-axis view. The two left frames are in diastole, the two right frames in systole. The latter show an abnormal disorganized systolic configuration of the mitral leaflets (*arrows*). In the lower right frame, the posterior mitral leaflet appears everted so that its free edge points into the LA rather than the LV.

data suggesting that patients with endocarditis who exhibit vegetations on echocardiography have a very poor prognosis if not subjected to surgery (Wann *et al.,* 1976). By comparison, those with endocarditis who were echo-negative for vegetations fared much better. More recent reports indicate that exceptions to the general rule certainly occur, i.e., one does see patients with large definite vegetations who respond well and uneventfully to medical therapy alone. Nonetheless, as a statement of statistical probabilities, the belief that patients with bacterial endocarditis who do have vegetations on echocardiography have a graver prognosis if not operated upon than those whose valves appear "clean" to ultrasound has served a useful purpose in influencing cardiologists to adopt a more

aggressive therapeutic policy. When faced with a patient in hemodynamic difficulties or assailed by valvular infection refractory to antibiotic drugs, the clinician tends to consider surgery to excise the infected valve more readily if he knows that that valve shows definite evidence of vegetations, perhaps with some degree of flail motion. The demonstration of large mobile mitral vegetations on 2-D echography has been considered in itself an indication for valve replacement as a prophylaxis against imminent embolism (Egeblad *et al.,* 1979). However, this is apt to be a controversial policy.

The M-mode characteristics of mitral valve vegetations (Figs. B-41 to B-45) include:

1. Abnormal echoes of variable size and density arise from the anterior or posterior mitral

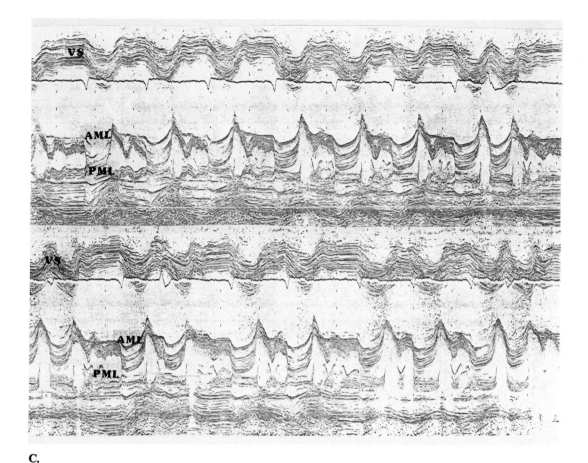

C.

Fig. B-39. *C.* The mitral valve in the same patient with a flail mitral valve, showing very abnormal appearances in the region of the posterior mitral leaflet. Note that the first few beats in the upper panel, at slightly different transducer angulation, show an apparently normal mitral valve motion pattern.

leaflet. The vegetation itself may be discernible as a definite small mass adherent to the leaflet and moving with it, or it merely may appear as a local nodular thickening of the cusp. The emphasis is on the word local: as the ultrasound beam transects that part of the leaflet that bears the vegetation, the leaflet appears very thickened, whereas other parts of the leaflet, recorded with slight shifts in transducer direction or from a different intercostal space, appear normal or almost normal in thickness. Textbook descriptions of mitral endocarditis often use the word shaggy in connection with the abnormal echo appearance of the valve leaflets. It should be noted that shagginess is not an essential element or criterion for the diagnosis. It is possible that irregular, rapid motion of a pedunculated or mobile vegetation is responsible for the shaggy effect; in other instances, abnormal diastolic flutter due to ruptured chordae or associated aortic regurgitation may cause the thickened leaflet with its adherent vegetation to vibrate or oscillate rapidly amid the diastolic turbulence. Boucher *et al.* (1977) emphasized the nonspecific nature of echoes from mitral vegetations in some cases and showed that calcification in a vegetation may contribute to its abnormal morphology on the echogram.

2. Diastolic motion of the mitral cusps usually is not restricted. Thus, the anterior or posterior mitral leaflet, although inordinately thick (because of the vegetation on it), does not exhibit abnormal motion of the type expected in a stenotic valve.

3. If chordae tendineae are ruptured secondary to the infection, part of the leaflet becomes

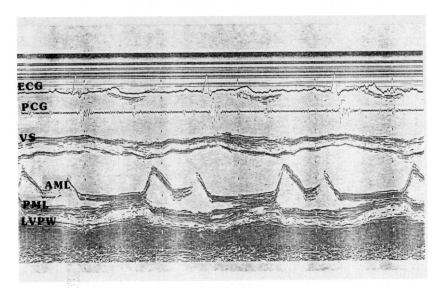

Fig. B-40. M-mode echogram of a young woman. The mitral cusps appear not to meet during the first half of systole. However, auscultation and phonocardiography revealed no evidence of mitral regurgitation. Thus, this pattern appears a normal variant, attributable to the ultrasound beam transecting the mitral cusps slightly above the plane of apposition.

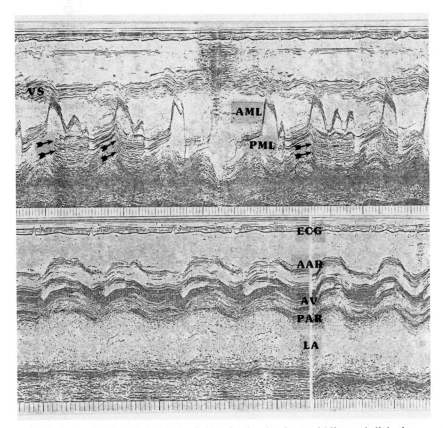

Fig. B-41. *Upper.* M-mode echogram of the mitral valve in a middle-aged diabetic man with *Pseudomonas* endocarditis of the mitral as well as aortic valve. A large vegetation is visible on the posterior mitral leaflet in diastole (*arrows*), but in systole it retreats completely into the LA. It could thus simulate a left atrial myxoma.

Lower. M-mode echogram of the aortic valve in the same patient with *Pseudomonas* endocarditis. Dense echoes can be seen in the center of the aortic root, and less dense echoes in its posterior portion. The appearances are not absolutely typical of aortic valve vegetations; somewhat similar appearances are seen in elderly patients with uncomplicated aortic valve sclerosis.

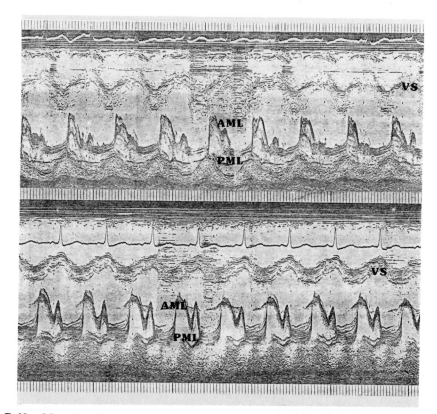

Fig. B-42. M-mode echogram of the mitral valve in a patient with mitral valve endocarditis resulting in flail leaflets and severe mitral regurgitation. In the upper panel, flail mitral motion and vegetations are evident, making the valve appear abnormal. In the lower panel, recorded on the same examination but at a slightly different transducer angulation, the mitral valve appears much less abnormal. However, systolic prolapse, not visible in the upper panel, is now apparent.

flail and shows abnormal diastolic motion of an exaggerated erratic nature, which may vary in degree from beat to beat. Such abnormal behavior of a mitral cusp, especially the posterior one, is often much more evident with one transducer direction than another. The valve may look normal or only slightly abnormal with slight alterations in transducer angulation. Sometimes the ruptured, loose chordae are seen as linear echoes streaking erratically across the left ventricular chamber, superimposed on the mitral valve echoes. The flail leaflet, with perhaps an attached vegetation, may appear in the LA in systole.

4. Systolic mitral flutter is a rather uncommon echocardiographic sign. Almost always, the patient has past or present bacterial endocarditis (Sze *et al.*, 1978). It may be seen in patients with healed calcified vegetations on a regurgitant mitral valve that is not flail (Fig. B-61). For reasons that are unclear, mitral re-

gurgitation due to rheumatic disease, mitral valve prolapse, or other etiologies is almost never associated with demonstrable systolic mitral flutter.

In an important recent M-mode study of 27 patients with mitral valve endocarditis, Sheikh *et al.* (1981) correlated the echographic appearances with various clinical aspects of the illness. They found that the size of the mitral vegetations did not predict accurately (1) the amount of cardiac change or dysfunction, (2) the type of infecting bacterium, or (3) whether a vegetation was "active" or healed. They reported that little or no change in size of the vegetation occurred during the first six weeks after diagnosis and start of antibiotic therapy, unless it broke off to embolize; the larger the vegetation, the more likely that it would embolize. Evidence of chordal rupture (flail leaflet) was a more important prognostic indicator than M-mode echographic morphology.

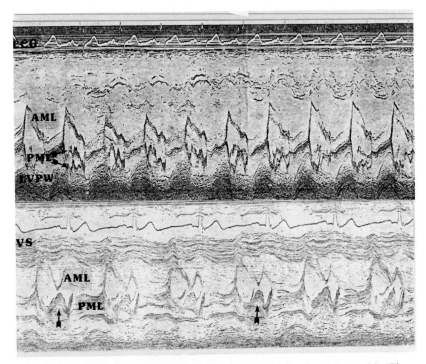

Fig. B-43. *Upper.* M-mode echogram of a patient with mitral valve endocarditis. The posterior mitral leaflet was flail and had a vegetation on it. On the tracing it has a very abnormal ragged contour and exhibits coarse irregular diastolic flutter. In some beats (second to sixth) it appears to show a double outline.

Lower. M-mode echogram of a patient who had recently recovered from bacterial endocarditis of the mitral valve. The posterior mitral leaflet appears thickened and exhibits a somewhat exaggerated diastolic motion (*arrows*).

2-D ECHOCARDIOGRAPHY IN MITRAL VEGETATIONS

The same abnormalities evident on the M-mode tracing—a localized thickening, nodule, or mass on either or both leaflets, with unrestricted leaflet motion—are visualized on 2-D echography, usually in long-axis, short-axis, and apical views. (Gilbert *et al.*, 1977; Mintz *et al.*, 1979; Wann *et al.*, 1979; Martin *et al.*, 1980). However, the size and shape of vegetations, and their precise location on the leaflet, are much better appreciated on 2-D than on M-mode echocardiography (Fig. B-46). The 2-D technique may also reveal the brief appearance in systole of a vegetation or a flail leaflet in the left atrium. Moreover, other 2-D characteristics of a flail mitral leaflet—eversion of the free edge of the affected cusp toward the left atrium and non-coaptation of the cusps—permit the diagnosis to be made with more confidence than is possible on M-mode tracings alone. Fenestration of the anterior mitral leaflet due to endocarditis

has been visualized on 2-D echography as a hiatus in the linear image of this leaflet in the long-axis view (Matsumoto *et al.*, 1982).

The differential diagnosis of mitral valve vegetations includes two dissimilar diagnostic situations:

1. When vegetations are small, they present on M-mode and 2-D recordings as a local or nodular thickening of the anterior or posterior mitral cusp, the cusp retaining its normal mobility. Somewhat similar appearances may be seen in (a) patients with old, healed lesions of previous endocarditis; (b) elderly persons with small sclerotic or calcified deposits in a mitral cusp (Fig. B-47); (c) occasional patients with old rheumatic valvar disease have local or nonuniform cusp scarring with normal or only slightly abnormal cusp motion. Much more often, rheumatic mitral valve sclerosis is accompanied by mitral stenosis or at least commissural fusion of the cusps, resulting in a distinctive pattern of abnormal motion on both M-mode and 2-D recordings.

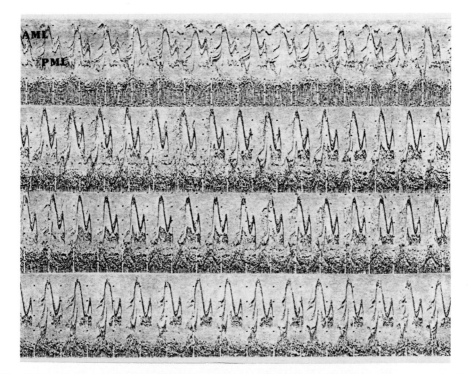

Fig. B-44. Segments from the M-mode echogram of a patient with severe mitral regurgitation secondary to mitral valve endocarditis, confirmed at surgery. The posterior mitral leaflet shows typical flail motion and appears to have a vegetation on it. Note the variety of echographic morphology that can be obtained with slight changes in transducer direction.

2. When mitral valve vegetations are large, they may have to be differentiated from other intracardiac masses: (a) left atrial myxomas, which are usually pedunculated and very mobile and retreat completely into the left atrium during systole; (b) posterior submitral (mitral annulus) calcification moves strictly with the LV posterior wall; these echoes have a typical

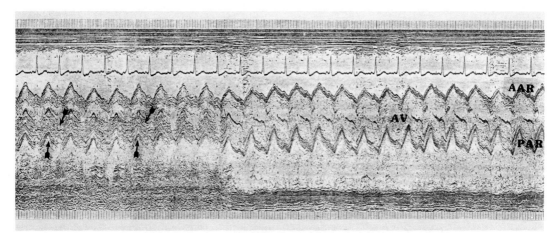

Fig. B-45. M-mode echogram scanning different parts of the aortic root, in a patient with mitral valve endocarditis and a ring abscess in the space between mitral and aortic valve rings (intervalvar space). The abscess appears as an ill-defined abnormal echo filling the posterior half of the aortic root (*left half of figure*). This abnormal echo is not due to a valvular vegetation because the aortic valve appears normal when the aortic root is scanned in a different direction (*right of figure*).

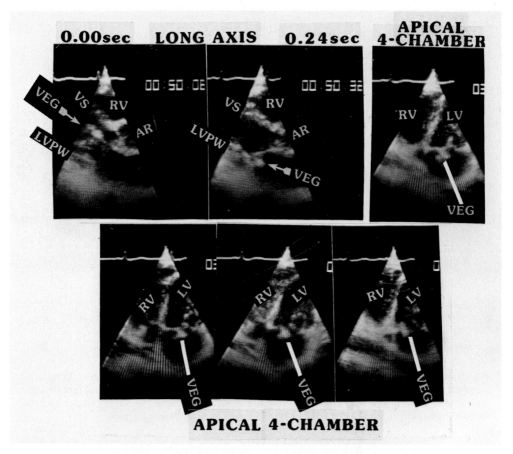

Fig. B-46. *Upper.* 2-D echogram of a patient with staphylococcal vegetations on the mitral valve. The left and center frames are in the long-axis view, the right frame in the apical 4-chamber view. Vegetations are seen on both mitral cusps; the one on the anterior mitral cusp appears to protude into the LA in systole.

Lower. 2-D echogram of the same patient in the apical 4-chamber view, obtained in slightly different planes. All frames are systolic. Note the malapposition of the mitral leaflets, and the vegetation on the anterior mitral leaflet.

dense quality as well as shape (round or oval in long axis, crescentic or bar-shaped in short axis); (c) left atrial or left ventricular mural thrombi are adherent to the subjacent atrial or ventricular wall and show little or no mobility; pedunculated mobile thrombi are exceptional; (d) exceptionally, vegetations may be located not on the mitral cusps but in the annulus region as in a patient reported by D'Cruz *et al.* (1982).

The cardiac entities that could, under certain conditions, be mistaken for mitral vegetations of bacterial endocarditis on the echocardiogram (Figs. B-48 to B-54) include:

1. *The thickened sclerotic or calcified valve of rheumatic heart disease* (mitral stenosis or combined stenosis and regurgitation). It can be differentiated from mitral valve vegetations because (a) Fibrous scarring and calcification produce very dense, well-defined, sharp echoes, whereas vegetations give rise to echoes which are less dense and may be shaggy. However, as mentioned above, shagginess is by no means invariable, or even very common, in valves of patients with endocarditis. On the other hand, healed vegetations have been shown to calcify rapidly (Stafford *et al.,* 1979). (b) Thickening of the fibrotic or calcified mitral valve affects the whole leaflet, so that *local* nodules on the leaflet, typical of vegetations, are not seen. It does sometimes happen in mitral stenosis that the anterior leaflet is very grossly calcified, while the posterior leaflet is of almost normal thickness; less commonly the reverse is true.

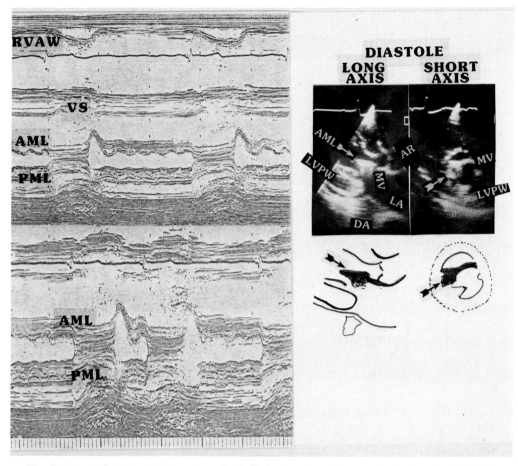

Fig. B-47. *Left.* M-mode echogram of an elderly woman with normal mitral motion but thick mitral cusp echoes. The lower panel displays an expanded image of the mitral valve. The echocardiographic appearances, probably due to senile sclero-calcific changes, would be compatible also with vegetations on both mitral cusps. There was no evidence for present or previous endocarditis.

    Right. 2-D echogram of a 95-year-old woman in long-axis (*left*) and short-axis (*right*) views. The anterior mitral leaflet is calcified at its free edge (*arrows*) but its mobility was normal and there was no mitral stenosis. This appearance can be mistaken for a vegetation, but there was no history or evidence of present or past bacterial endocarditis. Such anterior mitral calcification is an occasional and innocuous finding in very elderly women.

(c) The most important distinguishing feature between mitral stenosis and mitral vegetation is the abnormal diastolic motion of both leaflets typical of the former, in contrast to the normal leaflet motion in the latter case. If the posterior mitral leaflet is flail, it may be seen to move anteriorly during diastole, but this abnormal pattern differs from the abnormal anterior diastolic motion of mitral stenosis qualitatively in that cusp separation remains constant (i.e., the mitral leaflet echoes are flat and parallel) in mitral stenosis, whereas with a flail posterior leaflet this is not so. Exceptionally, a large mi-tral vegetation can cause severe mitral stenosis when superimposed on a preexisting mild mitral stenosis (Copeland *et al.,* 1979).

    2. *Prolapsed mitral valve.* The echocardiographic diagnosis of a vegetation on a prolapsed mitral valve is suggested by dense fuzzy echoes, and healing is suggested by transformation to a dense linear echo (Horowitz and Smith, 1977). In some patients with mitral valve prolapse syndrome, usually those with severe holosystolic prolapse and a holosystolic apical murmur of mitral regurgitation, thickened redundant folds of a large floppy mitral leaflet gather together

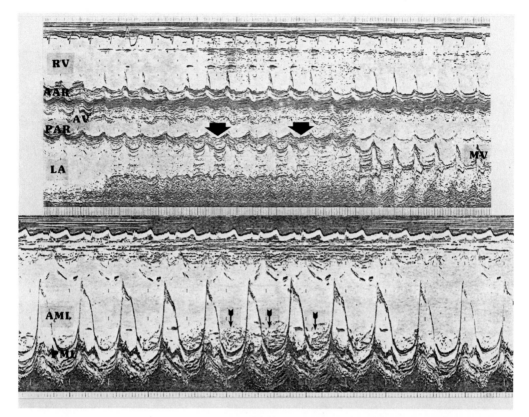

Fig. B-48. *Upper.* M-mode scan from aortic root to LV in a patient with cardiomyopathy. The aortic root and LA are clear at the beginning of the scan. The LV at mitral valve level is clearly visible at the end of the scan. In between, in the middle of the figure (*arrows*), the posterior aortic root and mitral valve echoes appear superimposed and indistinct, because the ultrasound beam width encompasses both structures. If only this segment were available, the erroneous diagnosis of mitral valve sclerosis or vegetation might have been considered; the true picture is easily revealed by a good LA-to-LV scan.

Lower. M-mode echogram of a young woman with mitral prolapse. There was no clinical evidence of bacterial endocarditis. At one particular setting of damping (reject) artefactual ill-defined echoes (*arrows*) appeared around the mitral valve in systole (*center of figure*). The nature of these nebulous echoes, which could possibly be confused with vegetations, remains uncertain. They could easily be suppressed by slight increase in damping (*right and left of figure*).

into a thick layered echo mass in diastole. In some instances, cusp thickening is attributable to myxomatous change. The thickened redundant posterior leaflet could easily be misinterpreted as a large vegetation, particularly since bacterial endocarditis is a well-known complication of mitral valve prolapse. Chandaratna *et al.* (1977) reported that 34 patients with mitral prolapse had thick shaggy echoes on either the anterior leaflet (11 cases) posterior leaflet (18 cases) or both (5 cases); yet only one patient had clinical evidence of bacterial endocarditis.

3. *Left atrial myxoma.* In practice, vegetations are seldom mistaken for myxomas and vice versa because (a) myxomas are usually of much larger size and (b) vegetations are very closely related to mitral valve leaflets. However, occasionally vegetations can grow to an unusually large size, especially when of fungal origin; such large vegetations have simulated myxomas (Pasternak *et al.,* 1976; Child *et al.,* 1979; Nicholson, *et al.,* 1980). A large vegetation on the posterior mitral leaflet can resemble a left atrial myxoma, inasmuch as it can be observed, on 2-D echocardiography, to move rapidly toward the left ventricle at the onset of diastole and toward the left atrium at the onset of systole. A large vegetation of this type can obstruct

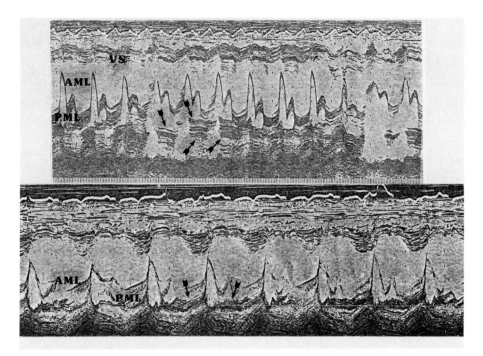

Fig. B-49. Submitral sclerosis simulating mitral vegetations in two different patients.

Upper. M-mode echogram of a 20-year-old woman who underwent mitral annuloplasty for severe mitral regurgitation a few years earlier. A dense echo (*arrows*) in the mitral annulus region (very near the posterior mitral leaflet) is due to the materials used in the annuloplasty sewing procedure and to postsurgical scarring. It should not be mistaken for a vegetation on the posterior mitral leaflet or for mitral annulus calcification, both of which commonly present as a dense echo in this region.

Lower. M-mode echogram in a 16-year-old boy who had suffered a stab wound in the cardiac region a month earlier. He had a murmur of mitral regurgitation. A dense echo is noted in the region of the posterior mitral cusp and annulus (*arrows*), on the M-mode as well as 2-D echogram. This is presumed to represent scarring from the previous trauma. It could be mistaken for a vegetation on the posterior mitral leaflet. However, there was no evidence for present or old endocarditis in this patient.

the mitral orifice (Prasquier *et al.,* 1978; Alam *et al.,* 1979). It should be kept in mind that infection can complicate a left atrial myxoma, in which case positive blood cultures and other septicemic manifestations may render a distinction from mitral endocarditis very difficult. (Rajpal *et al.,* 1979).

4. *Diastolic flutter on the anterior mitral leaflet* might sometimes be mistaken for thick, shaggy echoes, suggestive of a vegetation on this leaflet. Attention to technical details, such as adequate paper speed (50 mm per sec or more), expansion of the scale so as to obtain a large enough image of the mitral echo, and suitable gain or reject adjustment, will usually expose the rapid vibratory nature of mitral valve flutter.

5. *Nonbacterial thrombotic endocarditis* of

the mitral valve can present with repeated embolic episodes and progressive thickening of the mitral leaflets over a period of months (Estevez and Corya, 1976). Serial echocardiograms of this patient, a 34-year-old man, revealed increasing thickening and restriction of motion of the mitral valve; the diagnosis was established at surgery for mitral valve replacement. Kinney *et al.* (1979) described irregular thickening of the anterior mitral leaflet in a woman with long-standing scleroderma and mitral regurgitation; at autopsy nodular thickening of the mitral valve was seen, but no infection.

6. Submitral sclerosis as a result of mitral annuloplasty or old trauma (Fig. B-49).

7. Submitral (mitral annulus) calcification, very common in elderly persons (Fig. B-50).

8. Unusually dense echoes from the mitral

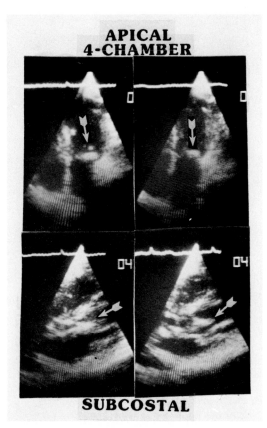

APICAL 4-CHAMBER

SUBCOSTAL

Fig. B-50. 2-D echogram in the apical 4-chamber view (*two upper frames*) of a patient with submitral mitral annulus calcification, which appears as a dense nodular mass (*arrows*) in the mitral valve region. This could mimic a vegetation on a single still frame, but when viewed in motion there should be no confusion: vegetations attached to mobile cusps show considerable mobility, whereas mitral annulus calcification manifests no mobility apart from that of the mitral annulus itself.

Subcostal 2-D echogram (*two lower frames*) of an old man with senile degenerative sclerosis of the mitral and aortic valves, shows the LA and LV in systole (*left*) and diastole (*right*). The thickened anterior mitral leaflet (*arrows*) is well visualized.

valve in patients with LV dilatation (Fig. B-51) as in dilated cardiomyopathy.

9. Superimposition of papillary muscle echoes on mitral leaflet echoes (Fig. B-52).

10. Thickened anomalous chordae tendineae in patients with cleft mitral valve and ostium primum atrial septal defects (Fig. B-53).

11. Artefacts due to the beam-width factor, superimposing echoes from neighboring structures on mitral leaflet echoes (Figs. B-54 and B-55).

12. A papillary fibroelastoma of the mitral

valve leaflet can present a 2-D echographic appearance very much like that of a vegetation (Shub *et al.,* 1981).

Apart from bacterial vegetations on the mitral leaflets, infective masses can also occur in the mitral annulus region. Thus a large sessile "vegetation" in the posterior mitral annulus region (D'Cruz *et al.,* 1982) and a ring abscess in the same general area (Nakamara *et al.,* 1982) have been reported recently. In both cases an echo mass was seen in the vicinity of the posterior mitral leaflet, but was relatively immobile. The abnormal echoes were somewhat similar to mitral annulus calcification in location, but were not as dense.

DIASTOLIC FLUTTER OF THE MITRAL VALVE (Figs. B-56 to B-59)

Rapid vibratory motion of the anterior mitral leaflet was first described in patients with aortic regurgitation (Joyner *et al.,* 1966; Dillon *et al.,* 1970; Gramiak and Shah, 1970; Pridie *et al.,* 1971). Polaroid recording techniques, in use at that time, could demonstrate gross, large-amplitude mitral flutter, but it was only with the introduction of fiberoptic strip-chart recorders that fine mitral flutter could be recorded. The incidence of mitral flutter in aortic regurgitation, as quoted in the earlier papers, was much lower than it was in the studies done after high-quality M-mode recording became available. In fact, M-mode tracings sometimes show a finely stippled or grainy texture of the mitral leaflets that should not be mistaken for true mitral flutter, which is characterized by a fairly regular, rapid vibratory pattern.

Aortic regurgitation remains the most important cause of mitral flutter in diastole. It is important to realize that, whereas mitral flutter in general is nonspecific inasmuch as it has been described in a variety of other entities (see below), mitral flutter of certain morphologies or patterns is virtually diagnostic of aortic regurgitation. Synonyms for such flutter have included the terms "vibration," "shudder," and even "fizz."

The echocardiographer is often called upon to verify the presence of an aortic leak when the auscultatory findings are equivocal. It is not rare to find definite mitral flutter in patients with very soft early diastolic murmurs and even

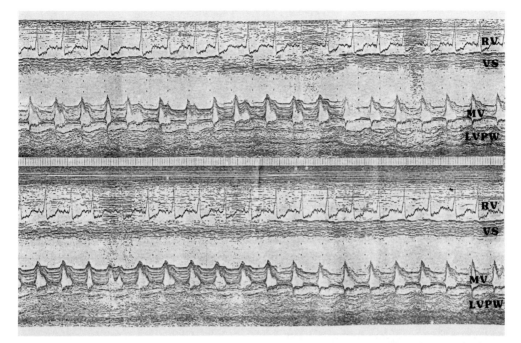

Fig. B-51. M-mode echogram of a patient with congestive cardiomyopathy, showing the LV at mitral valve level. At certain transducer angulations, the mitral valve appears surrounded by multiple linear echoes, especially in systole (*center of upper panel and right half of lower panel*). Such echoes are attributable to beam width and to the beam transecting the mitral valve obliquely. Elsewhere, at slightly different transducer angulation, these "perimitral" echoes are less conspicuous (*right and left of upper panel, right of lower panel*).

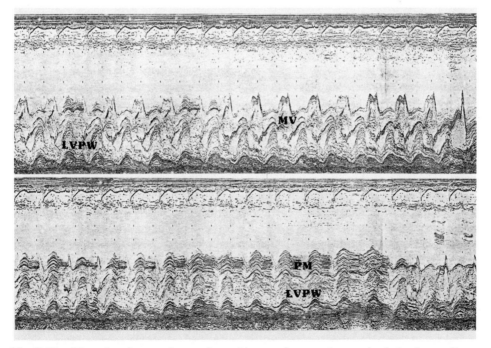

Fig. B-52. M-mode echogram in a patient with very short or absent mitral chordae tendineae. The papillary muscle is inserted almost directly on the mitral leaflets. Consequently, because of the beam-width effect, echoes arising from the papillary muscle tend to be superimposed on those of the mitral valve leaflets. This could simulate an LA myxoma pattern at places. The true diagnosis is easily recognized, and diagnosis of a myxoma excluded, by 2-D echography.

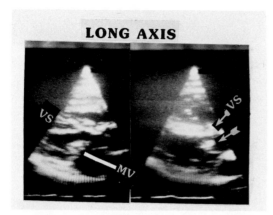

LONG AXIS

Fig. B-53. 2-D echogram of a 53-year-old woman with ostium primum atrial septal defect and cleft mitral valve, documented by hemodynamic studies and at surgery. Both frames are in the long-axis view. In systole (*left*) the chordae appear thick. In diastole (*right*) an abnormal dense echo, between the anterior mitral leaflet and septum, represents a thick anomalous chorda tendineae (confirmed at surgery). It could have been mistaken for a mitral vegetation.

in patients with no audible diastolic murmur but evidence of an aortic leak on aortography.

Diastolic mitral flutter in aortic regurgitation shows the following features:

1. Diagnostically reliable patterns include rapid, regular, large-amplitude vibration, with a "hair-on-end" appearance (Fig. B-56) and a fine, regular, small-amplitude flutter resembling the pile of a shag carpet (Fig. B-57). Other patients exhibit a less specific "minor" flutter pattern.

2. Flutter is always more conspicuous on the anterior leaflet, although frequently it may be discerned on the posterior leaflet also.

3. Flutter is usually visible through all of diastole, i.e., from the D point marking mitral opening to the subsequent C point when the valve closes. This is true even when the murmur is audible only in early diastole.

4. Mitral flutter is the rule in aortic regurgitation, unless the mitral valve is calcified or densely sclerotic. Thus it frequently is absent in patients with associated mitral stenosis. In some instances of mitral stenosis, mitral flutter may be evident in early to middiastole, but abruptly ceases at a constant duration after onset of diastole (D'Cruz *et al.,* 1976).

5. The severity of aortic regurgitation cannot

be predicted from the amplitude or any other characteristic of diastolic flutter. Severe acute aortic regurgitation can present with premature mitral closure but relatively minor flutter. Marked tachycardia, such as may accompany severe aortic regurgitation, can further mask mitral flutter by abbreviating diastole. It is possible that the degree of mitral flutter is dependent not on the quantity of regurgitant blood but on the velocity and site of impingement of the regurgitant jet.

6. When aortic regurgitation is caused by a flail (torn) aortic cusp, the latter appears as a fluttering echo anterior to the anterior mitral leaflet in diastole only (Fig. B-58).

On 2-D echography, careful scrutiny of the mitral valve in real time may confirm mitral flutter, especially when of large amplitude. Diastolic indentation of the anterior mitral leaflet echo, in the short-axis view, by the regurgitant jet, was described in 8 of 12 patients with severe aortic regurgitation (Rowe *et al.,* 1982).

SEPTAL FLUTTER IN AORTIC REGURGITATION

In a minority of patients with aortic regurgitation, the left border of the septum exhibits a fine, rapid flutter in diastole (Fig. B-59). In systole the septal echo is sharp and free of the fine "sawtooth" vibrations seen in diastole. In some patients, such septal flutter is manifest only in early diastole, while in others it is present throughout diastole, corresponding in duration and frequency to the flutter on the free edge of the subjacent anterior mitral leaflet. Septal flutter is attributable to an anteriorly directed regurgitant jet (D'Cruz *et al.,* 1976). Diastolic flutter of the septum is of particular diagnostic value in patients with mitral stenosis who often show no flutter on the sclerotic stiffened mitral cusps.

Caution: Technique is important in revealing the presence of mitral as well as septal flutter: (1) the scale is expanded to render the mitral valve image as large as possible, (2) fast paper speeds are used, (3) gain or reject settings are adjusted so as to suppress the mitral echo partly. Thus, if underdamped, cusp fluttering could be mistaken for cusp thickening.

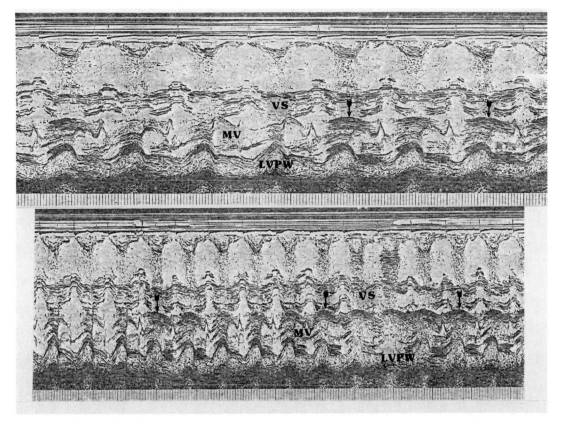

Fig. B-54. *Upper.* M-mode echogram showing the LV at mitral valve level. A dense echo between the mitral valve and LV posterior wall is due to posterior mitral annulus calcification. In addition, a dense echo (*arrows*) appears intermittently, partly superimposed on the anterior mitral leaflet echo. On cursory examination, this could be mistaken for a vegetation on the anterior mitral leaflet.

Lower. The scan from the mid-LV to mitral valve level shows the abnormal dense echo (*arrows*) in the anterior mitral leaflet become progressively more prominent. It is probably due to calcification in or near the attachment of the anterior mitral leaflet to the posterior aortic root.

MITRAL FLUTTER IN CONDITIONS OTHER THAN AORTIC REGURGITATION

1. Diastolic mitral flutter can occur in normal infants (Nanda and Gramiak, 1978) and occasionally in normal children and adolescents. It also may be observed in patients with increased mitral flow secondary to mitral regurgitation, anemia, left-to-right shunts, and so forth. Mitral flutter in a 23-year-old man with patent ductus arteriosus but no aortic leak was presumably of this nature (Mumford and Prakash, 1979). In a series of 34 anemic patients with chronic renal failure, 6 had "major" and 4 "equivocal" mitral diastolic flutter (Tye *et al.,* 1979).

Mitral flutter in rheumatic mitral regurgitation and other high mitral flow states differs from flutter due to aortic regurgitation in the following respects: (a) it is more prominent on the posterior than on the anterior mitral leaflet, (b) it is more evident in early diastole and gradually wanes in middiastole, (c) the flutter tends to be less rapid and regular.

2. Relatively slow diastolic undulations on the mitral valve commonly are seen in atrial flutter and fibrillation. In atrial flutter the frequency of mitral deflections is identical to the atrial rate; in atrial fibrillation too, the undulations are sometimes fairly regular (Prabhu *et al.,* 1978). Such undulations, sometimes re-

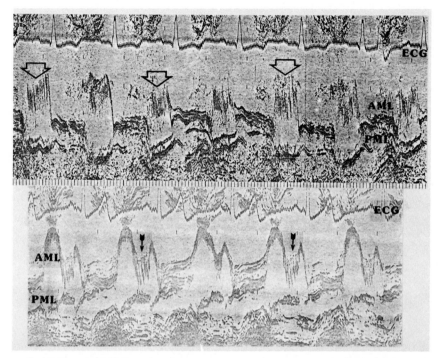

Fig. B-55. M-mode echogram of a patient with aortic regurgitation showing conspicuous rapid vibratory flutter of the anterior mitral leaflet in diastole (*arrows*). Note that flutter on the posterior mitral leaflet is trivial or absent.

M-mode echogram of a patient with aortic regurgitation showing a rapid diastolic flutter of the anterior mitral leaflet, conspicuous in middiastole (*arrows*).

ferred to as coarse flutter, are unlikely to be mistaken for the much faster mitral oscillations of aortic regurgitation, which are in the range of 35 to 135 cycles per sec (Nanda and Gramiak, 1978).

3. Diastolic mitral flutter is an important sign of a flail anterior or posterior mitral leaflet secondary to rupture of chordae tendineae or partial rupture of a papillary muscle. In such a situation, motion of the untethered leaflet is erratic and may vary from a slight tremulous vibration to a large flapping motion. A flail posterior leaflet may occupy an abnormal anterior position in diastole. Systolic mitral flutter also may be noted in some cases.

4. Mitral flutter has been described in certain varieties of cyanotic heart disease: (a) It has been seen in children with transposition of aorta and pulmonary artery who have had atrial septostomy by the balloon (Rashkind) procedure or by direct surgery (Blalock-Hanlon operation). It is also evident in children who have had the Mustard operation (Hagler *et al.*, 1975;

Aziz *et al.*, 1976; Silverman *et al.*, 1978). In Mustard's operation, the anatomy of the atria is altered by an intra-atrial baffle directing the blood from the vena cava to the mitral valve and the pulmonary venous blood flow to the tricuspid valve. The abnormal pattern of atrial flow inevitably leads to turbulence and mitral flutter. (b) Cor triatriatum, wherein a membrane or diaphragm in the left atrium above the mitral valve may engender turbulence, thus unduly agitating the mitral cusps. (c) Meyer *et al.* (1977) described mitral flutter in patients with pulmonary outflow tract obstruction and ventricular septal defects with right-to-left shunts. The mechanism of flutter in this hemodynamic situation seems uncertain.

5. Coarse flutter of the posterior mitral leaflet in a 69-year-old woman with acute myocardial infarction and a new systolic murmur was diagnosed initially as due to a flail mitral valve secondary to papillary muscle rupture, but hemodynamic study revealed instead an acquired defect in the muscular ventricular septum

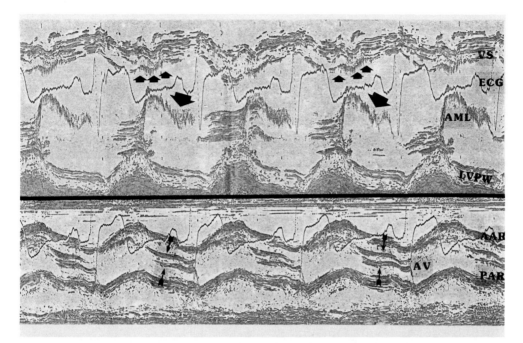

Fig. B-56. M-mode echogram of a young man with aortic regurgitation of rheumatic etiology. Rapid diastolic vibrations are apparent on the anterior mitral leaflet, in the upper panel (*large broad arrows*). Flutter also appears on the LV (posterior) aspect of the ventricular septum (*small broad arrows*) in early diastole.

In the lower panel, the aortic valve is slightly thickened and represented in diastole as a pair of parallel linear echoes. This is a frequent finding in rheumatic aortic regurgitation, though not diagnostic of it.

(Rosenthal *et al.,* 1979). There was no evidence of mitral regurgitation.

6. Diastolic mitral flutter was noted in a 68-year-old woman being investigated for crescendo angina. During coronary bypass surgery a mass was palpated in the left atrium, and on removal it was found to be a myxoma 4 to 5 cm in diameter. Mitral flutter was thus the only echocardiographic manifestation of the myxoma, which was itself "invisible" to ultrasound, presumably because of poor echo-reflecting properties. Another instance of mitral flutter accompanying LA myxoma, in a 54-year-old woman, was notable in that flutter was more prominent on the posterior mitral leaflet (Baird, 1981). I have seen flutter of the anterior mitral leaflet in a patient with a sarcomatous tumor of the left atrium protruding through the mitral orifice. Exceptionally, anterior mitral flutter accompanies massive posterior mitral annulus calcification. It seems probable that partial obstruction to mitral flow generates the turbulence that agitates the mitral leaflet.

7. Joswig *et al.* (1979) reported a perplexing case of diastolic mitral flutter (on M-mode echography) and an apical, early diastolic murmur (on auscultation and phonocardiography) in a 17-year-old man. No aortic regurgitation or any other abnormality was detected on cardiac catheterization or angiocardiography.

8. A 60-cycle regular disturbance on the echo signal could conceivably be mistaken for mitral flutter. It would, of course, continue throughout the cardiac cycle, whereas true mitral flutter due to aortic regurgitation is restricted to diastole.

FLAIL MITRAL VALVE

A flail mitral leaflet is one that is incompletely tethered to its papillary muscle attachments because of rupture of some of its chordae tendineae, or much less commonly of the papillary muscle itself. Either the anterior or the posterior leaflet or both may be flail; mitral regurgitation is inevitable and usually (but not always) severe, requiring mitral valve replacement. The echocardiographic identification of a flail mitral leaf-

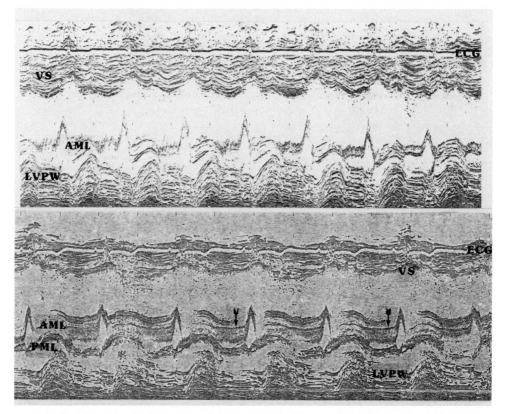

Fig. B-57. M-mode echograms of two patients with aortic regurgitation. In both, the anterior mitral leaflet shows very fine flutter and near-closure (*arrows*) until a brief full opening is achieved with atrial contraction (prominent "A" peak). The fluttering half-closed anterior mitral leaflet gives rise to unusual diastolic echoes that could be mistaken for a vegetation, especially in the lower panel. These patients had no evidence of bacterial endocarditis.

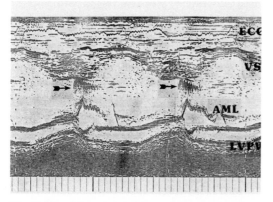

Fig. B-58. M-mode echogram of a patient with aortic regurgitation due to aortic valve endocarditis. The aortic valve was flail at surgery. Diastolic flutter can be seen on the anterior mitral leaflet, as well as on an abnormal structure (flail aortic leaflet) that prolapses down into the LV outflow tract in diastole only (*arrows*).

let is therefore an important task in patients presenting with the murmur of mitral regurgitation.

Normal motion of the mitral leaflets is so well controlled by the elaborate system of branching chordae tendineae attached to its ventricular surface that rupture of part of this chordal system results in abnormal exaggerated motion of the affected leaflet in both systole and diastole, which in turn can be viewed by reflected ultrasound. M-mode signs of a flail mitral valve (Figs. B-60 to B-62) include:

1. *Systolic flutter* of the flail leaflet (Meyer *et al.,* 1977; Sze *et al.,* 1978; Child *et al.,* 1979; Chandaratna and Aronow, 1979; Mintz *et al.,* 1980). Most reported cases have been associated with active or healed bacterial endocarditis, and it is these patients who have conspicuous or large-amplitude systolic flutter. Rapid oscilla-

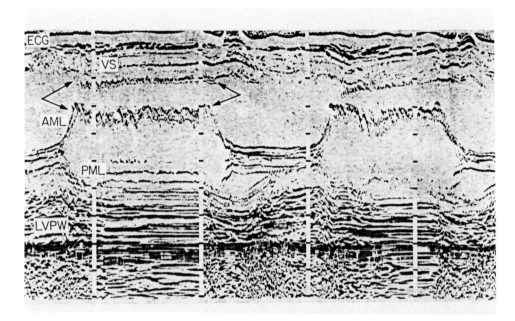

Fig. B-59. A combination of coarse and fine diastolic flutter is seen on the anterior mitral leaflet through all of diastole in this patient with aortic regurgitation. Simultaneously, fine diastolic flutter is also discernible on the left border of the ventricular septum.

tions of the flail leaflet in systole probably result from a combination of pliable leaflet, dense echo-reflecting nature of healing or healed vegetations, and physical properties of the affected leaflet that permit it to vibrate in the stream of the regurgitant jet. No convincing explanation is yet forthcoming as to why systolic flutter seldom if ever occurs in all other varieties of mitral regurgitation.

2. *Coarse diastolic fluttering* of the flail leaflet, especially in early diastole. This may vary from a barely perceptible, irregular quivering to a large, irregular, flapping motion so bizarre as to deserve the term chaotic (Humphries *et al.,* 1977; Child *et al.,* 1979; Chandaratna and Aronow, 1979; Mintz *et al.,* 1980). Such diastolic flutter usually is distinct morphologically from the regular fine flutter commonly seen in aortic regurgitation. Marked flutter of the posterior mitral leaflet has been reported in a patient with rupture of the posteromedial papillary muscle secondary to myocardial infarction; hypokinesis of the LV posterior wall, coupled with septal hyperkinesis, was a clue to the ischemic etiology of the mitral regurgitation (Ahmad *et al.,* 1978).

3. A flail posterior mitral leaflet may move to an *abnormally anterior position in diastole.* Thus instead of moving in a direction opposite to that of the anterior leaflet, it may in fact move parallel to the anterior leaflet (Sweatman *et al.,* 1972; Giles *et al.,* 1974; Humphries *et al.,* 1977; Child *et al.,* 1979; Mintz *et al.,* 1980).

4. *Systolic echoes within the left atrium,* posterior to the aortic root, may appear due to eversion of the flail mitral leaflet into the LA, and this can happen with either the anterior or posterior leaflet (Humphries *et al.,* 1977; Mintz *et al.,* 1980). Such an echo may appear only briefly within the LA and may show systolic flutter.

5. *Systolic mitral prolapse of the holosystolic type.* The flail leaflet moves abruptly to a posterior location against the posterior wall of the LV or atrioventricular junction, as in severe mitral prolapse, and remains there until the end of systole when it abruptly moves forward to its diastolic position (Humphries *et al.,* 1977; Child *et al.,* 1979).

6. *Early anterior systolic motion* of a partly flail anterior mitral leaflet has been documented in a patient with preexisting mitral valve prolapse, complicated by spontaneous chordal rupture (Kerin *et al.,* 1980).

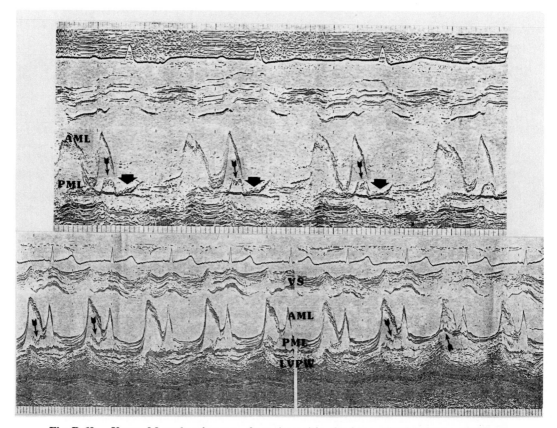

Fig. B-60. *Upper.* M-mode echogram of a patient with mitral regurgitation due to a flail poste-rior mitral leaflet. The ECG shows an abnormally long PR interval. The posterior mitral leaflet shows abnormal anterior motion (*thin arrows*) at the time of the "A" peak on the anterior mitral leaflet. Subsequent to apparent mitral closure, the posterior mitral leaflet moves posteriorly (*broad arrows*). Reference to the ECG reveals that this unusual motion (which should not be mistaken for mitral prolapse) precedes ventricular systole, because of the long PR interval.

    Lower. M-mode echogram of a patient with flail posterior mitral leaflet. Note that the posterior mitral leaflet appears to consist of two components in diastole, one of which occupies the normal position while the other moves to an abnormal anterior position near the anterior leaflet (*arrows*), with some variation from beat to beat.

    7. One instance of *systolic flutter of the LA anterior wall* (contiguous to the posterior aortic root) has been described in a patient who had a partly flail posterior mitral leaflet (Antman *et al.,* 1978). The patient had large, redundant mitral leaflets and thin, elongated chordae, some of which had spontaneously ruptured. The regurgitant mitral jet struck the left atrial wall adjacent to the aortic root, so that the pansys-tolic murmur of mitral regurgitation was re-markable in this patient for being well heard at the upper right sternal border, mimicking aortic stenosis.

    8. *Systolic flutter of the interatrial septum*

was noted in 5 of 10 patients with flail mitral leaflet (Tei *et al.,* 1980); the atrial septum was visualized by a right parasternal approach.

TWO-DIMENSIONAL ECHOCARDIOGRAPHY (Figs. B-62 and B-63)

In the long-axis view, flail mitral leaflets have been shown to exhibit a distinctive systolic be-havior that has proved a valuable diagnostic indicator of ruptured chordae, because it is not seen in any other condition (Child *et al.,* 1979; Mintz *et al.,* 1978, 1980). During systole, the

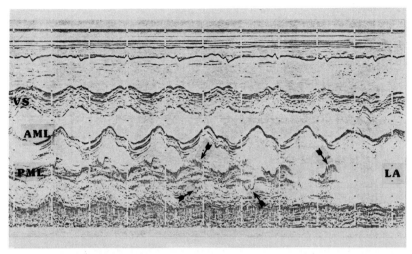

Fig. B-61. M-mode echogram of a 30-year-old man with chronic renal failure on hemodialysis, who had had successful chemotherapy for bacterial endocarditis four months previously. He presented on this admission with severe mitral regurgitation, revealed by hemodynamic studies. There is systolic flutter of both mitral leaflets (*arrows*), which extends into the LA. Other confusing dense linear echoes in the region of the posterior mitral leaflet are probably due to submitral (mitral annulus) calcification, which was noted in echograms done before onset of endocarditis.

tip (free edge) of the flail leaflet is seen to move rapidly into the left atrium, thus everting the leaflet and preventing its coaptation with the other leaflet. In some cases, because of scarring or superimposed vegetations, the flail leaflet may not be clearly seen in its entire length, but the untethered part of the cusp with perhaps attached severed chordae may be glimpsed darting swiftly into and out of the LV like a snake's tongue. These 2-D findings are often detected only after careful and painstaking slow-motion viewing or frame-by-frame scrutiny. Yet they are of much diagnostic value and so worth the effort.

Recently, attempts have been made to evaluate the diagnostic potentiality of M-mode echocardiography with regard to flail mitral leaflets and compare it to that of the 2-D technique. Humphries *et al.* (1977) stated that the presence of any one of the first four M-mode features listed above could suggest a flail mitral leaflet. These echographic abnormalities progressively augment the probability of the diagnosis. There seems no doubt that the 2-D echographic criterion of cusp eversion with noncoaptation is diagnostically superior to the M-mode criteria taken separately (Child *et al.*, 1979; Mintz *et al.*, 1980).

ECHOCARDIOGRAPHIC APPEARANCES THAT CAN SIMULATE FLAIL MITRAL LEAFLET

1. *In mitral prolapse* (with intact chordae), especially the severe holosystolic variety, systolic as well as diastolic motion of the posterior leaflet can mimic that of a flail leaflet. In fact, in a mechanical or hemodynamic sense, there may be little difference between a flail and an extremely elongated prolapsed mitral leaflet. However, systolic flutter is excessively rare with mitral prolapse; it is very common with a flail leaflet. On 2-D echography, the convexity of prolapsing mitral leaflets may bulge into the LA, but the tips (free edges) of the leaflets point normally toward the LV chamber. With a flail leaflet, it is the free edge of the affected cusp that everts and points toward the LA in systole. In prolapse, echographic coaptation of the mitral cusp is preserved; a flail valve fails to coapt.

Recently Cherian *et al.* (1982) have shown that "diastolic prolapse"—posterior motion of a flail mitral leaflet into the LA in late diastole—is a frequent finding on the long-axis 2-D echogram. These authors found that in true mitral prolapse the posterior motion began only after the QRS was inscribed.

[*Text continued on page 98.*]

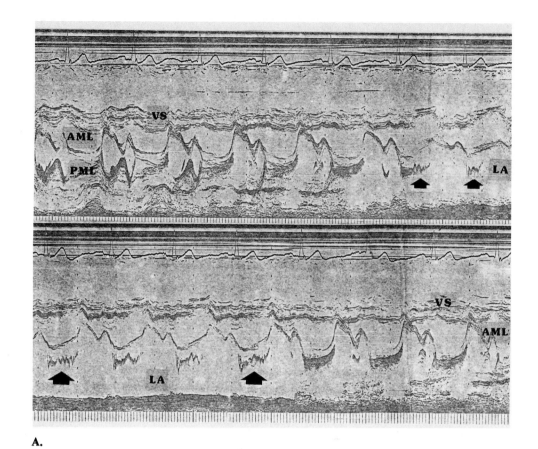

A.

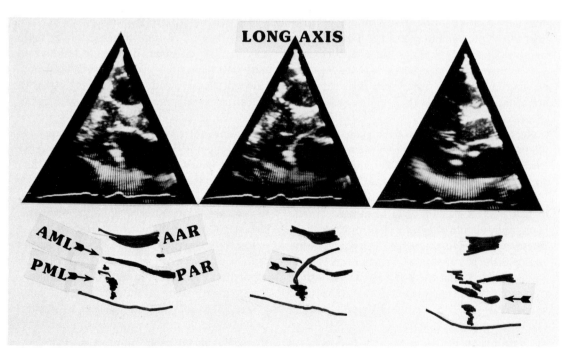

LONG AXIS

B.

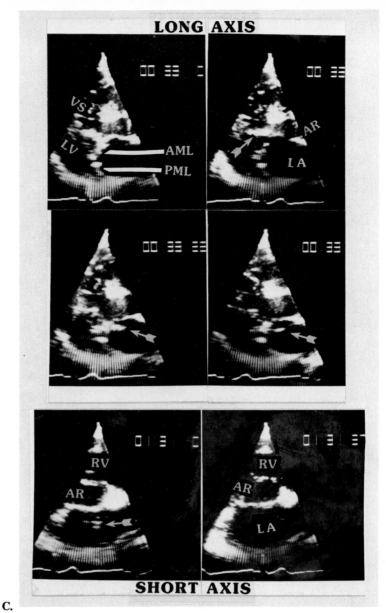

LONG AXIS

SHORT AXIS

C.

Fig. B-62. *A.* M-mode echogram of a man who had been successfully treated for bacterial endocarditis a year previously. He had residual mitral regurgitation. Healed vegetations account for the abnormal, dense thickening and peculiar motion in diastole as well as systole. The flail posterior mitral leaflet shows systolic flutter (*arrows*) as the transducer gradually scans toward the LA. Abnormally thick dense echoes from the posterior mitral leaflet, which exhibits exaggerated mobility, are also visible.

Fig. B-62. *B.* 2-D echogram of the same patient with a flail posterior mitral leaflet following bacterial endocarditis. All 3 frames are long axis. The first, near end-diastole, shows nodular thickening of the posterior mitral cusp. The second, at end-diastole, shows the torn chordae attached to the posterior mitral leaflet swinging across from LV toward LA; it is superimposed on the anterior mitral leaflet, which is still open. The third shows the typical configuration of a flail leaflet, with the free edge of the affected leaflet pointing into the left atrium.

Fig. B-62. *C.* 2-D echograms of the same patient. The four frames in the upper and middle are serial ones from the same cardiac cycle. The two in the upper row are in diastole; the two in the middle row are in systole. The main abnormal finding, typical of flail mitral leaflet, is a brief systolic protrusion of the edge or tip of the flail leaflet into the LA, which has been compared to the darting of a snake's tongue. The 2 frames in the lower row, in the short-axis view, show the aortic root and LA. In systole (*left*) the flail mitral leaflet appears as a small abnormal echo in the LA; in diastole this echo cannot be seen (*right*).

97

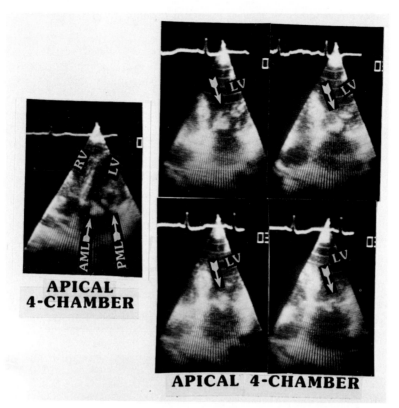

Fig. B-63. *Left.* 2-D echogram in the apical 4-chamber view of a patient with mitral valve endocarditis. The frame shown here is in systole and shows a vegetation on the anterior mitral leaflet. Note also that proper systolic coaptation of the mitral cusps does not occur; the anterior leaflet tends to evert into the LA.

Right. 2-D echogram of another patient with mitral valve endocarditis. At surgery, both mitral leaflets were partly flail and had healing vegetations. All four frames are in the apical 4-chamber view; the two upper frames are in diastole, the two lower frames in systole. Valvular vegetations are well visualized in the diastolic frames. An abnormal pattern of coaptation of the mitral cusps is present in the right lower frame.

2. Systolic flutter can occur with a *nonflail regurgitant mitral valve* (Sze *et al.,* 1978) in patients with healed scarring of previous endocarditis but intact chordae. Finer, less conspicuous systolic flutter rarely can occur with mitral prolapse, according to the same authors.

3. Abnormal anterior diastolic motion of the posterior mitral leaflet occurs with a flail posterior leaflet, as well as in *mitral stenosis.* However, in mitral stenosis, the mitral leaflets usually are densely sclerotic and do not flutter. Moreover, the pattern of mitral cusp motion on the 2-D echogram is very different from that of a flail mitral leaflet.

PAPILLARY MUSCLE DYSFUNCTION

Malfunction, malposition, and malalignment of LV papillary muscles have been implicated as a cause of mitral regurgitation in patients with ischemic heart disease for nearly two decades (Burch *et al.,* 1963), and several authors have described echocardiographic abnormalities in such cases (Tallary *et al.,* 1972; Burgess *et al.,* 1973; Ogawa *et al.,* 1979). In these studies and in the clinical practice of cardiology, it has been assumed that mitral incompetence occurring in patients with coronary disease is due to papillary muscle dysfunction, in the absence of any other obvious mitral pathology, especially if LV wall motion abnormality in the vicinity of the papillary muscle is demonstrable.

However, it is not always certain whether impairment of papillary muscle contraction exists or not, and if it does, whether such impaired contraction is the sole cause of mitral regurgitation in any given patient. For instance, it is very difficult to exclude a rheumatic origin of mitral valve incompetence; there may be little sclerosis and no stenosis in histologically proven rheumatic valves, and coronary disease, if present, may be coincidental.

Furthermore, some authors have used the term "papillary muscle dysfunction" perhaps too loosely to include not only instances of papillary muscle ischemia or infarction, but also mitral regurgitation accompanying congestive cardiomyopathy, myocarditis, endocardial fibrosis, and LV dilatation of any cause.

Ogawa et al. (1979) claimed to recognize two varieties of papillary muscle dysfunction on the basis of 2-D echographic appearances: (1) in three of their patients with akinetic inferoposterior wall akinesis but normal LV cavity size, papillary muscle fibrosis with lack of contractility was assumed to be the primary cause of late systolic mitral prolapse; (2) in nine other patients with LV dilatation or aneurysm formation, LV geometry and with it papillary muscle–chordal cusp alignment so altered with respect to the LV long axis and the mitral orifice, that mitral cusp coaptation was necessarily abnormal and the valve incompetent. These authors described six different patterns of LV anatomy as viewed in long axis, based on the LV dimension, motion of the LV posteroinferior wall, and systolic configuration of the anterior and posterior mitral leaflet echoes. A detailed exposition of all these echographic patterns and types of papillary muscle dysfunction will not be made here, since their diagnostic significance has yet to be established or widely accepted. It may seem reasonable, for the present, to consider papillary muscle dysfunction a possible basis of mitral regurgitation if: (1) the LV posterior wall at papillary muscle level is severely akinetic or (2) an abnormal, densely sclerotic area is seen on long- and short-axis views in the region of the posteromedial papillary muscle and adjacent LV wall, as in Case #2 of Ogawa et al. (1979).

Godley et al. (1981) recently described a new abnormal pattern of systolic mitral closure that they found highly specific for papillary muscle dysfunction in patients with mitral regurgitation following myocardial infarction: In the apical four-chamber view, one or both mitral leaflets were restrained or arrested within the LV during systole, so that the leaflets could not appose. The anterior mitral leaflet was more often affected. Almost all these patients showed dyskinetic LV wall motion adjacent to a papillary muscle. This new echographic sign could enhance the accuracy of the diagnosis of papillary muscle dysfunction, an improvement over its former vague status.

MITRAL VALVE MOTION AS INDICATOR OF LEFT VENTRICULAR FUNCTION

PREMATURE CLOSURE OF THE MITRAL VALVE

Normal closure of the mitral valve is effected by ventricular contraction, the mitral C point occurring 0.05 to 0.06 sec after the onset of inscription of the QRS complex (Mann et al., 1975). In two very different hemodynamic situations, the mitral valve closes before the onset of LV contraction, i.e., the mitral C point occurs before, at, or immediately after (within 0.04 sec) the onset of the QRS:

1. Acute severe aortic regurgitation (Fig. B-64), which is most commonly a complication of aortic valve endocarditis; less often acute dissection of the ascending aorta or trauma is responsible. First reported by Pridie et al. (1971), premature mitral closure was confirmed and studied in further detail by Mann et al. (1975) and Botvinick et al. (1975). The patient with this echographic finding is always in severe LV failure, often complicated by pulmonary edema or hypotension. The ventricular diastolic pressure rises to extremely high levels, and on cardiac catheterization it is observed to exceed the pulmonary wedge pressure. Thus, reversal of the left atrial–left ventricular pressure gradient ensues in late diastole, effecting premature closure of the mitral valve.

[Text continued on page 104.]

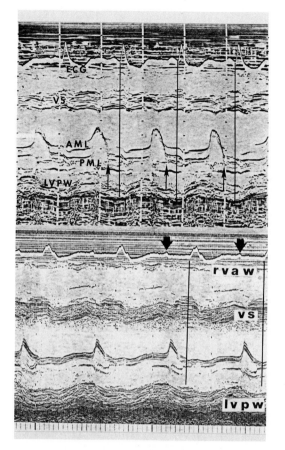

Fig. B-64. *Upper.* M-mode echogram of a 60-year-old man with severe aortic regurgitation. LV end-diastolic pressure was about 40 mmHg. The mitral valve closes (*arrows*) well before the onset of inscription of the QRS complex. Note that the PR interval is normal. At surgery for aortic valve replacement, the basis of aortic regurgitation appeared to be chronic rheumatic disease. There was no evidence of endocarditis or of a flail cusp. Note that diastolic mitral flutter is inconspicuous in this case.

Lower. M-mode echogram of a patient with premature mitral closure. The mitral valve closes (*vertical lines*) before the QRS is inscribed on the ECG. When the P wave is identified on the ECG (*arrows*) it is evident that the PR interval is prolonged. The "E" and "A" peaks of anterior mitral motion are superimposed, and followed by mitral closure because of reversal of the normal LA-LV gradient during the phase of atrial relaxation. This patient had no aortic regurgitation.

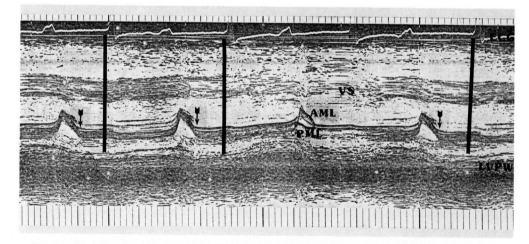

Fig. B-65. M-mode echogram showing the mitral valve in a patient with first-degree A-V block. The vertical lines indicate the onset of the QRS on the electrocardiogram. The mitral valve opens for only a brief interval, the atrial filling phase being superimposed on the rapid early filling phase; thereafter the valve closes (*arrows*) well before the QRS onset. This patient had no aortic regurgitation.

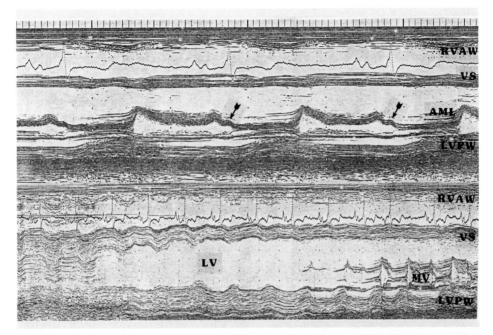

Fig. B-66. M-mode echogram of a patient with congestive failure and LV dilatation secondary to ischemic heart diseases. The upper panel, at fast paper speed, shows a prominent "bump" on the mitral valve AC slope (*arrows*), suggestive of significantly raised LV end-diastolic pressure. The lower panel, at slow paper speed, shows an LV scan from LV apex to papillary muscle and then chordae and mitral valve level. The LV overall performance is impaired, and regional disparities in systolic excursions of the LV wall and septum can be detected.

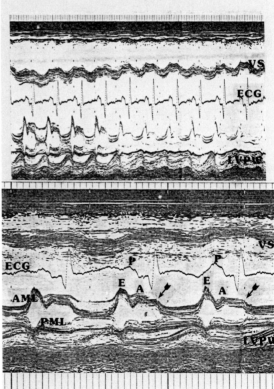

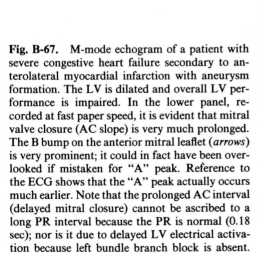

Fig. B-67. M-mode echogram of a patient with severe congestive heart failure secondary to anterolateral myocardial infarction with aneurysm formation. The LV is dilated and overall LV performance is impaired. In the lower panel, recorded at fast paper speed, it is evident that mitral valve closure (AC slope) is very much prolonged. The B bump on the anterior mitral leaflet (*arrows*) is very prominent; it could in fact have been overlooked if mistaken for "A" peak. Reference to the ECG shows that the "A" peak actually occurs much earlier. Note that the prolonged AC interval (delayed mitral closure) cannot be ascribed to a long PR interval because the PR is normal (0.18 sec); nor is it due to delayed LV electrical activation because left bundle branch block is absent.

101

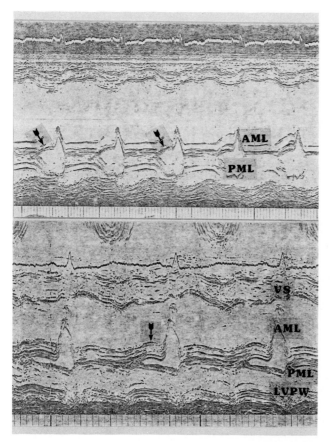

Fig. B-68. *Upper.* M-mode echogram of a 76-year-old man with congestive heart failure secondary to congestive cardiomyopathy. The LV is dilated and wide mitral-septal separation suggests poor LV overall performance. Initial mitral opening is gradual and incomplete (*arrows*), so that the EF slope is absent or even reversed. Further opening of the anterior mitral leaflet occurs after atrial contraction.

Lower. M-mode echogram of a patient with inferior wall infarction. The mitral valve opens to a very small extent in early diastole (*arrows*), and opens fully only with atrial contraction. This is one of the patterns associated with significantly elevated LV end-diastolic pressure.

Fig. B-69. M-mode echogram in a patient with Fallot's tetralogy. The anterior mitral leaflet shows an almost flat EF slope (*arrows*) in diastole. The RV anterior wall is not distinct, but appears considerably hypertrophied. The posterior mitral leaflet moves normally, with a W-shaped contour, making the diagnosis of mitral valve stenosis unlikely.

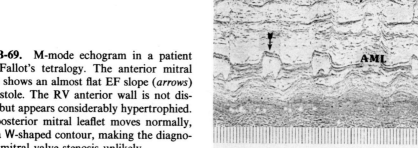

Fig. B-70. *A.* (*Opposite*) 2-D echogram in a patient with congestive cardiomyopathy. The LV is dilated and contracts poorly. The upper two frames are long axis; the lower two, short axis. The left frames are in diastole, the right frames in systole. The separation between the mitral cusps in diastole is unduly small because of the low mitral flow (low cardiac output). True mitral stenosis is not present.

Fig. B-70. *B.* (*Opposite*) Four successive frames from the same cardiac cycle, in the same patient. The mitral cusps are mildly thickened. The left upper frame and right lower frames are in systole; the two intervening frames, in diastole, show limited opening of the cusps, which would indicate mild mitral stenosis if the cardiac output were normal.

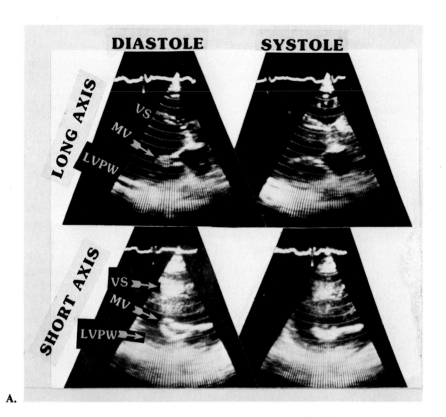

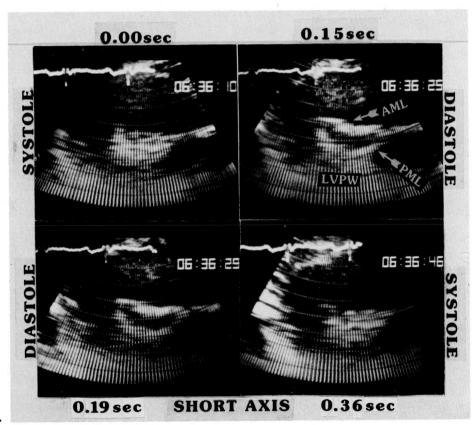

103

Premature mitral closure is very seldom seen in *chronic* aortic regurgitation, even if it is of severe degree. In such patients, the dilated and distensible left ventricle is presumed to accommodate a large regurgitant volume without too extreme a rise in diastolic pressure.

Caution. It must be added that acute severe regurgitation is not invariably accompanied by premature mitral closure. Therefore, the absence of this echographic sign should not be interpreted as indisputable evidence that the aortic regurgitation is not of critical severity, if other clinical findings suggest a more serious state of affairs. This point is not merely of academic interest, but also of crucial practical importance, because the detection of premature mitral closure in a patient with acute aortic regurgitation strongly influences a clinical decision in favor of prompt surgery for valve replacement, usually preceded by cardiac catheterization and aortography.

Arvan and Kleid (1976) reported an instance of *Candida* endocarditis of the aortic valve, in which premature mitral closure was not seen, in spite of the fact that two cusps of the aortic valve were perforated. It appears that the large bulky vegetations on the aortic cusps prevented hemodynamically important aortic regurgitation from developing. Thus, absence of premature mitral closure in a patient with aortic valve endocarditis does not entirely exclude the possibility of destructive lesions of the valve that would necessitate its replacement by a suitable prosthesis.

2. The other cause of premature mitral valve closure is an unduly long interval between atrial and ventricular contraction (Figs. B-64 and B-65). This could occur in first-, second-, or third-degree AV block. Normally atrial contraction is accompanied by an increase in mitral cusp separation ("A" peak), which is immediately followed by a closure motion of the valve (first half of the AC slope); final closure of the mitral leaflets is effected by ventricular contraction (second half of the AC slope). If, for any reason, atrial contraction is not followed by ven-

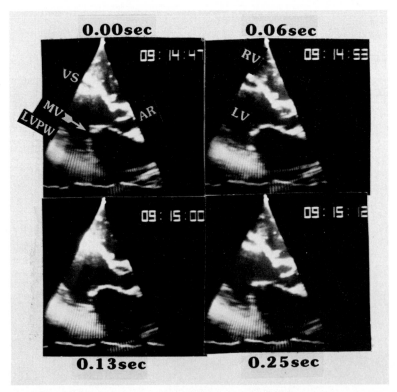

Fig. B-71. 2-D echogram in the long-axis view of a patient with congestive cardiomyopathy and poor LV performance. The four frames are serial ones from the same cardiac cycle. The lower left frame is in systole, the others in diastole. Note that the free edge of the anterior mitral leaflet shows only small excursions and does not reach near the septum. This is the 2-D equivalent of increased mitral E point–septal separation (IHSS).

tricular systole at the usual interval, the normal pressure gradient between left atrium and left ventricle may be reversed transiently (probably due to fall in atrial pressure caused by atrial relaxation), thus bringing about mitral valve closure.

Once atriogenic mitral closure has occurred, the valve may remain closed until the next ventricular contraction, or it may soon reopen and then reclose when the left ventricle contracts (Prabhu et al., 1978).

Unlike premature closure due to severe acute aortic regurgitation, "premature" mitral cusp apposition attributable to a long P-R interval has no ominous or adverse significance. Its importance lies in the possibility that it might be mistakenly thought to signify a very severe elevation of LV diastolic pressure, if the patient should happen to have aortic regurgitation or aortic valve endocarditis.

Other abnormalities of mitral valve motion, not due to intrinsic mitral disease but to impaired LV performance, include:

1. Delayed AC slope, with a bump or notch-bump on the AC slope. (Normally the AC slope is rapid, linear, and smooth.) This abnormality is a very useful sign of significantly impaired overall LV function. However, it may be missed easily unless the mitral valve image is sufficiently expanded and the paper speed fast enough (50 mm/sec or more). Examples are shown in Figures B-66 and B-67.

2. Incomplete mitral valve opening in early diastole (Fig. B-68) is another type of echographic pattern associated with poor LV performance and raised LV diastolic pressure. The mitral valve EF slope is a negative one, and the valve opens fully only with atrial contraction.

3. A flat EF slope is seen in some patients with RV systolic overload (Fig. B-69). This pattern, formerly called pseudo–mitral stenosis, should not be mistaken for that of true mitral stenosis.

4. Diminished diastolic opening excursion of the mitral valve is often seen in patients with advanced chronic LV failure (Figs. B-70 and B-71). The mitral valve is not structurally stenotic, but its amplitude of cusp separation in diastole is diminished because of the low stroke output. This pattern too should not be mistaken for true mitral stenosis.

REFERENCES

MITRAL STENOSIS

Akgun, G., and Layton, C.: Aortic root and left atrial wall motion: An echocardiographic study. Br. Heart J., 39:1082, 1977.

Biamino, G.; Wessel, H. G.; Schlag, W.; et al.: Echocardiographic pattern of motion of the aortic root as a correlate of left atrial volume changes. Am. Heart J., 100:191, 1980.

Chandaratna, P. A. N.; Aronow, W. S.; and Lurie, M.: Cross-sectional echocardiographic observations on the mechanism of preservation of the opening snap in calcific mitral stenosis. Chest, 78:822, 1980.

Cope, G. D.; Kisslo, J. A.; Johnson, M. L.: A reassessment of the echocardiogram in mitral stenosis. Circulation, 52:664, 1975.

Duchak, J. M.; Chang, S.; and Feigenbaum, H.: The posterior mitral valve echo and the echocardiographic diagnosis of mitral stenosis. Am. J. Cardiol., 29:628, 1972.

Edler, I.: Ultrasound cardiogram in mitral valve disease. Acta Chir. Scand. 111:230, 1956.

Effert, S.: Pre- and postoperative evaluation of mitral stenosis by ultrasound. Am. J. Cardiol., 19:59, 1967.

Elkayam, U.; Weiss, S.; and Landiado, S.: Pericardial effusion and mitral valve involvement in systemic lupus erythematosus. Echocardiographic study. Ann. Rheum. Dis., 36:349, 1977.

Feigenbaum, H.: Echocardiography, 2nd ed. Lea & Febiger, Philadelphia, 1976, p. 270.

Fisher, M. L.; Parisi, A. F.; Plotnik, G. D.; et al.: Assessment of severity of mitral stenosis by echocardiographic leaflet separation. Arch. Intern. Med., 139:402, 1979.

Flaherty, J. T.; Livengood, S.; and Fortuin, N. J.: Atypical posterior leaflet motion in echocardiogram in mitral stenosis. Am. J. Cardiol., 35:675, 1975.

Glasser, S. P., and Faris, J. V.: Posterior leaflet motion in mitral stenosis. Chest, 71:87, 1977.

Glover, M. U.; Warren, S. E.; Vieweg, W. V. R.; et al.: M-mode and two-dimensional echocardiographic correlation with findings at catheterization and surgery in patients with mitral stenosis. Am. Heart J. 105:98, 1983.

Goodman, D. J.; Harrison, D. C.; and Popp, R. L.: Echocardiographic features of primary pulmonary hypertension. Am. Heart J., 86:847, 1973.

Hall, R. J. C.; Clarke, S. E.; and Brown, D.: Evaluation of posterior aortic wall echogram in diagnosis of mitral valve disease. Br. Heart J., 41:522, 1979.

Heger, J. J.; Wann, L. S.; Weyman, A. E.; et al.: Long-term changes in mitral valve area after successful mitral commissurotomy. Circulation, 59:443, 1979.

Henry, W. L.; Maron, M. B.; and Griffith, M. S.: Measurement of mitral orifice area in patients with mitral valve disease by real-time two-dimensional echocardiography. Circulation, 51:827, 1975.

Joyner, C. R.; Reid, J. M.; and Bond, J. P.: Reflected ultrasound in the assessment of mitral valve disease. Circulation, 27:506, 1963.

Kelley, D. R.; Spotnitz, H. M.; Beiser, G. D.; et al.: Effects of chronic right ventricular volume and pressure loading on left ventricular performance. Circulation, 44:403, 1971.

Leutenegger, F.; Raeder, E. A.; Fromer, M.; et al.: Progression of mild mitral stenosis and incidence of restenosis after open commissurotomy: A study using echocardiography. Am. Heart J., 98:562, 1979.

Levisman, J. A.; Abbasi, A. S.; and Pearce, M. L.: Posterior mitral leaflet motion in mitral stenosis. Circulation, 51:511, 1975.

Martin, R. P.; Rakowski, H.; Kleiman, J. H.; et al.: Reliability and reproducibility of two-dimensional echocardiographic measurement of the stenotic mitral valve orifice area. Am. J. Cardiol., 43:560, 1979.

McLaurin, L. P.; Gibson, T. C.; Waider, W.; et al.: An appraisal of mitral valve echocardiograms mimicking mitral stenosis in conditions with right ventricular pressure overload. Circulation, 48:801, 1973.

Naccarelli, G. B.; Nomeir, A. M.; Watts, L. E.; et al.: Echocardiographic assessment of mitral stenosis by the left atrial emptying index. Chest, 76:668, 1979.

Naito, M.; Morganroth, J.; Mardelli, J.; et al.: Rheumatic mitral stenosis: Cross-sectional echocardiographic analysis. Am. Heart J., 100:34, 1980.

Nichol, P. M.; Gilbert, B. W.; and Kisslo, J. A.: Two-dimensional echocardiographic assessment of mitral stenosis. Circulation, 55:120, 1977.

Nicolisi, G. L.; Pugh, D. M.; and Dunn, M.: Sensitivity and specificity of echocardiography in the assessment of valve calcification in mitral stenosis. Am. Heart J., 98:171, 1979.

Palomo, A. R.; Quinones, M. A.; and Waggoner, A. D.: Echo-phonocardiographic determination of left atrial and left ventricular filling pressures with and without mitral stenosis. Circulation, 61:1043, 1980.

Quinones, M. A.; Gaasch, W. H.; and Waisser, E.: Reduction in the rate of diastolic descent of the mitral valve echogram in patients with altered left ventricular diastolic pressure-volume relations. Circulation, 49:246, 1974.

Raj, M. V. J.; Bennett, D. H.; Stovin, P. J. I.; et al.: Echocardiographic assessment of mitral valve calcification. Br. Heart J., 38:81, 1976.

Segal, B. L.; Likoff, W.; and Kingsley, B.: Echocardiography: Clinical application in mitral stenosis. JAMA, 193:161, 1966.

Shiu, M. F.: Mitral valve closure index. Echocardiographic index of severity of mitral stenosis. Br. Heart J., 39:839, 1977.

Shiu, M. F.; Crowther, A.; Jenkins, B. S.; et al.: Echocardiographic and exercise evaluation of results of mitral valvotomy operations. Br. Heart J. 41:139, 1979.

Shiu, M. F.; Jenkins, B.S.; and Webb-Peploe, M. M.: Echocardiographic analysis of posterior mitral leaflet movement in mitral stenosis. Br. Heart J., 40:372, 1978.

Snodgrass, R. P.; Kerber, R. E.; and Funk, D. C.: Echocardiography after reconstructive surgery for non-rheumatic mitral regurgitation. Br. Heart J., 39:1299, 1977.

Strunk, B. L.; Fitzgerald, J. W.; and Lipton, M.: The posterior aortic wall echocardiogram. Its relationship to left atrial volume change. Circulation, 54:744, 1976.

Strunk, B. L.; London, E. J.; and Fitzgerald, J.: The assessment of mitral stenosis and prosthetic mitral valve obstruction, using the posterior aortic wall echocardiogram. Circulation, 55:855, 1976.

Thomas, R. D.; Mary, D. A.; and Ionescu, M. I.: Echocardiographic pattern of posterior mitral leaflet movement after mitral valve repair. Br. Heart J., 41:399, 1979.

Toutouzas, P.; Karayannis, E.; Velimizis, A.; et al.: End-diastolic amplitude of mitral echogram in mitral stenosis. Br. Heart J. 39:73, 1977.

Vignola, P. A.; Walker, H. J.; and Gold, H. K.: Alteration of the left ventricular pressure-volume relationship in man and its effect on the mitral echocardiographic early diastolic closure slope. Circulation, 56:586, 1977.

Wann, L. S.; Weyman, A. E.; and Feigenbaum, H.: Determination of mitral valve area by cross-sectional echocardiography. Ann. Intern. Med., 88:337, 1978.

Weyman, A. E.; Rankin, R.; and King, H.: Loeffler's endocarditis presenting as mitral and tricuspid stenosis. Am. J. Cardiol., 40:438, 1977.

Weyman, A. E.; Heger, J. J.; Kronik, G.; et al.: Mechanism of paradoxical early diastolic septal motion in patients with mitral stenosis: A cross-sectional echocardiography study. Am. J. Cardiol., 40:891, 1978.

Wise, J. R.: Echocardiographic evaluation of mitral stenosis using diastolic posterior left ventricular wall motion. Circulation, 61:1037, 1980.

Zaky, A.; Nasser, W. R.; and Feigenbaum, H.: A study of mitral valve action recorded by reflected ultrasound and its application in the diagnosis of mitral stenosis. Circulation, 37:789, 1968.

Zanolla, L.; Marino, P.; Nicolisi, G. L., et al.: Two-dimensional echocardiographic evaluation of mitral value calcification. Chest 82:154, 1982.

CONGENITAL MITRAL STENOSIS

Chung, K. S.; Manning, J. A.; Lipchik, E. O.; et al.: Isolated supravalvar stenosing ring of left atrium: diagnosis before operation and successful surgical treatment. Chest, 65:26, 1974.

Driscoll, D. J.; Gutgesell, H. P.; and McNamara, D. G.: Echocardiographic features of congenital mitral stenosis. Am. J. Cardiol., 42:259, 1978.

Goodman, M. F.; Fiddler, G. I.; and Marquis, R. M.: Echocardiography in evaluation of congenital mitral valve disease in infants and children. Br. Heart J., 38:783, 1975.

LaCorte, M.; Harada, K.; and Williams, R. G.: Echocardiographic features of congenital left ventricular inflow obstruction. Circulation, 54:562, 1976.

Lundstrom, N. R.: Value of echocardiography in diagnosis of congenital mitral stenosis. Br. Heart J., 38:534, 1976.

Snider, A. R.; Roge, C. C.; Schiller, N. B.; et al.: Congenital left ventricular inflow obstruction evaluated by two-dimensional echocardiography. Circulation, 61:848, 1980.

MITRAL ANNULUS CALCIFICATION

Come, P. C., and Riley, M. F.: M-mode and cross-sectional echocardiographic recognition of fibrosis and calcification of the mitral valve chordae and left ventricular papillary muscles. Am. J. Cardiol. 49:461, 1982.

Curati, W. L.; Petitclerc, R.; and Winsberg, F.: Ultrasonic features of mitral annulus calcification. Radiology, 122:215, 1977.

Dashkoff, N.; Karacuschansky, M.; Come, P. C.; et al.: Echocardiographic features of mitral annulus calcification. Am. Heart J., 94:585, 1977.

D'Cruz, I. A.; Cohen, H. C.; Prabhu, R.; et al.: Clinical manifestations of mitral annulus calcification, with emphasis on its echocardiographic features. Am. Heart J., 94:367, 1977.

D'Cruz, I. A.; Panetta, F.; Cohen, H. C.; et al.: Submitral calcification or sclerosis in elderly patients: M-mode and two-dimensional echocardiography in "mitral annulus" calcification. Am. J. Cardiol., 44:31, 1979.

D'Cruz, I. A.; Devaraj, N.; Hirsch, L. J.; et al.: Unusual echocardiographic appearances attributable to submitral calcification simulating left ventricular masses. Clin. Cardiol., 3:260, 1980.

Fulkerson, P. K.; Beaver, B. M.; Auseon, J. C.; et al.: Calcification of the mitral annulus. Am. J. Med., 66:967, 1979.

Gabor, G. E.; Mohr, B. D.; Goel, P. C.; et al.: Echocardiographic and clinical spectrum of mitral annulus calcification. Am. J. Cardiol., 38:836, 1976.

Hammer, W. J.; Roberts, W. C.; and deLeon, A. C.: "Mitral

stenosis" secondary to combined "massive" mitral annular calcific deposits and small, hypertrophied left ventricles. *Am. J. Med., 64:*371, 1978.

Hirschfeld, D. S., and Emilson, B. B.: Echocardiogram in calcified mitral annulus. *Am. J. Cardiol., 36:*354, 1975.

Osterberger, L. E.; Goldstein, S.; Khaja, F.; *et al.:* Functional mitral stenosis in patients with massive mitral annular calcification. *Circulation, 64:*472, 1981.

Schott, C. R.; Kotler, M. N.; Parry, W. R.; *et al.:* Mitral annular calcification: Clinical and echocardiographic correlations. *Arch. Intern. Med., 137:*1143, 1977.

MITRAL VALVE PROLAPSE

Aranda, J. M.; Befeler, B.; Lazzara, R.; *et al.:* Mitral valve prolapse and coronary artery disease. *Circulation, 52:*245, 1975.

Bartall, H. Z.; Breed, C.; Benchimol, A.; *et al.:* Influence of Muller's maneuver on mitral valve prolapse. Correlation with external carotid pulse tracing and echocardiogram. *Chest, 74:*654, 1978.

Betriu, A.; Wigle, E. D.; Felderhof, C. H.; *et al.:* Prolapse of the posterior leaflet of the mitral valve associated with secundum *atrial* septal defect. *Am. J. Cardiol., 35:*363, 1975.

Brown, O. R.; DeMots, H.; Kloster, F. E.; *et al.:* Aortic root dilatation and mitral valve prolapse in Marfan's syndrome. *Circulation, 52:*651, 1975.

Chandaratna, P. A. N.; Lopez, J. M.; Littman, R. B.; *et al.:* Abnormal mitral valve motion during ventricular extrasystoles: An echocardiographic study. *Am. J. Cardiol., 34:*783, 1974.

Chandaratna, P. A. N.; Tolentino, A. O.; and Mutucumarana, W.: Echocardiographic observations on the association between mitral valve prolapse and asymmetric septal hypertrophy. *Circulation, 55:*622, 1977.

Chandaratna, P. A. N.; Vlahovich, G.; Kong, Y.; *et al.:* Incidence of mitral valve prolapse in one hundred clinically stable newborn baby girls: An echocardiographic study. *Am. Heart J., 98:*312, 1979.

Channick, B. J.; Adlin, E. V.; Marks, A. D.; *et al.:* Hyperthyroidism and mitral valve prolapse. *N. Engl. J. Med., 305:*497, 1981.

Cohen, M.: Double mitral leaflet prolapse: Echocardiographic-phonocardiographic correlation. *Am. Heart J., 91:*168, 1976.

Cohen, M. V.; Shah, P. K.; and Spindelo-Franco, H.: Angiographic-echocardiographic correlation in mitral valve prolapse. *Am. Heart J., 97:*43, 1979.

D'Cruz, I. A.; Shah, S. N.; Hirsch, L. J.; *et al.:* Cross-sectional echocardiographic visualization of abnormal systolic motion of the left ventricle in mitral valve prolapse. *Cathet. Cardiovasc. Diagn., 7:*35, 1981.

DeMaria, A. N.; King, J. F.; Hugo, B. G.; *et al.:* The variable spectrum of echocardiographic manifestations of the mitral valve prolapse syndrome. *Circulation, 50:*33, 1974.

DeMaria, A. N.; Neumann, A.; Lee, G.; *et al.:* Echocardiographic identification of the mitral valve prolapse syndrome. *Am. J. Med., 62:*819, 1977.

Devereux, R. B.; Perloff, J. K.; Reichek, N.; *et al.:* Mitral valve prolapse. *Circulation, 54:*3, 1976.

Dillon, J. C.; Haine, C. L.; Chang, S.; *et al.:* Use of echocardiography in patients with prolapsed mitral valve. *Circulation, 43:*503, 1971.

Feigenbaum, H.: *Echocardiography,* 2nd ed. Lea & Febiger, Philadelphia, 1976, p. 127.

Gardin, J. M.; Talano, J. V.; Stephanides, L.; *et al.:* Systolic anterior motion in the absence of asymmetric septal hypertrophy. A buckling phenomenon of the chordae tendineae. *Circulation, 63:*181, 1981.

Gilbert, B. M.; Schatz, R. A.; von Ramm, O. T.; *et al.:* Mitral valve prolapse. Two-dimensional echocardiographic and angiographic correlation. *Circulation, 54:*716, 1976.

Gottdiener, J. S.; Sherber, H. S.; and Harvey, W. P.: Midsystolic click and mitral valve prolapse following mitral commissurotomy. *Am. J. Med., 64:*295, 1978.

Higgins, C. B.; Reinke, R. T.; Gosink, B. B.; *et al.:* The significance of mitral valve prolapse in middle-aged elderly men. *Am. Heart J., 91:*292, 1976.

Kerber, R. E.; Isaeff, D. M.; and Hancock, E. W.: Echocardiographic patterns in patients with the syndrome of systolic click and late systolic murmur. *N. Engl. J. Med., 284:*691, 1971.

Levisman, J. A.; and Abbasi, A.: Abnormal motion of the mitral valve with pericardial effusion: Pseudo-prolapse of the mitral valve. *Am. Heart J., 91:*18, 1976.

Markiewicz, W.; Stoner, J.; London, E.; *et al.:* Mitral valve prolapse in one hundred presumably healthy young females. *Circulation, 53:*474, 1976.

Mathey, D. G.; DeCoodt, P. R.; Allen, H. N.; *et al.:* The determinants of onset of mitral valve prolapse in the systolic click–late systolic murmur syndrome. *Circulation, 53:*872, 1976.

Morganroth, J.; Mardelli, T. J.; Naito, M.; *et al.:* Apical cross-sectional echocardiography. Standard for the diagnosis of idiopathic mitral valve prolapse syndrome. *Chest, 79:*23, 1981.

Noble, L. M; Dabestani, A.; and Child, J. S.: Mitral valve prolapse. Cross-sectional and provocative M-mode echocardiography. *Chest 82:*158, 1982.

Ogawa, S.; Hagashi, J.; and Sasaki, H.: Evaluation of combined valvular prolapse syndrome by two-dimensional echocardiography. *Circulation 65:*174, 1982.

Owens, J. S.; Kotler, M. N.; and Segal, B. L.: Pseudoprolapse of the mitral valve in a patient with pericardial effusion. *Chest, 69:*214, 1976.

Popp, R. L.; Brown, O. R.; Silverman, J. F.; *et al.:* Echocardiographic abnormalities in the mitral valve prolapse syndrome. *Circulation, 49:*428, 1974.

Rippe, J. M.; Sloss, L. J.; Angoff, G.; *et al.:* Mitral valve prolapse in adults with congenital heart disease. *Am. Heart J., 97:*561, 1979.

Ruwitch, J. J.; Weiss, A. N.; and Fleg, J. L.: Insensitivity of echocardiography in detecting mitral valve prolapse in older patients with chest pain. *Am. J. Cardiol., 40:*686, 1977.

Sahn, D. J.; Allen, H. D.; Goldberg, S. J.; *et al.:* Mitral valve prolapse in children: A problem defined by real-time cross-sectional echocardiography. *Circulation, 53:*651, 1976.

Sahn, D. J.; Wood, J.; Allen, H. D.; *et al.:* Echocardiographic spectrum of mitral valve motion in children with and without mitral valve prolapse. The nature of false-positive diagnosis. *Am. J. Cardiol., 39:*422, 1977.

Schiller, N. B.; and Silverman, H. N.: Two-dimensional ultrasonic cardiac imaging. In: Kleid, J. J., and Arvan, S. B. (eds.): *Echocardiography: Interpretation and Diagnosis.* Appleton-Century-Crofts, New York, 1978, p. 399.

Smith, E. R.; Fraser, D. B.; Purdy, J. W.; *et al.:* Angiographic diagnosis of mitral valve prolapse: Correlation with echocardiography. *Am. J. Cardiol., 40:*165, 1977.

Strasberg, B.; Kanakis, C.; Dhingra, R. C.; *et al.:* Myotonia dystrophica and mitral valve prolapse. *Chest, 78:*845, 1980.

Udoshi, M. B.; Shah, A.; Fisher, V. J.; *et al.:* Incidence of mitral valve prolapse in subjects with thoracic skeletal abnormalities—a prospective study. *Am. Heart J.,* **97**:303, 1979.

Weinrauch, L. A.; McDonald, D. G.; and DeSilva, R. A.: Mitral valve prolapse in rheumatic mitral stenosis. *Chest,* **72**:752, 1977.

Weiss, A. N.; Mimbs, J. W.; and Ludbrook, P. A.: Echocardiographic detection of mitral valve prolapse. Exclusion of false positive diagnosis and determination of inheritance. *Circulation,* **52**:1091, 1975.

Winkle, R. A.; Goodman, D. J.; and Popp, R. L.: Simultaneous echocardiographic, phonocardiographic recordings at rest and during amyl nitrite administration in patients with mitral valve prolapse. *Circulation,* **51**:522, 1975.

Zerin, N. A.; Wajszczuk, W. J.; and Cascade, P. N.: Echocardiographic source of early anterior systolic motion in late systolic mitral valve prolapse. *Chest,* **77**:567, 1980.

SYNDROMES ASSOCIATED WITH MITRAL VALVE PROLAPSE

Muscular Dystrophy

Reeves, W. C.; Griggs, R.; Nanda, N. C.; *et al.:* Echocardiographic evaluation of cardiac abnormalities in Duchenne's dystrophy and myotonic muscular dystrophy. *Arch. Neurol.,* **37**:273, 1980.

Sanyal, S. K.; Leung, R. K.; Tierney, R. C.; *et al.:* Mitral valve prolapse syndrome in children with Duchenne's progressive muscular dystrophy. *Pediatrics,* **63**:116, 1979.

Progressive External Ophthalmoplegia

Darsee, J. R.; Miklozek, C. C.; Heymsfield, S. B.; *et al.:* Mitral valve prolapse and ophthalmoplegia: A progressive cardioneurologic syndrome. *Arch. Intern. Med.,* **92**:735, 1980.

Atrial Septal Defect

Schreiber, T. L.; Feigenbaum, H.; and Weyman, A. E.: Effect of atrial septal defect repair on left ventricular geometry and degree of mitral valve prolapse. *Circulation,* **61**:888, 1980.

Psychologic Abnormalities

Kantor, J. S.; Zitrin, C. M.; and Zeldis, S. M.: Mitral valve prolapse syndrome in agoraphobic patients. *Am. J. Psychiatry,* **137**:467, 1980.

Venkatesh, A.; Pauls, D. L.; Crowe, R.; *et al.:* Mitral valve prolapse in anxiety neurosis (panic disorder). *Am. Heart J.,* **100**:302, 1980.

Mitral Annulus Calcification

McLean, J.; Felner, J. M.; Whipple, R.; *et al.:* The echocardiographic association of mitral valve prolapse and mitral annulus calcification. *Clin. Cardiol.,* **2**:220, 1979.

Thoracic Skeletal Abnormalities

Udoshi, M. B.; Shah, S.; Fisher, V. J.; *et al.:* Incidence of mitral valve prolapse in subjects with thoracic skeletal abnormalities—a prospective study. *Am. Heart J.,* **97**:303, 1979.

Autonomic Disturbances

Bondoulas, H.; Reynolds, J. C.; Mazzaferri, E.; *et al.:* Metabolic studies in mitral valve prolapse syndrome. A neuroendocrine-cardiovascular process. *Circulation,* **61**:1200, 1980.

Gaffney, F. A.; Karlsson, E. S.; Campbell, W.; *et al.:* Autonomic dysfunction in women with mitral valve prolapse syndrome. *Circulation,* **59**:894, 1979.

Cerebrovascular Attacks

Barnett, H. J. M.; Boughner, D. R.; Taylor, D. W.; *et al.:* Further evidence relating mitral-valve prolapse to cerebral ischemic events. *N. Engl. J. Med.,* **302**:139, 1980.

Rice, G. P.; Boughner, D. R.; Stiller, C.; *et al.:* Familial stroke syndrome associated with mitral valve prolapse. *Ann. Neurol.,* **7**:130, 1980.

Watson, R. T.: TIA, stroke and mitral valve prolapse. *Neurology,* **29**:886, 1979.

MITRAL REGURGITATION

Akgun, G.; and Layton, C.: Aortic root and left atrial wall motion. An echocardiographic study. *Br. Heart J.,* **39**:1082, 1977.

Burgess, J.; Clark, R.; Masanolu, K.; *et al.:* Echocardiographic findings in different types of mitral regurgitation. *Circulation,* **48**:96, 1973.

Cosby, R. S.; Giddings, J. A.; and See, J. R.: The echocardiogram in nonrheumatic mitral insufficiency. *Chest,* **66**:642, 1974.

Fould, L.; and Reddy, R.: Severe mitral regurgitation with a normal sized left atrium. *Angiology,* **29**:174, 1978.

Frankl, W. S.; MacMillan, R.; and Smith, W. K.: Differential echocardiographic patterns in mitral regurgitation. *Angiology,* **23**:642, 1972.

Levisman, J. A.: Echocardiographic diagnosis of mitral regurgitation in congestive cardiomyopathy. *Am. Heart J.,* **93**:33, 1977.

Mintz, G. S.; Kotler, M. N.; Segal, B. L.; *et al.:* Two-dimensional echocardiographic evaluation of patients with mitral insufficiency. *Am. J. Cardiol.,* **44**:670, 1979.

Ogawa, S.; Hubbard, F. E.; Mardelli, T. J.; *et al.:* Cross-sectional echocardiographic spectrum of papillary muscle dysfunction. *Am. Heart J.,* **97**:312, 1979.

Patton, R.; Dragatakis, L.; Marpole, D.; *et al.:* The posterior left atrial echocardiogram of mitral regurgitation. *Circulation* **57**:1134, 1978.

Segal, B. L.; Likoff, W.; and Kingsley, B.: Echocardiography. Clinical application in mitral regurgitation. *Am. J. Cardiol.,* **19**:50, 1967.

Smallhorn, J. F.; DeLeval, M.; Stark, J.; *et al.:* Isolated anterior mitral cleft. Two-dimensional echocardiographic assessment and differentiation from "clefts" associated with atrioventricular septal defect. *Br. Heart J.* **48**:109, 1982.

Tei, C.; Tanaka, H.; Kashima, T.; *et al.:* Echocardiographic analysis of interatrial septal motion. *Am. J. Cardiol.,* **44**:473, 1979.

Wann, L. S.; Feigenbaum, H.; Weyman, A. E.; *et al.:* Cross-sectional echocardiographic detection of rheumatic mitral regurgitation. *Am. J. Cardiol.,* **41**:1258, 1978.

Winters, W.; Hafer, J.; and Soloff, L.: Abnormal mitral valve motion as demonstrated by the ultrasound technique in apparent pure mitral insufficiency. *Am. Heart J.,* **77**:196, 1967.

MITRAL VALVE VEGETATIONS

Alam, M.; Lewis, J. W.; Pickard, S. D.; *et al.:* Echocardiographic features of mitral obstruction due to bacterial endocarditis. *Chest,* **76**:331, 1979.

Andy, J. J.; Sheikh, M. U.; Ali, N.; *et al.:* Echocardiographic observations in opiate addicts with active infective endocarditis. *Am. J. Cardiol.,* **40**:17, 1977.

Boucher, C. A.; Fallon, J. T.; Myers, G. S.; *et al.:* The value and limitations of echocardiography in recording mitral valve vegetations. *Am. Heart J.,* **94**:37, 1977.

Chandaratna, P. A. N.; and Langevin, E.: Limitations of the echocardiogram in diagnosing valvular vegetations in patients with mitral valve prolapse. *Circulation,* **56:**436, 1977.

Child, J. S.; MacAlpin, R. N.; Moyer, G. H.; *et al.:* Coronary ostial embolus and mitral vegetation simulating a left atrial myxoma. *Clin. Cardiol.,* **2:**43, 1979.

Copeland, J. G.; Salomon, N. W.; Stinson, E. B.; *et al.:* Acute mitral valvular obstruction from infective endocarditis. *J. Thorac. Cardiovasc. Surg.,* **78:**128, 1979.

D'Cruz, I. A; Collison, H. K.; Gerrardo, L.; *et al.:* Two-dimensional echocardiographic detection of staphylococcal vegetation attached to calcified mitral annulus. *Am. Heart J.,* **103:**295, 1982.

DeLuce, I., and Colonna, L.: Echocardiographic diagnosis of mitral valve aneurysm. *Eur. J. Cardiol.,* **11:**325, 1980.

Dillon, J. C.; Feigenbaum, H.; Konecke, L. L.; *et al.:* Echocardiographic manifestatons of valvular vegetations. *Am. Heart J.,* **86:**698, 1973.

Egeblad, H.; Wennevold, A.; Berning, J.; *et al.:* Mitral valve replacement in infective endocarditis as prophylaxis against embolism. Identification of patients at risk by 2-dimensional echocardiography. *Eur. J. Cardiol.,* **10:**369, 1979.

Estebez, C. M.; and Corya, B. C.: Serial echocardiographic manifestations of valvular vegetations. *Chest,* **69:**801, 1976.

Gilbert, B. W.; Harvey, R. S.; Crawford, F.; *et al.:* Two-dimensional echocardiographic assessment of vegetative endocarditis. *Circulation,* **55:**346, 1977.

Horowitz, M. S.; and Smith, L. G.: Vegetative bacterial endocarditis on the prolapsing mitral valve. *Arch. Intern. Med.,* **137:**788, 1977.

Kinney, E.; Reeves, W.; and Zellis, R.: The echocardiogram in scleroderma endocarditis of the mitral valve. *Arch. Intern. Med.,* **139:**1179, 1979.

Martin, R. P.; Meltzer, R. S.; Chia, B. L.; *et al.:* Clinical utility of two-dimensional echocardiography in infective endocarditis. *Am. J. Cardiol.,* **46:**379, 1980.

Matsumoto, M.; Strom, J.; Hirose, H.; *et al.:* Preoperative echocardiographic diagnosis of anterior mitral valve leaflet fenestration associated with infective endocarditis. *Br. Heart J.* **48:**538, 1982.

Mintz, G. S.; Kotler, M. N.; Segal, B. L.; *et al.:* Comparison of two-dimensional and M-mode echocardiography in the evaluation of patients with infective endocarditis. *Am. J. Cardiol.,* **43:**738, 1979.

Nakamura, K.; Suguki, S.; Satomi, G.; *et al.:* Detection of mitral ring abscess by two-dimensional echocardiography. *Circulation* **65:**816, 1982.

Nicholson, M. R.; Roche, A. H.; Kerr, A. R.; *et al.:* Mitral valve vegetations in bacterial endocarditis resembling left atrial myxoma. *Aust. N.Z. J. Med.,* **10:**327, 1980.

Pasternak, R. C.; Cannom, D. S.; and Cohen, L. S.: Echocardiographic diagnosis of large fungal verruca attached to mitral valve. *Br. Heart J.,* **38:**1209, 1976.

Prasquier, R.; Gilbert, C.; Witchitz, S.; *et al.:* Acute mitral valve obstruction during infective endocarditis. *Br. Med. J.,* **1:**9, 1978.

Rajpal, R. S.; Leibsohn, J. A.; Liekweg, W. G.; *et al.:* Infective left atrial myxoma with bacteremia simulating infective endocarditis. *Arch. Intern. Med.,* **139:**1176, 1979.

Roy, P.; Tajik, A. J.; Giuliani, E. R.; *et al.:* Spectrum of echocardiographic findings in bacterial endocarditis. *Circulation,* **53:**474, 1976.

Sheikh, M. U.; Corarrubias, E. A.; Ali, N.; *et al.:* M-mode echocardiographic observations during and after healing of active bacterial endocarditis limited to the mitral valve. *Am. Heart J.,* **101:**37, 1981.

Shub, C.; Tajik, A. J.; Seward, J. R.; *et al.:* Cardiac papillary fibroelastomas: Two-dimensional echocardiographic recognition. *Mayo Clin. Proc.,* **56:**629, 1981.

Stafford, A.; Wann, L. S.; Dillon, J. C.; *et al.:* Serial echocardiographic appearance of healing bacterial vegetations. *Am. J. Cardiol.,* **44:**754, 1979.

Stewart, J. A.; Silimpert, D.; and Harris, P.: Echocardiographic documentation of vegetative lesions in infective endocarditis: Clinical implications. *Circulation,* **61:**374, 1980.

Wann, L. S.; Dillon, J. C.; Weyman, A.; *et al.:* Echocardiography in bacterial endocarditis. *N. Engl. J. Med.,* **295:**135, 1976.

Wann, L. S.; Hallam, C. C.; Dillon, J. C.; *et al.:* Comparison of M-mode and cross-sectional echocardiography in infective endocarditis. *Circulation,* **60:**728, 1979.

MITRAL FLUTTER

Ahmad, S.; Keliger, R. E.; and Connors, J.: The echocardiographic diagnosis of rupture of a papillary muscle. *Chest,* **73:**232, 1978.

Aziz, K. U.; Paul, M. H.; Muster, A. J.: Echocardiographic localization of interatrial baffle after Mustard's operation for dextrotransposition of the great arteries. *Am. J. Cardiol.,* **38:**67, 1976.

Baird, M. G.: Left atrial myxoma causing fluttering of the posterior mitral leaflet. *Am. Heart J.,* **101:**851, 1981.

Ciraulo, D. A.: Mitral valve fluttering. An echocardiographic feature of left atrial myxoma. *Chest,* **76:**95, 1979.

Cope, G. D.; Kisslo, J. A.; Johnson, M. L.; *et al.:* Diastolic vibration of the interventricular septum in aortic insufficiency. *Circulation,* **51:**589, 1975.

D'Cruz, I. A.; Cohen, H. C.; Prabhu, R.; Ayabe, T.; and Glick, G.: Flutter of left ventricular structures in patients with aortic regurgitation, with special reference to patients with associated mitral stenosis. *Am. Heart J.,* **92:**684, 1976.

Dillon, J. C.; Haine, C. C.; Chang, S.; *et al.:* Significance of mitral fluttering in patients with aortic insufficiency. *Clin. Res.,* **18:**304, 1970 (Abstr.).

Glasser, S. P.: Late mitral valve opening in aortic regurgitation. *Chest,* **70:**70, 1976.

Gramiak, R.; and Shah, P. M.: Echocardiography of the normal and diseased aortic valve. *Radiology,* **96:**1, 1970.

Hagler, D. J.; Tajik, A. J.; and Ritter, D. G.: Fluttering of atrioventricular valves in patients with *d*-transposition of the great arteries after Mustard operation, an echocardiographic observation. *Mayo Clin. Proc.,* **50:**69, 1975.

Joswig, B. C.; Pick, R. A.; Vieweg, W. V. R.; *et al.:* Flutter of the mitral valve associated with a diastolic murmur in the absence of disease. *Am. Heart J.,* **97:**635, 1979.

Joyner, C. R.; Dyrda, I.; and Reid, J. M.: Behavior of the anterior leaflet of the mitral valve in patients with the Austin-Flint murmur. *Clin. Res.,* **14:**251, 1966 (Abstr.).

Meyer, R. A.: *Pediatric Echocardiography.* Lea & Febiger, Philadelphia, 1977.

Mumford, M., and Prakash, R.: An unusual cause for mitral valve fluttering. *Chest,* **76:**599, 1979.

Nanda, N. C.; Stewart, S.; Gramiak, R.; *et al.:* Echocardiography of the intraatrial baffle in dextro-transposition of the great arteries. *Circulation,* **51:**1130, 1975.

Nanda, N. C.; and Gramiak, R.: *Clinical Echocardiography.* C. V. Mosby Co., St. Louis, 1978, pp. 144, 146.

Prabhu, R.; D'Cruz, I. A.; Cohen, H. C.; and Glick, G.: Echocardiographic correlates of atrial contraction in normal and abnormal atrial rhythm. *Prog. Cardiovasc. Dis.,* **20:**463, 1978.

Pridie, R. B.; Benham, R.; and Oakley, C. M.: Echocardiography of the mitral valve in aortic valve disease *Br. Heart J.,* **33**:296, 1971.

Rosenthal, R.; Kleid, J. J.; and Cohen, M. V.: Abnormal mitral valve motion associated with ventricular septal defect following acute myocardial infarction. *Am. Heart J.,* **98**:638, 1979.

Rowe, D. W.; Pechacek, L. W.; DeCastro, C. M.; *et al.:* Initial diastolic indentation of the mitral valve in aortic insufficiency *J. Clin. Ultrasound* **10**:53, 1982.

Silverman, N. H.; Payot, M.; Stranger, P.; *et al.:* The echocardiographic profile of patients after Mustard's operation. *Circulation,* **58**:1083, 1978.

Tingelstad, J. B.; and Robertson, C. W.: Fluttering of the interventricular septum. *Chest,* **69**:119, 1976.

Tye, K. H.; Desser, K. B.; and Benchimol, A.: Anemia producing mitral valve flutter on the echocardiogram. *Angiology,* **30**:291, 1979.

Winsberg, F.; Gabor, G. E.; and Heraberg, J. G.: Fluttering of the mitral valve in aortic insufficiency. *Circulation,* **41**:225, 1970 (Abstr.).

FLAIL MITRAL VALVE

Ahmad, S.; Kleiger, R. E.; Connors, J.; *et al.:* The echocardiographic diagnosis of rupture of a papillary muscle. *Chest,* **73**:233, 1978. ·

Antman, E. M.; Angoff, G. H.; and Sloss, L. J.: Demonstration of the mechanism by which mitral regurgitation mimics aortic stenosis. *Am. J. Cardiol.,* **42**:1044, 1978.

Bareiss, P.; Eisenmann, B.; Geitner, S.; *et al.:* Massive mitral insufficiency due to spontaneous and isolated rupture of a posterior papillary muscle. Echocardiographic study, treatment by assisted circulation and prosthetic valve replacement. *Arch. Mal. Coeur,* **70**:1213, 1977.

Chandaratna, P. A. N.; and Aronow, W. S.: Incidence of ruptured chordae tendineae in the mitral valvular prolapse syndrome. An echocardiographic study. *Chest,* **75**:334, 1979.

Cherian, G.; Tei, C.; Shah, P. M., *et al.:* Diastolic prolapse in the flail mitral valve syndrome. *Am. Heart J.* **103**:1074, 1982.

Child, J. S.; Skorton, D. J.; Taylor, R. D., *et al.:* M-mode and cross-sectional echocardiographic features of flail posterior mitral leaflets. *Am. J. Cardiol.,* **44**:1383, 1979.

Giles, T. D.; Burch, G. E.; and Martinez, E. R.: Value of exploratory "scanning" in the echocardiographic diagnosis of ruptured chordae tendineae. *Circulation,* **49**:678, 1974.

Humphries, W. G.; Hammer, W. J.; McDonough, M. T.; *et al.:* Echocardiographic equivalents of a flail mitral leaflet. *Am. J. Cardiol.,* **40**:802, 1977.

Kerin, N. Z.; Wajsczuk, W. J.; Cascade, P. N.; *et al.:* Echocardiographic source of early anterior systolic motion in late systolic mitral valve prolapse. *Chest,* **77**:567, 1980.

Meyer, J. F.; Frank, M. J.; Goldberg, S.; *et al.:* Systolic mitral flutter, an echocardiographic clue to the diagnosis of ruptured chordae tendineae. *Am. Heart J.,* **93**:3, 1977.

Mintz, G. S.; Kotler, M. N.; Segal, B. L.; *et al.:* Two-dimensional echocardiographic recognition of ruptured chordae tendineae. *Circulation,* **57**:244, 1978.

Mintz, G. S.; Kotler, M. N.; Parry, W. R.; *et al.:* Statistical comparison of M-mode and two-dimensional echocardiographic diagnosis of flail mitral leaflets. *Am. J. Cardiol.,* **45**:253, 1980.

Sweatman, T.; Selzer, A.; and Kamagaki, M.: Echocardiographic diagnosis of mitral regurgitation due to ruptured chordae tendineae. *Circulation,* **46**:580, 1972.

Sze, K. C.; Nanda, N. C.; and Gramiak, R.: Systolic flutter of the mitral valve. *Am. Heart J.,* **96**:157, 1978.

Tei, C.; Tanaka, H.; Nakao, S.; *et al.:* Motion of the interatrial septum in acute mitral regurgitation. Clinical and experimental echocardiographic studies. *Circulation,* **62**:1080, 1980.

PAPILLARY MUSCLE DYSFUNCTION

Burch, G. E.; DePasquale, N. P.; and Phillips, J. H.: Clinical manifestations of papillary muscle dysfunction. *Arch. Intern. Med.,* **12**:112, 1963.

Burgess, J.; Clark, R.; Kamigaki, M.; *et al.:* Echocardiographic findings in different types of mitral regurgitation. *Circulation,* **34**:97, 1973.

Godley, R. V.; Wann, L. S.; and Rogers, E. W.: Incomplete mitral leaflet closure in patients with papillary muscle dysfunction. *Circulation,* **63**:565, 1981.

Ogawa, S.; Hubbard, F. E.; Mardelli, T. J.; *et al.:* Cross-sectional echocardiographic spectrum of papillary muscle dysfunction. *Am. Heart J.,* **97**:312, 1979.

Tallary, V. K.; DePasquale, N. P.; and Burch, G. E.: The echocardiogram in papillary muscle dysfunction. *Am. Heart J.,* **83**:12, 1972.

PREMATURE MITRAL CLOSURE

Arvan, S. B.; and Kleid, J. J.: Echocardiographic findings in a patient with *Candida* endocarditis of the aortic valve. *Chest,* **70**:300, 1976.

Botvinick, E. H.; Schiller, N. B.; Wickramasekharan, R.; *et al.:* Echocardiographic demonstration of early mitral valve closure in severe aortic insufficiency. Its clinical implications. *Circulation,* **51**:836, 1975.

DeMaria, A. N.; King, J. F.; Salel, A. F.; *et al.:* Echography and phonocardiography of acute aortic regurgitation in bacterial endocarditis. *Ann. Intern. Med.,* **82**:329, 1975.

Mann, T.; McLaurin, L.; Grossman, W.; *et al.:* Assessing the hemodynamic severity of acute aortic regurgitation due to infective endocarditis. *N. Engl. J. Med.,* **293**:108, 1975.

Prabhu, R.; D'Cruz, I.; Cohen, H. C.; *et al.:* Echocardiographic correlates of atrial contraction in normal and abnormal atrial rhythm. *Prog. Cardiovasc. Dis.,* **20**:463, 1978.

Pridie, R. B.; Bonham, R.; and Oakley, C. M.: Echocardiography of the mitral valve in aortic valve disease. *Br. Heart J.,* **33**:296, 1971.

C

The Aortic Root

The ascending aorta appears as two parallel bandlike echoes representing the anterior and posterior aortic walls, respectively (Fig. C-1), between which may be seen delicate, thin, linear echoes of the aortic valve cusps (Gramiak and Shah, 1968, 1970). If the transducer is further angled upward (cephalad), the upper ascending aorta above aortic valve level can be visualized in most but not all patients.

The bandlike echo referred to by echocardiographers as the anterior aortic root includes not only the aortic wall in the region of the right coronary sinus of Valsalva, but also the adjacent connective tissue, pericardium, and even the posterior wall of the right ventricular outflow tract. Likewise, the posterior aortic root echo includes not only the aortic wall in the region of the noncoronary sinus of Valsalva, but also the anterior left atrial wall with intervening connective tissue, pericardium, and so forth.

Normally, the anterior and posterior aortic root echoes are no more than 5 to 7 mm thick. With decrease in gain or increase in reject (damping), only the strongest echoes persist, and the aortic root echoes can be attenuated to a more slender width.

M-MODE ECHOGRAPHIC MEASUREMENTS

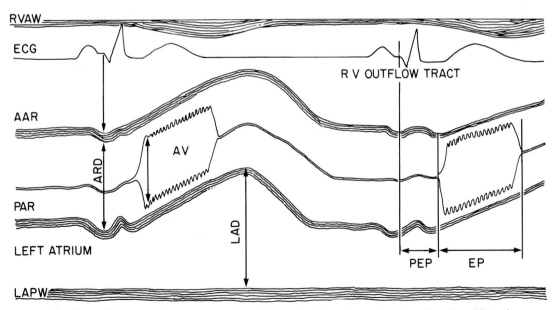

Fig. C-1. Diagrammatic representation of the normal aortic root and aortic valve. Note the RV outflow tract anterior to the aortic root, and the LA posterior to the root. The technique for measuring various distances and intervals is also shown (ARD = aortic root dimension; LAD = left atrial diameter; PEP = left ventricular pre-ejection period; EP = left ventricular ejection period).

It should be mentioned that echographic measurements of aortic root dimensions correlated poorly with surgical estimates in a series of 79 patients who had aortic valve replacement (Reeves *et al.*, 1979). The discrepancy was attributed to inclusion of the sinuses of Valsalva in the echographic measurements.

Normally, the anterior and posterior aortic root echoes are parallel to each other, or almost so, during the entire cardiac cycle. Systolic expansion of the ascending aorta is usually no more than 1 or 2 mm.

The width (diameter) of the aortic root is measured at end-diastole. In the past, it has been variously measured by different authors:

1. From inner (posterior) surface of anterior aortic root to inner (anterior) surface of posterior aortic root (Feigenbaum, 1976);

2. From outer (anterior) surface of anterior aortic root to outer (posterior) surface of posterior aortic root (Brown *et al.*, 1975);

3. From most anterior point (leading edge) on the anterior aortic root to most anterior point (leading edge) on posterior aortic root. The latter method now has been accepted as the standard one (Sahn *et al.*, 1978).

The different ways of measuring the diameter of the aortic root probably account for the diverse values quoted by different authorities as the upper normal limit, varying from 37 to 44 mm. Twenty-two mm/sq m body surface area is widely quoted as the upper limit of normal range.

AORTIC ARCH AND DESCENDING (THORACIC) AORTA

Suprasternal 2-D echography can image the aortic arch and proximal (upper) part of the descending aorta. The 2-D probe is placed in the suprasternal notch with the patient's head extended. The plane of scanning should be parallel to the plane of the aortic arch as it crosses over from the right parasternal region to the left paraspinal region. Since space between manubrium sternum and trachea is limited, 2-D ultrasound probes of smaller size are at an advantage for this purpose.

The aortic arch is recognizable as a curved echo-free band with the large arteries (brachiocephalic, left common carotid, and left subclavian) arising perpendicularly from its convexity. The right main pulmonary artery and bifurcation of the trachea can be clearly seen within the convexity of the aortic arch, just below it (Fig. C-2).

The following abnormalities can be detected:

1. Coarctation of the aorta can be visualized as a stenotic segment (Fig. C-2) interposed between the aortic arch and descending aorta. Poststenotic dilatation, when seen, emphasizes the coarcted segment above it.

2. Dilatation of the aortic arch itself may be obvious on 2-D suprasternal scanning and also evident on M-mode examination by the suprasternal approach (Fig. C-4).

3. Aneurysms of the large brachiocephalic arteries also may be detected. Thus 2-D echography in a patient presenting with a pulsating suprasternal mass revealed an aneurysm of the brachiocephalic artery (Fig. C-2).

THE DESCENDING AORTA (Fig. C-3)

The descending thoracic aorta remained ignored by echocardiographers until recently. Mintz *et al.* (1979) showed that it manifests on the M-mode tracing as an echo-free space just posterior to the junction of the left atrium and left ventricle. This space, about 1.5 to 2 cm wide, is rather localized and disappears if the ultrasound beam sweeps upward to the LA or downward to the LV. It easily can be overlooked also in 2-D echography but, if sought for, can be identified in most instances as a small circular space behind the atrioventricular junction in the long-axis view, 10 ± 1.4 mm (range 8 to 16) per M² in diameter. Mintz *et al.* (1979) also demonstrated that the descending aorta could be detected as a small round or oval space in the short-axis view, posterior to the LV and LA. Dilatation of the descending aorta was associated with enlargement of the circular echo-free space representing it to twice or even three times its normal diameter (Mintz *et al.*, 1979; Iliceto *et al.*, 1982). The descending aorta just below diaphragm level may be visualized in short axis (cross section) by subcostal scanning. Stephens *et al.* (1982) described a remarkable case of circumflex coronary artery aneurysm presenting as a round echo-free space in approximately the location of the descending aorta.

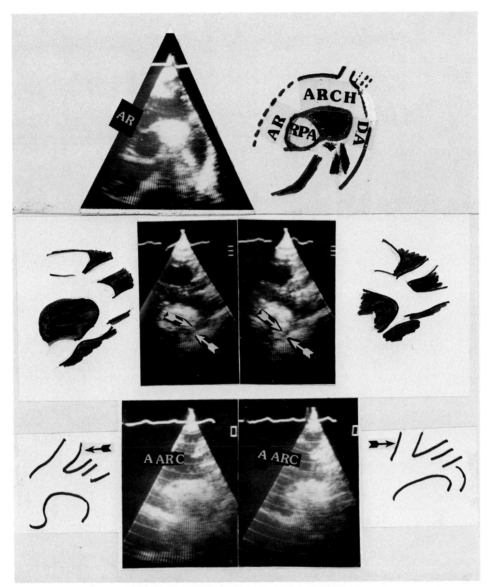

Fig. C-2. *Upper.* Suprasternal 2-D echogram in a normal individual showing the aortic arch and thoracic descending aorta. Inferior to the aortic arch, in its concavity, are the right pulmonary artery (RPA) anteriorly (echo-free space) and the left bronchus posteriorly (echo-dense space).

Center. Suprasternal echogram in a young woman with proven coarctation of the aorta. The aortic arch and area of coarctation (*arrows*) are demonstrated.

Lower. Suprasternal 2-D echogram showing the aortic arch (AARC) with origin of the brachiocephalic, left common carotid, and left subclavian arteries. The patient presented with a pulsatile suprasternal swelling, revealed by 2-D echography to be an aneurysm of the brachiocephalic artery (*arrows*).

DILATATION OF THE ASCENDING AORTA (Figs. C-4 to C-8)

Dilatation of the aortic root, scanning from the conventional left parasternal area, has been reported by numerous authors (Kronzon *et al.,* 1974; Brown *et al.,* 1975; DeMaria *et al.,* 1979; Chang, 1976; Feigenbaum, 1976; Atsuchi *et al.,* 1977; Come *et al.,* 1977). In some cases, the ascending aorta may be dilated from its origin, at sinus of Valsalva level, as is the rule in Marfan's syndrome, for instance. At this level the aortic cusps can be visualized within the dilated aortic root.

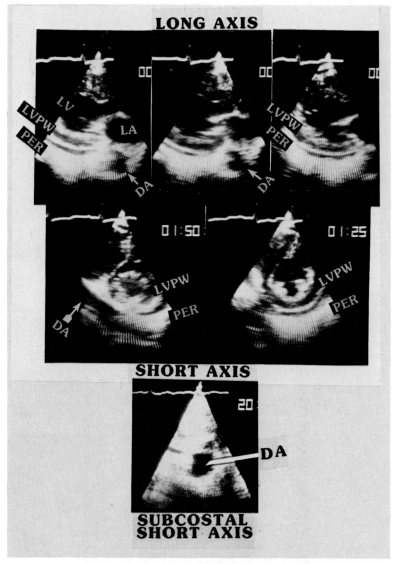

Fig. C-3. 2-D echogram of a patient with chronic renal failure and thickened pericardium. The descending aorta (DA) is visualized as a small echo-free space posterior to the atrioventricular junction, in the long-axis view (*upper left and middle*). It can be seen as an elongated space with parallel margins posterior to the LV in the short-axis view (*middle left*). However, the descending aorta is lost to view with a minor shift in probe direction (*upper and middle right*). The descending aorta can also be seen in transverse cross-section by the epigastric (subcostal) approach, as in the bottom frame.

In other instances the caliber of the aorta is of normal or almost normal dimension near its origin (at valve level) but dilated to wide or even aneurysmal proportions above the level of the aortic cusps (D'Cruz *et al.*, 1978). Repeated scans upward and medially from the aortic root at valve level should be made in any patient suspected to have aortic dilatation, otherwise this variety of upper ascending aorta di-

latation might be overlooked.* Syphilitic aneurysms, in particular, are apt to be saccular and of this type.

Normally, the heart and great vessels cannot be imaged by right parasternal scanning, be-

---

* *Caution:* Scanning upward from the aortic valve may produce an erroneous impression of aortic dilatation in thin patients with the straight-back syndrome and small AP thoracic diameter (Fig. C-9).

cause of the intervening edge of the right lung. However, an aneurysmally dilated ascending aorta tends to protrude toward the anterior chest wall in the second, third, or fourth right intercostal spaces near the sternal border. When this happens, aortic pulsations are palpable, and aortic systolic or diastolic murmurs are unduly well heard at this location. The chest x-ray re-veals an abnormal right mediastinal bulge. In such cases, it is worth attempting to scan the aortic root directly by positioning the ultra-sound transducer at the right parasternal border (D'Cruz et al., 1978; D'Cruz et al., 1981). The dilated ascending aorta is visualized as a large echo-free space immediately subjacent to the chest wall. The aortic diameter, thus visualized,

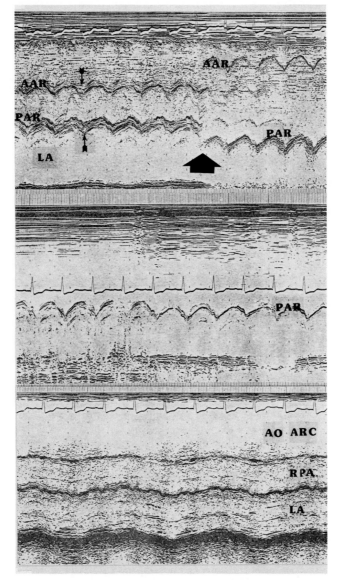

Fig. C-4. *Upper.* M-mode echogram in a 60-year-old woman from the left parasternal scanning site. The aortic root is of normal diameter at its origin (*arrows*) but abruptly doubles in caliber (*broad arrow*) as the ultrasound beam scans upward to the upper ascending aorta.

Center. M-mode echogram from the right parasternal region, with the transducer positioned over the dilated ascending aorta. Only the posterior aortic root is identifiable.

Lower. Suprasternal M-mode echogram showing a dilated aortic arch about 5 cm in diameter. The echo-free spaces inferior to that of the aortic arch represent the right pulmonary artery and LA.

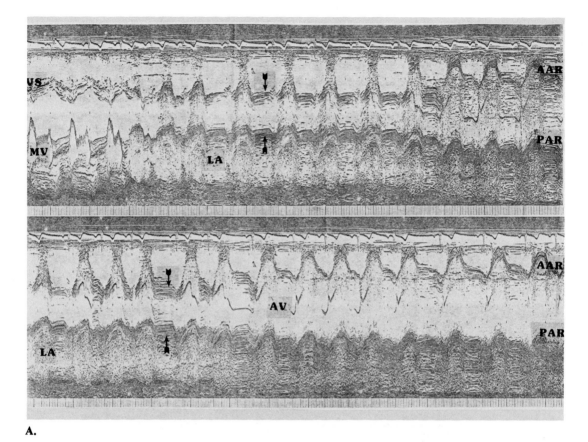

A.

Fig. C-5. *A.* M-mode echographic scan from LV to aortic root (*upper*) and from lower to upper ascending aorta (*lower*) in a 22-year-old woman. The aortic root is of normal caliber at its origin (*arrows*) but aneurysmally dilated just above (*right, both panels*). Aortography demonstrated a saccular type of aneurysm of the ascending aorta.

is a true measure of aortic caliber, since the ascending aorta is parallel to the chest wall at this level. Care must be taken to hold the transducer perpendicular to the chest wall; if the transducer beam transects the aorta eccentrically or obliquely (along its long axis) the aortic dimension recorded would not represent the true diameter. When feasible, aortic visualization by right parasternal scanning is probably as good as or better than conventional left parasternal scanning.

The echocardiographic appearances may have a role, albeit a limited one, in the differential diagnosis of dilatation of the ascending aorta.

In rheumatic aortic valve disease (regurgitation, stenosis, or a combination of both), aortic root dilatation is always of mild degree (diameter 40 to 45 mm); the aortic cusp echoes are thickened and dense due to sclerosis and per-

haps calcification. On the other hand, in aortic dilatation secondary to Marfan's syndrome, or luetic aortitis, the aortic diameter can vary from slightly to hugely increased; aortic regurgitation is a common complication, but the cusp echoes are thin and delicate with normal or increased amplitude of valve opening.

Echography of the aortic root has proven helpful not only in the diagnosis but also management of Marfan's syndrome (Donaldson *et al.,* 1980). A progressively dilating aorta and LV dilatation were considered indications for surgery in 11 symptom-free patients by these authors. Aortic root dilatation by echography in Takayasu's aortitis (Tanaka *et al.,* 1979) and the Ehlers-Danlos syndrome (Leier *et al.,* 1980) has been reported.

An important distinction, from a clinical viewpoint, is that of dissecting aortic aneurysm from aortic dilatation without dissection, of var-

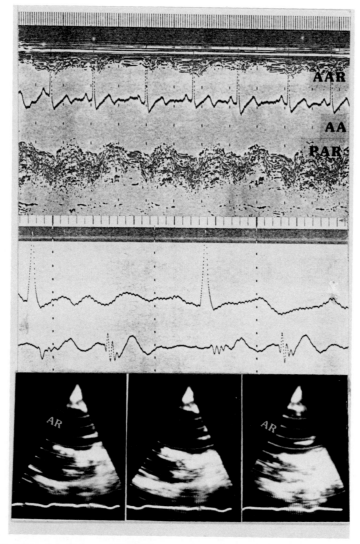

B.

Fig. C-5. *B.* M-mode echogram in another patient with dilated aortic root, with the transducer positioned over the second right intercostal space, showing the dilated ascending aorta just under the chest wall. A systolic pulsation was palpable at this site (*middle panel*). The lower panel shows the 2-D echogram, also obtained by the right parasternal approach, with the 2-D probe placed over the site of pulsation. The three frames are in slightly different planes, and show the dilated ascending aorta as a wide echo-free space anteriorly, with the aortic valve partly visible within it. The smaller echo-free space posterior to the aorta is the left atrium.

ious etiologies. The ultrasound features of dissecting aortic aneurysm are described in the next section, but they are not always evident. The classic finding of dissection—duplication of the aortic wall echo—is not always readily detected by echocardiography, even with 2-D scanning, in patients who have classic evidence of aortic dissection on aortography. Presumably there is echo dropout of the intimal flap separating the true from the false lumen, if it is a poor reflector of ultrasound.

In patients with aortic root dilatation, the anterior and posterior aortic root echoes usually move in a parallel manner. However, occasionally an excessive expansile movement of the aortic wall is manifest in systole. Thus, only the anterior aortic root echo may show exaggerated anterior systolic excursions; in other instances, the posterior aortic root echo may fail to move anteriorly in systole or may even move posteriorly (Atsuchi *et al.*, 1977). Such exaggerated expansile excursions of the aortic wall are at-

A.

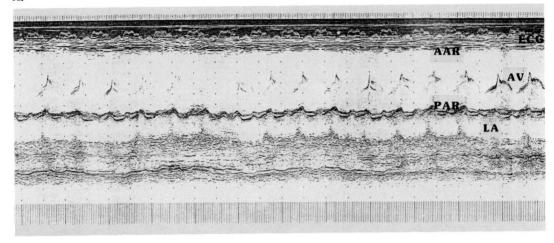

B.

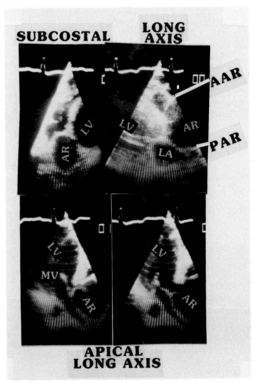

Fig. C-6. *A.* M-mode echogram of a 50-year-old man with Marfan's syndrome and pear-shaped dilatation of the ascending aorta (as seen on aortography). The aortic root is dilated to a caliber of 6 cm; the aortic valve can be seen within it toward the right.

Fig. C-6. *B.* 2-D echogram of the same patient in the parasternal long-axis view (*upper right*), subcostal view (*upper left*), and apical long-axis view (*lower frames*). In this patient, more extensive visualization of the aortic root could be obtained by the latter views than by the parasternal approach.

tributable to aortic regurgitation and the forceful systolic distention of a flaccid relatively empty aorta (at end-diastole).

Aneurysmal dilatation of the ascending aorta may be accompanied by gross dilatation of the aortic arch, which can be visualized by scanning downward from the suprasternal notch.

The 2-D echocardiographic appearances of ascending aorta aneurysm have recently been

described (DeMaria *et al.*, 1979; Imaizumi *et al.*, 1982). Although the M-mode technique in those patients did also detect aortic dilatation in these patients, 2-D imaging had the advantage of depicting the shape of the dilated aortic root in the long-axis view and presented a truer appreciation of the aortic caliber, which in the M-mode echogram was sometimes uncertain because of multiple parallel linear echoes repre-

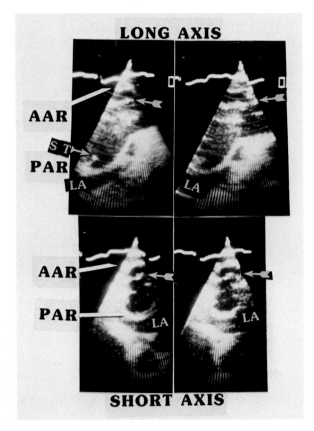

Fig. C-7. 2-D echogram of a patient with dilatation of the ascending aorta and Marfan's syndrome. The aortic valve was replaced with a porcine prosthesis because of severe aortic regurgitation. The wall of the ascending aorta was re-formed externally by a layer of Teflon. The true aortic wall, visualized within the "aortic root," might thus resemble the intimal flap of aortic dissection (*arrows*). The 2-D probe has been placed in the second right intercostal space, and visualizes the aortic root in its long axis (parasagittal plane) in the upper frames, in its short axis (horizontal plane) in the lower frames. The posterior wall of the dilated aortic root (AAR) bulges with convexity posteriorly. In the upper left frame a stent (ST) of the prosthetic aortic valve can be seen.

senting the aortic wall. DeMaria *et al.* (1979) found that in three of their patients with aortic dissection, the 2-D echogram correctly revealed the nature of the aneurysm, but not as easily as might be expected, because the intimal flaps separating the false and true aortic lumens appeared as a broken linear echo or suffered a dropout in part.

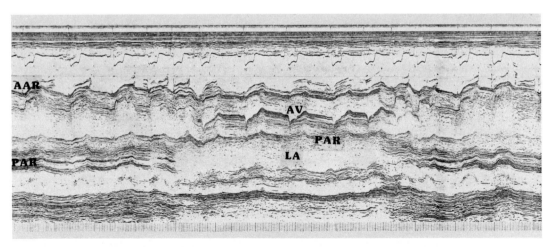

Fig. C-8. M-mode echographic scan from the upper ascending aorta (*left*) to the aorta at aortic valve level (*center*) and back to the upper ascending aorta (*right*), in a patient with dissecting aortic aneurysm. Marked thickening and multiple linear echoes in the posterior aortic root region are attributable to thrombus formation in the false lumen at this site.

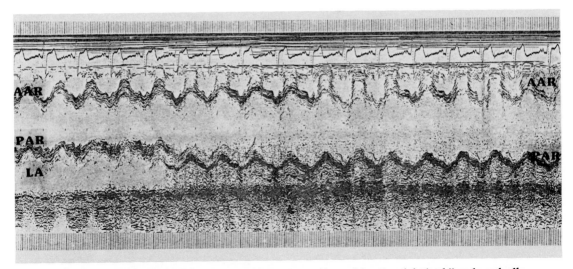

Fig. C-9. M-mode echogram of the aortic root in a patient with a "straight back" and markedly reduced anteroposterior diameter. The aortic root diameter at left appears normal. The transducer was then gradually angled upward to complete a scan of the ascending aorta, which appears progressively more dilated. On radiography the aorta appeared quite normal. It is probable that undue proximity of the transducer to the aortic root, in this patient, caused the ultrasound beam to transect the ascending aorta obliquely rather than perpendicularly, resulting in artefactual "widening" of the aortic root.

AORTIC DISSECTION (Figs. C-8, C-10, C-11)

Echocardiographic abnormalities in dissecting aneurysm of the aorta were first noted in a case report by Millward et al. (1972) and then described in fuller detail by Nanda et al. (1973). Other confirmatory reports by Kronzon and Mehta (1974), Yuste et al. (1974), Moothart et al. (1975), and Hirschfeld et al. (1976) followed. The result was that clinicians tended to overestimate the echocardiographer's ability to establish or exclude the diagnosis of aortic dissection. Brown et al. (1975) and Krueger et al. (1975) sounded a timely warning and demonstrated the limitations of the ultrasound criteria of dissecting aneurysm of the aorta.

The various echocardiographic abnormalities associated with aortic dissection are described below. They are based mainly on the work of Nanda et al. (1973). It should be borne in mind that one or even two criteria are not sufficient to establish the diagnosis. All the first three criteria must be present and, even so, must be considered in conjunction with the clinical features before a decision is made to proceed with aortography or other invasive procedures.

On the other hand, it is theoretically possible to have aortic dissection in such parts of the ascending aorta as do not manifest on routine echocardiography, i.e., at the upper end of the ascending aorta or the lateral aspect of the aortic root:

1. The aortic root diameter exceeds 42 mm. Sometimes the aortic dilatation is extreme, and values of 70 mm or more have been reported.

2. Either the anterior or posterior aortic root is widened or duplicated, the former by at least 16 mm and the latter by 10 mm. If the aortic dissection is circumferential, both anterior and posterior aortic root are abnormally widened.

3. The inner and outer borders of the affected widened aortic wall exhibit a parallel motion, the aortic valve cusps being visible only within the inner border. The space between the outer and inner boundaries of the dissected aortic wall may appear echo-free or contain stippled or linear echoes. In the latter case, it is probable that blood in the dissected area has organized into a solid or fibrosing thrombus.

4. Normally, in scans from aorta to left ventricle, the anterior aortic root becomes continuous with the ventricular septum, while the posterior aortic root is continued into the anterior mitral leaflet. In aortic dissection, the outer border of the affected aortic wall may not conform

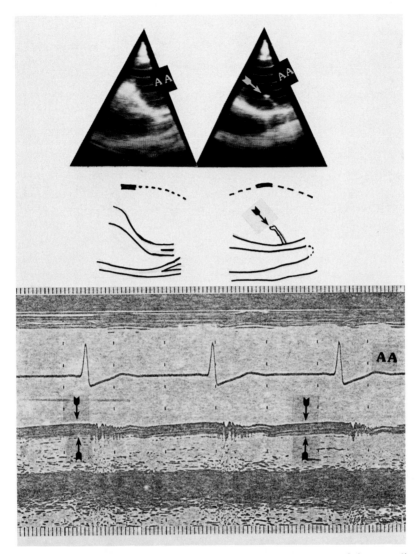

Fig. C-10. *Upper.* 2-D echogram of a patient with dissecting aneurysm of the ascending aorta and mild aortic stenosis, obtained from the right parasternal region in the long axis of the dilated ascending aorta. In the right frame the aorta is visualized at a slightly higher level than on the left frame. The intimal flap (*arrow*) can be seen as a small linear echo meeting the posterior aortic root.

Lower. M-mode echogram obtained from the right parasternal region in the same patient. It shows a wide echo-free space representing the aneurysmally dilated ascending aorta. A thick linear echo (*arrows*) traversing the posterior part of the dilated aorta arises from the intimal flap separating the true lumen (anterior) from the false lumen (posterior).

to this rule. Thus, in dissection of the posterior aortic root, the anterior, but not the posterior, border of the widened posterior root echo becomes continuous with the anterior mitral leaflet.

5. Nicholson and Cobbs (1976) described an oscillating linear echo *within* the area of aortic wall dissection, which they presumed was caused by an undulating flap of aortic intima.

An intimal flap can also hang into the true lumen of the aorta, giving rise to an undulating linear echo, which might be mistaken for echoes of the aortic valve (Nanda and Gramiak, 1978).

The echocardiographic differential diagnosis of dissecting aortic aneurysm includes other causes of (1) aortic root dilatation and (2) duplication or widening of the anterior and/or posterior aortic root.

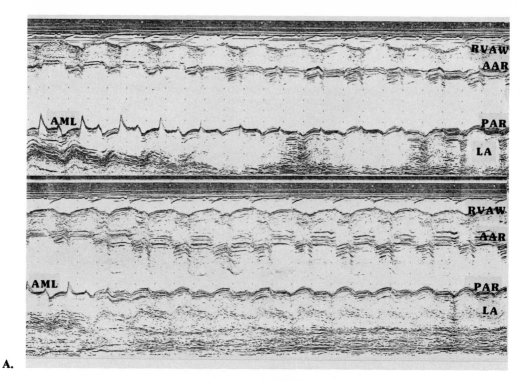

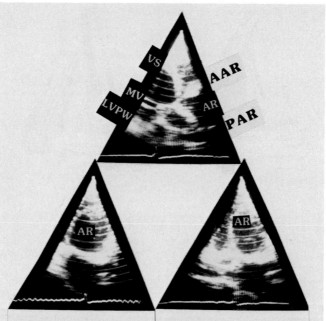

B.

Fig. C-11. *A.* M-mode echographic scans from LV to aortic root in a 50-year-old man with dissecting aneurysm of the ascending aorta. The diagnosis was made by aortography and confirmed at surgery. The patient had never experienced chest pain, and presented with chronic aortic regurgitation. The echogram shows aortic root dilatation and unusual appearances in the region of the anterior aortic root, especially in the lower panel. However, the classic pattern of aortic dissection, duplication of the aortic wall echo, is not visible.

Fig. C-11. *B.* 2-D echogram of the same man with proven aortic dissection. The upper frame is in the long-axis view and the lower frames are in the short-axis view. The aortic root is dilated to a width of about 6 cm. The intimal flap separating true from false lumen was clearly seen on aortography and at surgery, but was not evident on the 2-D echogram except for a fine linear echo within the dilated aorta (*right lower frame*).

1. Aortic dilatation of mild degree is common in aortic stenosis (poststenotic dilatation), rheumatic aortic regurgitation, or hypertension, but dilatation of severe or aneurysmal dimensions is usually due to syphilis or Marfan's syndrome. The echographic characteristics of aortic dilatation without dissection were discussed earlier in this chapter. Echocardiographic "windows" other than the conventional left parasternal one have a place in the detection of aortic dissection. Thus, Kasper *et al.* (1978) visualized a highly mobile intimal flap in the aortic arch by suprasternal scanning. D'Cruz *et al.* (1981) demonstrated a dissecting aneurysm of the aortic root by right parasternal 2-D as well as M-mode techniques (Fig. C-10). Systolic flutter of the intimal flap in this case was attributable to impingement on it of the jet issuing from a stenotic aortic valve.

2. Apparent widening, thickening, or duplication of the anterior or posterior aortic root echoes can be seen in a variety of conditions (Brown *et al.,* 1975; Krueger *et al.,* 1975; Kounis and Constantinidis, 1980):

a. A *bulging or outpouching of the right coronary sinus of Valsalva* can produce a double-contoured anterior aortic root. Similar dilatation of the noncoronary sinus of Valsalva could possibly manifest as duplication of the posterior aortic root. In both cases, it is presumed that the ultrasound beam is reflected from the annulus region as well as the convexity of the sinus of Valsalva (in a slightly anterior plane); in the M-mode echocardiogram the double reflection results in two parallel linear echoes. Two-D echography can demonstrate dilatation of the right or noncoronary sinus of Valsalva (Fig. C-12).

b. *Calcific sclerosis of the aortic wall* or large subintimal atheromatous plaques in the aorta just above aortic valve level could also manifest on the M-mode echogram as apparent

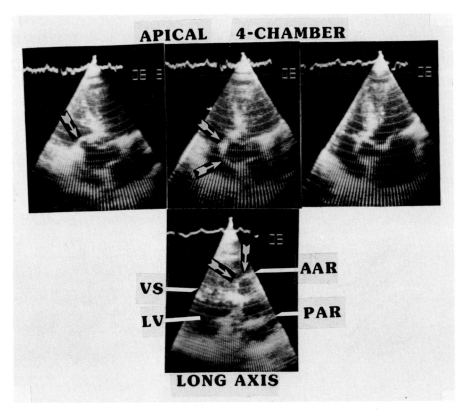

Fig. C-12. 2-D echogram of a man with dilatation of the right coronary sinus of Valsalva (*arrows*). The frames in the upper row are all in the apical 4-chamber view, but in slightly different planes, so that the dilated right side of the aortic root is visible in the left and middle frames, but not the right frame. In the lower frame (long axis) the dilated right sinus of Valsalva (*arrows*) bulges anterior to the plane of the ventricular septum.

duplication or thickening of the anterior and/or posterior aortic root. However, the aortic wall thickness in such cases seldom, if ever, exceeds 10 mm. Nevertheless, in some elderly persons, large accumulations of calcific deposits in the cardiac skeleton may be located in the intervalvar area (between aortic and mitral valve rings). Anatomically, anterior mitral annulus calcification is outside the aortic wall; however, echocardiographically it appears in or contiguous to the posterior aortic root (Fig. C-13).

c. *Calcification in the aortic valve cusps* usually is recognized easily as such because of its systolic opening motion as a component of the "box" pattern. However, a heavily calcified immobile aortic cusp may appear as a dense, linear or bandlike echo moving parallel to the aortic root and be mistaken for the inner boundary of a dissected aortic wall (Roller *et al.*, 1979).

d. The *transverse sinus,* a recess of the pericardial cavity, is normally only a potential space but may appear as a narrow, echo-free space behind the posterior aortic root if fluid in a large pericardial effusion should extend into it.

e. A *Swan-Ganz catheter* in the right ventricular outflow tract may be visualized as a dense linear echo anterior to the aortic root and therefore could conceivably mimic duplication of the aortic wall. However, catheters in the right ventricle usually have a typical pattern of motion imparted to them by ventricular contractions, which is not parallel to that of the aortic root.

f. *Ring abscesses* frequently occur in association with aortic valve endocarditis, because of direct extension of the bacterial infection from valve tissue via the aortic valve ring. If situated posterior to the aortic root (between it and the left atrium), it simulates posterior aortic dissection; if anterior to the right coronary sinus of the aortic root, it could resemble an anterior aortic dissection.

g. *Subannular aneurysm of the aorta,* opening into the ventricle just below the aortic valve, can present on the M-mode echogram as a space or chamber, just posterior to the posterior aortic root, that expands in systole (Alter *et al.,* 1978).

h. Open-heart surgery involving *incision of the ascending aorta* may result in local collection of blood or fluid in close proximity to the aortic wall, very similar to aortic dissection in echocardiographic appearance, during the early postoperative period.

i. *Prosthetic porcine aortic valves* (Fig. C-14) may simulate a double-barrelled aorta when the ultrasound beam transects the aortic root at valve level. The outer component of anterior and posterior aortic root echoes is

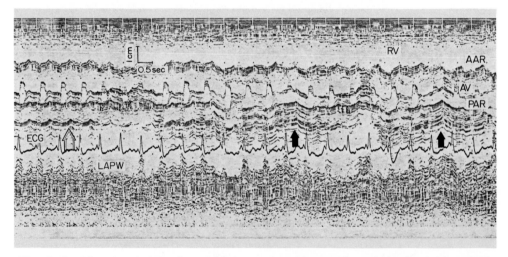

Fig. C-13. M-mode echogram in an elderly woman with extensive calcification in the mitral annulus region and also in the area between the aortic and mitral valve rings. The latter manifests as dense echoes adjacent to the posterior aortic root (*solid black arrows*). At a slightly different transducer angulation, it can produce a double outline of the posterior aortic root, simulating aortic dissection (*open arrow at left*). The aortic valve is mildly sclerotic but opens normally.

A.

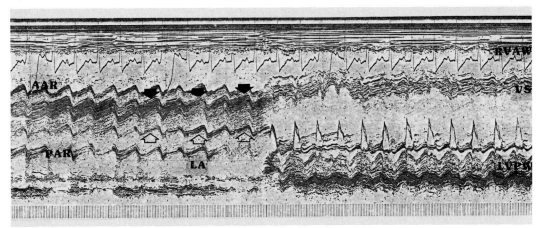

B.

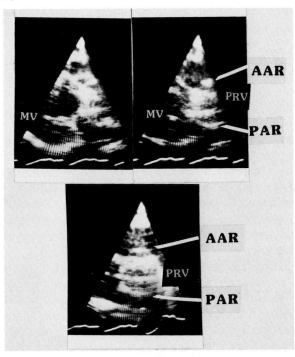

Fig. C-14. *A.* M-mode echographic scan from aortic root to LV in a patient with porcine heterograft replacement of the aortic valve. Dilatation of the aortic root and apparent duplication of its walls tend to simulate aortic dissection. The arrows indicate the stents of the prosthetic valve.

Fig. C-14. *B.* The 2-D echogram in the long axis (*upper*) and short axis (*lower*) likewise may simulate dissecting aortic aneurysm. The stents of the prosthetic valve cause abnormal dense parallel echoes within the aortic root, which could be mistaken for aortic wall duplication.

formed by the patient's normal aortic wall, while the inner aspect of the "duplicated" aortic root is formed by the stent of the prosthetic valve.

j. A *dilated right coronary artery,* anterior to the aortic root, has been responsible for abnormal echographic appearances in a patient with anomalous origin of the left coronary artery from the pulmonary artery (Yoshikawa *et al.,* 1978).

k. *Artefactual duplication* of the anterior aortic root, due to wide-beam factor, including ultrasound reflection from the upper end of the ventricular septum, and of the posterior aortic root, including reflection from the mitral annulus region, have been postulated as explanations for false-positive echographic diagnosis of aortic dissection (Brown *et al.*, 1975).

Most if not all the above entities that may, in certain circumstances, simulate aortic dissection by resembling thick or duplicated aortic walls, can be differentiated from dissecting aortic aneurysm and from each other by careful 2-D echocardiography in the long-axis view.

Two associated findings should be specifically sought in every suspected case of dissecting aneurysm of the aorta:

1. Pericardial effusion, signifying leakage of blood into the pericardial sac from the dissected area;

2. Diastolic flutter on the anterior mitral leaflet, of the type characteristic of aortic regurgitation.

The clinical significance of these important complications of acute dissection is obvious.

Dilatation of the aortic root can be viewed to even greater advantage by 2-D echocardiography than it is by the M-mode technique (DeMaria *et al.*, 1979). Although the two methods are comparable in diagnostic sensitivity, 2-D echocardiography provides better information inasmuch as it can depict the shape and distortion of the dilated aorta. The long-axis view demonstrates the anatomic relationship of the dilated aortic root to the aortic valve and annulus and to the sinuses of Valsalva. 2-D echographic visualization of the intimal flap is not always easy but is, of course, most valuable evidence of aortic dissection, especially in conjunction with conspicuous aortic root dilatation (DeMaria *et al.*, 1979; Victor *et al.*, 1981; Smuckler *et al.*, 1982). The intimal flap echo should not be mistaken for that of an aortic cusp (Cohen and Wharton, 1982).

ANEURYSM OF SINUS OF VALSALVA (Fig. C-12)

Several case reports documenting the echocardiographic diagnosis of this uncommon lesion have appeared (Rothbaum *et al.*, 1974; Cooperberg *et al.*, 1974; Weyman *et al.*, 1975; Matsu-

moto *et al.*, 1976; Nishimura *et al.*, 1976; Wong *et al.*, 1978; Oberhansli and Friedli, 1979; DeSa 'Neto *et al.*, 1979; Shulman *et al.*, 1980; Schatz *et al.*, 1981). The ultrasound appearances have not been stereotyped; the spectrum of M-mode findings has included:

1. An echo-free space parallel and adjacent to the anterior or posterior aortic root (Oberhansli and Friedli, 1979; Shulman *et al.*, 1981), in this respect resembling aortic wall dissection.

2. An abnormal linear echo adjacent to the aortic root but *not* parallel to it. The echo appears only in systole, corresponding to distention and protrusion of the sinus of Valsalva aneurysm at this phase of the cardiac cycle (Wong *et al.*, 1978).

3. More complex para-aortic echo patterns, varying to some extent with transducer angulation, have also been reported (Nishimura *et al.*, 1976).

4. The anterior aortic wall may appear broken or discontinuous in systole; this may be accompanied by protrusion of the right coronary cusp through the plane of the anterior aortic root.

5. The aneurysm may present as an abnormal echo mass in the right atrium (Weyman *et al.*, 1975) behind the tricuspid valve echo.

6. Exceptionally the aneurysm can dissect into the ventricular septum, the echo-free space anterior to the aortic valve extending into the thickness of the ventricular septum (Engel *et al.*, 1981).

Useful as all these M-mode manifestations are, most are not specific for aneurysms of the sinus of Valsalva, and visualization of the contours of the aneurysm itself by 2-D echocardiography, opening into the aortic root, is certainly more convincing diagnostic evidence.

The aneurysm as a fingerlike anterior protrusion of the anterior aortic root in the long-axis view has been illustrated by Nishimura *et al.* (1976), Matsumoto *et al.* (1976), Schulman *et al.* (1980), and Haaz *et al.* (1980). The aneurysm also may be well delineated in the short-axis view (Schatz *et al.*, 1981).

The differential diagnosis of aneurysms of the sinus of Valsalva includes:

1. Ring abscess associated with aortic valve endocarditis; aortic cusp vegetations serve as a clue to the diagnosis;

2. Aortic dissection, which is usually associated with impressive dilatation of the ascending aorta;

3. Aneurysms of the membranous ventricular septum (Gussenhoven *et al.*, 1980) protrude into the RV at a somewhat lower level than sinus of Valsalva aneurysms: the aortic root is intact; these aneurysms protrude during all of systole, whereas sinus of Valsalva aneurysms do so in early diastole;

4. Right heart tumors;

5. Coronary artery aneurysms and fistulas.

REFERENCES

NORMAL AORTIC ROOT

Brown, O. R.; Harrison, D. C.; and Popp, R. C.: An improved method for assessing aortic root diameter. *Br. Heart J.,* **37**:376, 1975.

Feigenbaum, H.: *Echocardiography.* 3rd ed. Lea & Febiger, Philadelphia, 1981.

Francis, G. S.; Hagan, A. D.; and Oury, J.: Accuracy of echocardiography for assessing aortic root diameter. *Br. Heart J.,* **37**:376, 1975.

Gramiak, R., and Shah, P. M.: Echocardiography of the aortic root. *Invest. Radiol.,* **3**:356, 1968.

Gramiak, R., and Shah, P. M.: Echocardiography of the normal and diseased aortic valve. *Radiology,* **96**:1, 1970.

Reeves, N. C.; Ettinger, U.; Thomson, K.; *et al.:* Limitations in the echocardiographic assessment of aortic root dimensions in the presence of aortic valve disease. *Radiology,* **132**:411, 1979.

Sahn, D. J.; DeMaria, A.; Kisslo, J., *et al.:* Recommendations regarding quantitation in M-mode echocardiography: Results of a survey of echocardiographic measurements. *Circulation,* **58**:1072, 1978.

AORTIC ARCH AND DESCENDING AORTA

Iliceto, S.; Antonelli, G.; Biasco, G.; *et al.:* Two-dimensional echocardiographic evaluation of aneurysms of the descending thoracic aorta. *Circulation,* **66**:1045, 1982.

Mintz, G. S.; Kotler, M. N.; Segal, B. L.; *et al.:* Two-dimensional echocardiographic recognition of the descending thoracic aorta. *Am. J. Cardiol.,* **44**:232, 1979.

Stephens, D. D.; Parrillo, J. E.; Dinsmore, R. D.; *et al.:* Circumflex coronary artery aneurysm visualized by real-time cross-sectional echocardiography. *Chest,* **81**:513, 1982.

AORTIC ROOT DILATATION

Atsuchi, Y.; Nagai, Y.; Komatsu, Y.; *et al.:* Echocardiographic manifestations of annulo-aortic ectasia: its "paradoxical" motion of the aorta and premature systolic closure of the aortic valve. *Am. Heart J.,* **93**:428, 1977.

Brown, O. R.; DeMots, H.; Kloster, F. E., *et al.:* Aortic root dilatation and mitral valve prolapse in Marfan's syndrome. An echocardiographic study. *Circulation,* **52**:651, 1975.

Chang, S.: *M-mode Echocardiographic Techniques and Patterns Recognition.* Lea & Febiger, Philadelphia, 1976, p. 52.

Come, P. C.; Bulkley, B. H.; and McKusick, V. A.: Echocardiographic recognition of silent aortic root dilatation in Marfan's syndrome. *Chest,* **72**:789, 1977.

D'Cruz, I. A.; Jain, D. P.; Hirsch, L.; *et al.:* Echocardiographic diagnosis of dilatation of the ascending aorta using right parasternal scanning. *Radiology,* **129**:465, 1978.

DeMaria, A. N.; Bommer, W.; Neumann, A.; *et al.:* Identification and localization of aneurysms of the ascending aorta by cross-sectional echocardiography. *Circulation,* **59**:755, 1979.

Donaldson, R. M.; Emanuel, R. W.; Olsen, E. G.; *et al.:* Management of cardiovascular complications in Marfan's syndrome. *Lancet,* **2**:1178, 1980.

Feigenbaum, H.: *Echocardiography,* 2nd ed. Lea & Febiger, Philadelphia, 1976, pp. 86, 218.

Imaizumi, T.; Orita, Y.; Koimaya, Y.; *et al.:* Utility of two-dimensional echocardiography in the differential diagnosis of aortic regurgitation. *Am. Heart J.,* **103**:887, 1982.

Kronzon, I.; Weisinger, B.; and Glassman, E.: Cystic medial necrosis with severe aortic root dilatation. *Chest,* **66**:79, 1974.

Leier, C. V.; Call, T. D.; Fulkerson, P. K.; *et al.:* The spectrum of cardiac defects in the Ehlers-Danlos syndrome, types I and III. *Ann. Intern. Med.,* **92**:171, 1980.

Tanaka, K.; Mihara, K.; Ookura, H.; *et al.:* Echocardiographic findings in patients with aortitis syndrome. *Angiology,* **30**:620, 1979.

AORTIC DISSECTION

Alter, B. R.; Treasure, R. L.; Martin, H. A.; *et al.:* Echocardiographic detection of a subannular aortic aneurysm. *Am. Heart J.,* **96**:525, 1978.

Brown, O. R.; Popp, R. C.; and Kloster, F. E.: Echocardiographic criteria for aortic root dissection. *Am. J. Cardiol.,* **36**:17, 1975.

Cohen, I. S., and Wharton, T. P.: Duplication of aortic cusp. *Br. Heart J.,* **47**:173, 1982.

D'Cruz, I. A.; Jain, M.; Campbell, C.; *et al.:* Ultrasound visualization of aortic dissection by right parasternal scanning including systolic flutter of the intimal flap. *Chest,* **80**:239, 1981.

DeMaria, A. N.; Bommer, W.; Neumann, A.; *et al.:* Identification and localization of aneurysms of the ascending aorta by cross-sectional echocardiography. *Circulation,* **59**:755, 1979.

Hirschfeld, D. S.; Rodriguez, H. J.; and Schiller, N. B.: Duplication of aortic wall seen by echocardiography. *Br. Heart J.,* **38**:943, 1976.

Kasper, W.; Meinertz, T.; Kersting, F.; *et al.:* Diagnosis of dissecting aortic aneurysm with suprasternal echocardiography. *Am. J. Cardiol.,* **42**:291, 1978.

Kounis, N. G.; and Constantinidis, K.: Comparison of echocardiography and radiology in the diagnosis of aortic root dilatation in Marfan's syndrome and in syphilis. *Thorax,* **35**:467, 1980.

Kronzon, I.; and Mehta, S. S.: Aortic root dissection. *Chest,* **65**:88, 1974.

Krueger, S. K.; Starke, H.; Forder, A. D.; *et al.:* Echocardiographic mimics of aortic root dissection. *Chest,* **67**:44, 1975.

Millward, D. K.; Robinson, N. J.; and Craig, E.: Dissecting aortic aneurysm diagnosed by echocardiography in a patient with rupture of the aneurysm into the right atrium. *Am. J. Cardiol.,* **30**:427, 1972.

Moothart, R. W.; Spangler, R. D.; and Blount, S. G.: Echocardiography in aortic root dissection and dilatation. *Am. J. Cardiol.,* **36**:11, 1975.

Nanda, N. C.; Gramiak, R.; and Shah, P. M.: Diagnosis

of aortic root dissection by echocardiography. *Circulation,* **48:**506, 1973.

Nanda, N. C., and Gramiak, R.: *Clinical Echocardiography.* C. V. Mosby, St. Louis, 1978, p. 180.

Nicholson, W. J., and Cobbs, B. W.: Echocardiographic oscillating flap in aortic root dissecting aneurysm. *Chest,* **70:**305, 1976.

Roller, D. H.; Muna, W. F.; and Ross, A. M.: Psoriasis, sacroiliitis and aortitis: An echocardiographic mimic of aortic root dissection. *Chest,* **75:**641, 1979.

Scanlan, J. G.; Seward, J. B.; and Tajik, A. J.: Valve ring abscess in infective endocarditis: Visualization with wide angle two-dimensional echocardiography. *Am. J. Cardiol.,* **49:** 1794, 1982.

Smuckler, A. L.; Nomeir, A. M.; Watts, L. E.; *et al.:* Echocardiographic diagnosis of aortic root dissection by M-mode and two-dimensional techniques. *Am. Heart J.,* **103:**397, 1982.

Victor, M. F.; Mintz, G. S.; Kotler, M. N.; *et al.:* Two-dimensional echocardiographic diagnosis of aortic dissection. *Am. J. Cardiol.,* **48:**1155, 1982.

Wong, C. M.; Oldershaw, P.; and Gibson, D. G.: Echocardiographic demonstration of aortic root abscess after infective endocarditis. *Br. Heart J.,* **46:**584, 1981.

Yoshikawa, J.; Owaki, T.; Kato, H.; *et al.:* Ultrasonic features of anomalous origin of the left coronary artery from the pulmonary artery. *Jpn. Heart J.,* **19:**46, 1978.

Yuste, P.; Minguez, A. I.; Cerezo, L.; and Bordiu, C. M.: Dissecting aortic aneurysm diagnosed by echocardiography. A pre- and postoperative study. *Br. Heart J.,* **36:**111, 1974.

SINUS OF VALSALVA ANEURYSM

Cooperberg, P.; Mercer, E. N.; Mulder, D. S.; *et al.:* Rupture of a sinus of Valsalva aneurysm. Report of a case diagnosed preoperatively by echocardiography. *Radiology,* **113:**171, 1974.

DeSa'Neto, A.; Padnick, M. B.; Desser, K. B.; *et al.:* Right sinus of Valsalva—right atrial fistula secondary to nonpenetrating chest trauma. *Circulation,* **60:**205, 1979.

Engel, P. J.; Held, J. S.; vander Bel-Kahn, J.; *et al.:* Echocardiographic diagnosis of congenital sinus of Valsalva aneurysm with dissection of the interventricular septum. *Circulation,* **63:**705, 1981.

Feigenbaum, H.: *Echocardiography,* 2nd ed. Lea & Febiger, Philadelphia, 1976, pp. 232–33.

Gussenhoven, W. J.; Riele, J. A. M.; Scherpenzeel, W.; *et al.:* Echocardiographic pattern of an aneurysm of the membranous interventricular septum. *Chest,* **77:**541, 1980.

Haaz, W. S.; Kotler, M. N.; and Mintz, G. S.: Ruptured sinus of Valsalva aneurysm: Diagnosis by echocardiography. *Chest,* **78:**781, 1980.

Matsumoto, M.; Matsuo, O.; Beppu, S.; *et al.:* Echocardiographic diagnosis of ruptured aneurysm of sinus of Valsalva. Report of two cases. *Circulation,* **53:**382, 1976.

Nishimura, H.; Hibi, N.; Koto, T.; *et al.:* Real time observation of ruptured right sinus of Valsalva aneurysm by high speed ultrasono-cardiotomography. *Circulation,* **53:**732, 1976.

Oberhansli, I., and Friedli, B.: Aneurysm of the left sinus of Valsalva draining into the right atrium. *Chest,* **76:**322, 1979.

Rothbaum, D. A.; Dillon, J. C.; Chang, S.; *et al.:* Echocardiographic manifestation of right sinus of Valsalva aneurysm. *Circulation,* **49:**768, 1974.

Schatz, R. A.; Schiller, N. B.; Tri, T. B.; *et al.:* Two-dimensional echocardiographic diagnosis of a ruptured right sinus of Valsalva aneurysm. *Chest,* **79:**584, 1981.

Shulman, R.; Khuri, S.; Ray, B. J.; *et al.:* Echocardiographic features of an unruptured aneurysm of the right sinus of Valsalva aneurysm. *Chest,* **77:**700, 1980.

Weyman, A. E.; Dillon, J. C.; Feigenbaum, H.; *et al.:* Premature pulmonic valve opening following sinus of Valsalva aneurysm rupture into the right atrium. *Circulation,* **51:**556, 1975.

Wong, B. Y. S.; Bogart, D. B.; and Dunn, M. I.: Echocardiographic features of an aneurysm of the left sinus of Valsalva. *Chest,* **73:**105, 1978.

D

The Aortic Valve

Normally the aortic valve cusps appear as a thin, short, sharp line in diastole running through the center of the aortic root, which in systole abruptly opens into a rectangular "box" form (Fig. D-1). The anterior component of the box represents the right coronary cusp, while the posterior component is generally presumed to reflect motion of the noncoronary cusp. Normally these two cusps open to almost the full width of the aortic lumen and may exhibit a small low-amplitude vibration (Fig. D-12, lower panel) during all of LV ejection. Abnormal aortic valve patterns of various types are shown diagrammatically in Figures D-1 and D-2.

Uniform mild thickening of the aortic valve, as may occur in patients with old rheumatic carditis or as a senile degenerative change in elderly persons, causes no alteration in the normal aortic valve pattern, except that the linear valve echoes are broader and heavier, as if drawn on the tracing with a thicker and darker pencil. Systolic flutter may be more marked and coarser. Typical patterns of the aortic valve in systole and diastole on 2-D echography are shown in Figures D-3, D-4, and D-5 (upper panel).

Leech et al. (1978) pointed out that the aortic valve could be visualized by placing the transducer at the cardiac apex and directing it medially and cephalad along the long axis of the LV, toward the aortic valve orifice. Normally aortic valve echoes can be seen only in diastole but not in systole, as normal aortic cusps withdraw completely from the ultrasound beam. In patients with bicuspid aortic valves, an aortic cusp remained in view in systole, inscribing a contour (on the M-mode tracing) somewhat like that of the usual pulmonic valve echo. All Leech's patients had early systolic ejection clicks, which coincided with the moment the aortic valve attained its full opening.

BICUSPID AORTIC VALVE (Fig. D-6)

Nanda et al. (1974) demonstrated that congenital bicuspid aortic valves could be detected by certain characteristics of the aortic valve echogram:

1. An eccentric line of diastolic closure. Normally the site of apposition of the aortic cusps in diastole appears as a sharp linear echo on the M-mode echogram, parallel to and equidistant from the anterior and posterior aortic root echoes. Should this line of diastolic closure be much closer to one wall of the aortic root than to the other, a bicuspid aortic valve is probably present. A ratio of the radius of the aortic root (half the aortic root diameter) to the smallest distance between the line of diastolic closure and the nearest aortic wall (also known as eccentricity index) of more than 1.5 is said to indicate a bicuspid aortic valve. Radford et al. (1976), who conducted a similar study, concluded that (a) an eccentricity index of 1.3 or more indicates a bicuspid aortic valve, and (b) three quarters of all patients with bicuspid aortic valves show this abnormality, i.e., a normal central closure line does not exclude the possibility of the valve being bicuspid.

The line of diastolic closure of the bicuspid aortic valve can vary to some extent according to the direction of the ultrasound beam. Thus when visualized with different transducer angulations or from different intercostal spaces, it can appear closer to the center of the aortic root (i.e., less eccentric) in some parts of the echo recording than in others.

2. Sometimes the aortic valve appears as an aggregation of several parallel lines rather than

AORTIC VALVE: M MODE PATTERNS

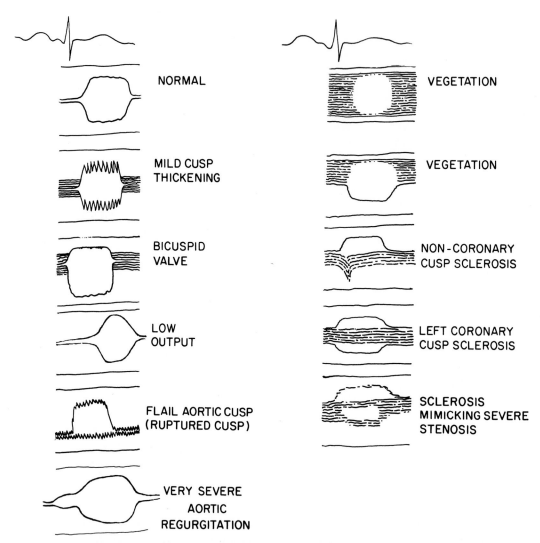

Fig. D-1. Diagram showing various M-mode patterns of aortic valve morphology and motion. The relationship of aortic valve motion to the electrocardiogram (*top of each row*) is also shown.

as a single linear echo—the so-called paintbrush sign.

Certain aortic valve echograms can be mistaken for that of a bicuspid aortic valve:

1. Linear echoes within the aortic root caused by calcification or dense sclerosis in an aortic cusp, or by a vegetation on a cusp, may be mistaken for the line of diastolic closure of the valve. The intimal (inner) layer of a dissecting aortic aneurysm or atheromatous plaque can also produce a dense linear echo that possibly could be erroneously labeled as the line of

diastolic aortic valve closure. Error can be avoided in all these cases by visualizing the aortic valve clearly and completely throughout the cardiac cycle; the true line of diastolic closure is identified by the fact that it is continuous with the box pattern of the aortic cusps in systole.

2. Destruction of one or more aortic cusps in bacterial endocarditis may be associated with an abnormal eccentric diastolic position of the flail cusp within the aortic root. This unusual echographic finding occurs in patients with very

AORTIC VALVE: M MODE PATTERNS

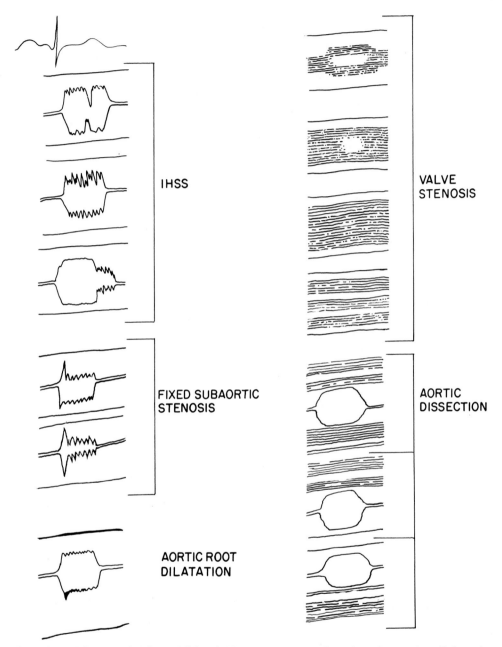

Fig. D-2. Diagram showing additional M-mode patterns of aortic valve motion (*left row*); aortic valve stenosis (*upper right*); aortic root dilatation (*bottom left*); and aortic root dissection (*lower right*).

severe aortic regurgitation; the patient may be moribund in pulmonary edema and cardiogenic shock.

Two-D echocardiography is helpful in strengthening the probability of diagnosis of a bicuspid aortic valve (Fowles *et al.,* 1979; Zema and Caccavono, 1982; Brandenburg *et al.,* 1982). Fowles *et al.* (1979) performed M-mode and 2-D echocardiograms in 19 patients with bicuspid aortic valves proven by aortography

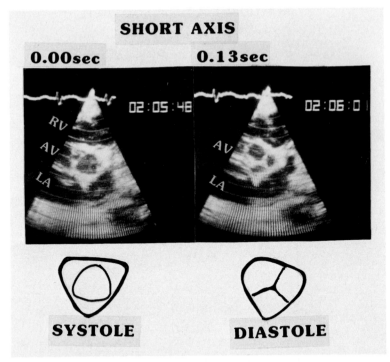

Fig. D-3. 2-D echogram in the short-axis view showing the aortic valve open in systole (*left*) and closed in diastole (*right*). The aortic cusps are distinct because they are slightly thickened.

and/or at surgery. Using an eccentricity index of 1.3 or more, 14 of the 19 cases could be identified by the M-mode technique. Two-D echocardiography in the short-axis view could diagnose the bicuspid nature of the aortic valve in 18 of the 19 patients. The abnormalities observed in this view included (1) two instead of three cusps seen during real-time opening

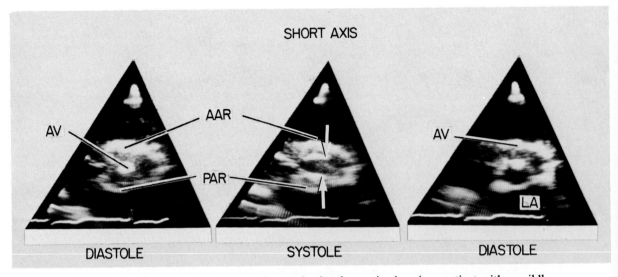

Fig. D-4. 2-D echogram of the aortic root in the short-axis view, in a patient with a mildly sclerotic aortic valve. In the left frame (early diastole) and the right frame (end-diastole) the valve is closed. A small dense central echo marks the site of apposition of the cusps. In the middle frame the lips of the thickened cusps define the valve orifice, which is at most only slightly stenotic.

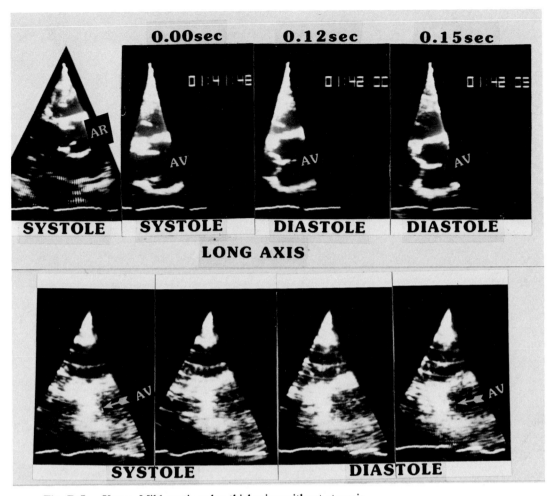

Fig. D-5. *Upper.* Mild aortic valve thickening without stenosis.

2-D echogram of the aortic root and valve in the long-axis view. The first frame shows the aortic root with left atrium. In the next three frames, which are serial frames from the same cardiac cycle, the aortic image has been expanded. The first frame shows the aortic valve open in systole. The last two frames, in diastole, show the aortic valve closed.

Lower. Aortic valve calcification and severe stenosis.

2-D echogram of an elderly man with calcific aortic valve stenosis (100 mm systolic gradient) showing four serial frames from the same cardiac cycle. There is almost no change between the first two frames (systole) and the last two (diastole). The heavy, calcified aortic cusps thus appear virtually immobile, and no valve orifice can be discerned.

and closing motion of the valve, (2) in diastole the cusp margins appeared redundant or folded into a sigmoid pattern, and (3) the location of commissural attachments in the circumference of the aortic root is different from that of a normal aortic valve. Doming of the aortic valve in the long-axis view provided additional important information by indicating which bicuspid valves were also stenotic, as in Figure D-7 (upper panel); these patients, aged 5 to 21 years, had gradients of 30 to 60 mm across the valve.

The ability to recognize a bicuspid aortic valve noninvasively is relevant to the common problem in clinical practice of ascertaining the nature of systolic murmurs at the base of the heart in young asymptomatic persons. Antibiotic prophylaxis for dental or surgical procedures usually is advised if a bicuspid aortic valve is diagnosed. Bicuspid aortic valves were detected by M-mode echography in as many as half of a series of 36 patients with coarctation of the aorta (Scovil *et al.*, 1976).

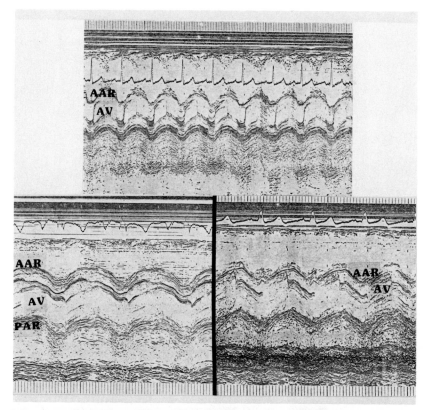

Fig. D-6. *Upper.* M-mode echogram of a patient with a bicuspid aortic valve. The line of diastolic closure is eccentric, much closer to the posterior than to the anterior aortic root.

　　Lower. M-mode echograms of two different patients with bicuspid aortic valves. In both, the line of diastolic closure of the mildly thickened valve is much closer to the anterior than to the posterior aortic root.

ABNORMAL AORTIC VALVE ECHOES

Abnormal echoes within the aortic root, arising from pathologic nodules or masses in or on the aortic valve cusps, can be of very different etiologies. The identification of their nature and the condition of the aortic valve are often of great diagnostic importance. It is an aspect of cardiology in which cardiac ultrasound is called upon to play a crucial investigative role.

Abnormal echoes originating from the aortic valve include:

1. Sclerotic changes or calcific deposits, either as a senile degenerative change in old persons or as a late end result of rheumatic valvulitis or a congenitally stenotic valve.

2. Recent or healed vegetations of bacterial endocarditis.

3. Bicuspid aortic valves sometimes produce multiple linear or "layered" echoes. The echo-cardiographic diagnosis of a bicuspid aortic valve is based mainly on an eccentric line of diastolic closure.

4. A technical artefact caused by viewing the aortic root at an undue improper angulation; when the ultrasound beam transects the aortic root tangentially, the latter may appear as a narrow mass of indistinct echoes. A properly recorded aortic root, on the other hand, is wider and bounded by two parallel, well-defined, bandlike echoes representing its anterior and posterior walls, respectively, within which normal or abnormal aortic cusps are clearly visualized. The identities of the anterior and posterior aortic root can be established by noting the continuity of the former with the ventricular septum and of the latter with the anterior mitral leaflet in aorta-to-left-ventricle scans.

5. Papillary fibroelastoma of the aortic valve can simulate an aortic valve vegetation very closely on the 2-D echogram (Shub *et al.*, 1981).

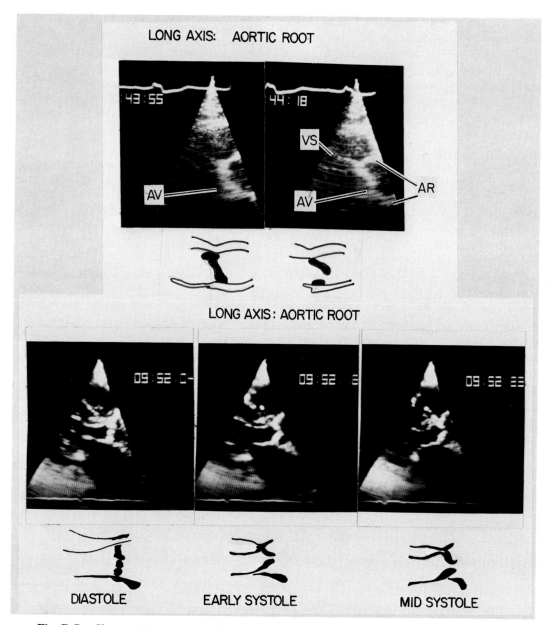

Fig. D-7. *Upper.* 2-D echogram of the aortic root in the long-axis view, of a patient with a thickened bicuspid stenotic valve. The left frame, in diastole, shows the aortic valve in closed position. The right frame, in systole, reveals a tendency to doming; the anterior (right coronary) cusp is much larger than the posterior (noncoronary) one.

Lower. The aortic valve is sclerotic and stenotic. The cusp outlines are well defined; cusp separation (valve orifice) is abnormally small in systole.

In actual practice, the important diagnostic issue is to differentiate the first two alternatives: to separate calcification or dense sclerosis of the aortic valve from vegetations of endocarditis. In both, abnormal dense echoes of varying size are seen within the aortic root.

A frequent but difficult problem in clinical practice is that of the patient with definite aortic valve calcification, on which one or more vegetations possibly may be superimposed. The patient is an elderly person, or one in chronic renal failure, with unexplained fever or stroke. The aortic root contains a mass of dense echoes that show a varying degree of motion; vegetations can neither be detected nor excluded, however carefully the abnormal valvular echoes within the aortic root are scrutinized.

Exceptionally, the anterior mitral leaflet echo appears superimposed on the aortic valve echo because of the beam-width factor on the M-mode echocardiogram, causing confusing patterns.

AORTIC VALVE ENDOCARDITIS
(Figs. D-8 to D-11)

Echocardiography has been of tremendous diagnostic help in this entity, because it can reveal not only the vegetations on the aortic cusps, but also the major life-threatening complications that result: flail (ruptured) cusp, ring abscess, and extreme elevation of LV diastolic pressure (reflected in premature mitral valve closure). Numerous published reports attest to the variety of echographic appearances encountered and to the intense interest echocardiographers have displayed in this disease (Dillon et al., 1973; Martinez et al., 1974; Gottlieb et al., 1974; Wray, 1975; DeMaria et al., 1975; Arvan et al., 1976; Yoshikawa et al., 1976; Hirschfeld and Schiller, 1976; Fox et al., 1977; Moorthy

et al., 1977; Mardelli et al., 1978; Pease et al., 1978; Kleiner et al., 1978; Mintz et al., 1979; Assey and Usher, 1979; Blair et al., 1980; Krivokapich et al., 1980; Bradsher et al., 1980; Rubenson et al., 1981).

The following echocardiographic features help in identifying aortic valve vegetations:

1. A full range of systolic motion of the affected cusps, in conjunction with abnormal dense echoes in the aortic root in diastole. The latter may appear as multiple or single, broad, linear or coalescent echoes moving parallel to the aortic root; sometimes the entire aortic lumen at valve level is filled with echo masses arising from large vegetations. Typically all these abnormal diastolic echoes abruptly clear to the full width of the aortic lumen after the onset of systole and abruptly reappear at end-systole (Figs. D-8 and D-10). On the other hand, sclerotic or calcified aortic valves show restriction of systolic mobility. In general, the more extensive the calcification, the less mobile the cusps, so that it is very unlikely that a very heavily calcified valve would open fully in systole.

Occasionally vegetations may be so attached to the cusps as to be more conspicuous in systole than diastole, but the normal motion (box pat-

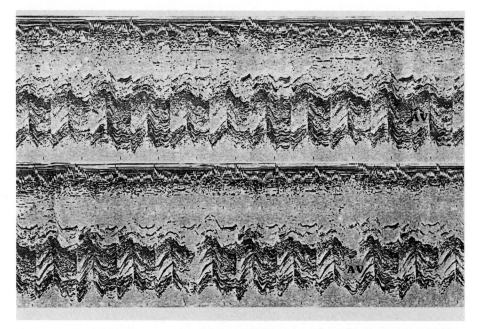

Fig. D-8. Segments from the M-mode echogram of a patient with proven aortic valve endocarditis. The aortic root fills with abnormal echoes arising from vegetations during diastole, but clears almost completely in systole (more evident in the upper panel).

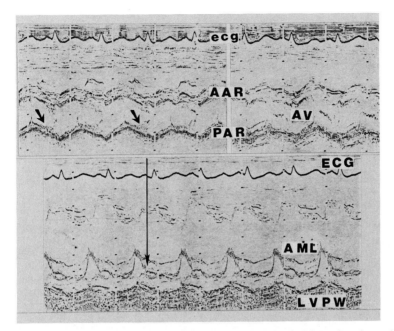

Fig. D-9. *Upper.* M-mode echogram of the aortic valve in a patient with aortic valve endocarditis resulting in wide-open aortic regurgitation and severe refractory LV failure. At surgery for aortic valve replacement, the aortic cusps were extensively destroyed and flail. No vegetations were visualized by echography; in fact, at first sight the aortic valve appeared normal (*right panel*). Closer scrutiny showed fine diastolic fluttering of the aortic valve echo, which occupied an abnormal eccentric position due to its flail nature.

Lower. M-mode echogram of the mitral valve in the same patient showing premature closure of the mitral valve (*arrow*) well before onset of the QRS complex.

tern) of contour is retained, as in patient No. 8 of Hirschfeld and Schiller (1976).

Caution: Frequently, an abnormal echo appears to be localized to a single aortic cusp. If bacterial endocarditis is being considered for clinical reasons, the question arises whether the local thickening or nodule on that cusp is a vegetation or not. In elderly patients, it may be difficult or impossible to distinguish a vegetation from a calcific nodule; both endocarditis and senile calcific change can affect one cusp with little or no obvious involvement of the other two.

In young patients a local nodular thickening of the aortic valve is more likely to be a vegetation, provided that the following are not present: (a) a congenitally bicuspid or stenotic aortic valve that has suffered degenerative sclerotic changes, or (b) healed vegetations from a previous episode of bacterial endocarditis. Unfortunately, addicts often continue to administer drugs to themselves intravenously after being cured of one or more attacks of bacterial endocarditis; when admitted for subsequent febrile illness, the echocardiographer is faced with the difficult task of ascertaining whether a suspected vegetation or valvular abnormality is new or old. When a patient with aortic valve vegetations is successfully treated by antibiotics, it is common for the healing vegetations to calcify rather than resolve completely without a trace (Stafford *et al.*, 1979).

2. Aortic valve endocarditis sometimes results in rupture of an aortic cusp, which prolapses into the left ventricular outflow tract and appears as a small fluttering echo near the left septal border in diastole only (Wray, 1975; Whipple *et al.*, 1977). It may be rather more conspicuous if the prolapsing shred of aortic cusp has a vegetation adherent to it (Fig. D-10). Repeated slow scans from aortic root to left ventricle may be necessary to document a prolapsed aortic leaflet; it is a valuable sign because it clinches the diagnosis of aortic valve endocarditis in a patient with echo appearances suspicious of vegetations in the aortic root. However, the visualization of an abnormal echo in the LV outflow tract does not necessarily

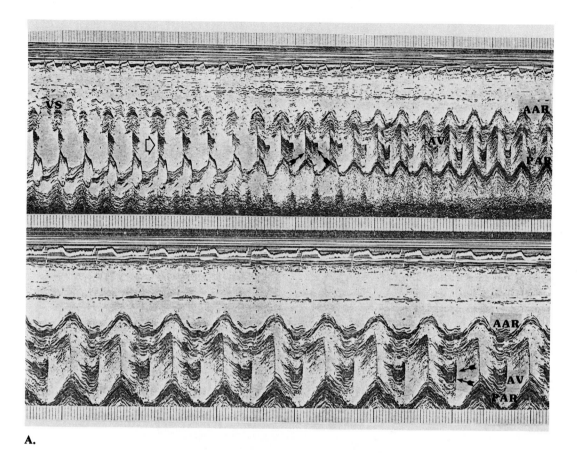

A.

Fig. D-10. *A.* The upper panel is an M-mode echographic scan from LV to aortic root in a patient with aortic valve endocarditis, confirmed at subsequent aortic valve replacement for severe residual aortic regurgitation. An abnormal echo (*arrow*) appears in diastole between septum and anterior mitral leaflet; this represents an aortic valve vegetation on a flail aortic cusp prolapsing into the LV outflow tract. The lower panel shows an expanded image of the aortic valve and its vegetations (*arrows*).

signify that an aortic cusp is flail. It is possible for a vegetation on an unruptured aortic valve to prolapse into the LV in diastole if the vegetation is elongated and highly mobile (Yoshikawa *et al.,* 1976; Blair *et al.,* 1980). The distinction is important because surgical replacement of the valve is usually unavoidable if the valve is flail.

3. Rapid flutter of the aortic valve echo in *diastole* (Fig. D-12) is a finding sometimes encountered in patients with healing or old aortic valve vegetations and aortic regurgitation (Srivastava and Flowers, 1978; Venkataraman *et al.,* 1979). For reasons that are unclear, this sign is very seldom, if ever, seen in aortic regurgitation of etiologies other than bacterial endocarditis. It occurs in patients with ruptured or perforated aortic leaflets, even in the absence

of vegetations (Das *et al.,* 1977; Whipple *et al.,* 1977).

4. Acute, severe aortic regurgitation is a frequent complication of bacterial endocarditis, resulting from perforation, rupture, or destruction of one or more aortic cusps. The very high LV diastolic pressure effects premature mitral valve closure (Fig. D-9), a well-known echocardiographic manifestation of this particular hemodynamic situation (Pridie *et al.,* 1976). On the other hand, calcification of the aortic valve secondary to congenital stenosis, rheumatic inflammation, or senile degeneration is never associated with acute, severe aortic regurgitation and thus rarely, if ever, presents with premature mitral valve closure.

5. Another complication of aortic valve endocarditis that can be detected by echocardiog-

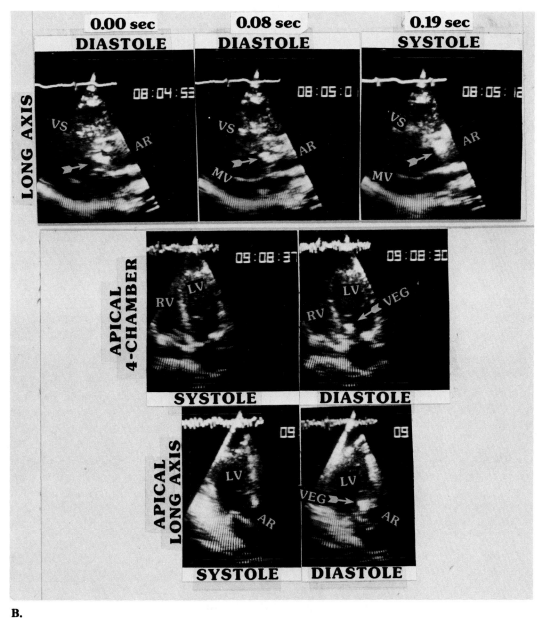

Fig. D-10. *B.* The upper panel is a 2-D echogram in the long-axis view of the same patient showing three serial frames from the same cardiac cycle. Vegetations (*arrow*) on the right and left coronary cusps fill most of the aortic root in diastole (*first two frames*) and exhibit a tendency to prolapse into the LV outflow tract in early to middiastole (*first frame*). During systole (*third frame*) the valve opens but the vegetation on the anterior (right coronary) cusp persists as a dense echo in the anterior aortic root.

2-D echogram in the apical 4-chamber view (*center frames*) and apical long axis view (*bottom frames*). The left frames are in systole and the right ones in diastole. The latter show an abnormal dense echo representing an aortic valve vegetation prolapsing into the LV outflow tract.

raphy is a para-aortic or "ring" abscess due to extension of infection from the valve (Mardelli *et al.,* 1978; Mintz *et al.,* 1979). If this abscess forms posterior to the aortic root, be-

tween it and the left atrium, it may be seen as a clear space behind the posterior root, or as duplication of the posterior aortic root (Fig. D-13). If the abscess forms anterior to the aorta,

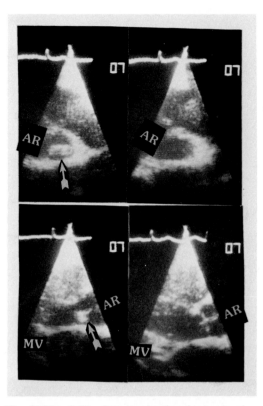

it may present in like manner as a narrow, echo-free space within or just in front of the anterior aortic root echo. In one instance of enterococcal endocarditis of the aortic valve, an abscess burrowed into the ventricular septum, causing progressive AV and bundle branch block and septal "thickening" (Mildvan *et al.*, 1977).

Two-D echocardiography has enhanced the diagnostic potentialities of ultrasound with regard to aortic valve endocarditis (Yoshikawa *et al.*, 1976; Mardelli *et al.*, 1978; Mintz *et al.*, 1979 a and b; Krivokapich *et al.*, 1980). Mintz *et al.* found that whereas 2-D echocardiography was not more sensitive than the M-mode technique in detecting aortic valve vegetations, it was more effective in revealing complications such as flail cusps.

Specifically, 2-D echography has the following advantages:

1. It provides better information about the shape and size of a vegetation than can be obtained on the M-mode tracing.

2. The mobility of an aortic valve vegetation is much better appreciated, which helps in distinguishing it from a calcified nodule in a sclerotic valve. In the long-axis view, vegetations are observed to move briskly up into the aortic root during systole and back into the plane of the aortic valve ring at the onset of diastole. Pedunculated vegetations show even more impressive flitting motion, scurrying alternately

Fig. D-11. 2-D echogram in the short-axis view (*upper*) and long-axis view (*lower*) in a patient with aortic valve endocarditis. A vegetation on the posterior aortic cusp (*arrow*) is evident in the frames on the left but is lost to view with slight changes in transducer direction (*right*). All four frames are diastolic.

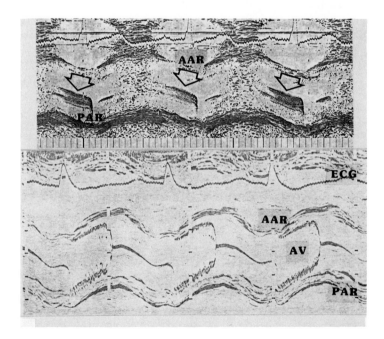

Fig. D-12. *Upper.* M-mode echogram of the aortic root 8 weeks after the onset of aortic valve endocarditis in a successfully treated patient with residual aortic regurgitation. The aortic valve is not well visualized in systole, but in diastole it manifests as a dense thick echo showing rapid fine flutter (*arrows*). Presumably the regurgitant jet set into vibration the cusp bearing a healed vegetation.

Lower. M-mode echogram of the aortic root, depicting normal motion of the aortic valve. Note that mild systolic flutter of the aortic cusps does not constitute an abnormal finding; no flutter is apparent in diastole.

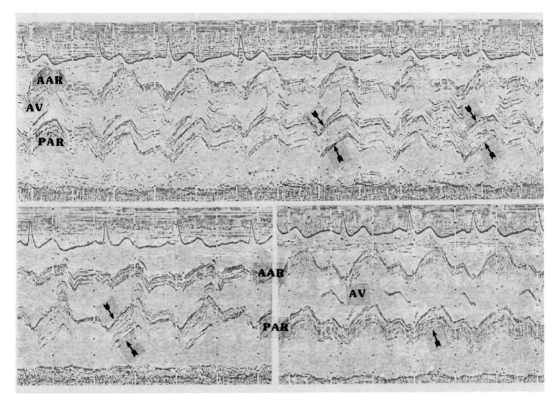

Fig. D-13. M-mode echogram in a young man with aortic valve endocarditis and a ring abscess (between the posterior aortic root and the anterior wall of the left atrium), proven at surgery. In the upper panel the para-aortic abscess appears as a double outline of the posterior aortic root enclosing a 1-cm echo-free space (*arrows*). With slight changes in transducer direction, the morphology of the abscess is altered to a double outline of the posterior aortic root in systole only (*lower left*) and a thickened but not sonolucent posterior aortic root (*lower right*).

into the aorta and the LV outflow tract. On the other hand, calcified nodules in a sclerotic aortic exhibit diminished or absent mobility in long- and short-axis views.

3. Krivokapich *et al.* (1980) pointed out that careful examination in the long-axis view can differentiate a pedunculated vegetation attached to an intact aortic cusp from a flail cusp with attached vegetation: the hinge point around which the mobile abnormal echo oscillated was the edge of the cusp in the former case, but was the aortic wall in the latter case. An unusual mobile, long, cordlike vegetation (3 cm long) was described by Yoshikawa *et al.* (1976); it was seen on M-mode but even better recognized on 2-D echocardiography.

4. Para-aortic ring abscesses may be seen well on 2-D echocardiography in the long-axis view. Such echo-free spaces just posterior to the posterior aortic root (Mardelli *et al.*, 1978; Mintz *et al.*, 1979b) are important to detect

because they may prompt a more aggressive surgical approach. (Fig. D-13).

Serial echocardiograms have been shown to be of great use in some patients with aortic valve endocarditis:

1. Assey and Usher (1979) reported a case of aortic valve endocarditis in whom serial echograms on the first and eighth days of hospital stay were normal, but one on the eleventh day showed typical vegetations. Arvan *et al.* (1976) described a patient with *Candida* endocarditis who showed increase in size of aortic valve vegetations over a two-week period.

2. Stafford *et al.* (1979) did serial echograms over an average period of about a year in six patients who had been successfully treated medically for bacterial endocarditis. They found that vegetations became smaller but denser (more echo-reflecting). Two patients had cerebral emboli associated with a striking decrease in size of aortic valve vegetations.

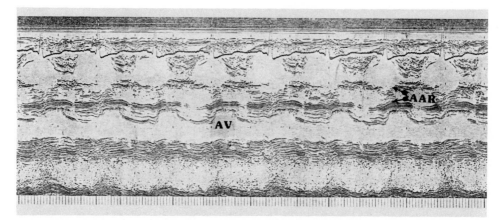

Fig. D-14. M-mode echogram of the aortic root showing a double echo of the anterior aortic root (AAR), attributable to a dilated right sinus of Valsalva. Its posterior border is discontinuous and contiguous to the anterior (right coronary) cusp of the aortic valve, simulating a vegetation. However, this abnormal echo does not follow cusp motion from systole to diastole, and this differentiates it from a vegetation attached to the right coronary cusp.

3. Wray (1975) reported a patient who exhibited marked diastolic flutter of the aortic valve who did not show this finding earlier in his illness. Presumably the fluttering cusp ruptured and became flail at some time during the intervening period.

4. Premature mitral valve closure as a new finding in a patient who had normal mitral motion previously would be accompanied by clinical deterioration and cause concern. Transfer to an intensive care area and surgical consultation then would be in order.

The differential diagnosis of aortic valve vegetations includes aortic valve sclerosis or calcification and calcified atheromatous plaques in the aortic root (Fig. D-14).

AORTIC VALVE STENOSIS (Figs. D-5, D-7, D-15)

During the early years of echocardiography, the diagnosis of aortic stenosis seemed simple: the normal aortic valve orifice diameter, measured as the width of the systolic box pattern, can be estimated precisely on the M-mode echocardiogram (the normal values vary from 15 to 27 mm); the extent to which the valve orifice is diminished may be expected to indicate the degree of stenosis. An aortic valve orifice diameter between 7 and 12 mm was considered moderate stenosis, and cusp separation less than 6 mm severe stenosis (Yeh *et al.,* 1973).

Whereas in some instances the size of a ste-

notic aortic orifice, measured thus on the M-mode echogram, may correctly represent the true dimension of the orifice, in actual clinical practice the accurate echocardiographic assessment of the presence of significant aortic valve stenosis and its severity is beset with many pitfalls and difficulties.

CALCIFIC OR SCLEROTIC AORTIC VALVE WITH OR WITHOUT STENOSIS IN MIDDLE-AGED OR ELDERLY PERSONS (Figs. D-5 and D-15)

In this age group, it is the rule for stenotic valves to be densely sclerotic and to some extent calcified. They are not dome shaped; on the contrary, the cusps may be so deformed by scarring or by deposition of calcific deposits as to lose their original shape and symmetric arrangement around a central orifice. In any particular case, the etiologic basis, very often uncertain, may be rheumatic, congenital bicuspid valve, or senile degenerative calcification.

Calcification and sclerosis are detected easily on the M-mode echogram of the aortic root; in this respect, ultrasound is far more sensitive than radiography or fluoroscopy. It is much less easy to state whether a calcified or sclerotic aortic valve is definitely stenotic and, if so, whether the stenosis is mild, moderate, or severe (Chang *et al.,* 1977).

It is very common for elderly patients with ejection systolic murmurs at the base of the

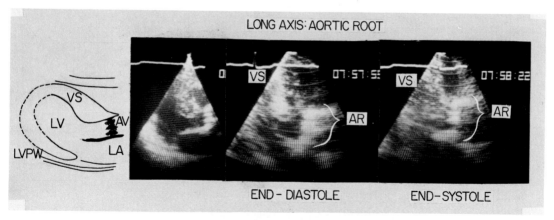

LONG AXIS: AORTIC ROOT

END - DIASTOLE   END-SYSTOLE

A.

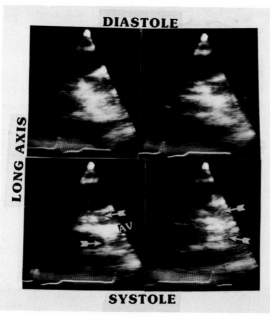

DIASTOLE

LONG AXIS

SYSTOLE

B.

Fig. D-15. *A.* 2-D echogram, in the long-axis view, of an elderly man with calcific aortic stenosis (systolic gradient 80 mm). The aortic root image has been expanded in the latter two frames. The end-diastolic frame shows the aortic root filled by dense echoes arising from a heavily calcified aortic valve. During systole the valve opens to a small extent posteriorly (*right*).

Fig. D-15. *B.* 2-D aortic valve echogram, in the long-axis view, of a different elderly man with a loud systolic murmur at the aortic area. The 4 frames are serial ones from the same cardiac cycle: the first (*top left*) in diastole, after atrial contraction, the third (*bottom left*) at the onset of systole, the fourth (*bottom right*) at midsystole. The aortic valve is heavily calcified; the cusps and valve orifice are not well defined. The immobile dense mass in the center of the aortic root is the left coronary cusp. However, there is considerable clearing or opening of the calcified cusps in systole (*arrows*), so that aortic stenosis was not hemodynamically severe in this patient.

heart to be referred for cardiac ultrasound with a request to confirm or exclude aortic stenosis. These patients have calcium in their valves but more often than not have no real stenosis (Fig. D-16). If they have symptoms or ECG abnor-

malities, other factors such as ischemic heart disease, hypertension, sinus node or conduction system disease, cardiomyopathy, and so forth could well explain them. In such circumstances, the clinician may rely heavily on the echocardi-

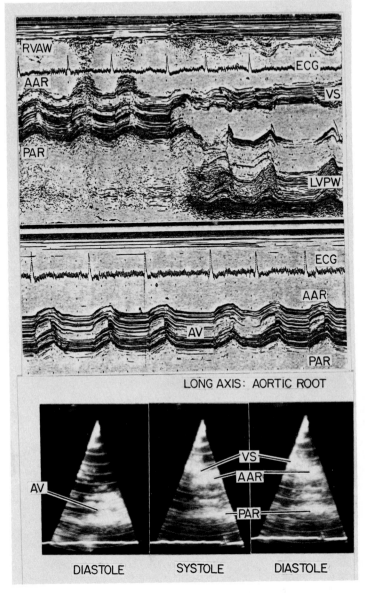

RVAW
ECG
AAR
VS

PAR

LVPW

ECG

AAR

AV

PAR

LONG AXIS: AORTIC ROOT

AV

VS
AAR
PAR

DIASTOLE   SYSTOLE   DIASTOLE

Fig. D-16. *Upper and Center.* M-mode echogram of an elderly man with an aortic ejection murmur. Aortic valve calcification manifests as multiple dense linear echoes, filling much of the aortic root. However, the systolic box pattern of the aortic valve is preserved, suggesting that there is no significant stenosis of the valve. No systolic pressure gradient was recorded across the aortic valve at catheterization.

Lower. 2-D echogram of the same patient, in the long-axis view. In diastole the aortic root is filled with dense echoes arising from the heavily calcified aortic valve, but in systole the dense echoes clear to a considerable degree, suggesting that the valve is not significantly stenotic.

ographer to tell him whether the aortic valve is significantly stenotic or not. If it appears stenotic, or probably so, cardiac catheterization with a view to possible surgical correction may be undertaken.

Some of the practical difficulties encountered on *M-mode echocardiography* are as follows:

1. It is possible for a valve to contain much calcium and yet not be stenotic, if the cusps retain sufficient mobility. Often large calcific nodules in one or two cusps generate impressive dense echoes, but the other cusp or cusps, mercifully spared from the calcific process, open

adequately so that only a minor gradient exists across the aortic valve.

On the other hand, if the aortic valve motion appears normal with linear cusp echoes opening in systole in a normal box pattern, the diagnosis of aortic stenosis is virtually ruled out. However, rare exceptions to this general rule do occur.

2. Deceptive echographic appearances can be produced by a calcified or sclerotic left coronary cusp. Normally this cusp is not visualized in systole but, if stiffened by sclerosis or rendered conspicuous by calcification, it may pre-

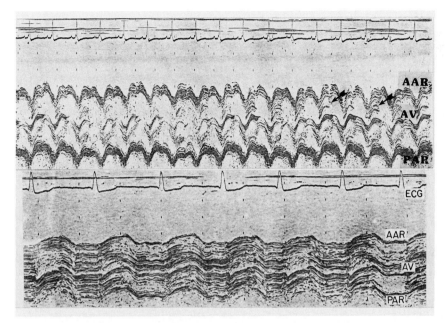

Fig. D-17. *Upper.* M-mode echogram of the aortic root in a young patient with aortic valve sclerosis but no significant stenosis. Slight changes in transducer direction result in varying echographic morphology of the valve. On the left of the figure, the aortic valve appears stenotic because only the left and noncoronary cusps are visualized. On the right, the anterior (right coronary) cusp (*arrows*) comes into view, revealing the true aortic valve orifice.

Lower. M-mode echogram of the aortic root in an elderly patient with calcific aortic stenosis. Multiple dense linear echoes filling most of the aortic root arise from calcified aortic cusps. The apparent aortic valve orifice shows considerable variation from beat to beat, with only slight alteration in transducer direction, at times seeming to open well (first and fifth beats) but elsewhere (third beat) appearing very narrow.

sent as a dense, thick, linear or bandlike echo in the middle of the aortic root. The rectangle formed by this abnormal cusp and one of the other two cusps (usually the right coronary) can easily be mistaken for the true aortic valve orifice, which is, of course, larger because the third remaining cusp is more mobile, though more easily overlooked (Fig. D-17, upper panel).

3. Large variations in the width of the aortic valve orifice can be produced sometimes by changes in transducer angulation or scanning site, presumably because of eccentric or irregular location of the valve orifice in the aortic root.

4. When the aortic valve is heavily calcified, no sharply defined valve orifice may be visible at all, in spite of the best efforts of a competent and experienced echographer. In the most extreme examples, the aortic root appears filled with dense, amorphous echoes that show little or no change with different phases of the cardiac cycle. In other instances, the echo mass within the aortic root reflected from the calcified valve shows a vague, ill-defined, partial clearing during systole. This clearing may not represent a true valve orifice but merely be a systolic shifting of calcified cusp tissue out of the path of the ultrasound beam (Fig. D-17, lower panel).

INDIRECT EVIDENCE OF AORTIC STENOSIS

Since inspection of the aortic valve echoes on the M-mode tracing was found unreliable in the assessment of aortic stenosis, echocardiographers sought other criteria of significant left ventricular outflow obstruction. They noted that the concentric hypertrophy accompanying aortic stenosis of moderate to severe degree manifested echocardiographically as increased diastolic and systolic thickness of the LV posterior wall and ventricular septum, and decrease in the LV chamber diastolic and systolic dimensions (Bennett *et al.,* 1975; Schwartz *et al.,* 1978). Various mathematical formulae combining these two measurements (LV wall thickness and LV dimension) were devised and shown to correlate well with LV peak systolic pressures or LV-aortic pressure gradients obtained at left-heart catheterization but others reported less satisfactory correlation. Reichek and Devereux (1982) found that a ratio of end-diastolic LV wall thickness to LV chamber radius > 0.45 was highly specific for predicting severe aortic valve stenosis, especially in the presence of aortic valve calcification and the absence of aortic regurgitation. Whereas the prediction of the severity of aortic stenosis on the basis of LV wall thickness and LV chamber size is reliable in most children and young adults with well-compensated aortic stenosis of congenital or rheumatic etiology, it can be misleading in certain special situations:

1. *When the LV fails,* in a patient with critical aortic stenosis, it dilates; wall thickness decreases and chamber size increases. Thus Schwartz *et al.* (1978) found that the severity of aortic stenosis was underestimated in all their patients with poor LV function, but correctly estimated in 30 patients with normal LV function. The formulae devised to predict severity of aortic stenosis would not hold, yet the prognosis in this type of patient is serious. Thus, these patients in urgent need of hemodynamic studies and surgical correction run the risk of being misdiagnosed as regards the severity of their aortic valve lesion.

2. *Elderly hypertensive patients* often have hypertrophied, small-chambered left ventricles. They are also unduly prone to aortic valve calcification. Thus, they may present with a short ejection systolic murmur, but if studied hemodynamically, have no real pressure gradient across the aortic valve. They are usually on hypotensive drugs and may have normal blood pressure at the time of echocardiography. These patients, too, could possibly be misdiagnosed as having severe aortic stenosis if only the criteria of LV wall thickness and chamber size are considered.

The pattern of LV posterior wall motion was found to correlate well with severity of aortic stenosis (Sheppard *et al.,* 1978). In patients with critical aortic stenosis requiring surgical correction, the anterior motion of the LV posterior

endocardium appears straight rather than curved, and the summit of endocardial motion (at or soon after end-systole) appears peaked or angular, whereas normally it is blunted or curved. This is a useful sign in clinical practice, although a subjective element enters into its evaluation and the endocardial contour changes are often subtle.

Initial experience with *2-D echographic* assessment of aortic valve stenosis was very promising. Thus, Weyman *et al.* (1975) studied 28 patients with stenotic aortic valves and found that maximum aortic valve opening was 4 to 11 mm (mean, 7.9) in severe stenosis, 9 to 15 mm (mean, 11.6) in moderate stenosis, 14 to 20 mm (mean, 16.9) in mild stenosis, and 15 to 26 (mean, 20.5) in a group of normal controls. Although there was some overlap among these four groups, a clear separation was evident between those with mild and severe aortic valve stenosis. Also, there was no overlap between those advised to have surgical therapy and those considered not severe enough to warrant surgery. All patients with aortic valve diameters of 11 mm or less were recommended surgery; valve diameters of 8 mm or less were always associated with hemodynamically severe stenosis. The same group (Godley *et al.,* 1981) extended their 2-D observations in the long-axis view to include a total of 81 adults. Maximal aortic cusp separation of less than 8 mm was 97 per cent predictive of severe stenosis. Cusp separation exceeding 12 mm was 96 per cent predictive of mild aortic stenosis. Prediction of severity of aortic stenosis was poor when cusp separation was between 8 and 12 mean (96 per cent) but improved to 86 per cent when the valve was viewed in short axis. Satisfactory recording and measurement of the aortic valve area in systole could be done in only 13 per cent of cases.

Recently DeMaria *et al.* (1980) published an important 2-D echographic study of 85 patients with stenotic aortic valves. Their assessment of aortic stenosis was based on measurement of maximum aortic cusp separation (in either long- or short-axis or apical views). This value was 15 to 23 mm (mean, 19.4) in a group of 20 normal controls, 3 to 15 mm (mean, 10.0) in patients with "noncritical aortic stenosis," and 1 to 11 mm (mean, 4.6) in those with "critical aortic stenosis." Maximal aortic cusp separation was more than 15 mm in all normal subjects and 11 mm or less in all patients with critical stenosis. Ninety per cent of patients with critical aortic stenosis had maximum aortic cusp separation of 8 mm or less, but so did 9 of 26 patients with noncritical stenosis. The sensitivity of this criterion was thus only 65 per cent.

Other observations of these authors are worth mentioning here, because they are of practical importance to echocardiographers confronted with the often difficult task of passing judgment on the presence and degree of aortic valve stenosis:

1. Completely normal systolic excursions of any of the three aortic cusps excludes critically severe aortic stenosis, however calcified and immobile the other two cusps may be.

2. No satisfactory statistical correlation could be demonstrated between maximum aortic cusp separation and either peak systolic pressure gradient across the aortic valve or calculated aortic valve area or index by cardiac catheterization.

3. Estimation of aortic stenosis by this method is not valid in patients with markedly impaired ventricular performance, as revealed by the echocardiogram.

4. Although theoretically the aortic valve orifice should be seen (and its area measurable) on the short-axis view, in actual practice the entire perimeter of the stenotic aortic valve seldom can be defined adequately.

5. Measurement of the aortic valve diameter was particularly difficult in patients with heavy calcific deposits in the aortic cusps.

The contours of the aortic cusp in the long-axis view and therefore the aortic valve diameter are particularly difficult to estimate in elderly persons with extensive senile degenerative calcification of the aortic valve. On the other hand, it is even more desirable in these older patients to have a reliable noninvasive means of separating those with calcification but little or no stenosis of the aortic valve from those with stenosis severe enough to require surgery. Patients with nonstenotic calcified aortic valves frequently have cardiac symptoms because of disorders of cardiac rhythm or conduction, or associated ischemic, hypertensive, or primary myocardial disease, whereas patients with critically stenotic valves have syncope, chest pain, or dyspnea attributable to the obstructed valve.

Since the calcific deposits in the aortic valve cusps usually appear on 2-D echography as multiple, dense nodules filling the aortic root, rather than well-defined diaphragm- or dome-like leaflets (as seen in calcified rheumatic valves in younger persons), accurate valve orifice diameter cannot be obtained. However, we have found that an echocardiologist experienced in echographic-hemodynamic correlation can generally distinguish between severe and mild aortic valve stenosis on the basis of the extent of systolic "clearing" of valvular calcific masses in the long-axis view.

CONGENITAL AORTIC VALVE STENOSIS IN CHILDREN AND ADOLESCENTS

M-mode echocardiography is of limited use in imaging congenitally stenotic aortic valves in children and young adults. In them the stenotic valve has the form of a pliable dome, the base of which is attached to the aortic annulus while the stenotic valve orifice is situated at the apex of the dome. The ultrasound beam transects the base of the dome and therefore records apparently normal cusps with normal cusp separation. The site of stenosis, at the apex of the dome, is not recorded easily on the echographic tracing, probably because its margins are tangential to the ultrasound beam. Multiple diastolic closure lines may be evident (Patel *et al.,* 1978).

If the valve is bicuspid, as it often is, the line of diastolic closure may be eccentric, i.e., not situated in or near the center of the aortic root. However, it must be added that recently Kececioglu-Draelos and Goldberg (1981) have cast doubt on the eccentricity index and the recording of multiple diastolic cusp lines as reliable indicators of a bicuspid stenotic valve.

Indirect M-mode data pertaining to LV wall thickness and LV internal dimension have been shown to be more useful than echographic morphology of the aortic valve itself in children with clinical signs of valvular aortic stenosis. The ratio of end-systolic LV posterior wall thickness to the end-systolic LV internal dimension correlates quite well with the LV peak systolic gradient across the aortic valve (Glanz *et al.,* 1976; Aziz *et al.,* 1977; Johnson *et al.,* 1977; Blackwood *et al.,* 1978; Bass *et al.,* 1979;

Gewitz *et al.,* 1979; Friedman *et al.,* 1979), with "r" values in the 0.80 to 0.90 range. This ratio is multiplied by a constant factor—225 according to Glanz *et al.,* 245 according to Blackwood *et al.*—to give the predicted LV peak systolic pressure in mmHg. The predicted aortic valve pressure gradient is obtained by subtracting the systolic arterial blood pressure, measured by the arm-cuff method, from the predicted LV peak systolic pressure.

It is worthy of note that prediction of LV systolic pressure by this noninvasive method is not reliable in patients who have been operated upon for the stenotic valve (Gewitz *et al.,* 1979), presumably because of incomplete regression of the LV wall hypertrophy in spite of adequate relief of the LV outflow obstruction. The more severe the aortic valve stenosis, the smaller the LV internal dimension and larger its systolic shortening fraction (Johnson *et al.,* 1976; Friedman *et al.,* 1979).

On 2-D echocardiography, in the long-axis view, the dome-shaped contour of the aortic valve in systole can be recognized as different from the normal appearance. The orifice diameter, corresponding to the distance between the edges of the thickened aortic cusps, can be measured and correlates well with the calculated aortic valve area and also with the peak systolic aortic valve gradient obtained at cardiac catheterization (Weyman *et al.,* 1977). These authors found that the ratio of the aortic valve orifice diameter to the aortic root diameter was 62 to 92 per cent (mean, 73) in normals, 42 to 62 per cent (mean, 53) in children with mild aortic stenosis, and 20 to 30 per cent (mean, 30) in those with moderate to severe stenosis.

ABNORMAL SYSTOLIC AORTIC VALVE PATTERNS (Figs. D-18 to D-23)

Deviations from the normal rectangular box pattern of aortic valve systolic opening can occur under a variety of circumstances. These can be divided into two main categories:

1. Where restricted opening motion of the cusps is caused by structural abnormalities of the cusps themselves, i.e., sclerosis or calcification resulting in increased stiffness. This situation is discussed in the section on aortic valve stenosis.

2. Where the aortic valve is intrinsically normal but the usual box systolic pattern is altered or modified because of abnormal characteristics of flow through the valve. Normally LV ejection is forceful and steady enough to hold the three aortic cusps fully open through the entire LV ejection period. Abnormal patterns of systolic flow, consequently of cusp motion, occur in:

a. *Idiopathic hypertrophic subaortic stenosis (IHSS).* In hypertrophic cardiomyopathy with LV outflow obstruction, the aortic valve opens normally during the first half of ejection, but then an abrupt notch is inscribed on one or both cusp echoes (Fig. D-18) in midsystole, i.e., the cusps approach each other transiently, sometimes referred to as *midsystolic closure* (Gramiak *et al.,* 1969; Rossen and Popp, 1975; Shah and Sylvester, 1977). Midsystolic near-closure of the aortic valve corresponds to the midsystolic notch on the arterial pulse and sharp midsystolic reduction in flow due to the muscular subvalvular narrowing attaining full severity at that moment of the cardiac cycle. During the remainder of ejection, the valve usually reopens to its initial extent; in a minority of instances, one or both cusps exhibit a somewhat attenuated amplitude of opening in late systole (Figs. D-19 and D-20). Although this pattern of partial late-systolic aortic closure is infrequent in uncomplicated IHSS, it is the most common pattern in IHSS with mitral annulus calcification in my experience (7 out of 10 cases).

Another aortic valve pattern seen in IHSS is an irregular, jagged, coarse flutter (Fig. D-18).

The finding of a normal rectangular box pattern does not rule out the diagnosis of IHSS. Nevertheless, the recording of midsystolic near-closure of the aortic valve is a reliable sign of significant and often large LV-aortic systolic pressure gradients (Glaser, 1975; Krajcer *et al.,* 1978; Chahine *et al.,* 1979; Doi *et al.,* 1980), therefore an important component of the echographic diagnosis of IHSS. It is particularly valuable in those patients with IHSS in whom the aortic root is well visualized but not the mitral valve or left ventricle because of emphysema, unfavorable thoracic shape, and so forth. However, midsystolic notching of the aortic valve systolic contour is not entirely specific for IHSS and may be seen rarely in association

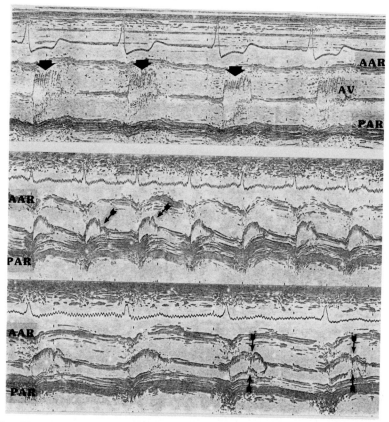

Fig. D-18.   *Upper.* Aortic valve systolic motion patterns in IHSS. M-mode echogram of the aortic valve in a patient with proven IHSS. The anterior aortic cusp shows marked systolic flutter (*arrows*) but no midsystolic "closure" notch. However, a gradual closure motion of the posterior aortic cusp does occur during the latter part of systole.

Center and Lower. Aortic valve echogram of a different patient with IHSS. Midsystolic near-closure of the aortic valve, typical of dynamic muscular subaortic stenosis, is well visualized in the last two beats of the lower panel (*arrows*). The center panel, at slower paper speed in the same patient, demonstrates considerable variation from beat to beat, but a conspicuous decrease in cusp separation in the latter third of LV ejection seems common to most beats.

with mitral regurgitation, ventricular septal defect, and so forth, as in Figure D-22.

b. *Discrete (fixed) subvalvular aortic stenosis.* The common form of this congenital anomaly in older children and young adults consists of a diaphragm-like membrane just below the aortic valve in the LV outflow tract. LV ejection occurs as a jet of blood through an aperture in the diaphragm, which enters the aortic root eccentrically or engenders eddies or turbulence of an asymmetric nature. The result is that the anterior (right coronary) or posterior (noncoronary) cusp, or rarely both, exhibits a characteristic pattern of motion (Fig. D-21): it opens normally at the onset of ejection but almost immediately closes, remaining fluttering

but closed during the rest of systole. This pattern is referred to as early systolic closure. Usually the other visible cusp shows normal systolic motion of the usual box pattern. (Popp *et al.,* 1974; Davis *et al.,* 1974).

Caution: Early- or midsystolic closure patterns of the aortic valve are seen on occasion in conditions other than IHSS or fixed subaortic stenosis: mitral prolapse (Howard *et al.,* 1977), mitral annulus calcification (Kanakis, 1979), aortic dissection (Candell-Riera *et al.,* 1980), subaortic stenosis produced by supernumerary mitral valve (Hatem *et al.,* 1981), and other entities (Wong *et al.,* 1980).

A common normal variant that should not be mistaken for the one diagnostic of fixed

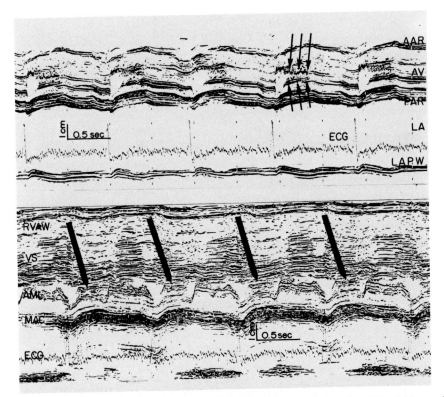

Fig. D-19. M-mode echogram of the aortic root (*upper*) and mitral valve (*lower*) in a patient with IHSS and submitral (mitral annulus) calcification. The aortic valve opens normally but the cusps move abruptly to a near-closed position (*arrows*) during the latter half of LV ejection. This phase of late systolic near-closure of the aortic valve corresponds to the phase during which abnormal systolic anterior motion (*arrows*) of the mitral valve (SAM) brings it against the ventricular septum. SAM and mitral annulus calcification are clearly visible in the lower panel; however, the right (anterior) aspect of the ventricular septum is not well defined.

subaortic stenosis is the mild overshoot that sometimes accompanies the initial opening motion of the right coronary cusp, especially when the aortic root is dilated. Following such normal overshoot, the cusp normally remains open during the rest of systole, whereas in discrete fixed subaortic stenosis it flutters in a closed position.

c. *Low cardiac output.* In patients with low cardiac output, as in cardiomyopathy with severe cardiac failure, the normal boxlike systolic pattern alters to one in which the cusps drift gradually together, instead of shutting abruptly. This pattern also sometimes is seen with mitral regurgitation and ventricular septal defect; it is presumed that reduction of forward flow into the aorta occurs in late systole because of a significant quantity of LV blood being lost through the regurgitant mitral valve or septal defect. Alternation in duration of LV ejection time may be manifest on the aortic valve motion (Fig. D-23).

d. *Irregular cardiac rhythm.* Irregular cardiac rhythm, whether due to premature beats, atrial fibrillation, or other causes, results in variable duration of aortic valve opening. The beats terminating long R-R intervals show unusually large ejection periods. Beats terminating unduly short R-R intervals show short and sometimes abnormally small (low amplitude) aortic valve opening. This should be kept in mind when aortic valve measurements are being made or the valve echo contour is being examined.

Premature opening of the aortic valve (in mid- to late diastole) has been reported in rare instances of extremely severe aortic regurgitation (Tajik and Giuliani, 1977; Pietro *et al.*, 1978; Cohen *et al.*, 1979; Nathan *et al.*, 1982).

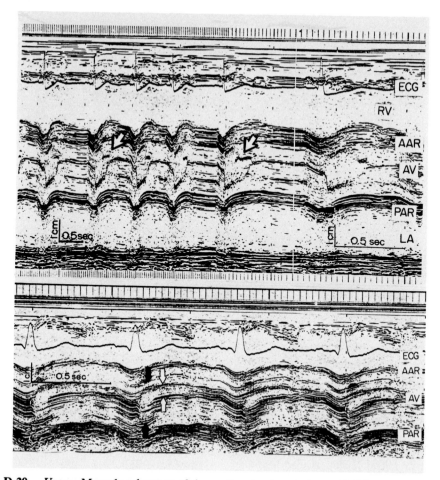

Fig. D-20. *Upper.* M-mode echogram of the aortic valve in a patient with IHSS and submitral (mitral annulus) calcification: paper speed has been increased in the right half of the figure. An unusual pattern of late systolic closure (*arrow*) of the anterior cusp is presented. Motion of the posterior aortic cusp is normal.

Lower. Aortic valve echogram in another patient with IHSS and submitral calcification. The aortic valve is sclerotic; it opens well in early systole (*solid arrows*), but the posterior cusp moves to a near-closed position in mid- to late systole (*small open arrows*).

The LV diastolic pressure rises so high that it exceeds the aortic pressure before the onset of ventricular contraction (Weaver *et al.*, 1977).

DISCRETE FIXED SUBAORTIC STENOSIS

The chief echocardiographic manifestation of this type of LV outflow obstruction is the peculiar systolic behavior of the aortic valve leaflets: (1) one or both aortic cusps seen in the M-mode echogram open well initially, but almost immediately return to the closed position (Fig. D-21). This early systolic closure motion dis-

torts the normal box pattern of the aortic valve in a very typical way, as mentioned above; (2) rapid systolic fluttering of the aortic cusps is the rule. These findings were first described in small groups of cases by Davis *et al.* (1974) and Popp *et al.* (1974) and then later confirmed to be a very consistent echographic characteristic by several other authors. Thus, abnormal aortic valve motion was noted in 19 of 20 patients of Krueger *et al.* (1979). However, these authors found that the amplitude of the early systolic closure motion varied widely (13 to 88 per cent of total aortic valve excursion) and did not correlate with the magnitude of the

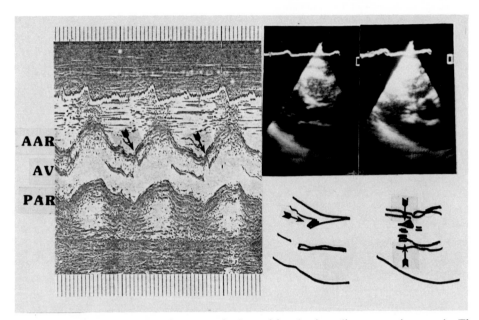

AAR

AV

PAR

Fig. D-21. M-mode and 2-D echograms of a boy with subvalvar discrete aortic stenosis. The M-mode echogram shows early systolic closure of the anterior aortic cusp. In the left frame of the 2-D echogram (long-axis view) part of the subvalvar membrane is attached to the septum (*arrow*). The right frame presents a better visualization of the stenotic subaortic area (*arrows*).

pressure gradient across the diaphragm-like site of stenosis.

Narrowing of the LV outflow tract, as measured from the ventricular septum to the base of the anterior mitral leaflet, is also found in most patients with fixed subaortic stenosis. Krueger reported that 19 of 22 patients in their series had LV outflow tracts less than 80 per cent as wide as the aortic root. For this purpose it is necessary to record a gradual scan from LV to aortic root or in the reverse direction; the LV outflow tract is measured from the C point of the anterior mitral leaflet (at the area of transition from posterior aortic root to typical anterior mitral M-shaped contour) to the left border of the ventricular septum.

Berry *et al.* (1979) also found LV outflow tract narrowing a reliable indicator of fixed subaortic stenosis and mentioned that the LV outflow width tended to be smaller in the patients with more severe gradients than in those with small gradients. Narrowing of the LV outflow region was also a conspicuous feature of patients with the unusual tunnel variety of fixed subaortic stenosis studied by Maron *et al.* (1976).

An abnormally narrow LV outflow tract is not usually seen in patients with aortic valve stenosis, but is (1) a well-known feature of hypertrophic cardiomyopathy, especially in those with LV outflow gradients. Diminished systolic space between anterior mitral leaflet and ventricular septum may also be observed in (2) patients with marked concentric hypertrophy and abnormally small LV chambers, and (3) in elderly individuals with large calcific deposits in the posterior mitral annulus region that displace the mitral leaflets anteriorly.

The early echocardiographic literature on fixed subaortic stenosis did not contain clear descriptions of the subaortic membrane or diaphragm itself. More recent reports have demonstrated abnormal linear echoes between anterior mitral leaflet and ventricular septum just below the aortic valve level, attributable to the stenosing diaphragm or membrane (Caudill *et al.,* 1976; Krueger *et al.,* 1979), but for some reason this abnormal structure tends to elude clear definition or depiction on the M-mode tracing. Krueger *et al.* could identify it in only 3 of their 20 patients.

Aortic regurgitation is a frequent accompaniment of a subaortic diaphragm. Diastolic flutter of the anterior mitral leaflet is consequently a common finding. Associated sclerosis of the aortic cusps does not prevent the characteristic

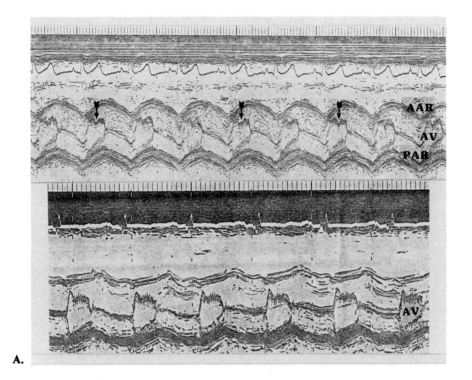

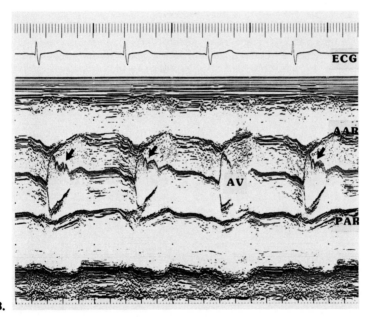

Fig. D-22. *A.* Aortic valve systolic patterns sometimes seen in patients with mitral regurgitation.

Upper. Aortic valve echogram in a patient with mitral regurgitation. A notch is visible on the systolic contour of the anterior (right coronary) cusp. On hemodynamic study there was no evidence of subaortic stenosis.

Lower. M-mode echogram of the aortic valve in a patient with mitral regurgitation following myocardial infarction and coronary bypass surgery. The anterior (right coronary) cusp shows early systolic partial closure and systolic flutter. Previous left heart catheterization for coronary disease evaluation showed that subaortic stenosis was absent.

Fig. D-22. *B.* M-mode echogram of a 14-year-old boy with pulmonary valve stenosis and a ventricular septal defect. No subvalvar aortic stenosis or IHSS was seen on catheterization or angiocardiography. The anterior aortic valve cusp echo shows midsystolic notching and coarse flutter, similar to that seen in IHSS.

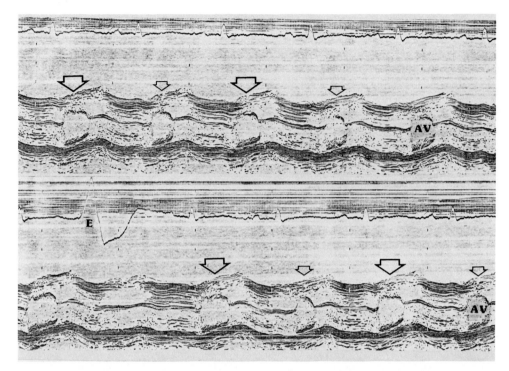

Fig. D-23. M-mode echogram showing the aortic valve in a patient with cardiomyopathy and chronic heart failure. The ECG shows regular sinus rhythm. Alternation of aortic valve ejection time is evident (mechanical alternans). Thus, in the upper panel, aortic valve opening is of greater duration in the first, third, and fifth beats than in the second and fourth. In the lower panel, the aortic valve fails to open in the premature ventricular beat (*E*), and thereafter the alternation in LV ejection time is accentuated.

early closure motion of discrete subvalvar stenosis (Hess *et al.*, 1977).

Prediction of the LV systolic pressure by means of a formula based on LV end-systolic wall thickness and LV internal dimension is usually reliable, as it is with aortic valve stenosis in young persons (Johnson *et al.*, 1977; Berry *et al.*, 1979).

Two-D echocardiographic visualization of the LV outflow tract (Fig. D-21) has succeeded in displaying anatomic detail of the LV outflow region superior to that obtained by the M-mode technique. Weyman *et al.* (1976) found linear echoes traversing this area in patients with the diaphragm type of subaortic stenosis, whereas those with the longer, more diffuse LV outflow tract narrowing showed an inward bowing of its anterior and posterior margins, or else an irregular protuberance that encroached upon the space between the septum and mitral valve. Roelandt and Van Dorp (1977) also demonstrated long-segment LV outflow tract narrowing by M-mode as well as 2-D echocardiogra-

phy in patients with "tunnel" subvalvar aortic stenosis. Shore *et al.* (1982) described 13 patients with ventricular septal defect complicated by LV outflow tract obstruction by a fibromuscular shelf, which was well visualized on 2-D echography.

SUPRAVALVAR AORTIC STENOSIS

The aortic root just above aortic valve level can be seen by M-mode as well as 2-D echography in almost all subjects, but scanning the aorta upward to visualize the upper ascending aorta is often unsuccessful. However, an attempt should be made to examine the aortic caliber at all possible levels in children or young adults with aortic systolic ejection murmurs to detect or exclude supravalvar aortic stenosis. An association with familial hypercholesterolemia has recently been documented by echocardiography (Allen *et al.*, 1980).

In supravalvar stenosis, the aortic root is of normal diameter at aortic valve level, but narrow above the sinus of Valsalva level. The ratio of the caliber of the narrow aortic segment to the aortic caliber at valve level has varied from slightly less than 1 to about 0.4 (Usher *et al.*, 1974; Bolen *et al.*, 1975; Nasrallah and Nihill, 1975). The length of the stenotic segment is also variable; when short (hourglass type of supravalvar aortic stenosis), it may be possible to demonstrate a normal aortic diameter above the level of stenosis.

Caution: The aortic diameter can appear artefactually narrow on M-mode echography if the ultrasound beam transects the ascending aorta eccentrically, i.e., records a chord rather than the true diameter.

Two-D echography can be used to image the aortic root and demonstrate its narrowing more convincingly than is possible by the M-mode technique. Again, viewing of the aortic root in inappropriate planes can easily produce a false impression of narrowing. Repeated scans and as thorough a visualization of the aortic root as possible are therefore essential to establish a firm diagnosis.

REFERENCES

BICUSPID AORTIC VALVE

Brandenburg, R. O.; Tajik, A. J.; Edwards, W. D.; *et al.*: Accuracy of two-dimensional echocardiographic diagnosis of bicuspid aortic valve. *Circulation,* **66:**1040, 1982 (Abstr.).

Fowles, R. E.; Martin, R. P.; Abrams, J. M., *et al.*: Two-dimensional echocardiographic features of bicuspid aortic valve. *Chest,* **75:**435, 1979.

Leech, G.; Mills, P.; and Leatham, A.: The diagnosis of a non-stenotic bicuspid aortic valve. *Br. Heart J.,* **40:**941, 1978.

Nanda, N. C.; Gramiak, R.; Manning, J.; *et al.*: Echocardiographic recognition of the congenital bicuspid aortic valve. *Circulation,* **49:**870, 1974.

Radford, D. J.; Bloom, K. R.; Izukawa, R.; *et al.*: Echocardiographic assessment of bicuspid aortic valves. *Circulation,* **53:**80, 1976.

Scovil, J. A.; Nanda, N. C.; Gross, C. M.; *et al.*: Echocardiographic studies of abnormalities associated with coarctation of the aorta. *Circulation,* **53:**953, 1976.

Zema, M. J., and Caccovano, M.: Two-dimensional echocardiographic assessment of aortic valve morphology: feasibility of bicuspid valve detection. *Br. Heart J.,* **48:**428, 1982.

AORTIC VALVE ENDOCARDITIS

Arvan, S.; Cagin, N.; Levitt, B.; *et al.*: Echocardiographic findings in a patient with *Candida* endocarditis of the aortic valve. *Chest,* **70:**300, 1976.

Assey, M. E., and Usher, B. W.: Development of aortic valvular vegetations during appropriate antibiotic therapy. Demonstration through serial echocardiogram. *Chest,* **76:**223, 1979.

Blair, T. P.; Waugh, R. A.; Pollack, M.; *et al.*: *Histoplasma capsulatum* endocarditis. *Am. Heart J.,* **99:**782, 1980.

Bradsher, R. W.; Wickre, C. G.; Savage, A. M.; *et al.*: *Histoplasma capsulatum* endocarditis cured by amphotericin B combined with surgery. *Chest,* **78:**791, 1980.

Das, G.; Lee, C. C.; and Weissler, A. M.: Echocardiographic manifestations of ruptured aortic valvular leaflets in the absence of valvular vegetations. *Chest,* **72:**464, 1977.

DeMaria, A. N.; King, J. F.; Salel, A. F.; *et al.*: Echography and phonography of acute aortic regurgitation in bacterial endocarditis. *Ann. Intern. Med.,* **82:**329, 1975.

Dillon, J. C.; Feigenbaum, H.; Konecke, L. L.; *et al.*: Echocardiographic manifestations of valvular vegetations. *Am. Heart J.,* **86:**698, 1973.

Fox, S.; Kotler, M. N.; Segal, B. L.; *et al.*: Echocardiographic diagnosis of acute aortic valve endocarditis and its complications. *Arch. Intern. Med.,* **137:**85, 1977.

Gottlieb, S.; Khuddus, S. A.; Salooki, H.; *et al.*: Echocardiographic diagnosis of aortic valve vegetations in *Candida* endocarditis. *Circulation,* **50:**826, 1974.

Hirschfeld, D. S., and Schiller, N. B.: Localization of aortic valve vegetations by echocardiography. *Circulation,* **53:**280, 1976.

Kleiner, J. P.; Brundage, B. H.; Ports, J. A.; *et al.*: Echocardiographic manifestation of flail right and noncoronary aortic valve leaflets. *Chest,* **74:**301, 1978.

Krivokapich, J.; Child, J. S.; and Skorton, D. J.: Flail aortic valve leaflets: M-mode and two-dimensional echocardiographic manifestations. *Am. Heart J.,* **99:**425, 1980.

Mardelli, F. J.; Ogawa, S.; Hubbard, F.; *et al.*: Cross-sectional echocardiographic detection of aortic ring abscess in bacterial endocarditis. *Chest,* **74:**576, 1978.

Martinez, E. C.; Burch, G. E.; and Giles, T. D.: Echocardiographic diagnosis of vegetative aortic bacterial endocarditis. *Am. J. Cardiol.,* **34:**845, 1974.

McManus, B. M.; Katz, N. M.; Blackbourne, B. D.; *et al.*: Acquired cor triatriatum (left ventricular false aneurysm): Complication of active infective endocarditis of the aortic valve with ring abscess treated by valve replacement. *Am. Heart J.* **104:**312, 1982.

Mildvan, D.; Goldberg, E.; Berger, M.; *et al.*: Diagnosis and successful management of septal myocardial abscess: a complication of bacterial endocarditis. *Am. J. Med. Sci.,* **274:**311, 1977.

Mintz, G. S.; Kotler, M. N.; Segal, B. L.; *et al.*: Survival of patients with aortic valve endocarditis. The prognostic implications of the echocardiogram. *Arch. Intern. Med.,* **139:**862, 1979a.

Mintz, G. S.; Kotler, M. N.; Segal, B. L.; *et al.*: Comparison of two-dimensional and M-mode echocardiography in the evaluation of patients with infective endocarditis. *Am. J. Cardiol.,* **43:**738, 1979b.

Moorthy, K.; Prakash, R.; and Aronow, N. S.: Echocardiographic appearance of aortic valve vegetations in bacterial endocarditis due to *Actinobacillus actinomycetem-comitans. J.C.U.,* **5:**49, 1977.

Pease, H. F.; Matsumoto, S.; and Cacchione, R. J.: Lethal obstruction by aortic valve vegetation. Echocardiographic studies of endocarditis without apparent aortic regurgitation. *Chest,* **73:**658, 1978.

Pridie, R. B.; Beham, R.; and Oakley, C. M.: Echocardiography of the mitral valve in aortic valve disease. *Br. Heart J.,* **33:**296, 1971.

Ramirez, J.; Guardiola, J.; and Flowers, N. C.: Echocardiographic diagnosis of ruptured aortic valve leaflet in bacterial endocarditis. *Circulation,* **57:**684, 1978.

Rubenson, D. S.; Tucker, C. R.; Stinson, E. B.; *et al.;* The use of echocardiography in diagnosing culture-negative endocarditis. *Circulation, 64:*641, 1981.

Shub, C.; Tajik, A. J.; Seward, J. B.; *et al.:* Valvular papillary fibroelastomas: Two-dimensional echocardiographic recognition. *Mayo Clin. Proc.,* **56:**629, 1981.

Srivastava, T. N., and Flowers, N. C.: Echocardiographic features of flail aortic valve. *Chest,* **73:**90, 1978.

Stafford, A.; Wann, A. S.; Dillon, J. C.; *et al.:* Serial echocardiographic appearance of healing bacterial vegetations. *Am. J. Cardiol.,* **44:**754, 1979.

Venkataraman, K.; Bornheimer, J. F.; Pontius, S.; *et al.:* Diastolic flutter of aortic valve in aortic regurgitation: a report of seven cases. *Angiology,* **30:**297, 1979.

Whipple, R. L.; Morris, D. C.; Feiner, J. M.; *et al.:* Echocardiographic manifestations of flail aortic valve leaflets. *J.C.U.,* **5:**417, 1977.

Wray, T. M.: Echocardiographic manifestations of flail aortic valve leaflets in bacterial endocarditis. *Circulation,* **51:**832, 1975.

Yoshikawa, J.; Tanaka, K.; Owaki, J.; *et al.:* Cord-like aortic valve vegetation in bacterial endocarditis: demonstration by cardiac ultrasonography, report of a case. *Circulation,* **53:**911, 1976.

AORTIC VALVE STENOSIS IN ADULTS

Bennett, D. H.; Evans, D. W.; and Raj, M. V.: Echocardiographic estimations of the systolic pressure gradients in aortic stenosis. *Br. Heart J.,* **37:**557, 1975.

Bennett, D. H.; Evans, D. W.; and Raj, M. V. J.: Echocardiographic left ventricular dimensions in pressure and volume overload: their use in assessing aortic stenosis. *Br. Heart J.,* **37:**971, 1975.

Chang, S.; Clements, S.; and Chang, J.: Aortic stenosis: echocardiographic cusp separation and surgical description of aortic valve in 22 patients. *Am. J. Cardiol.,* **39:**499, 1977.

DeMaria, A. N.; Bommer, W.; Joye, J.; *et al.:* Value and limitations of cross-sectional echocardiography of the aortic valve in the diagnosis and quantitation of valvular aortic stenosis. *Circulation,* **62:**304, 1980.

Feizi, O.; Symons, C.; and Yacoub, M.: Echocardiography of the aortic valve: studies of normal aortic valve, aortic stenosis, aortic regurgitation and mixed aortic valve disease. *Br. Heart J.,* **36:**341, 1974.

Godley, R. W.; Green, D.; Dillon, J. C.; *et al.:* Reliability of two-dimensional echocardiography in assessing the severity of valvular aortic stenosis. *Chest,* **79:**657, 1981.

Gramiak, R., and Shah, P. M.: Echocardiography of the normal and diseased aortic valve. *Radiology,* **96:**1, 1970.

Kececioglu-Draelos, Z., and Goldberg, S. J.: Role of M-mode echocardiography in congenital aortic stenosis. *Am. J. Cardiol.,* **47:**1267, 1981.

Reichek, N., and Devereux, R. B.: Reliable estimation of peak left ventricular systolic pressure by M-mode echographic determined end-diastolic relative wall thickness: Identification of severe valvular aortic stenosis in adult patients. *Am. Heart J.,* **103:**202, 1982.

Schwartz, A.; Vignola, P. A.; Walker, H. J.; *et al.:* Echocardiographic estimation of aortic valve gradient in aortic stenosis. *Ann. Intern. Med.,* **69:**329, 1978.

Sheppard, J. M.; Shah, A. A.; Sbarbaro, J. A.; *et al.:* Distinctive echocardiographic pattern of posterior wall endocardial motion in aortic stenosis. *Am. Heart J.,* **96:**9, 1978.

Weyman, A. E.; Feigenbaum, H.; Dillon, J. C.; *et al.:* Cross-sectional echocardiography in assessing the severity of valvular aortic stenosis. *Circulation,* **52:**828, 1975.

Williams, D. E.; Sahn, D. J.; and Friedman, W. F.: Cross-sectional echocardiographic localization of sites of left ventricular outflow tract obstruction. *Am. J. Cardiol.,* **37:**250, 1976.

Winsberg, F., and Mercer, E. N.: Echocardiography in combined valve disease. *Radiology,* **105:**405, 1972.

Yeh, H. C.; Winsberg, F.; and Mercer, E. M.: Echocardiographic aortic valve orifice dimension: Its use in evaluating aortic stenosis and cardiac output. *J.C.U.,* **1:**182, 1973.

AORTIC VALVE STENOSIS IN CHILDREN AND ADOLESCENTS

Aziz, K. U.; van Grondelle, A.; Paul, M. L.; *et al.:* Echocardiographic assessment of the relation between left ventricular wall and cavity dimensions and peak systolic pressure in children with aortic stenosis. *Am. J. Cardiol.,* **40:**775, 1977.

Bass, J. L.; Einzig, S.; Hong, C. Y.; *et al.:* Echocardiographic screening to assess the severity of congenital aortic valve stenosis in children. *Am. J. Cardiol.,* **44:**82, 1979.

Blackwood, R. A.; Bloom, K. R.; and Williams, C. M.: Aortic stenosis in children. Experience with echocardiographic prediction of severity. *Circulation,* **57:**263, 1978.

Friedman, M. J.; Sahn, D. J.; Burris, H. A.; *et al.:* Computerized echocardiographic analysis to detect abnormal systolic and diastolic left ventricular function in children with aortic stenosis. *Am. J. Cardiol.,* **44:**478, 1979.

Gewitz, M. H.; Werner, J. C.; Kleinman, C. S.; *et al.:* Role of echocardiography in aortic stenosis: Pre- and post-operative studies. *Am. J. Cardiol.,* **43:**67, 1979.

Glanz, S.; Hellerbrand, W. E.; Berman, M. A.; *et al.:* Echocardiographic assessment of the severity of aortic stenosis in children and adolescents. *Am. J. Cardiol.,* **38:**620, 1976.

Johnson, G. L.; Meyer, R. A.; Schwartz, D. C.; *et al.:* Left ventricular function by echocardiography in children with fixed aortic stenosis. *Am. J. Cardiol.,* **38:**611, 1976.

Johnson, G. L.; Meyer, R. A.; Schwartz, D. C.; *et al.:* Echocardiographic evaluation of fixed left ventricular outlet obstruction in children. *Circulation,* **56:**299, 1977.

Patel, R. G.; Freedom, R. M.; Bloom, K. R.; *et al.:* Truncal or aortic valve stenosis in functionally single arterial trunk. *Am. J. Cardiol.,* **42:**800, 1978.

Weyman, A. E.; Feigenbaum, H.; Hurwitz, R. A.; *et al.:* Cross-sectional echocardiographic assessment of the severity of aortic stenosis in children. *Circulation,* **55:**773, 1977.

ABNORMAL SYSTOLIC MOTION PATTERNS OF THE AORTIC VALVE

Candell-Riera, J.; Del Castillo, H. G.; and Rius, J.: Aortic root dissection. Another cause of early systolic closure of the aortic valve. *Am. J. Cardiol.,* **43:**579, 1980.

Chahine, R. A.; Raizner, A. E.; Nelson, J.; *et al.:* Mid systolic closure of aortic valve in hypertrophic cardiomyopathy. Echocardiographic and angiographic correlation. *Am. J. Cardiol.,* **43:**17, 1979.

Cohen, I. S.; Wharton, T. P.; Neill, W. A.: Pathophysiologic observations on premature opening of the aortic valve utilizing a technique for multiplane echocardiographic analysis. *Am. Heart J.,* **97:**766, 1979.

Davis, R. A.; Feigenbaum, H.; Chang, S.; *et al.:* Echocardiographic manifestations of discrete subaortic stenosis. *Am. J. Cardiol.,* **33:**277, 1974.

Doi, Y. L.; McKenna, W. J.; and Gehrke, J.: M-mode

echocardiography in hypertrophic cardiomyopathy: Diagnostic criteria and prediction of obstruction. *Am. J. Cardiol.,* **45**:6, 1980.

Elder, M.; Motro, M.; Rath, S.; *et al.:* Systolic closure of aortic valve in patients with prosthetic mitral valves. *Br. Heart J.,* **48**:48, 1982.

Glaser, J.: Mid systolic closure in IHSS. Letter to Editor. *Circulation,* **51**:1172, 1975.

Gramiak, R.; Shah, P. M.; and Kramer, D. H.: Ultrasound cardiography: Contrast studies in anatomy and function. *Radiology,* **2**:939, 1969.

Hatem, J.; Sade, R. M.; and Taylor, A.: Supernumerary mitral valve producing subaortic stenosis. *Chest,* **79**:483, 1981.

Howard, P. F.; Desser, K. B.; and Benchimol, A.: Systolic retraction of the aortic valve in mitral valve prolapse. *Chest,* **71**:659, 1977.

Kanakis, C.: Echocardiogram in idiopathic hypertrophic subaortic stenosis. Letter to Editor. *Am. J. Cardiol.,* **44**:581, 1979.

Krajcer, Z.; Orzan, F.; Pechacek, L. W.; *et al.:* Early systolic closure of the aortic valve in patients with hypertrophic subaortic stenosis and discrete subaortic stenosis. *Am. J. Cardiol.,* **41**:823, 1978.

Nathan, M.P.R; Arora, R.; and Rubenstein, H.: Mid-diastolic aortic valve opening in bacterial endocarditis of aortic valve. *Clin Cardiol,* **5**:294, 1982.

Pietro, D. A.; Davis, A. F.; Harrington, J. J.; *et al.:* Premature opening of the aortic valve: an index of highly advanced aortic regurgitation. *J.C.U.,* **6**:170, 1978.

Popp, R. L.; Silverman, F. J.; and French, J. W.: Echocardiographic findings in discrete subvalvular aortic stenosis. *Circulation,* **49**:226, 1974.

Rossen, R. M., and Popp, R. L.: Mid systolic AV closure in IHSS. *Circulation,* **51**:1172, 1975.

Shah, P. M., and Sylvester, L. J.: Echocardiography in the diagnosis of hypertrophic obstructive cardiomyopathy. *Am. J. Med.,* **62**:830, 1977.

Tajik, A. J., and Giuliani, E. R.: Diastolic opening of aortic valve: an echographic observation. *Mayo Clin. Proc.,* **52**:112, 1977.

Weaver, W. F.; Wilson, C. S.; Rourke, T.; *et al.:* Mid diastolic aortic valve opening in severe acute aortic regurgitation. *Circulation,* **55**:145, 1977.

Wong, P.; Cotter, L.; and Gibson, D. G.: Early systolic closure of the aortic valve. *Br. Heart J.,* **44**:386, 1980.

FIXED SUBVALVAR AORTIC STENOSIS

Berry, T. E.; Aziz, K. U.; and Paul, M. H.: Echocardiographic assessment of discrete subaortic stenosis in childhood. *Am. J. Cardiol.,* **43**:957, 1979.

Caudill, C. C.; Krueger, S. K.; and Wilson, C. S.: Membranous subaortic stenosis complicated by aneurysm of the membranous septum and mitral valve prolapse. *Circulation,* **53**:580, 1976.

Davis, R. A.; Feigenbaum, H.; Chang, S.; *et al.:* Echocardiographic manifestations of discrete subaortic stenosis. *Am. J. Cardiol.,* **33**:277, 1974.

Hess, P. G.; Nanda, N. C.; DeWesse, J. A.; *et al.:* Echocardiographic features of combined membranous subaortic stenosis and acquired calcific aortic valvulopathy. *Am. Heart J.,* **94**:349, 1977.

Johnson, G. L.; Meyer, R. A.; Schwartz, D. C.; *et al.:* Echocardiographic evaluation of fixed left ventricular outlet obstruction in children. Pre- and post-operative assessment of ventricular systolic pressures. *Circulation,* **56**:299, 1977.

Kronzon, I.; Schloss, M.; Danilowicz, D.; *et al.:* Fixed membranous subaortic stenosis. *Chest,* **67**:473, 1975.

Krueger, S. K.; French, J. W.; Forker, A. D.; *et al.:* Echocardiography in discrete subaortic stenosis. *Circulation,* **59**:506, 1979.

Maron, B. J.; Redwood, D. R.; Roberts, W. C.; *et al.:* Tunnel aortic stenosis: Left ventricular outflow tract obstruction produced by fibromuscular tubular narrowing. *Circulation,* **54**:404, 1976.

Popp, R. L.; Silverman, J. F.; French, J. W.; *et al.:* Echocardiographic findings in discrete subvalvular aortic stenosis. *Circulation,* **49**:226, 1974.

Roelandt, J., and Van Dorp, W. G.: Long segment (tunnel) subaortic stenosis. *Chest,* **72**:222, 1977.

Shore, D.F.; Smallhorn, J.; Stark, J.; *et al.:* Left ventricular outflow tract obstruction coexisting with ventricular septal defect. *Br. Heart J.,* **48**:421, 1982.

Weyman, A. E.; Feigenbaum, H.; Hurwitz, R. A.; *et al.:* Cross-sectional echocardiography in evaluating patients with discrete subaortic stenosis. *Am. J. Cardiol.,* **37**:358, 1976.

SUPRAVALVAR AORTIC STENOSIS

Allen, J. M.; Thompson, G. R.; Myant, N. B.; *et al.:* Cardiovascular complications of homozygous familial hypercholesterolemia. *Br. Heart J.,* **44**:361, 1980.

Bolen, J. L.; Popp, R. L.; and French, J. W.: Echocardiographic features of supravalvular aortic stenosis. *Circulation,* **52**:817, 1975.

Nasrallah, A., and Nihill, M.: Supravalvular aortic stenosis: Echocardiographic features. *Br. Heart J.,* **37**:662, 1975.

Usher, B. W.; Goulden, D.; and Murgo, J. P.: Echocardiographic detection of supravalvar aortic stenosis. *Circulation,* **49**:1259, 1974.

Weyman, A. E.; Feigenbaum, H.; Dillon, J. C.; *et al.:* Localization of left ventricular outflow obstruction by cross-sectional echocardiography. *Am. J. Med.,* **60**:33, 1976.

Weyman, A. E.; Caldwell, R. L.; Hurwitz, R. A.; *et al.:* Cross-sectional echocardiographic characterization of aortic obstruction. I—Supravalvular aortic stenosis and aortic hypoplasia. *Circulation,* **57**:491, 1978.

Williams, D. E.; Sahn, D. J.; and Friedman, W. F.: Cross-sectional echocardiographic localization of sites of left ventricular outflow obstruction. *Am. J. Cardiol.,* **37**:350, 1976.

E

The Tricuspid Valve

NORMAL TRICUSPID VALVE

Unlike the mitral valve, which is situated directly posterior to the left parasternal area, the tricuspid valve lies under the sternum and right parasternum. Whereas the mitral valve is the easiest cardiac structure to record by ultrasound, the tricuspid valve is visualized with difficulty, only by an oblique and rather awkward tilt of the transducer, positioned at the left sternal border, toward the right costal margin. With a little skill, the anterior tricuspid leaflet may be recorded through most or all of the cardiac cycle; at a slightly different transducer tilt the posterior tricuspid leaflet comes into view.

Should the heart be easier to scan because of a larger "bare area" uncovered by lung (as in children) or because of right ventricular dilatation, more of the tricuspid valve can be seen so that the anterior and septal leaflet motion is visualized in its entirety. When this is achieved, the characteristics of tricuspid motion, in both systole and diastole, are found to be very similar to those of mitral valve motion and, in fact, the same designations have been applied to its "E" and "A" peaks, as well as to its EF and AC slopes. Whereas there appears to be no question that the anterior component of the tricuspid valve echo represents the anterior leaflet, it is thought that the posterior tricuspid echoes could be either the septal or posterior (inferior) leaflet, depending on the direction of the ultrasound beam. When the interatrial septum is visualized posterior to the tricuspid valve, the septal leaflet of the tricuspid forms the "posterior" tricuspid cusp, whereas if the tricuspid valve is seen anterior to the right ventricular posterior wall, it is the posterior (inferior) leaflet.

In individuals whose hearts are accessible to subxiphoid scanning, an excellent view of tricuspid motion may be obtained, even better than that afforded by left parasternal scanning. Pulmonary emphysema, which so often thwarts the echocardiographer's efforts to obtain satisfactory cardiac echoes parasternally, can actually be a boon if it depresses the diaphragm, thus causing the heart to descend lower in the thorax and closer to the subxiphoid area. With the transducer positioned in the midline at the subcostal (subxiphoid) or epigastric region and directed superiorly and posteriorly, the right ventricular inflow tract and tricuspid valve are well visualized anterior to the aortic root (Fig. A-15). In such patients, with good subcostal windows, 2-D echocardiography too provides excellent views of tricuspid anatomy, in long-axis (coronal) and short-axis (sagittal) planes.

Normally, in the absence of gross mediastinal shift, the tricuspid valve cannot be recorded unless the ultrasound transducer is tilted toward the right. Should the right ventricle be very dilated, as in cor pulmonale, or both ventricles be enlarged, as in some cases of dilated cardiomyopathy, the tricuspid and mitral valves may be recorded simultaneously (Fig. E-1), with the transducer held perpendicularly at the left sternal border. These remarks about transducer position and tricuspid visualization are relevant because there is virtually only one cardiac condition in which the tricuspid valve can be well seen with the ultrasound probe held perpendicularly over the left anterior chest: Ebstein's anomaly.

Structures that could be mistaken for the tricuspid valve include (1) the mitral valve, if the LV posterior wall is not well defined and recognized for what it is. Strip-chart recording of

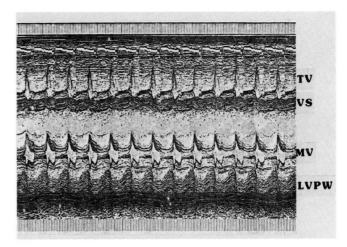

Fig. E-1. M-mode echogram of a patient with congestive cardiomyopathy and diffuse cardiac dilatation. The mitral and tricuspid valves are visualized simultaneously, as in Ebstein's anomaly and certain other congenital anomalies associated with right heart dilatation. However, unlike those anomalies, the amplitude of tricuspid valve opening is not unduly large, the RV is not unduly dilated, and LV function appears impaired.

the tricuspid valve should therefore always end with a scan to the mitral valve, establishing that the tricuspid is quite separate from the latter and on a more anterior plane; (2) Swan-Ganz catheters or pacemaker wires in the right-heart chambers (discussed later in this chapter); (3) rarely, the RV anterior wall can exhibit undue mobility in the presence of a pericardial effusion, so that it can simulate tricuspid motion, the anterior parietal pericardium being mistaken for the RV anterior wall (Fig. E-2).

TRICUSPID VALVE ENDOCARDITIS (Fig. E-3)

The echocardiographer is often called upon to examine the tricuspid valve for vegetations in patients who are known or suspected drug addicts and present with unexplained fever, lung opacities on x-ray, positive blood cultures, or some combination of these. In other cases, the patient is not an intravenous drug abuser but has thrombophlebitis, an infected arteriovenous shunt (for hemodialysis), or possible venous spread of some other source of bacterial infection.

Vegetations on the tricuspid valve are detectable by echocardiography, but by no means in every instance in which they exist (Andy *et al.,* 1977). By far the most common echographic manifestation is a shaggy thickening (Fig. E-3) of tricuspid leaflet echoes (Lee *et al.,* 1974; Kisslo *et al.,* 1976; Wann *et al.,* 1976; Andy *et al.,* 1977; Thomson *et al.,* 1977; Chandaratna and Aronow, 1979).

Occasionally other echocardiographic patterns have been noted in proven cases of tricuspid endocarditis. Thus, Chandaratna and Aronow found, in one patient, multilayered echoes resembling a myxoma related to the anterior tricuspid leaflet; in another, a fingerlike abnormal echo was seen anterior to normal-looking tricuspid leaflet echoes. Come *et al.* (1979) report two instances of tricuspid endocarditis in which a vegetation adherent to a tricuspid leaflet simulated a right atrial myxoma, appearing between anterior and posterior tricuspid leaflets in diastole. We have had a patient with large mobile masses of vegetations (up to 30 mm wide) in the tricuspid region completely replacing tricuspid leaflet echoes (Fig. E-4). At operation, large vegetations of this size were seen on all three cusps of the tricuspid valve, which was severely destroyed and disorganized.

CONDITIONS SIMULATING TRICUSPID VEGETATIONS

1. Whereas large, pedunculated tricuspid vegetations are easy to detect, in actual practice it is often difficult to differentiate a small sessile vegetation from *nonspecific thickening* or an old, healed vegetation resulting from a previous episode of endocarditis. Recurrent attacks of bacterial endocarditis are not uncommon among intravenous drug abusers who continue their addictive practices during the intervals between the bouts of valve infection.

2. Another possible source of error is technical *artefact* that may make the tricuspid echo appear unduly thick or as consisting of multiple, parallel, linear components (Fig. E-5). Reasons

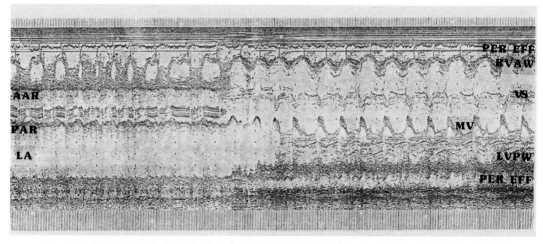

Fig. E-2. M-mode echographic scan from aortic root to LV, in a patient with pericardial effusion of moderate size. The RV outflow tract is seen in diastole only; in systole its cavity obliterates. The RV anterior wall therefore presents an unusual appearance at this level, which could be mistaken for the tricuspid valve but can be correctly identified by its continuity with the RV anterior wall at ventricular level.

for such confusing echographic appearances include the factor of beam width and the very oblique angulation "under the sternum" needed to scan the tricuspid valve from the left parasternal area.

3. Another type of artefact that could possibly be compared with tricuspid vegetations is the inadvertent microbubble effect produced by an intravenous drip (Fig. E-6).

4. In Ebstein's anomaly, the abnormal septal

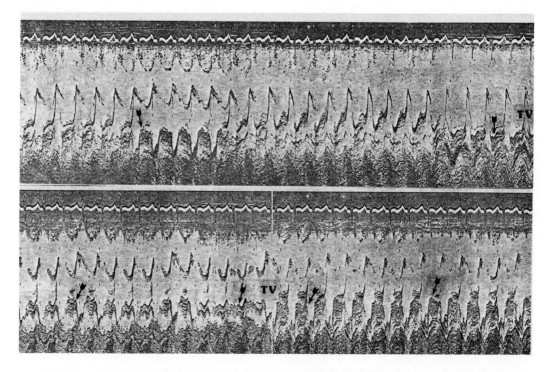

Fig. E-3. M-mode echogram in a young heroin addict with tricuspid valve endocarditis. The tricuspid valve has been visualized at slightly different transducer angulations, resulting in varying morphology of the valvular vegetation (*arrows*).

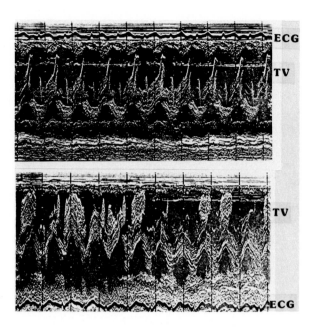

Fig. E-4. M-mode echograms of the tricuspid valve in a young heroin addict with *Streptococcus viridans* endocarditis. The upper panel shows the echogram on admission. Local cusp thickening suggestive of vegetations was noted. During the subsequent week, the infection became progressively more overwhelming and repeated pulmonary embolization occurred. The second echogram (*lower panel*), a week after the first, showed large mobile masses in the tricuspid area. Tricuspid valvectomy was successfully performed for cure of refractory endocarditis. Large vegetations (up to 2 to 3 cm in diameter) were found on all 3 tricuspid leaflets. The patient remains well 5 years later.

leaflet of the tricuspid valve is so intimately related to the ventricular septum that the echographic appearance could simulate a vegetation on this leaflet (Fig. E-7).

Fortunately, 2-D echocardiography, especially the apical four-chamber and subcostal views, permits adequate visualization of the tricuspid valve. First, vegetations or nodules on a tricuspid leaflet can be recognized with much more confidence and easily differentiated from right atrial myxoma (Come *et al.,* 1979); second, problems of artefact that beset the M-mode echographic technique are easily resolved.

How sensitive is echocardiography in diagnosing tricuspid vegetations, and is 2-D echocardiography superior to the M-mode technique in this regard? In this connection the experience of Berger *et al.* (1980) is worth noting: of 12 patients with right-heart endocarditis, 9 instances of tricuspid vegetations were visualized on 2-D echocardiography but only 6 by the M-mode technique. In the same study, follow-up echocardiograms in 7 patients after successful antibiotic therapy showed that vegetations appeared unchanged in 3, became smaller in 3, and were no longer seen in 1. In Ginzton *et al.*'s (1982) series of 16 patients with tricuspid endocarditis, all were diagnosed by 2-D echography but only 10 by the M-mode technique. Vegetations became small or disappeared in 7

of 8 patients followed by serial echocardiography.

In the relatively large series of Andy *et al.* (1977), including 20 patients with tricuspid endocarditis and regurgitation, the authors found that tricuspid vegetations tended to grow to a larger size than mitral regurgitations, but rupture of tricuspid chordae tendineae was much more difficult to diagnose than mitral chordal rupture.

TRICUSPID VALVE PROLAPSE (Fig. E-8)

Over the last decade, tricuspid valve prolapse has emerged as a definite entity, diagnosable by echocardiography and angiocardiography, but its clinical significance remains uncertain. The relationship of tricuspid prolapse to symptoms, ECG abnormalities, and arrhythmias is even more controversial than that of its mitral equivalent.

Reports of solitary cases of tricuspid valve prolapse, associated with a systolic click, murmur, or both, have appeared (Horgan *et al.,* 1975; Sasse and Froelich, 1978; Inoue *et al.,* 1979). These patients did not have mitral prolapse. It thus appears that tricuspid prolapse can, in rare instances, be responsible for auscultatory signs commonly associated in the clini-

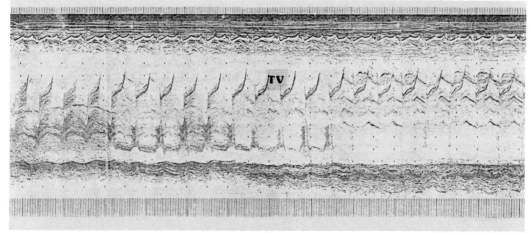

A.

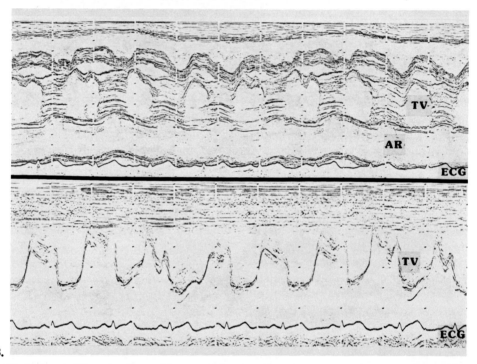

B.

Fig. E-5. *A.* M-mode echographic scan of the tricuspid valve in a normal person, demonstrating appearances that should not be mistaken for vegetations. At the left of the figure, apparent thickening of the tricuspid leaflets in systole is attributable to beam width and oblique relationship of the ultrasound beam to the apposed leaflets. In the center of the figure, the tricuspid valve appears normal. At the right of the figure, an additional echo arising from chordae is superimposed on that of the anterior tricuspid leaflet.

Fig. E-5. *B.* M-mode echogram of a patient with a history of rheumatic fever in childhood. In the upper panel (subcostal approach) the tricuspid valve exhibits multiple linear echoes in systole, which are attributable to oblique intersection of the valve leaflets by the ultrasound beam. This appearance should not be mistaken for vegetations. In the lower panel (parasternal approach) the tricuspid valve shows mild nonspecific thickening; multiple systolic echoes are not evident. Clinically there was no evidence of bacterial endocarditis.

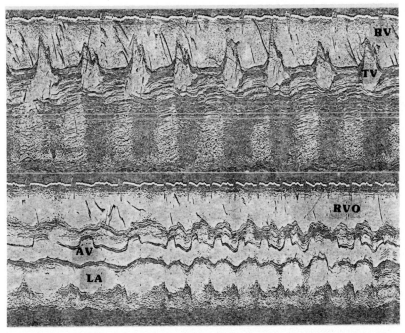

Fig. E-6. M-mode echogram in a patient with known tricuspid valve endocarditis. The multiple irregular short linear echoes near the tricuspid valve (*upper*) were thought by the cardiac fellow to be torn tricuspid chordae tendineae or mobile vegetations. This bizarre appearance was in fact caused by microbubbles caused by an intravenous antibiotic infusion the patient was receiving. The lower panel shows that the abnormal echoes were restricted to the RV outflow tract. They are not seen in the aortic root or LA.

cian's mind with mitral prolapse. The echocardiographer therefore should endeavor to seek or exclude tricuspid prolapse in patients with auscultatory evidence of Barlow's syndrome who do not show mitral prolapse.

Chandaratna *et al.* (1975) diagnosed tricuspid valve prolapse in a series of 12 patients, and Werner *et al.* (1978) in 15 patients. Both groups of authors found a very frequent association with mitral valve prolapse, which was present in 8 of 12 patients of Chandaratna, and all of Werner's 15 patients manifesting tricuspid prolapse. This is in accord with previous angiocardiographic studies (Ainsworth *et al.,* 1973). It is noteworthy that four of six patients in Werner's series with Marfan's syndrome and mitral prolapse had tricuspid prolapse; in contrast, none of 500 patients without mitral prolapse showed tricuspid prolapse. In a recent larger series (Schlamowitz *et al.,* 1982) tricuspid prolapse was found in 41 of 82 patients with mitral prolapse.

Strict echographic criteria for tricuspid prolapse have not yet been established. So-called holosystolic prolapse of the hammock or sagging contour has been described by Horgan *et al.* (1975), Chandaratna *et al.* (1975), and Werner *et al.* (1978), but it is uncertain as to whether a smooth posterior sagging of the apposed tricuspid leaflets is really an abnormal entity, and if so, what degree or amplitude of sagging or posterior bowing is to be considered pathologic. Moreover, it is possible that this sagging can be artefactually produced by certain angulations of the transducer, as may happen with the mitral valve. The diagnosis of tricuspid prolapse of the mid- to late systolic variety (Fig. E-8) is perhaps on firmer ground; the abrupt posterior motion of the posterior tricuspid leaflet during the middle third of systole constitutes a definite or even conspicuous deviation from the usual pattern (Fig. E-8). Eight of the 12 patients with tricuspid prolapse in Chandaratna's series showed this pattern.

M-mode echocardiographic appearances simulating tricuspid prolapse can occur in the following clinical situations:

1. Large pericardial effusions, wherein a pos-

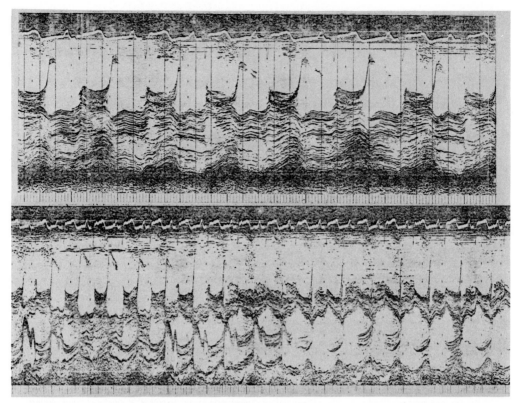

Fig. E-7. M-mode echogram, showing the tricuspid valve, in a patient with Ebstein's anomaly. At first sight the posterior (septal) tricuspid leaflet appears abnormally thickened and suggestive of a vegetation. This apparent cusp thickening is an illusion caused by the fact that this leaflet is abnormal and displaced or indistinguishable echographically from the ventricular septum itself. The lower panel shows a scan to the mid-LV (*right*).

terior systolic motion of the heart as a whole ("swinging heart") may produce tricuspid pseudoprolapse. Once the pericardial effusion subsides, the abnormal tricuspid pattern disappears.

2. Patients with dilated right ventricles, secondary to pulmonary hypertension or as part of a generalized cardiac enlargement in patients with severe cardiomyopathy or ischemic heart disease, often show a mild systolic sagging of the apposed tricuspid leaflets.

On 2-D echocardiography, tricuspid prolapse is suggested by bulging or convex contour of the tricuspid leaflets toward the right atrium during systole, above the tricuspid ring level, in the RV inflow tract (long-axis) view and apical four-chamber view (Morganroth *et al.,* 1980; Mardelli *et al.,* 1981; Schlamowitz *et al.,* 1982; Tei *et al.,* 1982).

FLAIL TRICUSPID VALVE

Flail tricuspid leaflets due to rupture of tricuspid chordae can simulate tricuspid prolapse inasmuch as abnormal systolic posterior displacement of a tricuspid leaflet may be evident in both conditions. In a patient reported by Mintz *et al.* (1978), excessive systolic separation of the anterior and posterior tricuspid leaflets was noted. In this patient as well as that of Kisslo *et al.* (1976), and of Bardy and Talano (1982), a very abnormal systolic motion of the flail leaflet or leaflets into the right atrium on 2-D echography was diagnostic of prolapse because in normal hearts and in tricuspid prolapse the free edges of the tricuspid leaflets should point in the opposite direction, i.e., into the RV. Pepper *et al.* (1980) recently have reported an instance of flail tricuspid valve in a child with a ventricular septal defect. Inadvertent recording of microbubble artefacts in patients with intravenous drips (Fig. E-6) should not be mistaken for loose chordae tendineae.

TRICUSPID VALVE FLUTTER (Fig. E-9)

Flutter of the tricuspid leaflets in *diastole* is a nonspecific finding and has been known to occur in a variety of cardiac conditions (Nanda and Gramiak, 1978). Because of its lack of specificity, flutter of the tricuspid valve is of limited diagnostic importance.

1. *Pulmonic valve incompetence.* Tricuspid flutter is not as constant an accompaniment of pulmonary regurgitation as mitral flutter is of aortic regurgitation, possibly because the regurgitant pulmonary jet is of lesser velocity and does not impinge as directly on the tricuspid cusps as the aortic jet does on the anterior mitral leaflet.

2. *Atrial septal defect.* Tricuspid flutter is believed to signify a relatively large left-to-right shunt; prominent flutter of the septal tricuspid leaflet is common in the ostium primum type of atrial septal defect (Nanda and Gramiak, 1978), as in Figure E-9.

3. *Transposition of the great vessels* after the Mustard operation or surgical creation of an atrial septal defect. Tricuspid as well as mitral flutter, in such situations, is attributable to turbulence caused by abnormal atrial patterns of blood flow (Nanda *et al.,* 1975b; Haggler *et al.,* 1975; Aziz *et al.,* 1976).

4. *Communication of sinus of Valsalva aneurysms with right atrium.* The tricuspid leaflets are agitated by torrential flow across the tricuspid valve (Weyman *et al.,* 1975).

5. *Rupture of tricuspid chordae tendineae.* This rupture tends to produce an erratic or bizarre type of tricuspid flutter, perhaps associated with vegetations because bacterial endocarditis is usually the underlying cause and the

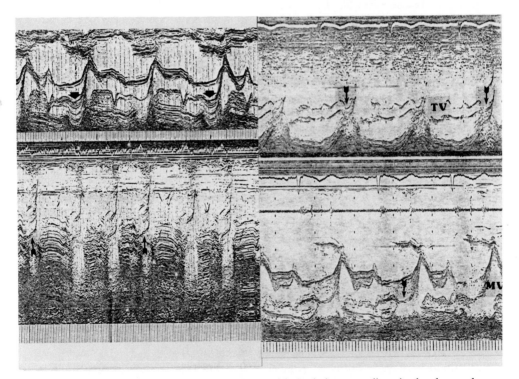

Fig. E-8. M-mode echograms of two patients with both late systolic mitral valve prolapse and late systolic tricuspid valve prolapse.

Left. M-mode echogram showing late systolic mitral prolapse (*arrows*) in the upper panel, and late systolic tricuspid prolapse (*arrows*) in the lower panel.

Right. M-mode echogram of a young woman with a mid-systolic click. Both the tricuspid valve (*upper panel*) and mitral valve (*lower panel*) show late systolic prolapse.

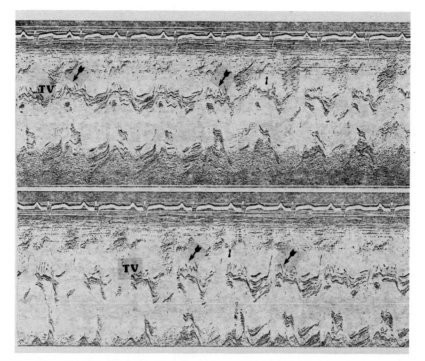

Fig. E-9. M-mode echogram of a 15-year-old boy with Down's syndrome and an endocardial cushion defect of incomplete type. Diastolic flutter of the septal leaflet of the tricuspid valve is revealed.

patient a drug addict (Chandaratna and Aronow, 1979).

Atrial flutter may be associated with regular diastolic deflections and atrial fibrillation with less regular and smaller undulations of the tricuspid leaflets, but these are qualitatively different from rapid vibratory motion of flutter. Electrocardiographic depiction of the abnormal atrial rhythm confirms the nature of the tricuspid undulations.

Flutter of tricuspid leaflets in *systole* is rare but has been noted in only a very few uncommon conditions and is therefore of some diagnostic value.

1. Nanda *et al.* (1975a) reported high-frequency low-amplitude vibration of the tricuspid valve in systole in two patients with congenital *left ventricle–right atrial communication*. The authors attributed tricuspid flutter to passage of the left ventricular jet of blood into the right atrium through a defect in the tricuspid valve, the margins of which are fibrotic and fused to the margins of the defect in the membranous ventricular septum. In both cases, the clinical presentation was that of an uncomplicated ven-

tricular septal defect; tricuspid flutter was the only clue to the unusual nature of the septal defect. Two further instances of systolic tricuspid flutter in this type of septal defect were reported by Mills *et al.* (1977). Bourgin *et al.* (1980) have also confirmed this finding in a series of ten patients with this unusual anomaly.

2. Recently Alam *et al.* (1980) demonstrated systolic tricuspid flutter in four patients with *ventricular septal defects;* they explained the flutter "on the basis of the tricuspid leaflets lying in the turbulent stream of blood flowing through a high ventricular septal defect." The incidence of systolic tricuspid flutter in uncomplicated ventricular septal defects of the usual type is unknown.

3. Snider *et al.* (1979) described peculiar fluttering, linear, curved echoes in systole, appearing just anterior to the tricuspid valve, in nine children with *aneurysms of the ventricular septum* confirmed by angiography. The aneurysms could be visualized by 2-D echocardiography in the long-axis and apical four-chamber views. It is probable that such septal aneurysms represented a transitional stage leading eventually to spontaneous closure of ventricular septal defects, explaining perhaps why the entity has not yet been reported in adults.

4. Systolic tricuspid flutter also can occur if a *tricuspid leaflet is flail* secondary to a destructive endocarditis (Kisslo *et al.,* 1976).

In conclusion, it appears that systolic flutter of the tricuspid valve is not entirely specific for any particular anatomic defect, but its presence should direct the echocardiographer's attention not only to the tricuspid valve itself but also to the region of the membranous ventricular septum, which should be closely examined by 2-D echocardiography in all possible views.

TRICUSPID REGURGITATION

Tricuspid regurgitation is probably the most common type of right ventricular volume overload in adult practice, often associated with generalized cardiac dilatation and congestive failure as in cardiomyopathy or coronary disease. However, in such cases, the echographic picture is dominated by the left ventricular dilatation, and there is little doubt that the primary important pathology is in the left heart.

Tricuspid regurgitation, presenting with right ventricular dilatation and a normal to small left ventricle can be due to:

1. *Severe pulmonary hypertension,* secondary to cor pulmonale, Eisenmenger's syndrome, primary pulmonary hypertension or severe mitral stenosis (possibly "silent" in the sense that the diastolic murmur is absent or very localized or soft), or cor triatriatum.

2. *Malformations of the right heart* such as Ebstein's anomaly of the tricuspid valve or the much rarer Uhl's anomaly wherein the right ventricular wall is thin, devoid of myocardium and contractile power.

3. *Tricuspid valve destruction* by bacterial endocarditis, usually in drug addicts.

Of these several entities causing tricuspid incompetence, some are eminently detectable by echocardiography, although hemodynamic studies are needed to establish a definitive diagnosis:

1. Mitral stenosis;
2. Vegetations on the tricuspid leaflets;
3. Tumor masses in the right heart;
4. Ebstein's anomaly;

5. Tricuspid valve prolapse.

On the M-mode echocardiogram, tricuspid regurgitation manifests RV dilatation and paradoxic (anterior) systolic motion of the ventricular septum. These features are not specific and occur with other forms of RV overload such as atrial septal defect. Nevertheless, the echographic demonstration of RV enlargement and abnormal septal motion has been useful in suggesting damage to the tricuspid apparatus, leading eventually to remedial surgery. Under such circumstances the diagnosis of tricuspid regurgitation has been correctly made (Mary *et al.,* 1973), even when the diagnosis is not obvious on other clinical grounds (Kessler *et al.,* 1976).

More subtle M-mode signs such as a fine rapid flutter or erratic "notching" on tricuspid leaflet contour in diastole may strengthen the case for traumatic tricuspid regurgitation as in the patient of Bardy *et al.* (1979). These authors also noted abnormal motion of the anterior tricuspid leaflet, especially a posterior movement toward the right atrium in systole, suggestive of a flail tricuspid cusp. Avulsion of the anterior papillary muscle in the RV was found at surgery.

Two-D echocardiography, using contrast methods involving dye or saline injection into an antecubital vein to opacify the right-heart chambers, has an important role to play in the demonstration of tricuspid regurgitation (Lieppe *et al.,* 1978), as follows:

1. Scanning in the xiphisternal or epigastric region, in the sagittal plane, the probe is inclined to the right to visualize the right atrium and inferior vena cava entering it, the latter as an echo-free cylindric space behind the left lobe of the liver, widening into the larger spherical cavity of the right atrium.

2. Saline or green dye is injected into an antecubital vein.

3. A few seconds later, microbubbles appear in the right atrium, but normally never in the inferior vena cava. Such microbubbles, moving rapidly and swirling as an aggregation of stippled echoes, are soon washed out by unopacified blood entering the right atrium.

In the presence of severe tricuspid regurgitation, microbubbles regurgitate into the inferior vena cava or even hepatic veins in systole and for the space of a few seconds ebb and flow within these vessels (Fig. E-10). Moreover, the right-heart chambers do not empty of micro-bubbles for an unduly long period because in severe tricuspid incompetence a considerable amount of blood moves back and forth between right ventricle and atrium, while relatively little moves forward into the pulmonary circulation. Chen et al. (1980) required the presence of microbubbles in both the inferior vena cava and the hepatic veins for at least three consecutive cardiac cycles to establish a diagnosis of tricuspid regurgitation. Close observation of the pattern of linear reflux contrast echo lines in the right atrium, and in the inferior vena cava and hepatic vein, on the M-mode tracing (obtained by cursors on the 2-D echogram) enhances the diagnostic potential of contrast echography in tricuspid regurgitation (Tei et al., 1982).

Caution: Contrast can appear in the inferior vena cava in the absence of tricuspid regurgitation if the patient is breathing or in the left lateral position; it can also appear during certain arrhythmias. Tricuspid regurgitation can be diagnosed reliably only if (1) contrast appears only in systole, (2) the patient is lying flat, and (3) the patient has held his breath.

The scope for this rapid bedside means of confirming or excluding the diagnosis of tricuspid regurgitation is considerable, especially since physical signs of this valve lesion may be equivocal, and even cardiac catheterization and angiocardiography have shortcomings, such as the possibility that the catheter itself is producing an artefactual incompetence of the valve. In patients with tricuspid regurgitation secondary to carcinoid heart disease, the tricuspid leaflets appeared abnormally rigid and stumplike in the four-chamber view on 2-D echography (Baker et al., 1981; Howard et al., 1982; Callahan et al., 1982).

TRICUSPID STENOSIS

Like mitral stenosis, stenosis of the tricuspid valve presents with a thickened anterior mitral leaflet that exhibits a flat EF slope and diminished anterior diastolic excursion (Edler et al., 1961; Joyner and Reid, 1963; Joyner et al., 1967). In most cases, typical findings of mitral stenosis are also present.

As with mitral stenosis, the posterior tricuspid leaflet is believed to move abnormally (anteriorly) during diastole in tricuspid stenosis, but in actual practice it is difficult to visualize adequately.

A low or flat tricuspid EF slope is not conclusive evidence of tricuspid valve stenosis because it has been reported in patients with diminished right ventricular compliance of various etiologies such as severe pulmonic stenosis, Bernheim's syndrome, and so forth (Gramiak and Shah, 1971; Feigenbaum 1976).

On the other hand, normal tricuspid diastolic motion of the usual M-shaped configuration is very helpful in excluding tricuspid stenosis, should this diagnosis be considered as a possibility for one reason or another in patients with mitral valve disease.

Unlike stenotic mitral valves, stenotic tricuspid valves are seldom if ever heavily calcified. Although slightly thicker and denser than normal, tricuspid leaflets do not exhibit the massive calcific deposits sometimes encountered in rheumatic mitral valves.

A rheumatic etiology is presumed in tricuspid stenosis presenting in adults, unless proven otherwise. At least one report of tricuspid and mitral stenosis secondary to Loeffler's endocarditis, diagnosed echocardiographically and successfully operated upon, has appeared (Weyman et al., 1977).

Fig. E-10. *A.* M-mode echogram of a patient with severe cor pulmonale, tricuspid regurgitation, and florid right heart failure. The RV is extremely dilated and larger than the LV, at both mitral valve and chordae levels. The ventricular septum shows paradoxical septal motion, attributable to tricuspid regurgitation.

Fig. E-10. *B.* 2-D echogram of the same patient, by the subcostal approach in a parasagittal plane, showing the liver, and the inferior vena cava (IVC) entering the RA. The top left frame is just before the injection of contrast. Microbubbles are seen in the RA (*top center*) and then in the IVC (*top right*). The three lower frames, in a slightly different plane, show the right superior hepatic vein joining the IVC, which in turn enters the RA. Note that the microbubbles from the RA regurgitate into the IVC as well as the hepatic vein, confirming the presence of tricuspid regurgitation.

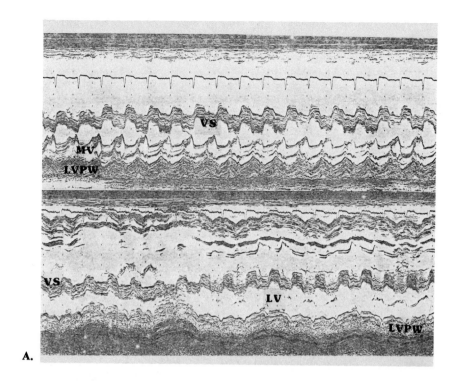

A.

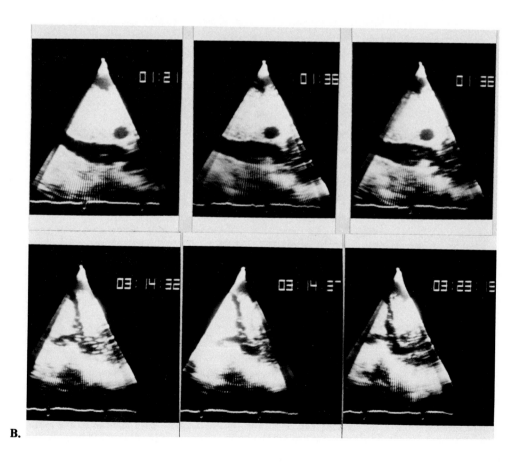

B.

A thickened anterior tricuspid leaflet with flat EF slope can be mimicked by a Swan-Ganz catheter or pacemaker wire within the right ventricle (Fig. E-11). Echoes emanating from such objects are denser and more evocative of intense reverberations than normal or even thickened tricuspid leaflets. In fact, the gain setting suitable for recording the catheter echoes is often too low to obtain tricuspid leaflet echoes, which are therefore easily overlooked, thus contributing to the fallacy of mistaking catheter or pacemaker wire for tricuspid valve echoes.

Swan-Ganz catheter or pacemaker wire echoes can be recognized (and distinguished from tricuspid valve echoes) by:

1. Their dense nature;

2. Frequently dense, parallel reverberations posterior to the main linear echo;

3. The knowledge of a catheter or pacemaker lying in the right ventricle. If the catheter is withdrawn from the right heart, the abnormal echoes abruptly disappear, and reappear if the catheter is reintroduced into the right ventricular chamber.

4. Careful scanning and gain adjustment can reveal the true tricuspid cusp echoes with normal M-shaped contour, which are obviously different from (though perhaps superimposed on) the denser, more rectangular ones of the catheter.

5. The right atrial segment of the catheter or wire may be seen as a dense, thick, linear echo between the tricuspid valve and right atrial posterior wall.

6. The right ventricular outflow segment may likewise appear between aortic root and right ventricular anterior wall.

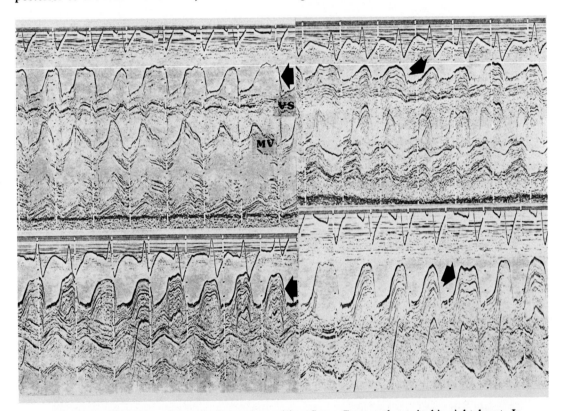

Fig. E-11. M-mode echogram of a patient with a Swan-Ganz catheter in his right heart. In the upper right panel, the catheter echoes tend to merge with the septal echo at times, making the septum appear thicker than it really is. In the lower right panel, the catheter motion resembles that of the tricuspid valve, and reverberations immediately behind the main echo mimic a right atrial myxoma.

In the upper left panel, Swan-Ganz catheter echoes mimic those of a stenotic tricuspid valve. In the lower left panel, the catheter can be seen in the RV outflow tract anterior to the aortic root. Catheter reverberations are particularly numerous and dense, possibly simulating an RV mass.

On 2-D echography, stenotic tricuspid valves exhibit a typical pattern of diastolic doming and restricted motion (Daniels *et al.,* 1983; Nanna *et al.,* 1983).

INTRACARDIAC CATHETERS AND PACEMAKER WIRES (Figs. E-11 to E-14)

A Swan-Ganz flotation catheter passes successively through the right atrium, tricuspid valve, RV body (inflow region), RV outflow tract, pulmonary trunk, and right or left pulmonary artery. It can be visualized therefore echocardiographically in several anatomic locations or relationships:

1. Posterior to tricuspid valve echo (in right atrium);

2. Between anterior and posterior tricuspid leaflets (within tricuspid orifice);

3. Within RV chamber at LV chordae tendineae level (RV body);

4. Anterior to aortic root (RV outflow tract);

5. Anterior to atriopulmonary sulcus, in usual site of pulmonic valve (within pulmonary trunk);

6. Within right pulmonary artery, as viewed by suprasternal scanning.

Pacemaker wires are similar to Swan-Ganz catheters in caliber and ultrasound-reflecting properties, as well as in anatomic location insofar as they lie within the right atrium, tricuspid valve, and RV body. In addition, a pacemaker wire placed in the coronary sinus can be recorded on the M-mode echocardiogram as a low-amplitude, undulating, dense, linear echo posterior to the tricuspid valve (Reeves *et al.,* 1978).

In actual practice, however, Swan-Ganz catheters and pacemaker wires may appear on the M-mode tracing in only some or even none of these locations, since they are rather slender sinous structures that may elude the ultrasound beam. On the other hand, as good reflectors of ultrasound, Swan-Ganz catheters and pacemaker wires are capable of producing not only dense, sharp echoes but also echo reverberations that can potentially simulate a large variety of normal and abnormal cardiac structures (Charuzi *et al.,* 1977; Reeves *et al.,* 1978):

1. The anterior tricuspid leaflet catheter or pacemaker wire echoes often tend to form rect-

angular contours with low or flat diastolic slopes, simulating *tricuspid stenosis.*

2. *Right atrial myxoma.* This effect is caused by multiple parallel reverberations of the catheter or pacemaker wire. Such reverberatory echoes are evident throughout the cardiac cycle, whereas actual myxomas would appear as multilayered echoes behind the anterior tricuspid leaflet echo in diastole only. Such examples have been described also by Kendrick *et al.* (1977) and Yarnal and Smiley (1978).

3. *Right ventricular anterior wall.* If the catheter or pacemaker in the RV has only a small amplitude of motion, it could be mistaken for the RV wall, if the true RV wall echoes are not recorded because of oversuppression of near gain. In this case, the RV space anterior to the catheter echo could be mislabeled an anterior pericardial effusion.

4. *Anterior aortic root.* If the thick, linear catheter echo in the RV outflow tract moves parallel to the true anterior aortic root echo, it may be mistaken for the latter. Thus the aortic root may be thought dilated when it is not, and the space between catheter and anterior aortic root be misdiagnosed as a false lumen of aortic dissection.

5. *Pulmonic valve.* Catheter motion can occasionally mimic that of the posterior cusp of the pulmonic valve. Since catheter motion contour tends to be rectangular with no "a" dip, the erroneous diagnosis of pulmonary hypertension could be made.

6. Right border of the *ventricular septum.* The septum therefore appears thicker than it really is, leading to the false diagnosis of asymmetric septal hypertrophy (ASH) (Fig. E-12).

7. Occasionally, the reverberations of a catheter or pacemaker wire in the RV can appear in the LV chamber. If not recognized for what they are, they possibly could be taken for *LV mural thrombi, mitral valve vegetations, or mitral annulus calcification.*

The distinctive strong nature of the echoes produced by Swan-Ganz catheters can be turned to the clinician's advantage by using echocardiography to guide the passage of such a catheter into position in the pulmonary artery (Kasper *et al.,* 1980). These authors showed that M-mode scanning from parasternal, subxiphoid (Fig. E-13), and suprasternal sites can be useful in ascertaining catheter position. In

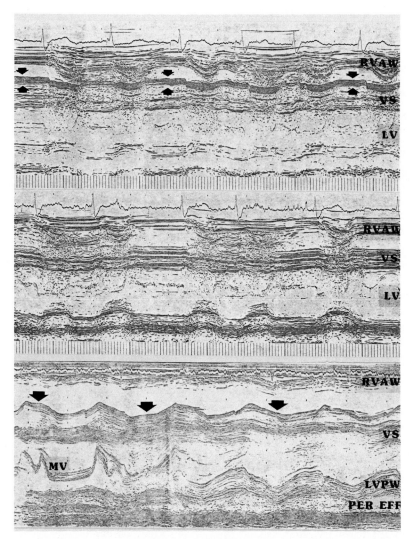

Fig. E-12. Pacemaker wire in RV simulating increased septal thickness in two different patients:
   Upper and center. M-mode echogram of a patient with a permanent endocardial pacemaker in the RV. The pacemaker wire can be recognized as a dense bandlike echo (*arrows*) in the RV (*upper panel*). However, because of its localized nature, it is no longer visible after a small change in transducer direction (*center panel*).
   Lower. M-mode echogram revealing a pacemaker wire (*arrows*) within the RV chamber. In the center of the figure this abnormal echo tends to merge with the septal echo, and could therefore lead to a false impression that the septum is hypertrophied, if this were the only segment available. Elsewhere in the tracing it could be mistaken for part of the tricuspid apparatus.

particular, they demonstrated that the Swan-Ganz catheter can be visualized in the right pulmonary artery by the suprasternal approach as a linear echo with a typical pattern of motion, which becomes rather damped as the balloon is inflated (Kasper *et al.,* 1980).

The simultaneous use of M-mode echocardiography and phonocardiography has elucidated the mechanism of systolic clicks in a patient with a Swan-Ganz catheter (Isner *et al.,* 1979). Nanda and Barold (1982), Drinkovic (1981), and Meier and Felner (1982) have recently described how 2-D echography can be used to confirm normal position or to diagnose dislodgement or perforation of the pacemaker wire through the RV wall or septum; the path of

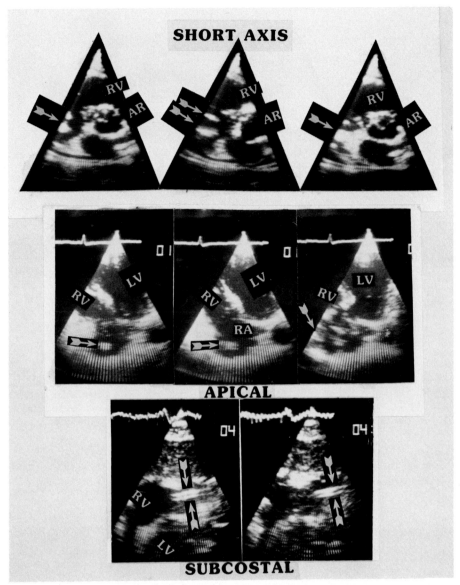

SHORT AXIS

APICAL

SUBCOSTAL

Fig. E-13. Echographic visualization of Swan-Ganz catheter or pacemaker wire in the right heart in 3 different patients.

Upper. 2-D echograms in the short-axis view of a patient with a Swan-Ganz catheter in the right heart chambers. The aortic root is visualized in the center of the field, with the LA posterior to it and the RA to its right. The catheter (*arrows*) has probably formed a loop in the RA because it is seen as two discrete dense small echoes in the left and middle frames. In the right frame, the catheter echoes appear larger and more complex, simulating a right atrial mass.

Center. 2-D echogram in the apical 4-chamber view in a patient with a large apicoseptal ventricular aneurysm and a Swan-Ganz catheter in place. The LV apex appears dilated with the adjacent septum deviated toward the RV. The catheter (*arrows*) appears as a single dense small echo in the RA, in the left and middle frames. In the right frame, the catheter has produced multiple echoes, extending into the RV.

Lower. Subcostal 2-D echogram showing the RV chamber. The pacemaker wire appears as a double linear dense echo (*arrows*) within the RV, directed toward the RV apex. The image has been expanded so that the LV is not completely visible.

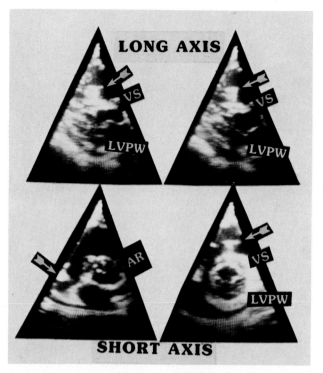

Fig. E-14. 2-D echogram of a patient with a Swan-Ganz catheter in place in the right heart chambers. The upper frames (long axis) show the catheter echo as a dense echo in the RV adjacent to the ventricular septum. The left lower frame (short axis) shows the catheter echo in the RA near the atrial septum. In the right lower frame (short axis) the catheter echo appears in the RA as well as anteriorly in the RV just in front of the septum.

the wire through these myocardial structures could be visualized clearly, especially in the subcostal view.

REFERENCES

TRICUSPID VALVE ENDOCARDITIS

Andy, J. J.; Sheik, H. M. U.; Ali, N.; *et al.:* Echocardiographic observations in opiate addicts with active infective endocarditis. *Am. J. Cardiol.,* 40:17, 1977.

Berger, M.; Delfin, L. A.; Jelveh, M.; *et al.:* Two-dimensional echocardiographic findings in right sided infective endocarditis. *Circulation,* 61:855, 1980.

Chandaratna, P. A. N., and Aronow, W. S.: Spectrum of echocardiographic findings in tricuspid valve endocarditis. *Br. Heart J.,* 42:528, 1979.

Come, P. C.; Kurland, G. S.; and Vine, H. S.: Two-dimensional echocardiography in differentiating right atrial and tricuspid valve mass lesions. *Am. J. Cardiol.,* 44:1207, 1979.

Crawford, F. A.; Wechsler, A. S.; and Kisslo, J. A.: Tricuspid endocarditis in a drug addict: detection of tricuspid vegetations by two-dimensional echocardiography. *Chest,* 74:473, 1978.

Dillon, J. C.: Endocardiography in valvular vegetations. *Am. J. Med.,* 62:856, 1977.

Gilbert, B. W.; Haney, R. S.; Crawford, F., *et al.:* Two-dimensional echocardiographic assessment of vegetative endocarditis. *Circulation,* 55:346, 1977.

Ginzton, L. E.; Siegel, R. J.; and Criley, J. M.: Natural history of tricuspid valve endocarditis: A two-dimensional echocardiographic study. *Am. J. Cardiol.,* 49:1853, 1982.

Kisslo, J.; van Ramm, O. T.; Haney, R.; *et al.:* Echocardiographic evaluation of tricuspid valve endocarditis. *Am. J. Cardiol.,* 38:502, 1976.

Lee, C. C.; Ganguly, S. N.; Magnisalis, K.; *et al.:* Detection of tricuspid valve vegetations by echocardiography. *Chest,* 66:432, 1974.

Thomson, K. E.; Nanda, N. C.; and Gramiak, R.: The reliability of echocardiography in the diagnosis of infective endocarditis. *Radiology,* 125:473, 1977.

Wann, L. S.; Dillon, J. C.; and Weyman, A. E.: Echocardiography in bacterial endocarditis. *N. Engl. J. Med.,* 295:135, 1976.

TRICUSPID VALVE PROLAPSE

Ainsworth, R. P.; Hartman, A. F.; Aker, U.; *et al.:* Tricuspid valve prolapse with late systolic tricuspid insufficiency. *Radiology,* 107:309, 1973.

Baker, B. J.; McNee, V. D.; Scovil, J. A.; *et al.:* Tricuspid insufficiency in carcinoid heart disease: an echocardiographic description. *Am. Heart J.,* 101:107, 1981.

Chandaratna, P. A. N.; Lopez, J. M.; Fernandez, J. J.; *et al.:* Diagnosis of tricuspid valve prolapse by echocardiography. *J.C.U.,* 2:225, 1974.

Chandaratna, P. A. N.; Lopez, J. M.; Fernandez, J. J.; *et al.:* Echocardiographic detection of tricuspid valve prolapse. *Circulation,* 51:823, 1975.

Chandaratna, P. A. N.; Littman, B. B.; and Wilson, D.: The association between atrial septal defect and prolapse of the tricuspid valve. *Chest*, **73**:839, 1978.

Horgan, J. H.; Beachley, M. C.; and Robinson, F. D.: Tricuspid valve prolapse diagnosed by echocardiogram. *Chest*, **68**:822, 1975.

Inoue, D.; Furukawa, K.; Matsukubo, H.; *et al.:* Subxiphoid two-dimensional echocardiographic detection of tricuspid valve prolapse. *Chest*, **76**:693, 1979.

Maranhao, V.; Gooch, A. S.; Yang, S. S.; *et al.:* Prolapse of the tricuspid leaflets in the systolic murmur-click syndrome. *Cathet. Cardiovasc. Diagn.*, **1**:81, 1975.

Mardelli, T. J.; Morganroth, J.; Chen, C. C.; *et al.:* Tricuspid valve prolapse diagnosed by cross-sectional echocardiography. *Chest*, **79**:201, 1981.

Morganroth, J.; Jones, R. H.; Chen, C. C.; *et al.:* Two-dimensional echocardiography in mitral aortic and tricuspid valve prolapse. *Am. J. Cardiol.*, **46**:1164, 1980.

Nanda, N. C.; Gramiak, R. G.; and Gross, C.: Echocardiography of cardiac valves in pericardial effusion. *Circulation*, **54**:500, 1976.

Sasse, L., and Froelich, C. R.: Echocardiographic tricuspid prolapse and nonejection systolic click. *Chest*, **73**:869, 1978.

Schlamowitz, R. A.; Gross, S.; Keating, E.; *et al.:* Tricuspid valve prolapse: A common occurence in the click-murmur syndrome. *J. C. U.*, **10**:435, 1982.

Tei, C.; Shah, P. M.; Cherian, G.; *et al.:* Tricuspid valve prolapse: A two-dimensional echographic study of annular and leaflet abnormalities. *Circulation*, **49**:1009, 1982 (Abstr.).

Werner, J. A.; Schiller, N. B.; and Prasquier, R.: Occurrence and significance of echocardiographically demonstrated tricuspid valve prolapse. *Am. Heart J.*, **96**:180, 1978.

FLAIL TRICUSPID VALVE

Bardy, G. H., and Talano, J. V.: Right ventricular failure in a young man after chest trauma. *Arch. Intern. Med.*, **142**:615, 1982.

Kisslo, J.; von Ramm, O. T.; and Thurstone, F. L.: Cardiac imaging using a phased-array ultrasound system. II. Clinical technique and application. *Circulation*, **53**:262, 1976.

Mintz, G. S.; Kotler, M. N.; Segal, B. L.; *et al.:* Two-dimensional echocardiographic recognition of ruptured chordae tendineae. *Circulation*, **57**:244, 1978.

Pepper, J. R.; Joseph, M. C.; and Deverall, P. B.: Severe heart failure in child with ventricular septal defect and acute tricuspid regurgitation. *Br. Heart J.*, **43**:700, 1980.

TRICUSPID VALVE FLUTTER

Alam, M.; Folger, G. M.; and Goldstein, S.: Tricuspid valve fluttering. Echocardiographic features of ventricular septal defect. *Chest*, **77**:517, 1980.

Aziz, K. U.; Paul, M. H.; and Muster, A. J.: Echocardiographic localization of interatrial baffle after Mustard operation for dextro-transposition of the great arteries. *Am. J. Cardiol.*, **38**:67, 1976.

Bourgin, J. H.; Rey, C.; Piot, C., *et al.:* Apport de l'echocardiographie au diagnostic des communications ventricule gauche-oreillette droite. A propos de 10 observations. *Arch. Mal. Coeur*, **73**:438, 1980.

Chandaratna, P. A. N., and Aronow, W. E.: Spectrum of echocardiographic findings in tricuspid valve endocarditis. *Br. Heart J.*, **42**:528, 1979.

Haggler, D. J.; Tajik, A. J.; and Ritter, D. G.: Flutter of atrio-ventricular valves in patients with *d*-transposition

of the great arteries after Mustard operation. *Mayo Clin. Proc.*, **50**:69, 1975.

Mills, P.; McLaurin, L.; Smith, C.; *et al.:* Echocardiographic findings in left ventricular to right atrial shunts. *Br. Heart J.*, **39**:594, 1977.

Nanda, N. C., and Gramiak, R.: *Clinical Echocardiography.* C. V. Mosby, St. Louis, 1978, p. 213.

Nanda, N. C.; Gramiak, R.; and Manning, J. A.: Echocardiography of the tricuspid valve in congenital left ventricular-right atrial communication. *Circulation*, **51**:268, 1975a.

Nanda, N. C.; Stewart, S.; Gramiak, R.; *et al.:* Echocardiography of the intra-atrial baffle in dextro-transposition of the great vessels. *Circulation*, **51**:1130, 1975b.

Snider, A. R.; Silberman, N. H.; Schiller, N. B.; *et al.:* Echocardiographic evaluation of ventricular septal aneurysms. *Circulation*, **59**:920, 1979.

Weyman, A. E.; Dillon, J. C.; Feigenbaum, H.; *et al.:* Premature pulmonic valve opening following sinus of Valsalva aneurysm rupture into the right atrium. *Circulation*, **51**:556, 1975.

TRICUSPID REGURGITATION

Bardy, G. H.; Talano, J. V.; Meyers, S.; *et al.:* Acquired cyanotic heart disease secondary to traumatic tricuspid regurgitation. Case report with a review of the literature. *Am. J. Cardiol.*, **44**:491, 1979.

Callahan, J. A.; Wroblewski, E. M.; Reeder, G. S.; *et al.:* Echocardiographic features of carcinoid heart disease. *Am. J. Cardiol.*, **50**:762, 1982.

Chen, C. C.; Morganroth, J.; Mardelli, T. J.; *et al.:* Tricuspid regurgitation in tricuspid valve prolapse demonstrated with contrast cross-sectional echocardiography. *Am. J. Cardiol.*, **46**:983, 1980.

Howard, R. J.; Drobac, M.; Rider, W. D.; *et al.:* Carcinoid heart disease: Diagnosis by two-dimensional echocardiography. *Circulation*, **66**:1059, 1982.

Kessler, K. M.; Foianini, J. E.; Davia, J. E.; *et al.:* Tricuspid insufficiency due to nonpenetrating trauma. *Am. J. Cardiol.*, **37**:442, 1976.

Lieppe, W.; Behar, V. S.; Scallion, R.; and Kisslo, J. A.: Detection of tricuspid regurgitation with two-dimensional echocardiography and peripheral vein injections. *Circulation*, **57**:128, 1978.

Mary, D. A.; Day, J. B.; Pakrashi, B. C.; *et al.:* Tricuspid insufficiency after penetrating trauma. *Am. J. Cardiol.*, **31**:792, 1973.

Seides, S. F.: Echocardiographic findings in isolated surgically created tricuspid insufficiency. *Am. J. Cardiol.*, **47**:597, 1973.

Tei, C.; Shah, P. M.; and Ormiston, J. A.: Assessment of tricuspid regurgitation by directional analysis of right atrial systolic linear reflex echoes with contrast M-mode echocardiography. *Am. Heart J.*, **103**:1025, 1982.

TRICUSPID STENOSIS

Daniels, S. J.; Mintz, G. S.; and Kotler, M. N.: Rheumatoid tricuspid valve disease: Two-dimensional echocardiographic, hemodynamic and angiographic correlations. *Am. J. Cardiol.*, **51**:492, 1983.

Edler, I.; Gustafson, A.; Karlefors, T.; *et al.:* Ultrasound cardiography. *Acta Med. Scand. (Suppl.)*, **379**:68, 1961.

Feigenbaum, H.: *Echocardiography*, 2nd ed. Lea & Febiger, Philadelphia, 1976, p. 169.

Gramiak, R., and Shah, P. M.: Cardiac ultrasonography: A review of current applications. *Radiol. Clin. North Am.*, **9**:469, 1971.

Joyner, C. R., and Reid, J. M.: Applications of ultrasound in cardiology and cardiovascular physiology. *Prog. Cardiovasc. Dis.,* **5**:482, 1963.

Joyner, C. R.; Hey, E. B.; Johnson, J.; and Reid, J. M.: Reflected ultrasound in the diagnosis of tricuspid stenosis. *Am. J. Cardiol.,* **19**:66, 1967.

Nanna, M.; Chandaratna, P. A.; Reid, C.; *et al.:* Value of two-dimensional echocardiography in detecting tricuspid stenosis. *Circulation,* **67**:221, 1983.

Weyman, A. E.; Rankin, R.; and King, H.: Loeffler's endocarditis presenting as mitral and tricuspid stenosis. *Am. J. Cardiol.,* **40**:438, 1977.

CATHETERS AND PACEMAKER WIRES IN THE RIGHT HEART

Charuzi, Y.; Kraus, R.; and Swan, H. J. C.: Echocardiographic interpretation in the presence of Swan-Ganz intracardiac catheters. *Am. J. Cardiol.,* **40**:989, 1977.

Drinkovic, N.: Subcostal echocardiography to determine right ventricular pacing catheter position and control advancement of electrode catheters in intracardiac electrophysiologic studies. *Am. J. Cardiol.,* **47**:1260, 1981.

Isner, J. M.; Horton, J.; and Ronan, J. A.: Systolic click from a Swan-Ganz catheter: Phonoechocardiographic depiction of the underlying mechanism. *Am. J. Cardiol.,* **43**:1046, 1979.

Kasper, W.; Meinertz, T.; and Kerstin, F.: Echocardiographic control of Swan-Ganz catheters. *Chest,* **77**:380, 1980.

Kendrik, M. H.; Harrington, J. J.; Sharma, G. V. R. K.; *et al.:* Ventricular pacemaker wire simulating a right atrial mass. *Chest,* **72**:649, 1977.

Meier, B., and Felner, J. M.: Two-dimensional echocardiographic evaluation of intracardiac pacemaker leads. *J. C. U.,* **10**:421, 1982.

Nanda, N. C., and Barold, S. S.: Usefulness of echocardiography in cardiac pacing. *Pace,* **5**:22, 1982.

Reeves, W. C.; Nanda, N. C.; and Barold, S. S.: Echocardiographic evaluation of intracardiac pacing catheters: M-mode and two-dimensional studies. *Circulation,* **58**:1049, 1978.

Yarnal, J. R., and Smiley, W. H.: Right atrial mass simulated echocardiographically by a Swan-Ganz catheter. Letter to Editor. *Chest,* **74**:478, 1978.

F

The Pulmonic Valve

Unlike the other three cardiac valves, the pulmonic valve is only visible in part by reflected ultrasound; nor can its orifice be defined or measured on the M-mode tracing. Only one of the three semilunar cusps (the posterior one) usually is visualized; at best its motion is recorded through the whole cardiac cycle, but more often it is only in late diastole and early systole that the cusp motion is glimpsed. From fragmentary evidence of this nature a surprising amount of information has been obtained, and surmises can be made about the presence or absence of pulmonary hypertension, pulmonary stenosis, and certain other aspects of right heart pathology (Weyman, 1977; Heger and Weyman, 1979; Lew and Karliner, 1979).

Visualization of the pulmonic valve (Gramiak et al., 1972) requires oblique angulation of the transducer from the left sternal border superiorly and to the left (toward the left shoulder). The best method to follow is to (1) first visualize the aortic root from as high an intercostal space in the left parasternal region as possible; (2) then gradually angle the transducer in the direction of the left shoulder until the parallel echoes of the anterior and posterior aortic root merge into a thick amorphous band or echoes, called the atriopulmonary sulcus by Gramiak et al. (1972); (3) anterior to the atriopulmonary sulcus a wide echo-free space is evident within which a linear echo with a characteristic pattern of motion may be apparent. If not seen initially, it should come into view after slight exploratory alterations of transducer direction. This is the posterior cusp of the pulmonic valve.

An attempt should be made to record the pulmonic valve echo continuously through both systole and diastole. This is often possible in young children and patients with very enlarged hearts. However, in patients with hearts of normal size, it is common to see the valve only in the latter portion of diastole and the beginning of systole.

When the pulmonary artery is markedly dilated and its pulsation palpable in the second left intercostal space, it may be possible to obtain a pulmonary valve echo by holding the transducer perpendicularly over this location. In such circumstances, the anterior pulmonic cusp may also come into view.

In elderly patients, those with pulmonary emphysema, obesity, or large anteroposterior thoracic diameters, it is the exception rather than the rule to record satisfactory pulmonic valve echoes, unless the heart is dilated.

NORMAL PULMONIC VALVE MOTION (Figs. F-1 to F-4)

The normal pattern of pulmonic valve motion is as shown in Figure F-1. Although various points on it have been given alphabetical designations and a range of normal values for the slopes of certain segments have been established, these are not widely used in the actual practice of clinical echocardiography.

The only features of pulmonic valve motion found to be of real diagnostic importance are the "a" wave and the systolic contour during right ventricular ejection.

The "a" wave follows the onset of the P wave on the ECG by 72 to 130 msec and has a duration of 120 to 200 msec (Hada et al., 1977b). Its maximal amplitude is normally 2 to 7 mm. However, the depth of the "a" wave varies considerably with (1) the phase of respiration: maximum during inspiration and minimum during expiration; (2) the length of diastole: the longer the diastolic period, the deeper the "a" wave;

PULMONIC VALVE: M MODE PATTERNS

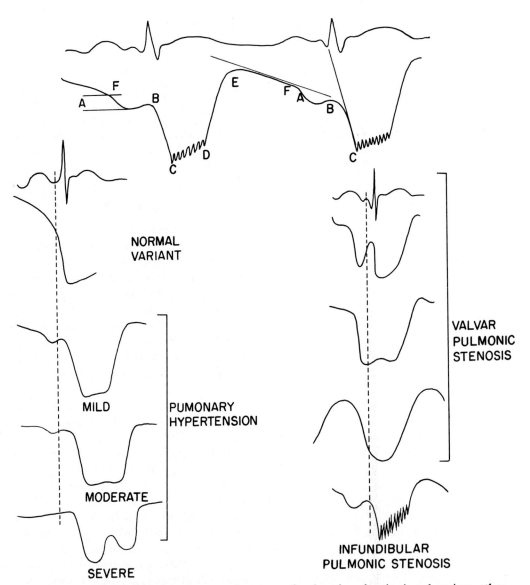

Fig. F-1. Diagram showing the normal pattern of pulmonic valve (*top*) and various other patterns associated with pulmonary hypertension and pulmonic stenosis.

(3) the length of the P-R interval: a long P-R interval causes the atrial contraction to occur earlier than usual in ventricular diastole, and the "a" wave is smaller in amplitude than it would have been if it had come later in diastole.

It has recently been pointed out (Doi *et al.,* 1981) that extreme respiratory variation in depth of the "a" wave is seen in constrictive pericarditis.

The pulmonic valve "a" wave reflects a billowing or "upward doming" motion of the valve toward the pulmonary artery in response to the transient rise in right ventricular pressure resulting from right atrial contraction. This

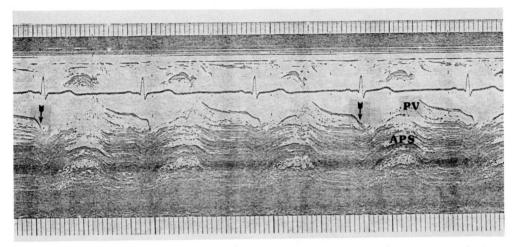

Fig. F-2. The M-mode echogram of the pulmonic valve. The "a" amplitude is 3 mm in the second, third, and fifth beats, but much deeper in the first and fourth (*arrows*), attributable to respiratory variation. If the precise relationship to the ECG were not carefully ascertained, the "a" wave could be mistakenly thought absent in these latter beats.

"atriogenic" motion of the pulmonary cusps depends upon (1) the extent of rise in right ventricular diastolic pressure, which in turn is determined by the force of right atrial contraction and the resistance to right ventricular fill- ing (reciprocal of compliance), and (2) the pulmonary artery pressure at this phase of diastole. Respiration, the length of diastole, the point in diastole at which atrial contraction occurs, and abnormally high or low pulmonary artery

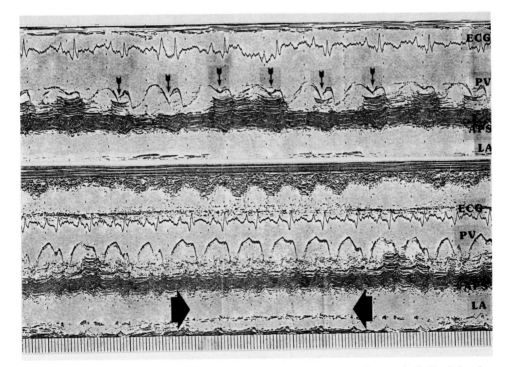

Fig. F-3. *Upper.* M-mode echogram of the pulmonic valve in a normal young individual showing marked respiratory variation in the "a" wave amplitude (*arrows*) from beat to beat.

Lower. Pulmonic valve echogram in the same patient, showing that variations in "a" wave amplitude cease to occur during periods of apnea. Deep "a" waves are not seen during apnea (*broad horizontal arrows*).

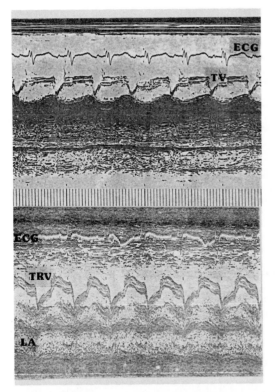

Fig. F-4. Structures simulating the pulmonic valve.
Upper. M-mode echogram showing the posterior leaflet of the tricuspid valve (TV). Its pattern of motion could possibly be mistaken for that of the pulmonic valve. However, a glance at the ECG will show that the opening of the valve takes place in diastole, whereas the pulmonic valve opening would of course be in systole.
Lower. M-mode echogram showing the truncal semilunar valve in a patient with proven common truncus arteriosus. It could easily be mistaken for a pulmonic valve echo, because at this transducer angulation the anterior cusp was not visualized. The diagnostic relevance of such an error is that demonstration of a pulmonic valve excludes the diagnosis of a common truncus arteriosus (TRV = truncal valve).

pressures influence the amplitude of the pulmonic valve "a" wave by affecting this interplay or balance between right ventricular pressure and pulmonary artery pressure (Figs. F-2 and F-3).

Pocoski *et al.* (1978) have presented evidence that the M-mode contour of pulmonic valve motion is affected not only by pressure differences between right ventricle and pulmonary artery, but also by atrial events, since the left atrium lies immediately posteroinferior to the main pulmonary artery. This might explain why

the pulmonic valve "a" wave and diastolic (EF) slope are not always reliable indicators of pulmonary hypertension.

The diagnostic value of the pulmonic valve "a" wave has been further questioned by Hada *et al.* (1977a) who showed that its amplitude can vary with transducer position; the "a" wave becomes smaller when the transducer is angulated downward and medially from an unusually high intercostal space.

Caution: Motion of the posterior tricuspid leaflet possibly could be mistaken for pulmonic valve motion in contour, but not in timing (Fig. F-4).

On 2-D echocardiography (Fig. F-5), the posterior cusp of the pulmonic valve can be seen anteriorly and to the left of the aortic root in the short-axis view (Heger and Weyman, 1979). Once the aortic root is visualized in this view, slight alterations of angulation of the 2-D probe may be necessary until the pulmonic valve reveals itself as a small linear echo just outside the aortic root (Fig. F-5), flicking back and forth a little anterior to the region of the left main coronary artery. The "a" dip and systolic opening of the valve manifest as a posterior motion of the cusp echo as it falls back against the adjacent posterior wall of the pulmonary trunk; during diastole the small linear echo representing the posterior pulmonic cusp hangs or projects into the lumen of the artery.

The main uses of the pulmonic valve echogram in the clinical practice of cardiology are in the detection of pulmonary hypertension and pulmonary stenosis:

PULMONARY HYPERTENSION
(Figs. F-6 to F-8)

Several abnormalities of pulmonary valve echo contour have been described in patients with raised pulmonary artery pressure. Of these, two have proven more reliable than others:

1. The normal U- or V-shaped systolic contour alters to a W-shaped one with a midsystolic "partial closure" motion (Figs. E-6 and E-7). This sign is by no means present in every patient with raised pulmonary artery pressure. It tends to be associated mainly with severe pulmonary hypertension. However, it is fairly specific for pulmonary hypertension; it is seldom, if ever, seen in individuals with normal pulmonary artery pressures, except for idiopathic dilatation

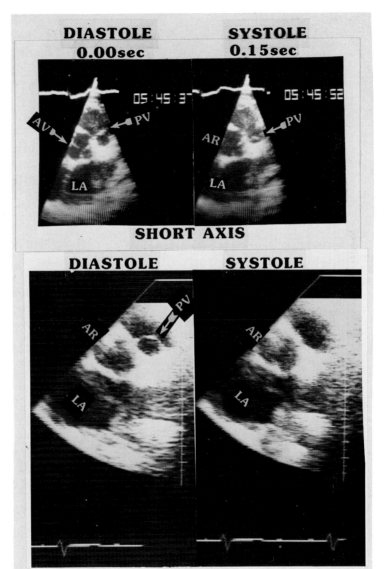

Fig. F-5. 2-D echogram of a normal pulmonic valve in the short-axis view. It occupies a position anterior and to the left of the aortic root. The left atrium is visible as a large echo-free space posterior to the aortic and pulmonic valves. Both frames are from the same cardiac cycle. The left frame, in diastole, shows the pulmonic valve cusp in an anterior position. The right frame, in systole (0.15 sec later), shows that the valve cusp has moved to a posterior position against the posterior wall of the pulmonary artery.

2-D echogram in the short-axis view in a normal adult. The pulmonic valve is presented in somewhat unusual plane, so that two of its cusps are seen, in a closed position, forming a thin arch anterior to the aortic root and atriopulmonary sulcus (*left*). Later in the same cardiac cycle (*right*) the pulmonic valve is open.

of the pulmonary artery (Bauman *et al.,* 1979) and dynamic subpulmonary stenosis with tetralogy of Fallot (Caldwell *et al.,* 1979).

2. Absent or shallow (less than 2 mm) "a" wave (Figs. F-6 to F-8). Presumably the high pulmonary artery diastolic pressure renders the atriogenic rise in right ventricular pressure ineffective with respect to displacing or moving the pulmonic valve. Small "a" waves (2 mm or less) are associated with mild to moderate pulmonary hypertension (mean pulmonary artery pressure 20 to 40 mmHg), whereas in more severe pulmonary hypertension the "a" wave is absent.

Pitfalls: (1) An obvious but important error to avoid in this regard is that absence of the "a" wave is to be expected in atrial fibrillation (Fig. F-9) or other arrhythmia which causes the atria to contract during ventricular systole; (2) early ectopic beats can result in an "abortive" pulmonic opening, resulting in a brief dip or notch that should not be mistaken for an "a" wave (Fig. F-9); (3) an "a" wave of normal size may be observed with pulmonary hypertension if cardiac failure is present; (4) if the aorta and pulmonary arteries are transposed, the "pulmonic" valve is really the aortic (Fig. F-10).

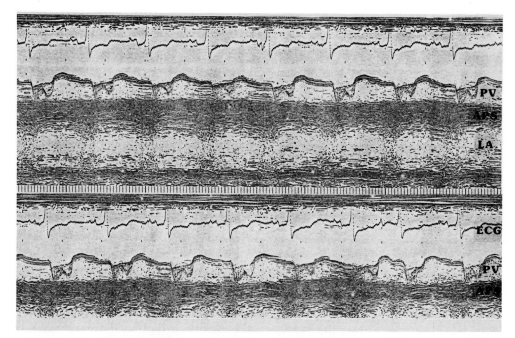

Fig. F-6. M-mode echogram in a patient with severe pulmonary hypertension showing absence of the pulmonic valve "a" wave and a midsystolic notch on the pulmonic valve systolic contour (midsystolic "closure" with subsequent reopening). This pattern is somewhat altered in a premature beat (second to last beat in lower panel).

Less reliable indicators of pulmonary hypertension include:

3. *A flat diastolic (EF) slope* of the pulmonic valve. The normal range for this measurement is very wide, 6 to 115 mm/sec, the average being 37 ± 25 mm/sec (Weyman *et al.*, 1974). In pulmonary hypertension this diastolic EF segment of the pulmonic valve echo becomes

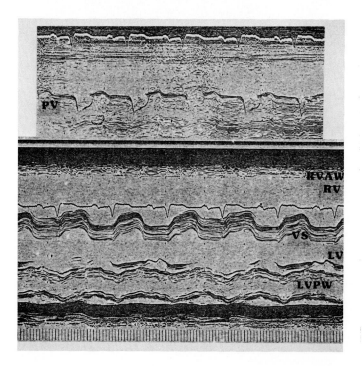

Fig. F-7. M-mode echogram in a patient with cor pulmonale (*upper*) suggesting pulmonary hypertension because of absence of the "a" wave. The lower panel shows RV anterior wall hypertrophy, RV dilatation, and paradoxic septal motion (attributable to tricuspid regurgitation).

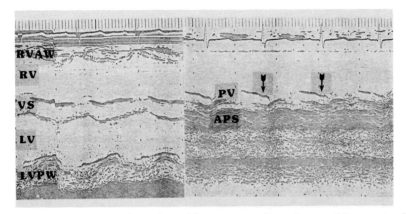

Fig. F-8. M-mode echogram of a patient with acute cor pulmonale caused by recent pulmonary embolism (documented by lung scans). RV dilatation of mild degree is apparent in the left panel; an abnormally small "a" wave (*arrows*) on the pulmonic valve echo can be seen in the right panel, suggesting mild to moderate pulmonary hypertension.

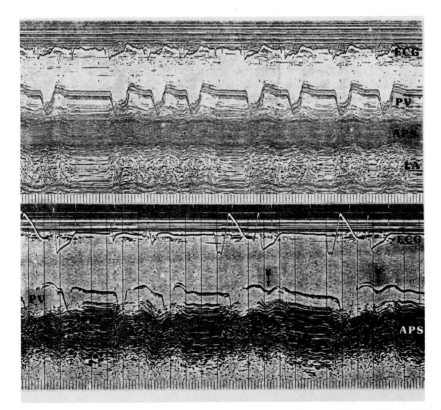

Fig. F-9. M-mode echograms of the pulmonic valve in two different patients with atrial fibrillation.

Upper. Nonspecific cusp thickening in a patient with congestive cardiomyopathy.

Lower. Note absence of "a" waves preceding systolic opening of the pulmonic valve. The ECG reveals ventricular bigeminy. In the last two pairs of beats, the second beat of each pair does not produce full opening of the pulmonic valve; there results instead a small undulation (*arrow*) not unlike that of a normal "a" wave. The ECG demonstrates that this undulation is not due to atrial contraction.

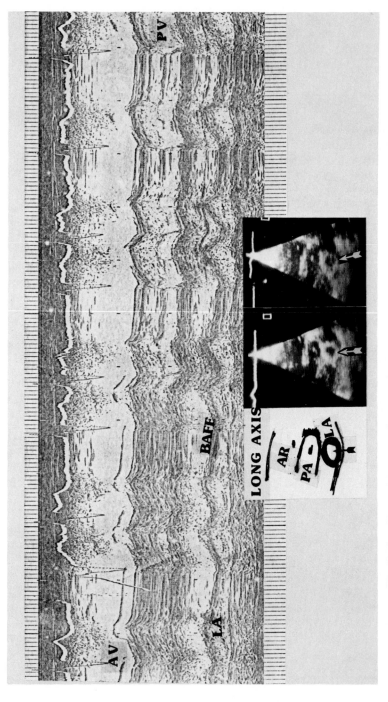

Fig. F-10. *Upper.* M-mode echogram of a patient with transposition of great vessels in whom a Mustard operation had been done. A scan has been made from the anterior large vessel, the aorta, containing the aortic valve, to the posterior great vessel, the pulmonary artery, containing the pulmonic valve. The baffle (BAFF) can be seen within the atrial chamber.

Lower. 2-D echogram in the long-axis view at the level of origin of the great vessels. The aortic root is visible anterior to the pulmonary artery. The baffle is apparent (*arrows*) posterior to the pulmonary artery, in the left atrial region.

184

horizontal (zero EF slope) or even slopes upward (negative EF slope).

4. *Rapid systolic opening* of the pulmonic valve, manifesting as a steep EF slope. The absent "a" wave, horizontal EF diastolic segment, and almost vertical opening motion combine to form a characteristic "right angle" contour, easily recognizable as different from the normal pattern.

5. *Prolonged right ventricular preejection period* (RVPEP), which is the interval between onset of the QRS complex and opening of the pulmonary valve. As the pulmonary arterial resistance and pressure rise, the RVPEP increases while the RVEP (right ventricular ejection period) decreases (Nanda *et al.*, 1974; Hirschfeld *et al.*, 1975; Riggs *et al.*, 1978; Pocoski *et al.*, 1978). Because of considerable overlap between values in normal and pulmonary hypertensive patients, the RVPEP is of limited value in practice as an indicator of pulmonary hypertension. However, the RVPEP/RVEP ratio is more reliable. In normal subjects this ratio is 0.30 or less; in patients with pulmonary hypertension it is above 0.35.

Pitfalls: (1) The apparent onset of the QRS complex may not coincide with the true onset if the initial inscription of the QRS is isoelectric or almost so. The RVPEP would then appear erroneously short; (2) right bundle branch block might delay right ventricular electrical activation and thus unduly prolong the RVPEP; (3) the pulmonic valve opening contour may be rounded rather than sharp, so that the precise moment of valve opening is difficult to pinpoint; (4) in the presence of myocarditis, the RVPEP/RVEP ratio would tend to be prolonged at normal pulmonary artery pressures and therefore could not be valid as an indicator of pulmonary hypertension.

It must be emphasized that the reliability of the pulmonic valve echogram as an indicator of pulmonary hypertension is very controversial. Whereas most earlier published reports agreed that some features, such as the pulmonic valve "a" wave and the RVPEP/RVEP ratio, are dependable in predicting pulmonary hypertension, some recent authors have found unsatisfactory correlation between the ultrasound criteria and hemodynamic data, using simultaneous high-fidelity catheterization-echographic

recordings (Aquatella *et al.*, 1979; Silverman *et al.*, 1980). The only definite criterion (specific though insensitive) of pulmonary hypertension accepted by all is a combination of absent "a" wave and midsystolic notching.

It may be added that studies correlating M-mode echocardiographic measurements with hemodynamic data continue to appear and claim success in the use of new echographic parameters to predict elevated pulmonary pressure or vascular resistance. Thus Spooner *et al.* (1978) found that the ratio of the PEP/EP of the RV to that of the LV correlates very closely with the ratio of the pulmonary arteriolar resistance to the systemic arteriolar resistance. Mills *et al.* (1980), using dual echocardiography, measured the RV isovolumic contraction time (interval from tricuspid valve closure to pulmonic valve opening, recorded simultaneously). They found that a value of less than 0.025 sec suggested a normal pulmonary artery pressure, but a reliable quantitative relationship between the RV isovolumic contraction time and raised pulmonary artery pressures could not be obtained.

Green and Popp (1981) recently studied pulmonic valve motion by 2-D as well as dual echography, in normal as well as pulmonary hypertensive subjects, and concluded that the pulmonic valve "a" wave does not represent independent valvar displacement but rather reflects motion of the entire cardiac base including the pulmonary artery.

PULMONIC STENOSIS

Unduly deep "a" waves are seen in patients with stenosis of the pulmonic valve. Weyman *et al.* (1974) found that patients with moderate to severe pulmonic valve stenosis (gradients over 50 mm) have "a" waves averaging about 10 mm, range, 6 to 18 mm. However, in pulmonary stenosis of milder severity (gradient below 50 mm) the "a" wave ranged from 2 to 10 mm, average, 6 mm. Thus, the latter group overlapped the range of normal values to a large extent.

Pitfall: In some normal persons, especially young children and those with slow heart rates, such as athletes, marked respiratory fluctuation in "a" wave amplitude is observed (Figs. F-2 and F-3), such that during inspiration it may exceed 6 or even 8 mm.

PREMATURE PULMONIC VALVE OPENING

A variant of the deep "a" wave pattern is one in which ventricular ejection begins before the pulmonic valve has time to return to its closed position; the "a" wave merges with systolic opening, and the phenomenon may be referred to as premature pulmonary valve opening. There is evidence that under certain circumstances the pulmonic valve not only bulges upward during atrial contraction but actually opens to allow forward flow across the valve. This pattern is seen in patients with severe pulmonic valve stenosis, gradients over 65 mmHg (Weyman et al., 1974), and may be associated with a presystolic click coinciding with full presystolic (atriogenic) pulmonic valve opening (Flanagan and Shah, 1977). It has also been reported in certain other hemodynamic situations: rupture of a sinus of Valsalva aneurysm into the right atrium or ventricle, Uhl's anomaly, Ebstein's anomaly, and severe tricuspid regurgitation (Fig. F-11).

Common to most of these hemodynamic entities are either a high diastolic pressure in the right ventricle or increased right ventricular stroke volume and a normal or low pulmonary artery diastolic pressure.

The differential diagnosis between pulmonic stenosis and the other conditions capable of causing premature pulmonary valve opening depends on associated physical, electrocardiographic, and radiologic signs, a detailed discussion of which is beyond the scope of this book. However, associated echocardiographic findings may be of help; for example, delayed tricuspid closure and an unduly leftward location of the tricuspid valve suggest Ebstein's anomaly; dense thickened pericardial echoes might raise the possibility of constrictive pericarditis.

Weyman et al. (1977) found 2-D echocardiography a great improvement over the M-mode technique in the diagnosis of pulmonic valve stenosis. The pulmonic valve could be visualized in 20 of their 22 patients with stenotic pulmonic valves as a distinctive dome-shaped curved echo very different from the linear normal one. In contrast, the pulmonic valve could

be recorded in only 12 of these patients on M-mode echocardiography; a definitely abnormal contour, characterized by an unduly deep "a" dip, was noted in only 5 of the 12.

Abrupt anterior motion of the dome valve at onset of diastole and abrupt posterior motion at onset of systole, as viewed in real time, are very typical of pulmonic valve stenosis.

Normally only the posterior pulmonary cusp is visible, both by M-mode and 2-D echocardiography. However, by the 2-D method the dome-shaped valve with anterior as well as posterior leaflets (Fig. F-12) and the narrow orifice at the apex of the dome can be discerned (Weyman et al., 1977) in some cases. Both anterior and posterior valve leaflets were recognized on M-mode by Rey and LaBlanche (1979) in 3 of their 16 patients; all 3 had severe pulmonic stenosis.

Associated echographic findings in patients with moderate to severe pulmonic stenosis include (1) increased right ventricular dimension, (2) increased right ventricular anterior wall thickness, (3) a ventricular septum that is mildly hypertrophied but shows normal (not paradoxic) systolic motion. Patients with isolated pulmonic stenosis (with intact ventricular septum) have (1) no aortic root dilatation, (2) no aortic overriding, and (3) no septal-anterior aortic root discontinuity in scans from left ventricle to aortic root.

The bifurcation of the main pulmonary artery into right and left branches can sometimes be visualized by parasternal and suprasternal approaches, thus making it possible to diagnose pulmonary artery branch stenosis (Tinker et al., 1982).

TETRALOGY OF FALLOT AND RELATED ANOMALIES (Fig. F-12)

Fallot's tetralogy is perhaps the most common variety of cyanotic heart disease seen in older children or adults, and it is fortunate that all its four components lend themselves to echocardiographic recognition: right ventricular hypertrophy, aortic overriding, ventricular septal defect, and right ventricular outflow tract narrowing. Another important aspect of this entity is that it is important for the clinician to distinguish it from pulmonary valvular stenosis with intact ventricular septum.

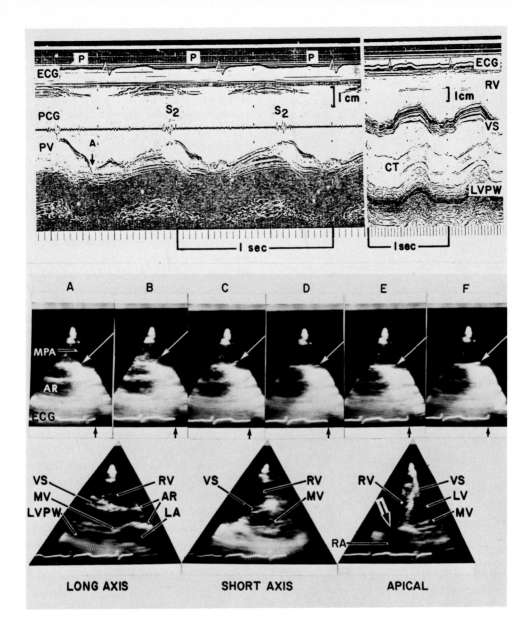

Fig. F-11. Echograms of a young man with absent tricuspid valve (surgically removed for refractory endocarditis).

Upper. M-mode echocardiogram. In the left panel, the pulmonary valve (PV) can be seen to open fully after the onset of the P wave (large "a" wave), well before the onset of QRS (ECG, electrocardiogram; PCG, phonocardiogram; S₂, second heart sound). The right panel shows, the left ventricle at chordae tendineae (CT) level. The right ventricle (RV) is dilated and the ventricular septum (VS) shows paradoxic anterior systolic motion. (LVPW, left ventricular posterior wall).

Lower. 2-D echocardiogram. The upper row of six frames shows the posterior cusp of the pulmonary valve in different phases of the cardiac cycle, which are indicated on the electrocardiogram by the small black upward arrows. The cusp is in an open position in systole (*frame A*), then closes in early to middiastole (*B and C*), but opens in late diastole (*D and E*) after onset of the P wave. (MPA, main pulmonary artery.) The lower three frames, in the long-axis, short-axis, and apical views, were all taken during systole. They show that the right ventricle (RV) is dilated, while the left ventricle (LV) is of normal size. The arrow in the apical view indicates where the tricuspid valve would have been seen if it were present.

(Reproduced from D'Cruz, I, A.; Shah, S. N.; Levinsky, R.; *et al.:* Premature pulmonary valve opening in a patient with absent tricuspid valve. *Br. Heart J.,* **44:**714, 1980 with permission of the publishers.)

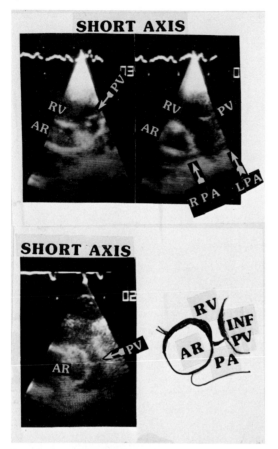

Fig. F-12. 2-D echogram of a child with stenosis of both the pulmonic valve and the right and left pulmonary arteries at their origin, a frequent association. The diagnosis was proven by catheterization and angiocardiography. In the left frame the stenotic cusps with a central orifice present an appearance different from that in normals, in whom only one (posterior) cusp can be seen. The left atrium can be seen posterior to the aortic root. The right frame depicts a slightly higher plane, which passes through the pulmonary trunk and its bifurcation into right and left pulmonary arteries; the pulmonary arteries appear narrow at their origin.

2-D echogram, in the short-axis view, of a patient with tetralogy of Fallot. Infundibular pulmonic stenosis was prominent (gradient over 100 mmHg across the infundibulum). The scanning plane, which passes through the RV outflow tract, pulmonic valve, and main pulmonary artery, demonstrated the narrow RV outflow tract.

The following three echocardiographic features are easily recognizable in tetralogy of Fallot but absent in isolated pulmonary valve stenosis (Gramiak and Shah, 1971; Tajik *et al.,* 1973; Sahn *et al.,* 1974; Morris *et al.,* 1975): (1) abnormal narrowing of the right ventricular

outflow tract (Fig. F-12), (2) an abnormally wide aortic root, which (3) overrides or straddles the ventricular septum, with which it is discontinuous (normally the ventricular septum is continuous with the anterior aortic root).

Other echographic findings of lesser specificity commonly encountered in Fallot's tetralogy are right ventricular enlargement and increased thickness of the right ventricular anterior wall.

All these ultrasound characteristics detectable by the M-mode technique are even more obvious on the 2-D echocardiogram. Thus, Caldwell *et al.* (1979) showed that this technique demonstrated (1) narrowing of the RV outflow tract, (2) a ventricular septal defect, and (3) the presence of a pulmonic valve in 90 per cent or more of their 29 patients with tetralogy; on the other hand, M-mode echocardiography was less effective in detecting RV outflow tract narrowing and ventricular septal defect and capable of recording the pulmonic valve in only a quarter of the patients.

The importance of recognizing the existence of a functioning pulmonic valve is that it enables the clinician to exclude persistent truncus arteriosus and pseudotruncus (pulmonary atresia with ventricular septal defect) which can otherwise closely resemble Fallot's tetralogy, clinically as well as echographically. The 2-D echographic differentiation can be made by imaging the origin of the pulmonary artery from the truncus in patients with true persistent truncus, and by identifying a blind RV outflow tract and perhaps an atretic pulmonary artery in patients with psuedotruncus (Barron *et al.,* 1983). Another diagnostic clue to persistent truncus is that dilatation of the aortic root is of more impressive proportions that it is in tetralogy (Morris *et al.,* 1975).

Caution: The "anterior aortic root" echo of a truncus may easily drop out, so that the "posterior aortic root" and adjacent posterior cusp of the truncal valve can be mistaken for a pulmonic valve (Meltzer *et al.,* 1980), as in Figure F-4.

Double-outlet RV and Taussig-Bing anomaly also have several clinical and echographic features in common with Fallot's tetralogy, but can be distinguished by lack of normal mitral-aortic continuity (more than 10 mm difference in the levels of the mitral attachment and the posterior aortic root).

PREMATURE PULMONIC VALVE OPENING (Figure. F-11)

Weyman *et al.* (1975) described echographic visualization of pulmonic valve opening well before the onset of ventricular systole in a patient with rupture of a sinus of Valsalva aneurysm into the right atrium. The same group (Wann *et al.*, 1977) later reported another five patients who also exhibited premature pulmonic valve opening, each with a different variety of cardiac pathology. This echocardiographic sign has been documented in association with Uhl's anomaly (French *et al.*, 1975) and tricuspid valvectomy for endocarditis (D'Cruz *et al.*, 1980).

Wann *et al.* (1977) pointed out that these diverse cardiac conditions fall into one of the two pathophysiologic situations: (1) Restriction of right ventricular diastolic filling, with diastolic pressure rise transiently exceeding pulmonary artery pressure. Constrictive pericarditis and Loeffler's endocarditis belong to this group. (2) Increased volume of blood entering the RV. This applies to severe tricuspid regurgitation associated with Ebstein's anomaly, tricuspid valve destruction, or surgical removal, and also to atrial septal defect associated with pulmonic regurgitation (Wann *et al.*, 1977).

Under these circumstances, vigorous right atrial contraction can generate a pressure exceeding pulmonary artery diastolic pressure so that the pulmonic valve opens and is still open when RV contraction continues forward flow into the pulmonary artery.

In rupture of sinus of Valsalva aneurysm into the right heart, pulmonic valve opening may actually precede atrial contraction (Weyman *et al.*, 1975), in which case it is attributable to torrential diastolic flow from aorta to the right heart, independent of the motive force of right atrial contraction.

Premature pulmonic valve opening recently has been reported in a patient with acute inferior myocardial infarction who had a mean RA pressure of 20 mmHg and RV dilatation, presumably due to RV infarction (Coma-Canella *et al.*, 1981).

PULMONIC VALVE VEGETATIONS

Of the four cardiac valves, the pulmonic is by far the least frequently involved in bacterial endocarditis. The first reported instance (Kramer *et al.*, 1977) was that of a heroin addict who succumbed to *Pseudomonas* endocarditis and had vegetations on all four valves at the time of death. In another case (Dzindzio *et al.*, 1979), the endocarditis was gonococcal; pulmonic valve vegetations and cusp destruction were found at surgery.

Pulmonic valve vegetations presented on echocardiography as shaggy or granular abnormal echoes in diastole attached to the posterior aspect of the pulmonic valve echo. Pulmonic valve motion is normal, except that premature valve opening can appear if pulmonic valve regurgitation becomes severe.

Abnormally broad or thick pulmonary valve echoes are seen in some patients (especially adults) with sclerotic or calcified stenotic valves. The stenotic state of the valve may be suspected on the basis of physical signs (typical murmur and thrill), exaggerated "a" dip, and the distinctive curved-dome shape on the short-axis 2-D echocardiogram. Nonspecific thickening of the pulmonic valve is not uncommon in patients with chronic congestive cardiomyopathy (Fig. F-9), chronic renal failure, and so forth. Thick, stubby, relatively immobile pulmonic valve cusps have been described in patients with carcinoid heart disease; the tricuspid valve is similarly affected (Howard *et al.*, 1982; Callahan *et al.*, 1982).

Further instances of pulmonic valve vegetations, well visualized as nodular densities on the valve by 2-D echocardiography and as a shaggy thickening on M-mode, have been reported (Sheikh *et al.*, 1979; Berger *et al.*, 1980; Nakamura *et al.*, 1983; Chiang *et al.*, 1981; Mehlman *et al.*, 1982; Weiss *et al.*, 1982; Dander *et al.*, 1982; Nakamura *et al.*, 1983).

PULMONIC VALVE FLUTTER (Fig. F-13)

SYSTOLIC FLUTTER

A minor degree of vibratory motion of the pulmonic valve in systole is not abnormal, just as a similar fine, low-amplitude flutter of systolic aortic valve motion is considered within normal limits. However, a gross large-amplitude flutter or "chaotic" systolic motion of the pulmonic valve has been described in (1) infun-

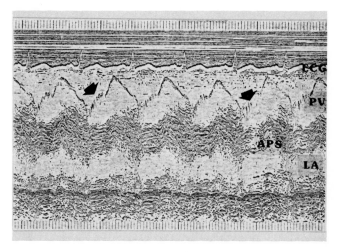

Fig. F-13. M-mode echogram of the pulmonic valve showing systolic flutter (*arrows*), in a patient with an unusually high (subpulmonic) ventricular septal defect. The valve flutters because the jet through the septal defect impinges directly on it.

dibular pulmonic stenosis (with intact ventricular septum) by Weyman *et al* (1975) and in (2) subpulmonic ventricular septal defects by Glasser and Baucum (1977).

In both situations, the mechanism of pulmonic valve flutter appears to be the impingement on it of a high-velocity jet of blood emerging through a narrow orifice, in one case at the site of infundibular stenosis and in the other at the unusual high subpulmonic defect in the ventricular septum. Defects at other sites in the septum are not associated with such pulmonic valve flutter.

Weyman *et al.,* (1975) pointed out that gross flutter of the pulmonic valve in their three patients with infundibular stenosis continued well beyond the end of RV systole and discussed the various possible explanations for this interesting, though puzzling, finding.

Ayasama *et al.* (1977) described systolic pulmonic valve flutter in a patient with idiopathic dilatation of the pulmonary artery. The cusp flutter in this case was fine and rather inconspicuous as compared to the violent chaotic flutter associated with infundibular pulmonic stenosis and subpulmonic ventricular septal defect. The dilated pulmonic trunk manifested as an unusually wide, echo-free space just posterior to the chest wall.

DIASTOLIC FLUTTER

Nanda and Gramiak (1978) demonstrated diastolic flutter on the pulmonic valve of a patient with tetralogy of Fallot and stenosis of the pulmonic valve as well as pulmonary artery branches; pulmonic valvotomy had rendered the valve incompetent. Diastolic flutter of the pulmonic valve has been reported in a patient with patent ductus arteriosus (Fisher *et al.,* 1982).

Diastolic undulations on the pulmonic valve may be noted in patients with atrial fibrillation or flutter (Prabhu *et al.,* 1978), perhaps because of transmission of atrial fibrillatory contractions from the adjacent left atrial anterior wall.

MIDSYSTOLIC NEAR-CLOSURE OF THE PULMONIC VALVE

Midsystolic notching of the pulmonic valve echo (sometimes referred to as premature closure) is a valuable sign of severe pulmonary hypertension, as discussed above.

However, it has been described in certain other situations:

1. Congenital infundibular pulmonic stenosis (Weyman *et al.,* 1975; Haddad *et al.,* 1980).

2. Subvalvar muscular pulmonic stenosis in hypertrophic cardiomyopathy; the very thickened ventricular septum encroaches on RV as well as LV outflow tracts (Asin-Cardiel *et al.,* 1978; Haddad *et al.,* 1980).

3. Idiopathic dilatation of the pulmonary trunk, with normal pulmonary artery pressure (Bauman *et al.,* 1979).

Thus it appears that midsystolic near-closure of the pulmonic valve depends not only on abnormal flow patterns across the valve but also on the capacitance of the main pulmonary artery and its branches and the resistance of the distal vascular bed.

PULMONARY ARTERY

Visualization of the main pulmonary artery by 2-D echography, in a somewhat superiorly angled short-axis view, has made it possible to diagnose pulmonary artery dilatation (Bauman et al., 1979; Bloch et al., 1977), narrowing, surgical banding (Weyman, 1982) as well as a neoplastic mass within the vessel (Wright et al., 1983).

REFERENCES

NORMAL PULMONIC VALVE

Gramiak, R.; Nanda, N. C.; and Shah, P. M.: Echocardiographic detection of pulmonic valve. *Radiology*, 103:153, 1972.

Hada, Y.; Sakamoto, T.; Hayashi, T.; *et al.:* Echocardiogram of the pulmonary valve. Variability of the pattern and the related technical problems. Jpn. Heart J., 18:298, 1977a.

Hada, Y.; Sakamoto, T.; Hayashi, T.; *et al.:* Echocardiogram of the normal pulmonary valve. Physiologic data and the effect of atrial contraction on the valve motion. *Jpn. Heart J.,* 18:421, 1977b.

Heger, J. J., and Weyman, A. E.: A review of M-mode and cross-sectional echocardiographic findings of the pulmonary valve. *J.C.U.,* 7:98, 1979.

Lew, H., and Karliner, J. S.: Assessment of pulmonary valve echogram in normal subjects and in patients with pulmonary arterial hypertension. *Br. Heart J.,* 42:147, 1979.

Meltzer, R. S.; Sunderland, C. O.; and Roelandt, J.: Truncus arteriosus with apparent pulmonary valve echocardiogram. *Chest,* 78:632, 1980.

Pocoski, D. J.; Shah, P. M.; and Sylvester, L.: Physiological correlates and echocardiographic pulmonary valve motion in diastole. *Circulation,* 58:1064, 1978.

Weyman, A. E.: Pulmonary valve echo motion in clinical practice. *Am. J. Med.,* 62:843, 1977.

PULMONARY HYPERTENSION

Aquatella, H.; Schiller, N. B.; Sharpe, D. N.; *et al.:* Lack of correlation between echocardiographic pulmonary valve morphology and simultaneous pulmonary arterial pressure. *Am. J. Cardiol.,* 43:496, 1979.

Green, S. E., and Popp, R. L.: The relationship of pulmonary valve motion to the motion of surrounding cardiac structures: A two-dimensional and dual M-mode echocardiographic study. *Circulation,* 64:107, 1981.

Gutgesell, H. P.: Echocardiographic estimation of pulmonary artery pressure in transposition of the great arteries. *Circulation,* 57:1151, 1978.

Hirschfeld, S.; Meyer, R.; and Schwartz, D. C.: The echocardiographic assessment of pulmonary artery pressure and pulmonary vascular resistance. *Circulation,* 52:642, 1975.

Hirschfeld, S. S.; Fleming, D. G.; Doershuk, C.; *et al.:* Echocardiographic abnormalities in patients with cystic fibrosis. *Chest,* 75:350, 1979.

Johnson, G.; Meyer, R. A.; Korfhagen, J.; *et al.:* Echocardiographic assessment of pulmonary arterial pressure in children with complete right bundle branch block. *Am. J. Cardiol.,* 41:1264, 1978.

Mills, P.; Amara, I.; McLaurin, L. P.; *et al.:* Noninvasive assessment of pulmonary hypertension from right ventricular isovolumic contraction time. *Am. J. Cardiol.,* 46:273, 1980.

Nanda, N. C.; Gramiak, R.; Robinson, T. I.; *et al.:* Echocardiographic evaluation of pulmonary hypertension. *Circulation,* 50:575, 1974.

Riggs, T.; Hirschfeld, S.; Borket, G.; *et al.:* Assessment of the pulmonary vascular bed by echocardiographic right ventricular systolic time intervals. *Circulation,* 57:939, 1978.

Silverman, N. H.; Snider, A. R.; and Rudolph, A. M.: Evaluation of pulmonary hypertension by M-mode echocardiography in children with ventricular septal defect. *Circulation,* 61:1125, 1980.

Spooner, E. W.; Perry, B. C.; Stern, A. M.; *et al.:* Estimation of pulmonary/systemic resistance ratios from echocardiographic systolic time intervals in young patients with congenital or acquired heart disease. *Am. J. Cardiol.,* 42:811, 1978.

Weyman, A. E.; Dillon, J. C.; Feigenbaum, H.; *et al.:* Echocardiographic patterns of pulmonary valve motion with pulmonary hypertension. *Circulation,* 50:905, 1974.

PULMONIC STENOSIS

Flanagan, W. H., and Shah, P. M.: Echocardiographic correlate of presystolic pulmonary ejection sound in congenital valvular pulmonary stenosis. *Am. Heart J.,* 94:633, 1977.

Mills, P.; Wolfe, C.; Redwood, D.; *et al.:* Noninvasive diagnosis of subpulmonary outflow tract obstruction. *Br. Heart J.,* 43:276, 1980.

Nanda, N. C.; Gramiak, R.; Manning, J. A.; *et al.:* Echocardiographic features of subpulmonic obstruction in dextro-transposition of the great vessels. *Circulation,* 51:515, 1975.

Rey, C., and LaBlanche, J. M.: Pulmonary valve motion in valvular pulmonary stenosis in childhood. *Acta Med. Scand. (Suppl.),* 627:185, 1979.

Tinker, D. D.; Nanda, N. C.; Harris, J. P.; *et al.:* Two-dimensional echocardiographic identification of pulmonary artery branch stenosis. *Am. J. Cardiol.,* 50:814, 1982.

Weyman, A. E.; Dillon, J. C.; Feigenbaum, H.; *et al.:* Echocardiographic patterns of pulmonic valve motion in valvular pulmonary stenosis. *Am. J. Cardiol.,* 36:644, 1974.

Weyman, A. E.; Dillon, J. C.; Feigenbaum, H.; *et al.:* Echocardiographic differentiation of infundibular from valvar pulmonary stenosis. *Am. J. Cardiol.,* 36:21, 1975.

Weyman, A. E.; Hurwitz, R. A.; Girod, D. A.; *et al.:* Cross-sectional echocardiographic visualization of the stenotic pulmonary valve. *Circulation,* 56:769, 1977.

TETRALOGY OF FALLOT AND RELATED ANOMALIES

Barron, J. V.; Sahn, D. J.; Attie, F.; *et al.:* Two-dimensional echocardiographic study of right ventricular outflow and great artery anatomy in pulmonary atresia with ventricular septal defects and in truncus arteriosus. *Am. Heart J.,* 105: 281, 1983.

Caldwell, R. L.; Weyman, A. E.; and Hurwitz, R. A.: Right ventricular outflow tract assessment by cross-sectional echocardiography in tetralogy of Fallot. *Circulation,* 59:395, 1979.

Gramiak, R., and Shah, P. M.: Cardiac ultrasonography: A review of current applications. *Radiol. Clin. North Am.,* 9:469, 1971.

Morris, D. C.; Felner, J. M.; Schlant, R. C.; *et al.:* Echocardiographic diagnosis of tetralogy of Fallot. *Am. J. Cardiol.,* **36:**908, 1975.

Sahn, D. J.; Terry, R.; O'Rourke, R.; *et al.:* Multiple crystal cross-sectional echocardiography in the diagnosis of cyanotic congenital heart disease. *Circulation,* **50:**230, 1974.

Tajik, A. J.; Gau, G. T.; Ritter, D. G.; *et al.:* Echocardiogram in tetralogy of Fallot. *Chest,* **64:**107, 1973.

PREMATURE PULMONIC VALVE OPENING

Coma-Canella, I.; Lopez-Sendon, J.; and Oliver, J.: Premature pulmonic valve opening and inverted septal convexity in acute ischemic right ventricular dysfunction. *Am. Heart J.,* **101:**684, 1981.

D'Cruz, I. A.; Shah, S. N.; Levinsky, R.; and Goldbarg, A.: Premature pulmonary valve opening in a patient with absent tricuspid valve. *Br. Heart J.,* **44:**714, 1980.

Doi, Y. L.; Tetsuro, S.; and Spodick, D. H.: Motion of pulmonic valve and constrictive pericarditis. *Chest,* **80:**513, 1981.

French, J. W.; Baum, D.; and Popp, R. L.: Echocardiographic findings in Uhl's anomaly. *Am. J. Cardiol.,* **36:**349, 1975.

Wann, L. S.; Weyman, A. E.; Dillon, J. C.; *et al.:* Premature pulmonary valve opening. *Circulation,* **55:**128, 1977.

Weyman, A. E.; Dillon, J. C.; Feigenbaum, H.; *et al.:* Premature pulmonic valve opening following sinus of Valsalva aneurysm rupture in the right atrium. *Circulation,* **51:**556, 1975.

PULMONIC VALVE VEGETATIONS AND SCLEROSIS

Berger, M.; Delfin, L. A.; Jelveh, M.; *et al.:* Two-dimensional echocardiographic findings in right-sided infective endocarditis. *Circulation,* **61:**855, 1980.

Callahan, J. A.; Wroblewski, E. M.; Reeder, G. S.; *et al.:* Echocardiographic features of carcinoid heart disease. *Am. J. Cardiol.,* **50:**762, 1982.

Chiang, C. W.; Lei, Y. S.; Chang, C. H.; *et al.:* Preoperative and postoperative echocardiographic studies of pulmonic valvular endocarditis. *Chest,* **80:**232, 1981.

Dander, B.; Righetti, B.; and Poppi, A.: Echocardiographic diagnosis of isolated pulmonic valve endocarditis. *Br. Heart J.* **47:**298, 1982.

Dzindzio, B. S.; Meyer, L. R.; Osterholm, R.; *et al.:* Isolated gonococcal pulmonary valve endocarditis: Diagnosis by echocardiography. *Circulation,* **59:**1319, 1979.

Howard, R. J.; Drobac, M.; Rider, W. D.; *et al.:* Carcinoid heart disease: Diagnosis by two-dimensional echocardiography. *Circulation,* **66:**1059, 1982.

Kramer, N. E.; Gill, S. S.; Patel, R.; *et al.:* Pulmonary valve vegetations detected with echocardiography. *Am. J. Cardiol.,* **39:**1064, 1977.

Mehlman, D.; Furey, W.; Phair, J.; *et al.:* Two-dimensional echocardiographic features diagnostic of isolated pulmonic valve endocarditis. *Am. Heart J.,* **103:**137, 1982.

Nakamura, K.; Satomi, G.; Sakai, T.; *et al.:* Clinical and echocardiographic features of pulmonary valve endocarditis. *Circulation,* **67:**198, 1983.

Sheikh, M. J.; Ali, N.; Covarrabias, E.; *et al.:* Right-sided infective endocarditis: an echocardiography study. *Am. J. Med.,* **66:**283, 1979.

Weiss, R. J.; LeMire, M. S.; Bajor, M.; *et al.:* Two-dimensional echocardiographic detection of pulmonic valve endocarditis. *J. C. U.,* **10:**451, 1982.

PULMONIC VALVE FLUTTER

Ayasama, J.; Matsuura, T.; Endo, N.; *et al.:* Echocardiographic findings of idiopathic dilatation of the pulmonary artery. *Chest,* **71:**671, 1977.

Fisher, E. A.; Sepehri, B.; Barron, S.; *et al.:* Echocardiographic diastolic flutter of the pulmonary valve in isolated patent ductus arteriosus. *Chest,* **81:**74, 1982.

Glasser, S. P., and Baucum, R. W.: Pulmonary valve fluttering in subpulmonic ventricular septal defect. *Am. Heart J.,* **94:**3, 1977.

Nanda, N. C., and Gramiak, R.: *Clinical Echocardiography.* C. V. Mosby, St. Louis, 1978, p. 240.

Prabhu, R.; D'Cruz, I.; Cohen, H.; *et al.:* Echocardiographic correlates of atrial contraction in normal and abnormal atrial rhythms. *Prog. Cardiovasc. Dis.,* **20:**463, 1978.

Weyman, A. E.; Dillon, J. C.; Feigenbaum, H.; *et al.:* Echocardiographic differentiation of infundibular from valvular pulmonary stenosis. *Am. J. Cardiol.,* **36:**21, 1975.

MIDSYSTOLIC PULMONARY VALVE CLOSURE IN OTHER THAN PULMONARY HYPERTENSION

Asin-Cardiel, E.; Alonso, M.; Delean, J. L.; *et al.:* Echocardiographic sign of right-sided hypertrophic obstructive cardiomyopathy. *Br. Heart J.,* **40:**1321, 1978.

Bauman, W.; Wann, L. S.; Childress, R.; *et al.:* Midsystolic notching of the pulmonary valve in the absence of pulmonary hypertension. *Am. J. Cardiol.,* **43:**1049, 1979.

Haddad, A. K.; Lebeau, R.; and Tremblay, G.: Midsystolic notching of the pulmonary valve. Letter to Editor. *Am. J. Cardiol.,* **46:**525, 1980.

Mills, P., and Craige, E.: Echocardiography. *Prog. Cardiovasc. Dis.,* **20:**337, 1978.

Weyman, A. E.; Dillon, J.; Feigenbaum, H.; *et al.:* Echocardiographic differentiation of infundibular from valvular pulmonary stenosis. *Am. J. Cardiol.,* **36:**21, 1975.

PULMONARY ARTERY

Bauman, W.; Wann, L. S.; Childress, R.; *et al.:* Midsystolic notching of the pulmonary valve in the absence of pulmonary hypertension. *Am. J. Cardiol.,* **43:**1049, 1979.

Bloch, A.; Terrapon, M.; and Bopp, P.: Echocardiographic diagnosis of pulmonary artery aneurysm. *Eur. J. Cardiol.,* **6:**33, 1977.

Weyman, A. E.: *Cross-sectional Echocardiography.* Lea & Febiger, Philadelphia, 1982, p. 377.

Wright, E. C.; Wellons, H. A.; and Martin, R. P.: Primary pulmonary artery sarcoma diagnosed noninvasively by two-dimensional echocardiography. *Circulation,* **67:**459, 1983.

G
Right Heart Chambers

In the normal M-mode echocardiogram, recorded by parasternal scanning, the left ventricle is on an average three times as wide as the right ventricle. The upper limit of right ventricular internal diameter (RVID) to left ventricular internal diameter (LVID) is 0.47 (Laurenceau and Dumesnil, 1976). According to Feigenbaum (1976), the mean RVID in normal adults is 15 mm (range, 7 to 23 mm) with the patient lying flat, and 17 mm (range, 9 to 26 mm) in the left lateral position. With the patient turned to his left side, the ultrasound beam traverses the right ventricular chamber more obliquely and so records a larger diameter.

By the subxiphoid approach the right ventricular dimension appears larger than in the parasternal view. With the transducer positioned in the epigastric region in the midline, the ultrasound beam is directed posteriorly and superiorly to transect the right ventricular inflow tract at its widest. Scanning leftward toward the left shoulder, the left ventricle comes into view, and at this level the right ventricular dimension appears smaller.

On the other hand, by the parasternal approach, the right ventricle appears widest at its outflow tract level (anterior to the aortic root), less wide at mitral valve level, and narrows farther as the left ventricle is scanned toward its apex. The upper normal limit of RV dimension, as observed by other authors (Kleid and Arvan, 1978; Haft and Horowitz, 1978), is also about 25 mm. In terms of body surface area, the upper normal limit is 15 mm/M^2 (Popp et al., 1969; Diamond et al., 1971).

The M-mode estimation of right atrial and right ventricular size is beset with several problems that do not apply to estimation of left atrial and left ventricular size:

1. The right atrium can be visualized only by oblique and variable angulation of the ultrasound beam, which has to be directed rightward from the left parasternal area, under the sternum. Consequently the right atrium, when it can be recorded at all, may vary widely in dimension depending on where the beam transects the chamber.

2. Unlike the LV shape, which is generally acknowledged to be that of a prolate ellipse, the RV shape is irregular and does not lend itself to simple geometric characterization. Therefore, the RV dimension cannot be extrapolated easily by mathematical formulae to yield an estimate of RV volume.

3. The RV anterior wall sometimes lacks sharp definition so that the anterior boundary of the RV is open to question.

Fortunately these problems have been surmounted by the ability to visualize the RV and RA quite well by 2-D echocardiography, using the short-axis and apical four-chamber view (Bommer et al., 1979). These authors have published normal values for RV and RA dimensions (Table G-1). Patients with RV volume overload had much larger right atrial dimensions: short-axis, 60 ± 3 mm; long-axis, 65 ± 3 mm. The overlap with normal values was greater for the long-axis than short-axis dimension. The planed right atrial area in patients

Table G-1. Range of Normal Values for Right Atrial (RA) and Right Ventricular (RV) Dimensions (Data from Bommer et al., 1979)

	LONG AXIS (mm)	SHORT AXIS (mm)	PLANED AREA (sq cm)
RA	42 ± 1	36 ± 1	13.9 ± 0.7
RV	74 ± 3	35 ± 2 (maximal)	18.0 ± 1.2
		28 ± 2 (mid-LV level)	

with RV overload was about two and one half times that of normal subjects.

With RV volume overload, the RV long-axis dimension did not increase significantly (78 ± 2 mm) as compared to normal (74 ± 3 mm), but the RV short-axis dimension almost doubled. Thus the maximal RV short-axis dimension was 61 ± 3 mm; the mid-RV short-axis dimension (short axis midway between tricuspid ring and RV apex) was also 61 ± 4 mm.

Recently attempts have been made to estimate RV volume from the 2-D echogram using the apical views (Watanabe *et al.,* 1982) and the subcostal view (Starling *et al.,* 1982). It is claimed that RV volumes and ejection fractions thus derived correlated well with the corresponding values obtained by invasive or by radionuclide ventriculography.

THE RIGHT VENTRICULAR ANTERIOR WALL

The RV wall echo appears in the M-mode echogram as a narrow band just behind the dense,

flat, chest wall echo. Anteriorly, the RV wall is related to the pericardium and posteriorly to the echo-free space of the RV chamber. With sufficient attention to technique, the RV wall can be recognized as such in most patients. Inability to visualize any RV wall echoes at all can result from oversuppression of near echoes; on the other hand, the obscuration of the RV wall by dense, amorphous echoes due to too high near gain is a common form of imperfect technique in practice.

Under various circumstances, several other structures can be mistaken for the RV wall:

1. The commonest error is to mistake reverberations of the chest wall for the RV wall. Such echoes are strictly linear and parallel to the chest wall echo ("main bang"); they lack the systolic thickening and endocardial contour of the true RV wall.

2. Thickened or calcified anterior pericardium.

3. Components of the tricuspid valve apparatus, especially chordae.

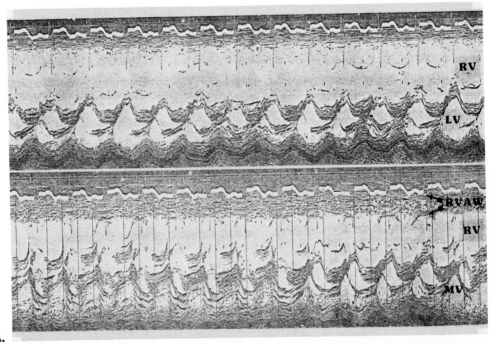

Fig. G-1. *A.* M-mode echogram in a child with transposition of great vessels. The upper panel shows both ventricles at the level of mitral chordae. The RV, hugely dilated, is much larger than the small LV. The ventricular septum shows normal systolic motion. In the lower panel the ultrasound beam transects the ventricles at a different level. The tricuspid valve can be partly seen at left. At right the ventricular septum and anterior mitral leaflet together form an appearance that could be mistaken for the mitral valve, in which case the RV may erroneously be taken for part of the LV. The hypertrophied RV anterior wall is evident.

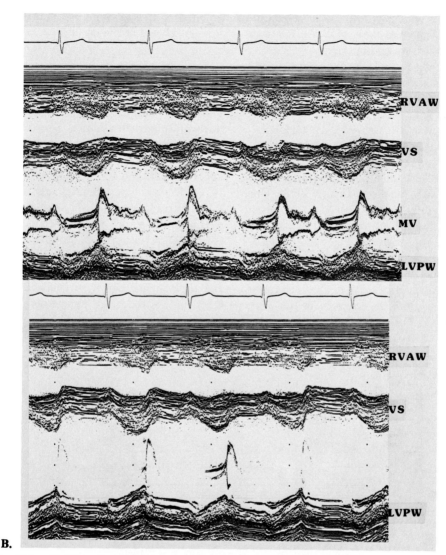

Fig. G-1. *B.* M-mode echogram showing the LV at mitral valve level (*above*) and chordae level (*below*). The patient was a 14-year-old boy with pulmonary valve stenosis (gradient 80 mmHg). The RV anterior wall and ventricular septum are hypertrophied in response to the RV pressure overload. The LV posterior wall is of normal thickness and much less thick than the ventricular septum.

4. Trabeculae or muscular bands traversing the RV chamber.

5. Swan-Ganz catheter or pacemaker wire.

6. The right septal border, the thickness of the ventricular septum (especially a thick one) being mistaken for the RV cavity.

7. Large pericardial effusions producing tamponade may be associated with diminished RV internal dimension, so that the RV anterior wall and ventricular septum may appear merged on the M-mode tracing into what seems to be the septal echo; the anterior pericardial effusion could then be mistaken for the RV chamber. However, a small pericardial effusion is a boon to the echocardiographer because it makes the anterior surface of the RV wall more conspicuous and better defined than usual; moreover, the systolic excursions of the RV wall are augmented, facilitating the identification of this structure.

Optimal visualization of the RV wall requires careful adjustment of the near gain so as to obtain echoes just posterior to the chest wall but at the same time keep the RV area free of amorphous background echoes or reverberatory echoes from the chest wall; the RV wall can be identified by noting that:

1. It increases in thickness during systole just after the QRS complex on the ECG.

2. It contains an intramural pattern of echoes that shows a typical sequence of changes during the cardiac cycle (D'Cruz *et al.,* 1976): a parallel linear morphology in middiastole, which alters to a discontinuous stippled pattern during ventricular contraction, and also during early and late (atrial) rapid ventricular filling. One can thus distinguish the RV wall echo from pericardium, chest wall reverberations, tricuspid chordae, and so forth. Likewise, in subxiphoid scans, the RV wall intramural pattern changes enable the echocardiographer to separate it from a variable width of stratified linear echoes arising from the left lobe of the liver,

which do not show changes synchronous with different phases of the cardiac cycle.

RIGHT VENTRICULAR WALL THICKNESS (Figs. G-1 and G-2)

The average diastolic thickness of the RV anterior wall in normal adults is 3 to 3.5 mm; 3.4 mm according to Matsukubo *et al.* (1977), 3.2 mm in the series of Child *et al.* (1979). The upper normal limit is 5 mm (Matsukubo *et al.,* 1977). The M-mode echographic assessment of RV wall thickness has been found to correlate well with the actual anatomic thickness, measured at open heart surgery (Arcilla *et al.,* 1976) and at autopsy (Prakash, 1978). Prakash found that echocardiography could successfully separate the patients with hypertrophied RV walls from those without RV hypertrophy. The im-

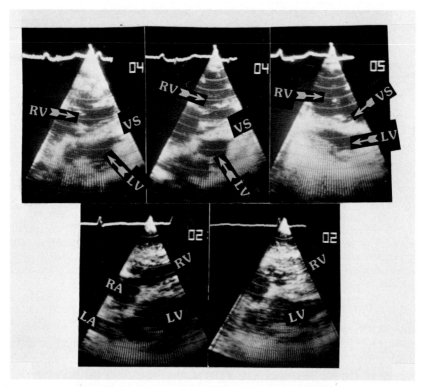

Fig. G-2. *Upper.* 2-D echogram in a patient with RV dilatation due to cor pulmonale. The left frame, in the subcostal view, shows the RV and RA anteriorly. The aortic root arises from the LV posteriorly. The center frame, also in the subcostal view but in a slightly more posterior plane, shows the RA and RV anteriorly and the LA and LV posteriorly. The right frame, in the short-axis view, shows a very dilated RV anteriorly, separated by the ventricular septum from a rather small LV posteriorly.

Lower. Subcostal 2-D echogram in another patient with cor pulmonale and RV hypertrophy on the ECG. The anterior wall, as well as the ventricular septum, appears hypertrophied in diastole (*left*). The wall thickens impressively in systole (*right*).

portance to the clinical cardiologist of RV wall thickness measurements, and the echocardiographic identification of RV hypertrophy, lies in the finding of Matsukubo *et al.* (1977) that RV hypertrophy is more reliably diagnosed by cardiac ultrasound than by electrocardiography. These authors found the subcostal approach particularly suitable for assessment of RV wall thickness and demonstrate a good correlation between RV wall thickness and peak systolic RV pressure.

Child *et al.* (1979) have called attention to a new diagnostic application of RV anterior wall thickness. They found abnormally thick RV walls in six patients with infiltrative amyloid cardiomyopathy. In patients with the triad of echographic LV abnormalities (symmetric increase in LV wall and septal thickness, diffuse hypokinesis and small to normal LV internal diastolic dimension) suggestive of cardiac amyloidosis, an abnormally thick RV wall further supports this diagnosis. On the other hand, patients with concentric LV hypertrophy due to hypertension or aortic stenosis could exhibit this triad of LV echocardiographic findings, but would not have an abnormally thick RV wall. Examples of RV hypertrophy in the M-mode echogram (Fig. G-1) and 2-D echogram (Fig. G-2) are shown.

Increased RV anterior wall thickness has also been described in the entity of endomyocardial fibrosis (Candell-Riera *et al.,* 1982; George *et al.,* 1982).

RIGHT VENTRICULAR WALL MOTION

Normally the RV anterior wall thickens in systole, so that its endocardial echo moves posteriorly in the same direction as the left border of the ventricular septum. When it can be identified, the RV anterior wall epicardium normally shows little or no motion. When an anterior pericardial effusion is present, the normal motion of the RV wall is exaggerated, the increase in amplitude being proportional to the extent of pericardial fluid. In the presence of tamponade, an abnormal posterior motion may be evident in diastole (Schilt *et al.,* 1980).

In patients with myocardial infarction involving the RV, 2-D echography might reveal wall motion abnormalities of the RV when particular care is taken to image this chamber as thoroughly as possible in different views. The RV anterior wall—the only part of the RV visible in the M-mode echogram—is the least commonly affected. Thus normal motion of this structure does not exclude RV infarction.

DILATATION OF THE RIGHT VENTRICLE (Figs. G-3 to G-11)

An increased RVID on the M-mode echogram is often part of a diffuse or generalized cardiac dilatation, most typically in an advanced congestive cardiomyopathy, or left ventricular dilatation and failure secondary to ischemic heart disease. In such situations, the left ventricle is dilated to the same degree, or to an even greater degree, than the right ventricle.

This section, however, deals with the differential diagnosis of quite a different echocardiographic appearance: that of a dilated right ventricular chamber that approaches, equals, or even exceeds in dimension a left ventricle that is normal to small in size.

Most instances of dilatation of the right heart chambers are caused by diastolic overload of this chamber, the most common causes of which, in adult cardiology, are tricuspid regurgitation, pulmonary hypertension of various etiologies, atrial septal defect, Ebstein's anomaly, and RV infarction.

ATRIAL SEPTAL DEFECT (Figs. G-3 and G-4)

Although not specific, the M-mode echographic features of atrial septal defect are encountered in a high percentage of patients with this anomaly, the most common form of congenital heart disease in adults. The clinical diagnosis of an atrial septal defect is certainly strengthened by the ultrasound detection of RV dilatation and abnormal systolic motion of the ventricular septum (Diamond *et al.,* 1971; McCann *et al.,* 1972; Tajik *et al.,* 1972a and b; Meyer *et al.,* 1972; Kerber *et al.,* 1973; Hagan *et al.,* 1974; Weyman *et al.,* 1976; Wanderman *et al.,* 1978; St. John Sutton *et al.,* 1979).

The RVID is almost always increased in patients with left-to-right atrial shunts; less than 5 per cent have a normal right ventricular dimension (Radtke *et al.,* 1976).

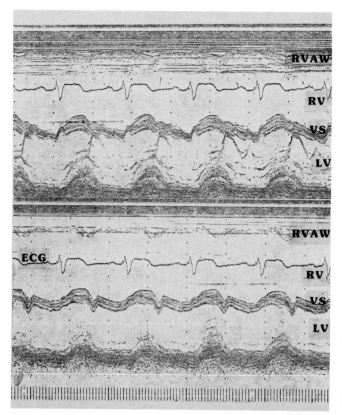

Fig. G-3. M-mode echogram in a young man with an atrial septal defect showing the RV and LV at mid-LV level. The upper panel depicts a slightly higher ventricular level than does the lower panel. The RV is markedly dilated, and in fact much larger than the LV. The ventricular septum shows abnormal anterior paradoxic systolic motion, but normal septal systolic thickening.

Slightly less common is abnormal systolic motion of the ventricular septum (Fig. G-3). The incidence of abnormal septal motion in various reported series has varied from 54 to 94 per cent; an average of all these series taken together would be in the range of 85 to 90 per cent, which is in accord with the experience of most echocardiographers.

Laurenceau and Dumesnil (1976) demonstrated a strong correlation between the degree of RV dilatation and abnormality of systolic septal motion: when the RV/LV internal end-diastolic dimension exceeds 0.65 (normal average, 0.33; upper normal limit, 0.47), ventricular septal motion is usually abnormal.

The mechanism of systolic anterior motion of the ventricular septum in RV volume overload, and in atrial septal defects in particular, has been the subject of much speculation (Hagan *et al.*, 1974; Weyman *et al.*, 1976; Lieppe *et al.*, 1977). Some of these hypotheses invoke an abnormal geometric configuration or behavior of the ventricular septum during systole, or in systole as well as diastole. Others postulate that the net systolic anterior movement of the

septum is caused by an exaggerated systolic anterior motion of the main body of the RV.

The large variation in the reported incidence of ventricular septal motion abnormalities in different series could be attributed to the following:

1. Abnormal systolic septal motion is not an all-or-none phenomenon, but includes in fact a broad spectrum of contour changes. In most pronounced form (also known as type A) the entire septum exhibits a large anterior excursion during systole, followed by a corresponding posterior motion returning it to a baseline position in early diastole. A lesser degree of septal abnormality, sometimes known as flat or type-B motion, is that in which the ventricular septum moves neither anteriorly nor posteriorly in systole.

2. Radtke *et al.* (1976) pointed out that systolic thickening of the septum, usually well marked in atrial septal defects, results in divergent motion of the left and right surfaces of the septum. Thus it is not uncommon to see the right septal border sloping toward the transducer (anteriorly), while the left septal margin

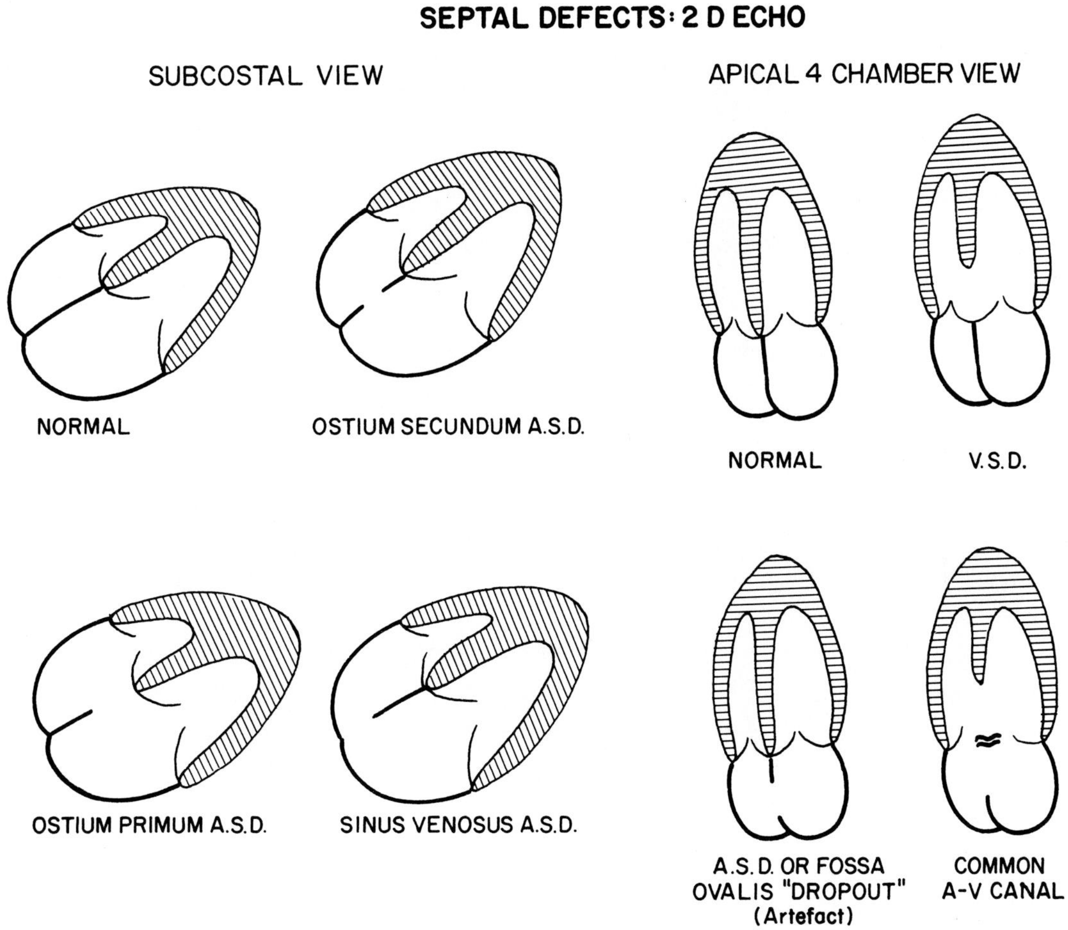

SEPTAL DEFECTS: 2 D ECHO

SUBCOSTAL VIEW · · · · · · · · · · APICAL 4 CHAMBER VIEW

NORMAL · · · · OSTIUM SECUNDUM A.S.D.

NORMAL · · · · V.S.D.

OSTIUM PRIMUM A.S.D. · · · · SINUS VENOSUS A.S.D.

A.S.D. OR FOSSA OVALIS "DROPOUT" (Artefact) · · · · COMMON A-V CANAL

Fig. G-4. Diagram showing 2-D echographic appearances of atrial and ventricular septal defects in the subcostal view (*left*) and apical 4-chamber view (*right*). Atrial septal defects are best seen in the subcostal view, ventricular septal defects in the apical 4-chamber and subcostal views.

has a flat (type-B) contour or even a gentle posterior motion. The identical tracing would be variously interpreted by different observers as abnormal type A, abnormal type B, or normal, depending on whether the echocardiographer's attention focused on left or right septal border.

3. Septal motion must be noted below the level of the mitral cusps. Abnormal anterior septal motion tends to be most pronounced at mitral valve level, least obvious near the ventricular apex.

CAVEATS FOR THE ECHOGRAPHIC DIAGNOSIS OF ATRIAL SEPTAL DEFECT

1. Both right and left septal borders should be defined clearly, as the ventricular septum

is visualized at the level of mitral chordae. Often it may be necessary to place the transducer many centimeters left of the sternum to do so; the altered alignment of the mitral and tricuspid valves and of the two ventricles with respect to the chest wall is a consequence of the considerable right ventricular dilatation in most instances of atrial septal defect.

2. A prominent posterior septal motion in early diastole should not be mistaken for systolic motion; end-systole can be ascertained at the moment the ventricular septum and left ventricular posterior wall reach maximum thickness, which is a trifle before the peak of the latter structure's endocardial motion.

3. Ten to fifteen per cent of all patients with left-to-right atrial shunts have genuinely normal systolic septal motion. These comprise (a) small

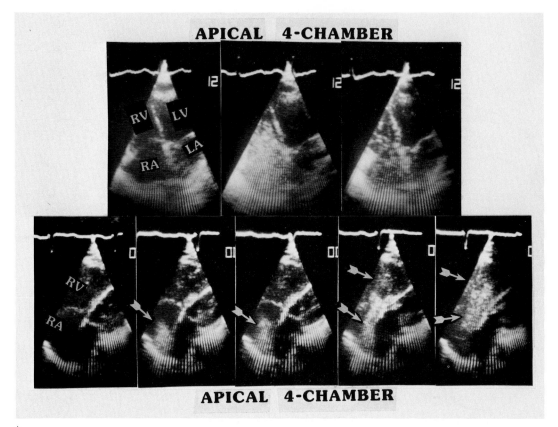

APICAL   4-CHAMBER

A.

Fig. G-5. *A. Upper.* 2-D echogram of a 15-year-old girl with a midsystolic ejection murmur at the left upper sternal border. The clinician wanted to exclude the possibility of an atrial septal defect. The left frame shows the ventricular and atrial septa separating the right from the left heart chambers. Intravenous saline was then injected into an arm vein, causing the microbubble bolus to opacify the RA and RV. If an atrial septal defect were present, a stream of unopacified blood would have appeared as a "filling defect" in the RA. No such shunting was seen; neither were a few microbubbles seen moving across the atrial septum to the LA or LV (as frequently seen with atrial septal defects of the usual type). In the right frame, a few seconds later, unopacified blood from the vena cavae has started "washing out" the microbubble-opacified blood in the right heart chambers.

    Lower. Panel. A different individual, also in the apical 4-chamber view, showing the passage of a bolus of contrast into the RA and RV (*arrows*). Note apparent streaming effect.

(less than 2:1 QP/QS ratio) shunts (Tajik *et al.,* 1972c); (b) associated mitral regurgitation which tends to normalize septal motion because the enhanced left ventricular stroke volume balances the effect of right ventricular diastolic overload; (c) a very small percentage of patients with uncomplicated large left-to-right atrial shunts.

4. The diagnosis of an uncomplicated atrial septal defect in a patient with a normal-size right ventricle and/or a dilated left ventricle is highly unlikely, even if physical signs or electrocardiogram have suggested it.

5. Following repair of atrial septal defects, the RVID usually decreases but very often does not return to normal for reasons yet unclear. In the Pearlman *et al.* (1978) series of 31 patients, the RV remained dilated in 77 per cent and septal motion abnormal in 68 per cent after surgical closure of atrial septal defects. Ventricular septal motion may return to normal or it may not. It has been shown that the presence of these echographic abnormalities after surgical closure of an atrial septal defect does *not* imply improper closure or reopening (Pearlman *et al.,* 1978).

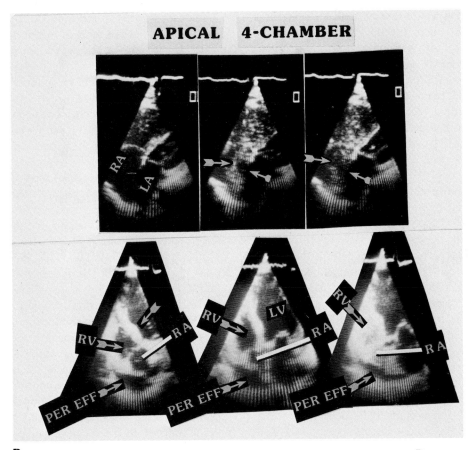

B.

Fig. G-5. *B.* Two important applications of contrast echocardiography.

Upper. 2-D echogram in the apical 4-chamber view, in a patient with atrial septal defect of secundum type. The first frame was recorded just before injection of saline into an arm vein. The second and third frames show contrast microbubbles in the right atrium and ventricle. A negative filling defect in the right atrium (*arrows*) is caused by the stream of unopacified blood from the left atrium across the atrial septal defect.

Lower. 2-D echogram of a patient with a pericardial effusion. The left and middle frames are in the apical 4-chamber view, in slightly different planes. An intra-atrial band appears to be dividing the RA into two. Injection of saline into an arm vein caused opacification of the RA and RV. The "band" or "septum" in the RA is thus shown to be the RA wall. The unopacified space behind it represents an accumulation of pericardial fluid.

6. The tricuspid valve is worth looking at in a patient with suspected atrial septal defect. If both tricuspid leaflets can be visualized easily throughout the whole cardiac cycle, that in itself is good evidence that the right ventricle is dilated. Diastolic flutter on the tricuspid leaflets is suggestive of a large left-to-right atrial shunt—a QP/QS ratio over 2.3 to 1 or more, according to Nanda and Gramiak (1978).

7. Very exceptionally, the right ventricle may be dilated and septal motion paradoxic for no detectable hemodynamic reason (Bahler *et al.,* 1976).

2-D ECHOCARDIOGRAPHIC FINDINGS IN ATRIAL SEPTAL DEFECTS (Figs. G-4 and G-5)

The long-axis, short-axis, and apical four-chamber views all show right ventricular dilatation with a normal to small left ventricle.

Close observation of the contour of the ventricular septum in the short-axis view at successive phases of the cardiac cycle reveals interesting changes that are not found in persons without right ventricular overload. Normally the left ventricle appears circular in this view in systole as well as diastole, and the ventricular septum is convex toward the right ventricular cavity. In right ventricular diastolic overload, the ventricular septum becomes flat or even convex toward the left ventricle in diastole, but in systole resumes its circular contour. It is worth noting that a similar change in septal curvature has been described in patients with high PEEP (positive end-expiratory pressure) by Jardin *et al.* (1981).

Mirro *et al.* (1979) demonstrated that rotational change or displacement of the LV, as manifested by angular displacement of a line joining the bases of the two LV papillary muscles in the short-axis view, is much more in individuals with atrial septal defects (mean, 17°; range, 9 to 29°) than in normal subjects (mean, 3°; range, 2 to 5°) or patients with other forms of heart disease. Such exaggerated rotation of the LV around its long axis disappeared after surgical closure of the atrial septal defect and constitutes yet another 2-D echographic sign of RV volume overload.

The atrial septum is best visualized by 2-D echocardiography (Fig. G-4) by subxiphoid scanning (Lange *et al.,* 1979; Bierman and Williams, 1979); it consistently appears as a well-defined echo, the ultrasound beam striking it more perpendicularly than tangentially. Secundum-type atrial septal defects, as well as balloon-created atrial septal openings at the fossa ovalis site (Rashkind procedure), are clearly seen.

Caution: The atrial septum normally tends to drop out in the fossa ovalis region, in individuals with perfectly intact atrial septa, in the apical four-chamber view. This is the thinnest part of the septum, which is tangential or parallel to the scanning plane in this view and so reflects ultrasound poorly. In the short-axis view, likewise, the atrial septum can easily drop out of the 2-D image (Dillon *et al.,* 1977), partly or entirely. Defects in the atrial septum should not be diagnosed on the basis of these views. The subcostal view is more reliable and contrast echography should be performed if possible (see below).

Sinus venosus types of atrial septal defect can be recognized by 2-D echography in the subcostal view by a deficiency at the *superior* end of the atrial septum, i.e., at a level above the fossa ovalis (Nasser *et al.,* 1981; Shub *et al.,* 1982).

Lieppe *et al.* (1977) found an exceptionally high incidence (95 per cent) of mitral prolapse in patients with atrial septal defects and claimed that a distinctive feature of the prolapse was predominant involvement of the anterior mitral leaflet. Schreiber *et al.,* (1980) encountered mitral prolapse in 7 of 14 patients with atrial septal defects; postoperatively the prolapse was diminished or abolished in 6 of the 7; concomitantly, the changes in LV geometry (septal curvature changes in diastole and systole) were normalized partly or entirely, suggesting that mitral prolapse in patients with atrial septal defects is secondary to altered LV shape and therefore tends to disappear once the defect is closed.

Contrast echocardiography (Figs. G-5A and B) has proven useful in the detection of atrial septal defects (Bourdillon *et al.,* 1980). Free or massive transfer of contrast microbubbles from RA to LA is obvious in patients with right-to-left atrial shunts, as for instance in patients with the Eisenmenger syndrome. However, a small but definite transfer of contrast from RA to LA is detectable in most patients with left-to-right atrial shunts. In such cases (usual ASD) streaming of unopacified LA blood into the contrast-filled RA causes a filling defect confirming the pressure and site of LA-to-RA shunt.

THE ECHOCARDIOGRAPHIC DISTINCTION BETWEEN ATRIAL SEPTAL DEFECTS OF THE OSTIUM PRIMUM AND OSTIUM SECUNDUM TYPES

The key to this important differential diagnosis is the echographic morphology of the mitral valve (Figs. B-37 and B-38). In ostium secundum type of defect the mitral cusps appear normal and display normal motion characteristics in systole and diastole. In ostium primum defects, on the other hand, the anterior mitral leaflet is cleft and anomalous chordae tendineae tether the cleft leaflet to the rim of the ventricular septum. Consequently, the planes of motion of the two components of the cleft leaflet are somewhat different from that of the normal anterior mitral leaflet. With cleft leaflet:

1. The normal M-shaped contour of the anterior mitral leaflet in diastole is often difficult or impossible to record; after the initial opening motion (DE segment) the leaflet may be lost to view.

2. The distance from mitral closure (C) point to ventricular septum is decreased, corresponding to the "gooseneck" narrowing of the left ventricular outflow tract on angiocardiography.

3. The amplitude of anterior diastolic excursion (DE) of the anterior mitral leaflet is diminished.

4. In systole the apposed mitral cusps appear multilayered and thick, 1 cm or more wide.

5. Undue close and prolonged contact of the anterior mitral leaflet with the left septal surface in diastole is noted.

6. Abnormal diastolic motion of the posterior mitral leaflet is common.

Since the extent to which the anterior mitral leaflet is cleft and tethered by anomalous chordae is variable from case to case, all of the above findings may not be evident in every patient.

Ostium primum atrial septal defects also demonstrate distinctive appearances on 2-D echocardiography (see Figs. B-37 and B-38). The separation of the anterior mitral leaflet into two components by the cleft, with attached adventitious chordae tendineae, results in the following abnormalities:

1. In the short-axis view, the anterior mitral leaflet splits into two parts as it whips open in diastole, i.e., it appears as two short, linear echoes, one on either side, rather than one continuous, curved, linear echo (Beppu *et al.,* 1980).

2. The separation of the anterior mitral leaflet into two components also may be evident on the long-axis view. Additional small mobile echoes in the anterior mitral region or in the space between mitral valve and ventricular septum represent anomalous chordae.

3. In the subcostal and apical 4-chamber views, the atrial septum is seen to be deficient in its lowermost part, with tricuspid and mitral valves inserted on the crest of the intact ventricular septum (Hynes *et al.,* 1982).

DIFFERENTIAL DIAGNOSIS BETWEEN COMPLETE AND PARTIAL A-V CANAL DEFECTS (Fig. G-6)

The differentiation of partial from complete A-V (atrioventricular) canal is important to the clinician. In the former the ventricular septum

is intact; closure of the ostium primum atrial septal defect and repair of a cleft mitral leaflet can be successfully carried out with very low risk. On the other hand, persistent common A-V canal in complete form is a very formidable defect, not only in a hemodynamic sense but also because its surgical correction is much more complex and difficult and fraught with high risk.

Adults or adolescents with endocardial cushion defects are likely to have a partial A-V canal variety. Infants with the complete form of common A-V canal seldom survive the first year or two of life; however, some do so if they have severe pulmonary hypertension (Eisenmenger syndrome) or pulmonary stenosis. In the latter case, they run the hazard of being mistaken for tetralogy of Fallot or double-outlet RV, even after hemodynamic study, a surgical catastrophe if recognized only at open-heart surgery.

The following features (Bass *et al.,* 1978) help in distinguishing partial from complete A-V canal on the M-mode echocardiogram: paradoxic systolic motion of the ventricular septum, a normal or only slightly abnormal pattern of mitral motion, absence of tricuspid or mitral motion crossing the plane of the ventricular septum, and visualization of the ventricular septum intervening between mitral and tricuspid valves in all scans favor the partial form of A-V canal. Normal septal systolic motion, a severely abnormal or "disorganized" pattern of mitral motion, absence of septal echoes between mitral and tricuspid valve echoes when scanning from LV to aorta, and especially large-amplitude "mitral" echoes crossing into the RV in diastole (Fig. G-6A) would support the diagnosis of complete A-V canal defect. *Caution:* In patients with partial A-V canal defects, the DE slopes of separate tricuspid and mitral valves may appear almost continuous with each other so as to simulate crossing of an abnormal A-V leaflet across the septal defect and thus falsely indicate a complete A-V canal defect, on cursory inspection. Fast paper speeds and careful scrutiny of the A-V valve echoes may be necessary to determine whether they originate from two separate (mitral and tricuspid) valves or anomalous valve tissue traversing a large common A-V canal.

However, the anatomic and echographic spectrum of endocardial cushion defects is so

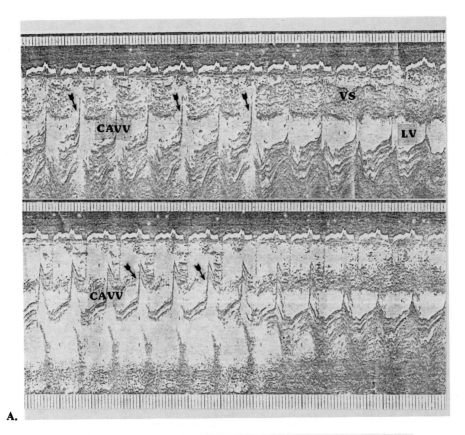

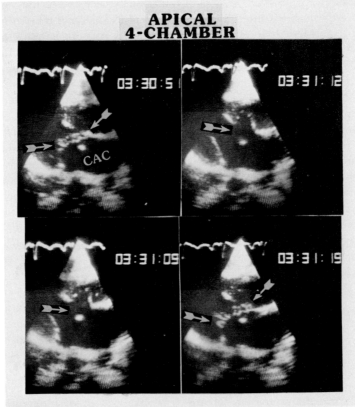

wide and varied (Williams and Rudd, 1974; Pieroni *et al.,* 1975) that the M-mode differentiation of partial from complete form is often difficult and no infallible criterion has yet been established. Two-dimensional echocardiography, using the apical or (when possible) subcostal four-chamber view, depicts the anatomy of the crucial central area of the heart where the atrial and ventricular septa meet and where the tricuspid and mitral valves are attached. In the partial A-V canal type of defect, with intact ventricular septum, the attachments of the septal tricuspid leaflet and the anterior mitral leaflet to the crest of the septum, with the hiatus caused by ostium primum atrial septum just above it, present a distinctive appearance. In complete A-V canal defects, the septal gap is obviously larger, and leaflet components of the common A-V valve may be seen interposed or traversing this hiatus (Hagler *et al.,* 1979). These authors have shown that even subvarieties of common A-V canal (A, B, and C of Rastelli's classification) can be recognized. The important question of the presence and size of a ventricular component of an endocardial cushion defect can be answered by contrast echocardiography; indocyanine green and/or saline is injected into the LV during left-heart catheterization and the flow of "microbubble opacification" into the right heart chambers is recorded in the apical four-chamber view (Hagler *et al.,* 1979).

In the subcostal view, endocardial cushion defects (of partial as well as complete types) show a distinctive LV outflow tract contour: elongated, narrow, and somewhat horizontally inclined (Yoshida *et al.,* 1980), similar to the gooseneck deformity on the angiogram. During systole the mitral valve echoes appear thickened, jagged, and irregular in the same view, corresponding to the scalloped outline of this region in the LV angiogram.

PARTIAL ANOMALOUS PULMONARY VENOUS DRAINAGE

This anomaly is usually associated with atrial septal defects, and the echographic findings are no different from those usually found in patients with large left-to-right atrial shunts, as described above. A minority of patients with drainage of one or more right pulmonary veins into the right atrium have intact atrial septa; these would behave echocardiographically like small atrial septal defects, presenting with mildly dilated right ventricles and partly or slightly abnormal systolic motion of the ventricular septum.

Danilowicz and Kronzon (1979) have demonstrated that contrast echocardiography could have a useful diagnostic role during the cardiac catheterization of patients with atrial septal defects. Cardiogreen or the patient's own blood is injected into the left atrium, as well as into the pulmonary vein or veins entered by the catheter. If clouding (microbubbles) is seen in both right and left heart chambers after left atrial as well as pulmonary venous injection, an atrial septal defect with normal pulmonary venous drainage is indicated. On the other hand, if the left atrial injection shows clouding of both right- and left-side chambers, but injection into a right pulmonary vein produces clouding of only right atrium and ventricle, it suggests that the vein drains anomalously into the right atrium.

Bourdillon *et al.* (1980) described a very unusual congenital anomaly in a 64-year-old

Fig. G-6. *A.* M-mode echogram of a child with an endocardial cushion defect of the complete type (common A-V canal). In the upper panel, the mitral valve appears abnormal and clearly crosses the plane of the ventricular septum (*arrows*), which is deficient at this level. The valve seen is part of the common A-V valve (CAVV) spanning the common A-V defect. In the lower panel, this valve is viewed from a different direction and could be mistaken for a normal tricuspid valve. However, it too crosses the septal defect (*arrows*).

Fig. G-6. *B.* 2-D echogram in the apical 4-chamber view, of a child with common atrioventricular (A-V) canal of the complete type. The four frames are serial ones from the same cardiac cycle. There is an almost common atrial chamber (CAC) as well as deficiency of the upper ventricular septum. Abnormal A-V valve tissue straddles the common A-V canal in systole (*top left and bottom right*). In diastole (*top right and bottom left*) the RV and LV components of the common A-V valve can be seen to open widely.

woman presenting with cardiac failure and physical signs like those of atrial septal defect. A persistent left superior vena cava drained into a large coronary sinus, which entered the right atrium normally but also communicated with the left atrium. A large left-to-right shunt existed at atrial level through the coronary sinus, the atrial septum and pulmonary veins being quite normal. The dilated coronary sinus was demonstrated on M-mode as well as 2-D echography as an abnormal "chamber" posterior to the LA and opening into it. Injection of green dye into a right brachial vein did not result in the appearance of microbubbles in the LA. However, injection into the left brachial vein produced opacification by microbubbles of the dilated coronary sinus and of the LA itself.

TOTAL ANOMALOUS PULMONARY VENOUS DRAINAGE

The patient is usually an infant or young child. Echocardiographically it resembles atrial septal defect, with the additional finding that an echo-free space posterior to the left atrium may be seen by M-mode as well as 2-D echography, which represents the anomalous venous channel conveying pulmonary venous blood to the right atrium (Tajik *et al.*, 1972; Aziz *et al.*, 1978; Orsmond *et al.*, 1979; Sahn *et al.*, 1979). In particular, a dilated coronary sinus, conveying pulmonary venous blood entering a persistent left superior vena cava, presents as a wide sonolucent space behind the left atrium. Injection of saline or green dye into a left antecubital vein results in microbubbles opacifying the anomalous pulmonary venous vessel and coronary sinus, thus validating the identity of these structures.

Sahn *et al.* (1979) pointed out that the 2-D echographic visualization of one or more pulmonary veins entering the LA would exclude the diagnosis of total anomalous pulmonary venous drainage. They correctly diagnosed this entity in 7 infants; in 125 other infants without anomalous pulmonary veins, at least two normally draining pulmonary veins could be detected in 96, and at least one in 118.

EBSTEIN'S ANOMALY (Figs. G-7 and G-8)

Ebstein's anomaly of the tricuspid valve is one of the common varieties of congenital heart disease encountered in adults. Fortunately, it is unusually rich in echocardiographic manifestations (Lundstrom, 1973; Yuste *et al.*, 1974; Milner *et al.*, 1976; Farookhi *et al.*, 1976; Matsumato *et al.*, 1976; Hirschklau *et al.*, 1977; Monibi *et al.*, 1978).

On M-mode echography (Fig. G-7), the two most important (virtually pathognomonic) abnormal findings are:

1. Delayed tricuspid valve closure, which follows mitral valve closure by an interval of 0.03 (Farookhi *et al.*, 1976) or 0.04 sec or more (Nanda and Gramiak, 1978). Others require that this interval be 0.05 (Milner *et al.*, 1976) or 0.06 sec. Values as high as 0.10 sec have been reported. Simultaneous recording of tricuspid and mitral valves, at least of the closure (C) point, is necessary to accurately measure the tricuspid delay (Fig. G-7). If preexcitation of the RV is present (a finding well known to be associated with Ebstein's anomaly), there may be no delay in tricuspid closure (Koiwaya *et al.*, 1979). Marked delay in tricuspid valve closure has been reported in a patient with corrected transposition and Ebstein's anomaly of the systemic ventricle (Henry *et al.*, 1979).

2. The tricuspid valve is easily and well visualized with the ultrasound transducer held perpendicular to the chest wall and placed several centimeters to the left of the midline. Apart from gross shift of the mediastinum to the left, this can never happen in normal persons and very seldom in cardiac disease, including congenital defects, of any kind other than Ebstein's. It is attributable to displacement of the tricuspid valve downward and to the left toward the right ventricular apex and the huge right atrial cavity that incorporates the upper "atrialized" portion of the right side of the ventricular septum. The tricuspid valve, especially its anterior leaflet, thus is situated directly anterior to the mitral valve or almost so, whereas in normal hearts the tricuspid is some distance to the right of the mitral valve. Hence, it is usually not too difficult to find a precordial site from which both valves are seen on the echographic tracing at the same time, a feat that would otherwise be beyond the skill of any echocardiographer.

In Ebstein's anomaly the anterior tricuspid leaflet exhibits an unusually large amplitude of diastolic opening motion, and often its EF slope appears unduly flat. This large, conspicuous

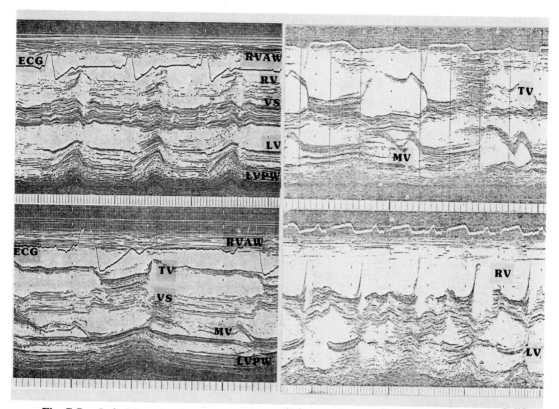

Fig. G-7. *Left.* M-mode echogram in a patient with Ebstein's anomaly and the Wolff-Parkinson-White syndrome. The left upper panel shows the RV and LV at LV chordae level. The dilated RV is wider than the LV. The ventricular septum thickens normally in systole, but fails to move posteriorly; abnormal septal motion is attributable to tricuspid regurgitation. The tricuspid and mitral valves are visualized simultaneously in the left lower panel. Tricuspid closure follows mitral closure by more than 0.06 sec, a finding that is virtually pathognomonic of Ebstein's anomaly.

Right. M-mode echogram in a different patient with Ebstein's anomaly. The upper right panel was recorded at twice the speed of the lower panel. The tricuspid valve closure follows mitral valve closure by an appreciable interval. In the lower right panel, at mitral chordae level, the RV appears dilated. In both panels, the tricuspid valve presents an unusual appearance, the posterior or septal leaflet being absent or seeming to merge with the ventricular septum. This configuration, very suggestive of Ebstein's anomaly, is due to the anomalous insertion of the septal leaflet.

rectangular tricuspid echo tends to dwarf the small, more delicate M-shaped mitral diastolic echo behind it. Abnormal morphology of the expansive floppy sail-like tricuspid anterior cusp is an essential feature of the anomaly Ebstein described.

Right ventricular dilatation, paradoxic systolic septal motion, and a small left ventricle are the rule in Ebstein's anomaly. These are, of course, nonspecific features, but if absent, the diagnosis of Ebstein's disease is unlikely. Premature pulmonic valve opening, as a result of abnormally powerful right atrial contractions, has been reported in Ebstein's anomaly.

Two-D echocardiography has proven of particular value in the diagnosis of Ebstein's anomaly by allowing visualization of its basic anatomic abnormality: the displacement of septal and posterior tricuspid leaflets toward the RV apex (Fig. G-8), with atrialization of the RV between these leaflets and the tricuspid valve ring. Initial observations in this regard were made by Matsumato *et al.* (1976) and Hirschklau *et al.* (1977) but for various technical reasons were not entirely successful in depicting the abnormal RV anatomy of Ebstein's disease. They were improved upon by Ports *et al.* (1978) who used the apical four-chamber view and by

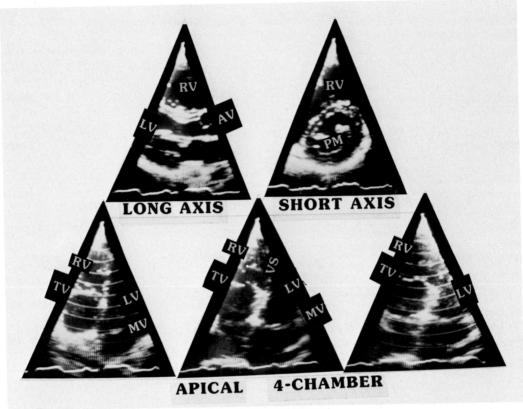

Fig. G-8. 2-D echogram of a patient with Ebstein's anomaly. The two upper frames, in the long- and short-axis views, show RV dilatation. In the three lower frames, in the apical 4-chamber view, the tricuspid valve leaflet is not at the same level as the mitral valve. The tricuspid valve is about 3 cm closer to the apex than the mitral valve.

Kambe *et al.* (1980) who visualized the right heart chambers by apical as well as subcostal approaches.

Since the sites of attachment of the tricuspid and mitral valves to the ventricular septum can be well seen, as well as the levels of the tricuspid and mitral valve rings with reference to the entire length of the ventricular septum, the extent of downward displacement of the tricuspid valve toward the RV apex, i.e., the extent of atrialized RV, can be measured precisely. This distance was found to be 2 to 7 cm by Ports *et al.,* and 1.4 to 3.2 cm by Kambe *et al.* The discrepancy may be explained by a preponderance of more severe tricuspid abnormality in the former series.

Another way of expressing the downward displacement of the tricuspid valve quantitatively is by the ratio: mitral-to-apex distance/tricuspid-to-apex distance, as measured in the apical four-chamber view. Ports *et al.* (1978) found this ratio to be 1 to 1.2:1 in normals, whereas in Ebstein's anomaly it is increased to 1.8 to 3.2:1.

In Ebstein's disease the tricuspid leaflets not only are displaced to an abnormal location in the RV but may also be thickened, relatively immobile, redundant, or partly adherent to the adjacent RV wall or ventricular septum. Such abnormalities can often be appreciated by careful 2-D scanning in the apical four-chamber or subcostal view.

RIGHT VENTRICULAR DYSPLASIA

RV dilatation is a prominent echographic feature of Uhl's anomaly (Perrenoud *et al.,* 1982) and of arrhythmogenic RV dysplasia (Marcus *et al.,* 1982; Rossi *et al.,* 1982; Baran *et al.,* 1982). In the latter, peculiar bulgings or diverticula of the RV wall may be seen on 2-D echography.

RIGHT VENTRICULAR INFARCTION

It has recently been recognized that right ventricular infarction is not rare; it may accompany inferior wall myocardial infarction and manifest with hypotension and RV failure. Sharpe *et al.* (1978) reported six patients with RV infarction on the basis of abnormal radionuclide uptake localized to the RV wall on infarct scintigraphy or segmental akinesis of the RV wall on gated radioangiography, or both, who had increased RV dimensions and RL/LV end-diastolic dimension ratios on echocardiography. The RV dilatation was of mild to moderate degree (RV internal dimension, 20 to 36 mm, RV/LV dimension ratio, 0.32 to 0.82). Massive RV dilatation was not seen. Mild to moderate RV dilatation was a frequent finding in patients with inferior infarction who had ECG, hemodynamic, and scintigraphic evidence of RV infarction (Candell-Riera *et al.*, 1981; Butman *et al.*, 1982). Lorell *et al.* (1979) reported 12 patients with acute inferior wall infarction associated "with jugular venous distention, clear lungs to auscultation, and arterial hypotension." Some of the patients were initially misdiagnosed as having cardiac tamponade. Echocardiography was helpful in excluding a pericardial effusion and in demonstrating RV dilatation.

Regional akinesia, dyskinesia, and even aneurysm of the RV free wall have been visualized on 2-D echography in patients with inferior wall myocardial infarction and associated RV infarction (D'Arcy and Nanda, 1982), as well as in contusion of the RV wall following blunt chest trauma (Miller *et al.*, 1982).

IDIOPATHIC RIGHT VENTRICULAR DILATATION

Bahler *et al.* (1976) described two patients with heart murmurs, electrocardiograms, and chest x-rays suggestive of atrial septal defect who exhibited RV dilatation and paradoxic systolic septal motion on echocardiography, but had no demonstrable left-to-right shunt or any other abnormality on hemodynamic study. The abnormal findings remain a mystery.

ECHOCARDIOGRAPHIC APPEARANCES SIMULATING A DILATED RV

An anterior pericardial effusion, especially if large but loculated, could easily be mistaken for the RV chamber, especially if the true RV cavity is compressed so that the RV anterior wall cannot be distinguished easily from the ventricular septum. Anterior mediastinal cysts or masses likewise can simulate RV dilatation (D'Cruz *et al.*, 1982) if the true RV chamber is not readily identifiable (Fig. G-9). A hydatid cyst in the ventricular septum has simulated RV enlargement on the M-mode echogram (Farookhi *et al.*, 1977).

RIGHT VENTRICULAR PRESSURE OVERLOAD

Right ventricular dilatation is a common feature of pulmonary hypertension and pulmonary stenosis. Apart from left heart disease, the most frequent cause of pulmonary hypertension in adults is chronic pulmonary disease; Eisenmenger syndrome, various forms of diffuse interstitial pulmonary fibrosis and arteritis, and primary pulmonary hypertension are much rarer. In children and young adults pulmonic valve stenosis, tetralogy of Fallot (Fig. G-10), various transposition complexes (Fig. G-10), double-outlet right ventricle, and other less frequent anomalies present echocardiographically with

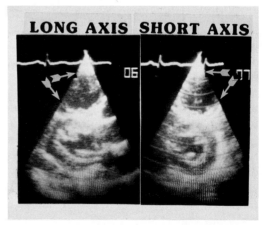

Fig. G-9. 2-D echogram of a 10-year-old girl with an anterior mediastinal cyst (*arrows*) compressing the RV. The cavity of the cyst simulates the RV chamber. At thoracotomy a rigid cystic chondroma was found to be compressing the RV.

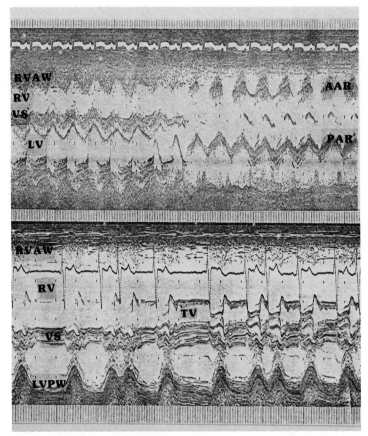

Fig. G-10. *Upper.* M-mode echographic scan from LV to aortic root level, in a patient with Fallot's tetralogy. The ventricular septum is not continuous with the anterior aortic root, which is on a more anterior plane; thus, overriding of the aorta is present.

Lower. M-mode echogram of a child with transposition of great vessels and congestive cardiac failure. The RV is dilated to twice the diameter of the LV. The tricuspid valve is visible in the right third of the figure. The tricuspid valve was competent in this patient, so that the RV overload was due to pressure only, and the ventricular septum exhibits normal motion.

increased RV and normal or decreased LV dimension. RV enlargement is only of mild to moderate degree in pressure overload states, seldom attaining the huge dimensions often seen in patients with atrial septal defect and large left-to-right shunts or with severe tricuspid regurgitation. Thus the RV/LV dimension ratio (average, 0.33 in normals) was an average of 0.93 in patients with RV diastolic overload and an average of 0.44 (but not more than 0.6) in patients with RV systolic overload (Laurenceau and Dumesnil, 1976).

The main echocardiographic difference between right ventricular pressure and volume overload is that ventricular septal systolic motion is normal in pressure overload, but usually abnormal (paradoxic) in volume overload states. In the latter situation, the right ventricular stroke volume is twice or more the left ventricular stroke volume, causing a net motion of the septum toward the transducer in systole. On the other hand, in right ventricular pressure overload, the two ventricles eject the same stroke volume, and there is little reason for the septum to move anteriorly in systole.

Another difference between right ventricular pressure and volume overload is that the right ventricular anterior wall may be unduly thick in pressure overload.

If pulmonary hypertension and pulmonary stenosis are severe enough, right ventricular dilatation and tricuspid regurgitation supervene sooner or later, and the hemodynamic as well as echocardiographic picture becomes mixed, one of both pressure and volume overload.

COR PULMONALE

Several M-mode echographic studies in children and young adults suffering from cystic fibrosis have demonstrated that this technique is very useful in detecting RV enlargement and an abnormal increase in the RV/LV dimension ratio (Ryssing, 1977; Rosenthal et al., 1976; Gewitz et al., 1977; Hirschfeld et al., 1979; Allen et al., 1979). Furthermore, the degree of RV dilatation correlated with severity of pulmonary function impairment. Hirschfeld et al. also showed that the ratio of RV preejection period to RV ejection time, as measured on the pulmonic valve echo, correlates well with the pulmonary artery diastolic pressure and also correlates with the extent of pulmonary function deterioration. However, the pulmonic valve echo cannot be recorded in most older patients with cor pulmonale whose hearts are impenetrable to ultrasound anteriorly because of emphysematous overlying lung. From the echocardiographer's viewpoint, patients with right ventricular dilatation (and usually failure) form a special group. Because of pulmonary emphysema, it is common for the heart to be inaccessible to ultrasound scanning from the parasternal region. However, the diaphragm and with it the heart may be situated unusually low in the thorax. The heart is thus beneath the xiphisternum and subxiphoid area, and in fact right ventricular pulsations may be well palpable at this site. The cardiac chambers therefore are visualized easily by subcostal M-mode scanning (Fig. G-11) and even better appreciated by 2-D echocardiography from this approach (Fig. G-12).

The relative sizes of the left and right ventricles are well demonstrated in the coronal plane (subcostal four-chamber view), with the 2-D probe held firmly down on the epigastrium in the midline and directed upward, posteriorly and leftward. The shape and size of all four cardiac chambers are evident, as are also the motion and thickness of the mitral, aortic, and tricuspid valves.

The visualization of a huge right ventricular chamber, occupying all of the anterior and right bulk of the heart, is convincing and valuable evidence that congestive heart failure in a given patient is right sided; cor pulmonale rather than left heart pathology of an ischemic or cardiomyopathic nature is the basis for the cardiac decompensation. When of moderate to severe degree, right ventricular dilatation is perceived easily in the apical four-chamber view as well as subxiphoid, long-axis, and short-axis views.

RV dilatation and an abnormally high RV/LV dimension ratio have been reported in

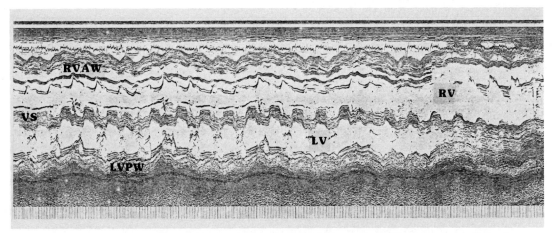

Fig. G-11. M-mode echogram by the subcostal approach in a patient with severe cor pulmonale secondary to chronic bronchitis. A scan has been made from mitral valve level toward the cardiac apex. The RV dimension exceeds that of the LV. Note that the RV anterior wall is closer to the transducer than it usually is in subcostal scans; this is due to the low diaphragm bringing the heart closer to the abdominal wall in the epigastrium.

SUBCOSTAL

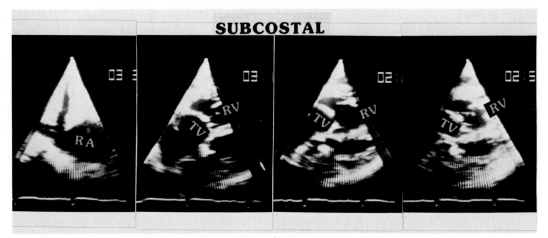

Fig. G-12. Subcostal 2-D echogram of a elderly man with cor pulmonale. A scan of the cardiac chambers has been made as follows: with the 2-D probe placed in the midline and at first directed to the right, the probe is gradually rocked across the midline toward the left. The probe is also rotated so that it moves from a sagittal to a coronal plane. The dilated RA and RV and tricuspid valve are well visualized. Thus the RA only, with entry of inferior vena cava into it, is visible in the first frame; the tricuspid valve and part of the RV and LV come into view in the second frame; the ventricles are more completely visible in the third and fourth frames.

patients with acute pulmonary hypertension caused by pulmonary embolism (Alpert *et al.,* 1977; Kasper *et al.,* 1980) as well as in chronic pulmonary hypertension of the primary type or secondary to repeated pulmonary emboli (Krayenbuehl *et al.,* 1978). Thus echocardiography may have a diagnostic role in the evaluation of patients presenting with acute or subacute dyspnea of uncertain etiology.

The status of LV function in patients with pulmonary hypertension and RV dilatation or failure, and cor pulmonale in particular, has intrigued clinicians, pathologists, and physiologists for many years. M-mode abnormalities of LV size, function, and wall thickness have been described (Krayenbuehl *et al.,* 1978) and are of much theoretical interest; however, they are usually of mild degree and of little practical diagnostic value.

Certain changes in LV geometry pertaining to the configuration of the ventricular septum are rather characteristic of RV diastolic overload states and may have a bearing on interaction between the two ventricles (Tanaka *et al.,* 1980). These interesting abnormalities of septal contour are seen best in the 2-D short-axis view, although also manifest to a lesser degree in the other 2-D views; they correspond to the abnormal paradoxic septal motion on M-mode tracings.

The normal convexity of the ventricular septum toward the RV may become flattened and in extreme cases actually concave toward the RV. This contour change is most pronounced in early diastole; during systole the LV, including its septal segment, returns to its circular outline, or almost so. The LV chamber in fact may be flattened and compressed to a narrow slit in extreme cases (Jacobstein *et al.,* 1981).

One echocardiographic implication of these alterations in LV shape is that the LV diastolic shape ceases to be that of a prolate ellipsoid and therefore calculations of LV volume and ejection fraction based on the LV internal dimension are no longer valid.

RIGHT ATRIUM (Figs. G-13 to G-15)

The right atrium (RA) was the last of the four cardiac chambers to be studied quantitatively. Because of its relatively inaccessible location (to ultrasound scanning) to the right of the sternum, it was not routinely recorded on M-mode echocardiography. To echocardiographers it remained a vague uncharted area posterior to the tricuspid valve until 2-D echocardiography demonstrated that the RA could be viewed as clearly and completely as the other three chambers. The shape and size of the RA are best appreciated in the apical and subcostal four-chamber views and to a somewhat lesser extent in the short-axis view (Figs. G-13 and G-14).

Using the apical four-chamber view, Reeves *et al.* (1981) found that the RA area varied from 11.4 to 24 cm² (mean, 16 cm²) in normal subjects; RA area over 25 cm² was considered dilatation. Correlating the electrocardiographic findings with echocardiographic RA dilatation, they found P-wave criteria poor indicators of increased RA size; a qR pattern in V1, however, was consistently associated with RA dilatation.

Kushner *et al.* (1978) measured the right and left atrial dimensions in the apical four-chamber view "from the AV valve rings (tricuspid and mitral valve insertions) to the posterosuperior atrial roofs at end-systole." These authors found the average LA dimension, thus measured, to be the same as the average PA dimension in normal subjects (35 mm, range, 30 to 40 mm for RA; 35 mm, range, 23 to 40 mm for LA).

All five of their patients with atrial septal defects had dilatation of the RA (mean, 54 mm). Ten of 11 patients with mitral stenosis and pulmonary hypertension had dilated right atria (mean, 54 mm). The measurement of RA dimension in the apical four-chamber view therefore may be of some diagnostic help in patients suspected to have atrial septal defect or pulmonary hypertension. Enormous dilatation of the RA is encountered sometimes in Ebstein's anomaly (Seward *et al.*, 1979; Desimone and Kronzon, 1981). Both the patients described in these case reports were elderly, 85 and 65 years, respectively. The gigantic RA chamber (12 × 14 cm in Desimone's case, in the apical four-chamber view) was far greater in size than the other three chambers combined.

Idiopathic dilatation of the right atrium is a rare entity first described by Pastor and Forte (1961), wherein the RA is markedly dilated in comparison with the other cardiac chambers, and all other known causes of RA enlargement have been excluded. The M-mode echographic findings in such a case have been reported (Asayama, 1977). Scanning in a rightward direction from the aortic root–left atrial region revealed an enormous expanse of echo-free space, 11.6 cm wide, representing the huge RA.

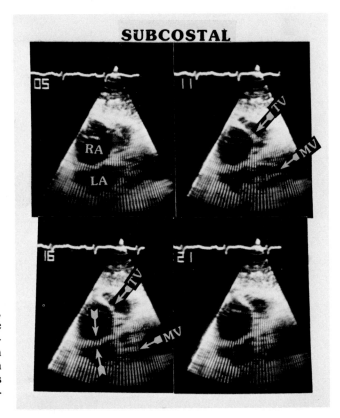

SUBCOSTAL

Fig. G-13. Subcostal 2-D echogram, demonstrating good visualization of the right and left atria and of the atrial septum (*arrows, left lower frame*) between them. The tricuspid and mitral valves can also be seen. Right atrial dilatation in this patient was secondary to chronic lung disease.

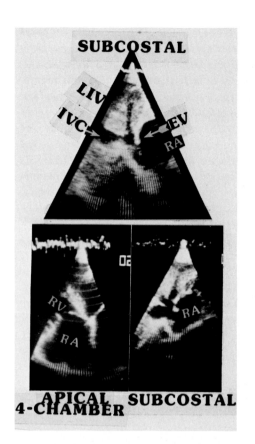

Fig. G-14. 2-D echogram showing salient features of right atrial anatomy. The upper frame, in a right parasagittal plane in the subcostal view, shows the inferior vena cava (IVC) entering the right atrium (RA). In its course through the liver (LIV), the inferior vena cava is joined by a hepatic vein. The Eustachian valve (EV) is seen at the junction of the cava and right atrium.

The two lower frames, in another patient, demonstrate the right atrium in the apical 4-chamber view (*left*) and subcostal parasagittal view (*right*).

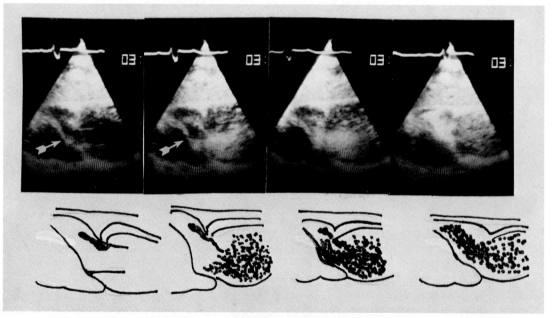

Fig. G-15. 2-D echographic frames in a child who had had a Mustard operation for transposition of the great vessels. The arrows indicate the intra-atrial baffle. The first frame was recorded just before the injection of saline into a forearm vein. The second frame shows the arrival of contrast in the left ventricle via the superior vena cava. In the third and fourth frames the contrast appears in the systemic atrium. The pulmonary venous atrium remains unopacified.

In the *Mustard operation* for transposition of great vessels, an intra-atrial baffle radically alters atrial anatomy. The baffle and the new pathways of atrial flow it produces can be visualized by 2-D echography (Fig. G-15).

INFERIOR VENA CAVA (Figs. G-16 to G-18)

The inferior vena cava, a large vessel 1 to 2 cm in diameter, runs vertically upward to enter the lower end of the right atrium. It is about 8 to 10 cm from the epigastric surface, separated from it by the thickness of the liver, to the posterior surface of which it is intimately related. It can be visualized by placing the M-mode transducer on the epigastrium at about the midline and directing it posteriorly and slightly to the right: the inferior vena cava (IVC) appears as an echo-free space with parallel borders (Fig. G-16), posterior to the stratified linear echoes of the liver, that collapses

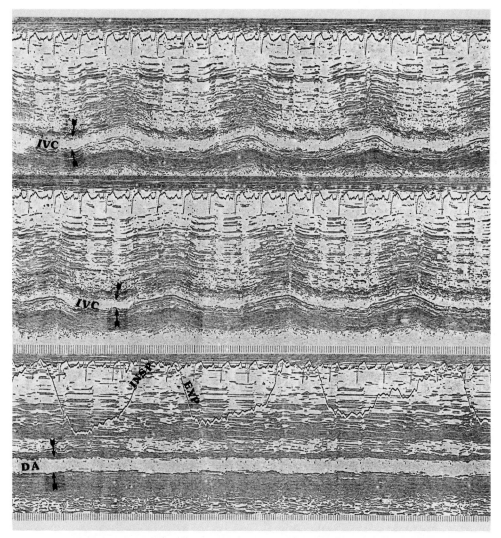

Fig. G-16. M-mode echogram, by the subcostal approach, with the transducer directed posteriorly. The echo-free space posterior to the liver (*upper and center*) represents the inferior vena cava (IVC). During inspiration the IVC moves toward the transducer and during expiration away from it. Note that the IVC caliber narrows in inspiration, especially in the center panel. With a slight leftward shift, the descending aorta was brought into view (*lower*). Note that the aorta does not show significant respiratory variation in position or caliber. Phases of respiration are recorded in this panel by means of a transducer strapped to the thorax.

(narrows) during a rapid brief inspiration. It can be differentiated from the descending aorta (Wise *et al.,* 1981), which lies beside it in the epigastrium, by (1) inspiratory collapse (Fig. G-16) and (2) lack of systolic pulsation. An IVC width greater than 24 mm was seen only in patients with tricuspid regurgitation, whereas a width of less than 16 mm was incompatible with tricuspid regurgitation, but values in between were seen in both groups (Meltzer *et al.,* 1981).

Having located the IVC, an M-mode sweep should be made from the RA down toward the confluence of the IVC with the common hepatic vein. This is the proper level to watch for appearance of contrast (dextrose, saline, or green dye) injected into an antecubital vein, during which the patient lies supine and is asked to hold his breath. Tricuspid regurgitation is present if contrast appears in the IVC during ventricular systole (Wise *et al.,* 1981). In pericardial constriction, contrast may appear in the

IVC before the QRS complex inscription. It is important to know that contrast may appear in the IVC in the absence of tricuspid regurgitation, and even in normal persons, if the patient is breathing at the time or lying on the left lateral position (Wise *et al.,* 1981) and also during certain arrhythmias (Meltzer *et al.,* 1982).

The IVC can also be visualized by 2-D echography (Figs. G-17 and G-18) by the subcostal approach, the plane visualized being slightly to the right of the midline. The IVC can be identified readily by the fact that it receives the right superior hepatic vein and that it enters the RA. The entry of contrast into the IVC in tricuspid regurgitation can be well seen; the temporal relationship of such phasic tides of flow into the IVC can be appreciated on the 2-D echogram as well as the M-mode tracing. Systolic collapse of the IVC during a sharp inspiration may not occur if the RA pressure is considerably elevated.

The right superior hepatic vein itself has been

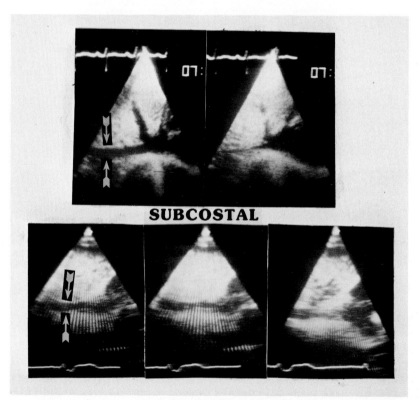

SUBCOSTAL

Fig. G-17. *Upper.* Subcostal 2-D echogram showing the inferior vena cava of normal caliber (*arrows*) traversing the liver to enter the right atrium. A hepatic vein can be seen entering the inferior vena cava. The plane visualized is a parasagittal one, slightly to the right of the midline.
 Lower. Subcostal echogram in another individual, showing respiratory variation in caliber of the inferior vena cava (*arrows*).

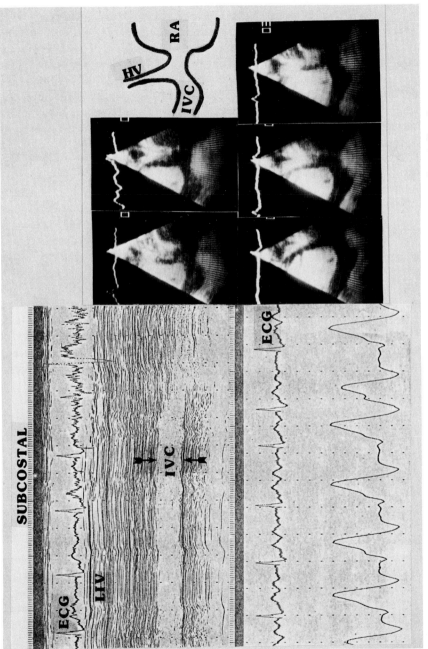

Fig. G-18. *Left.* Subcostal M-mode echogram showing the liver (LIV) and dilated inferior vena cava (IVC), in a patient with congestive cardiomyopathy and tricuspid regurgitation. Systolic hepatic pulsations, typical of tricuspid regurgitation, were recorded on the epigastrium (*lower panel*).

Right. Subcostal 2-D echogram in a right parasagittal plane, showing the dilated inferior vena cava emerging from the liver to enter the right atrium. A hepatic vein can be seen entering the inferior vena cava.

217

studied by Reeves *et al.* (1981). They found it dilated in all patients with tricuspid regurgitation to a maximum width of 18 mm or more. Patients without tricuspid regurgitation almost always had hepatic vein widths less than 18 mm. These authors also found that dilatation of the right superior hepatic vein was a useful reflection of raised central venous pressure. Hepatic vein dilatation would be expected also with the Budd-Chiari syndrome; obstruction of the upper inferior vena cava in this rare condition would be evident on the 2-D echogram.

Quantitative observations on IVC dimension have recently been made by Mintz *et al.* (1981) as follows: taking the end-diastolic IVC dimension as a baseline (100 per cent), the normal "A" wave consists in slight dilatation (to not more than 125 per cent), the normal "V" wave in dilatation (to not more than 140 per cent); inspiration was associated with a 50 per cent decrease in IVC width. A large "A" wave and overall IVC dilatation indicate right atrial hypertension; a large "V" wave suggests significant tricuspid regurgitation; lack of inspiratory IVC narrowing is encountered in RV dysfunction and also in pericardial constriction.

MASSES IN THE RIGHT HEART

Abnormal echoes due to space-occupying lesions within the right heart chambers are rarely encountered in practice but are important because most are life-threatening and yet amenable to surgical excision. Two-D echocardiography is superior to all other diagnostic methods for this purpose, and that is perhaps why such a large number of case reports on the topic have appeared (Goldschlager *et al.*, 1972; Waxler *et al.*, 1972; Harbold and Gau, 1973; De Maria *et al.*, 1975; Yuste *et al.*, 1976; Farooki *et al.*, 1976; Fitterer *et al.*, 1976; Chandaratna *et al.*, 1977; Covarrubias *et al.*, 1977; Meyers *et al.*, 1977; Ports *et al.*, 1977; Nanda *et al.*, 1977; Roelandt *et al.*, 1977; Pernod *et al.*, 1978; Jaffe *et al.*, 1978; Balk *et al.*, 1979; Battle-Diaz *et al.*, 1979; Come *et al.*, 1979; Frishman *et al.*, 1979; Hamer *et al.*, 1979; Mahoney *et al.*, 1979; Malcolm *et al.*, 1979; Mori *et al.*, 1979; Powers *et al.*, 1979; Snider *et al.*, 1979; Attar *et al.*, 1980; Caralis *et al.*, 1980; Hada *et al.*, 1980; Lutz *et al.*, 1980; Mills *et al.*, 1980; Mil-

ner *et al.*, 1980; Steffens *et al.*, 1980). Right heart tumors should be excluded in any patient presenting with unexplained right heart failure or unexplained pulmonary embolism (see Fig. G-22).

Myxomas are perhaps the most common of right heart tumors. Myxomas arising in the right atrium are commonly pedunculated and mobile so that they move down into the right ventricle in diastole, where they are visualized more easily by M-mode echocardiography. Hence, it is perhaps more convenient and practical to consider the echographic diagnosis of right atrial and right ventricular tumors together.

Right atrial myxomas are much less frequent than left atrial myxomas and resemble them in their motion characteristics and therefore in the echocardiographic patterns they produce. They usually are attached to the right aspect of the interatrial septum by a pedicle of variable length; they move forward into the right ventricle in diastole and back into the right atrium soon after the onset of right ventricular systole. Correlation of the pathologic anatomy and echocardiographic appearances in the published reports suggests that variation in ultrasound findings can be explained by differences in shape and size of myxomas and in length and site of attachment of their pedicles.

1. The most frequent pattern on M-mode echocardiography is that of a large, dense echo mass appearing just posterior to the anterior tricuspid leaflet, with a time lag after tricuspid valve opening, i.e., an echo-free space may be evident between the DE segment of the tricuspid anterior leaflet and the tumor echo mass. During systole this mass disappears from view because it has retreated back into the right atrium.

2. The tumor mass may appear intermittently in the body of the RV, at a level beyond the tricuspid leaflets, as a mass of dense, mottled or stippled echoes. Most published illustrations indicate that the myxoma abruptly appears here in early systole.

3. Sometimes the myxoma may be seen in the RV outflow tract, anterior to the aortic root (De Maria *et al.*, 1975; Pernod *et al.*, 1978; Mills *et al.*, 1980) and may even cause obstruction to RV outflow, associated with a substantial pressure gradient between RV and pulmonary artery.

4. Exceptionally, a right atrial myxoma can grow to a very large size, filling the RV chamber not only in diastole, but also retaining some of its bulk there in systole and interfering with function of tricuspid as well as pulmonic valves (Frishman *et al.*, 1979). This patient presented with severe right heart failure; at surgery a huge myxoma, attached by a short stalk to the right atrial wall, was removed successfully.

5. When visible, the pedicle or stalk of the tumor may be seen on the M-mode tracing as a linear or narrow band echo that whips forward into the RV in diastole and back into the right atrium in systole (Yuste *et al.*, 1976). The tumor mass itself may appear as a large cloud of stippled echoes.

Right ventricular myxomas have been diagnosed by echocardiography, but are of great rarity (Chandaratna *et al.*, 1977; Nanda *et al.*, 1977; Ports *et al.*, 1977). Typically, the RV myxoma is a rather small pedunculated tumor, attached to the RV endocardium in its infundibular (outflow) region; it tends to move into the pulmonary valve orifice during systole. Thus both hemodynamically and by auscultation, it can easily mimic pulmonic valve stenosis. On the M-mode tracing, the tumor echo mass is seen in the RV outflow tract (anterior to the aortic root) especially in systole, and also may be seen anterior to the pulmonary cusp echo when the pulmonic valve is scanned.

All right heart tumors are not myxomas. Rarely, malignant neoplasms elsewhere can result in secondary deposits within the right atrium or ventricle. Farooki *et al.* (1976) described the extension of a Wilms' tumor of the

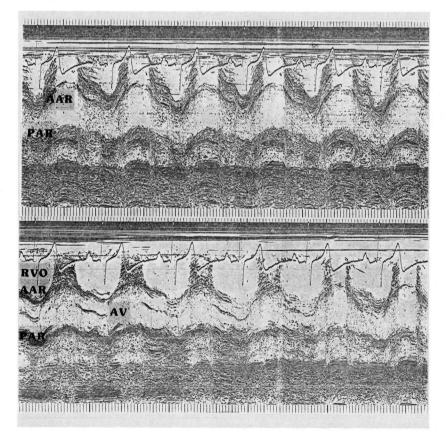

Fig. G-19. M-mode echogram showing the aortic root. Improper transducer angulation distorts the anterior aortic root echo producing an artefact that possibly could be mistaken for a mass in the RV outflow tract (*upper*). More suitable transducer angulation can minimize the artefact (*lower left*).

kidney into the right atrium via the inferior vena cava; the M-mode echocardiographic appearances resembled those of a right atrial myxoma. The patient of Ports *et al.* (1977) had a huge metastatic mass from a malignant melanoma filling the entire RV and completely obscuring tricuspid leaflets on the echocardiogram. In the patient of Fye and Molina (1980) a right atrial tumor was diagnosed by 2-D echography and surgery was performed without further invasive tests; an angiosarcoma of the RA was removed. Metastases from a rectal adenocarcinoma (Henuzet *et al.*, 1982) and from an invasive uterine leiomyoma (Maurer and Nanda, 1982) have been detected by 2-D echography.

The echocardiographic differential diagnosis of right heart tumors includes:

1. Large tricuspid valve vegetations as in Fig. E-4 (Come *et al.*, 1979). Two-D echocardiography in the apical or subcostal four-chamber view is helpful in demonstrating the attachment of the abnormal echo mass to the tricuspid valve with which the mass moves in the case of vegetations. On the other hand, a right atrial myxoma would show a larger to-and-fro motion between RA and RV.

2. a. Artefacts caused by improper angulation of the ultrasound beam so that normal anatomic components of the right heart such as tricuspid annulus or chordae, atrial septum or anterior aortic root (Fig. G-19) intercept

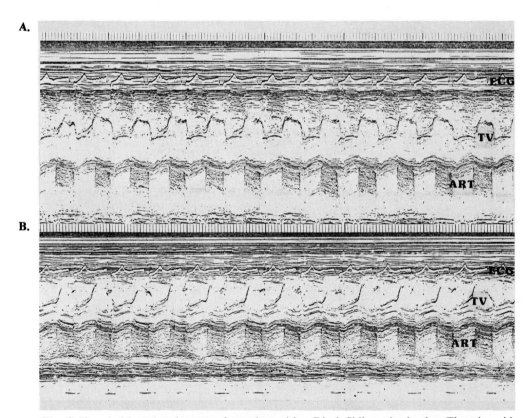

Fig. G-20. *A.* M-mode echogram of a patient with a Bjork-Shiley mitral valve. The tricuspid valve is visualized in both panels, at slightly different rightward angulations of the transducer. An abnormal echo appears behind the tricuspid valve, in the RA region, in diastole only. This patient has no RA mass; the apparent echo mass was an ultrasonic illusion, caused by the periphery of the ultrasound beam picking up echoes from the prosthetic disk.

Fig. G-20. *B.* M-mode echographic scan from tricuspid valve–RA region to aortic root–LA region. Similar echoes from the prosthetic disk are seen in both the RA and LA areas because the edge of the disk falls within the width of the ultrasound beam in diastole.

the ultrasound beam at some part of the cardiac cycle and appear as a pseudomass in the RV.

b. Another kind of artefact arises from reverberations of the chest wall echo (main bang), and these can be quite conspicuous on M-mode as well as 2-D echocardiograms.

c. Inadequate suppression of near gain can result in the RV appearing continuously full of amorphous echoes of variable density. These artefacts can be eliminated, or at least recognized for what they are, by careful attention to technique, including scanning from different sites and with changes in transducer angulation, near-gain adjustment, and so forth.

d. Prosthetic mitral valves artefactually can produce echoes in the RV or RA areas (Fig. G-20).

e. Pacemaker wires in the RA or RV also can be mistaken for intracardiac masses (Fig. G-21).

3. Thrombi in the right heart chambers, on their way to the pulmonary arteries from the systemic veins, may be seen in the right atrium or ventricle (Starkey and deBono, 1982; Rosenzweig and Nanda, 1982). Such an instance of "impending pulmonary embolism" was described by Corvarrubias et al. (1977); multiple shaggy echoes were visualized just posterior to the anterior mitral leaflet. The patient died soon after, and at autopsy a large saddle embolus was found, obstructing the bifurcation of the main pulmonary artery. Detection of large mobile RA or RV thrombi is thus an emergency situation.

4. Aneurysms of the membranous ventricular septum can present echocardiographically as linear convex echoes, perhaps finely fluttering, anterior to the tricuspid valve (Snider et al., 1979). Such an appearance might seem perplexing until 2-D echocardiography demonstrates the aneurysmal upper ventricular septum protruding into the RV just below tricuspid valve level.

5. Persistence of the right sinus venosus valve as a large membranous septum within the right atrium appeared on the M-mode echoes in a newborn infant (Battle-Diaz et al., 1979). Lesser degrees of this anomaly, consisting of incomplete membranes or "Chiari network" within the right atrium, are known to occur at any age as incidental findings at autopsy in 2 to 3 per cent of cases. On the M-mode echogram the Chiari network appears as highly mobile linear echoes in the right atrium, posterior to the tricuspid valve, with the transducer tilted acutely to the right. On 2-D echography it is represented by curvilinear echoes in the RA, located in its inferior part and quite separate from the tricuspid valve (Werner et al., 1981; Orita et al., 1982; Gussenhoven et al., 1982). It should not be mistaken for tricuspid vegetations or right atrial tumors or thrombi.

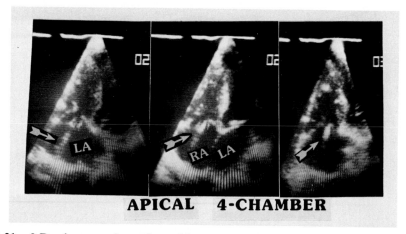

APICAL   4-CHAMBER

Fig. G-21. 2-D echogram of a patient with an endocardial pacemaker in the RV. All three frames shown are in the apical 4-chamber view, in diastole. The tricuspid valve is open, and the pacemaker wire is visualized passing through it.

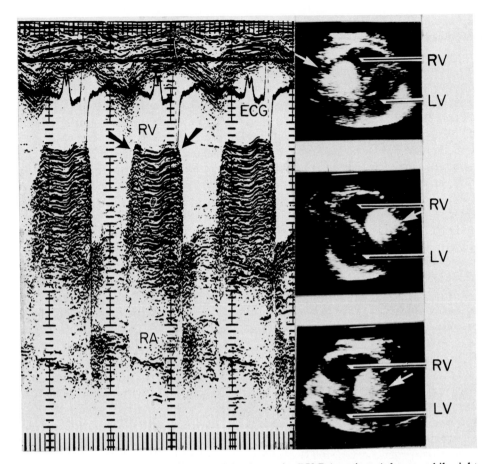

Fig. G-22. The M-mode echocardiogram (*left*) shows the RV-RA region. A large mobile right atrial mass (*arrows*) appears in the RV area in diastole only. The 2-D echogram is shown at right. The large right atrial mass (*arrows*) is visualized protruding into the RV, in the parasternal short-axis view (*upper*), as well as in the RV long-axis parasternal view (*center and lower*). A diagnosis of RA myxoma was made in this middle-aged woman, but at surgery the neoplasm was found to have originated in a kidney and extended upward through the inferior vena cava into the RA.

REFERENCES

NORMAL RIGHT VENTRICLE

Bommer, W.; Weinert, L.; Neumann, A.; *et al.:* Determination of right atrial and right ventricular size by two-dimensional echocardiography. *Circulation,* **60:**91, 1979.

D'Cruz, I.; Hirsch, L.; Prabhu, R; *et al.:* Intramural myocardial echographic patterns during the cardiac cycle. *Circulation,* **54:** Suppl II:84, 1976 (abstr).

Diamond, M. A.; Dillon, J. C.; Haine, C. L.; *et al.:* Echocardiographic features of atrial septal defect. *Circulation,* **43:**129, 1971.

Feigenbaum, H.: *Echocardiography.* Lea & Febiger, Philadelphia, 1976.

Gramiak, R.; Shah, P. M.; and Kramer, D. H.: Ultrasound cardiography: Contrast studies in anatomy and function. *Radiology,* **92:**939, 1969.

Haft, J. I., and Horowitz, M. S.: *Clinical Echocardiography.* Futura Publishing Co., New York, 1978.

Kleid, J. J., and Arvan, S. B.: *Echocardiography: Interpretation and Diagnosis.* Appleton-Century-Crofts, New York, 1978.

Laurenceau, J. L., and Dumesnil, J. G.: Right and left ventricular dimensions as determinants of ventricular septal motion. *Chest,* **69:**388, 1976.

Popp, R. L.; Wolfe, S. B.; and Hirata, T.: Estimation of right and left ventricular size by ultrasound. A study of echoes from the interventricular septum. *Am. J. Cardiol.,* **24:**523, 1969.

Starling, M. R.; Crawford, M. H.; Sorensen, S. G.; *et al.:* A new two-dimensional echocardiographic technique for evaluating right ventricular size and performance in patients with obstructive lung disease. *Circulation,* **66:**612, 1982.

Watanabe, T.; Katsume, H.; Matsukubo, H.; *et al.:* Estimation of right ventricular volume with two-dimensional echocardiography. *Am. J. Cardiol.,* **49:**1946, 1982.

RIGHT VENTRICULAR WALL

Arcilla, R. A.; Mathew, R.; Sodt, P.; *et al.:* Right ventricular mass estimation by angio-echocardiography. *Cathet. Cardiovasc. Diag.,* **2:**125, 1976.

Candell-Riera, J.; Permanyer-Mizalda, G.; and Soler-Soler, J.: Echocardiographic findings in endomyocardial fibrosis. *Chest,* **82:**88, 1982.

Child, J. S.; Krivokapich, J.; and Abbasi, A. S.: Increased right ventricular wall thickness on echocardiography in amyloid infiltrative cardiomyopathy. *Am. J. Cardiol.,* **44:**1391, 1979.

George, B. O.; Gaba, F. E.; and Talabi, A. I.: M-mode echocardiographic features of endomyocardial fibrosis. *Br. Heart J.,* **48:**222, 1982.

Matsukubo, H.; Matsuura, T.; Endo, N.; *et al.:* Echocardiographic measurement of right ventricular wall thickness. A new application of subxiphoid echocardiography. *Circulation,* **56:**278, 1977.

Prakash, R.: Determination of right ventricular wall thickness in systole and diastole. Echocardiographic and necropsy correlation in 32 patients. *Br. Heart J.,* **40:**1257, 1978.

Prakash, R., and Lindsay, P.: Determination of right ventricular wall thickness by echocardiogram. *JAMA,* **239:**638, 1978.

Schilt, B. F.; Feigenbaum, H.; and Weyman, A. E.: A new echocardiographic sign for cardiac tamponade. *Circulation,* **62,** Suppl. III:100, 1980 (Abstr.).

Tsuda, T.; Sawayama, T.; Kawai, N.; *et al.:* Echocardiographic measurement of right ventricular wall thickness in adults by anterior approach. *Am. J. Cardiol.,* **44:**55, 1980.

RIGHT ATRIUM

Asayama, J.; Matsuura, T.; Endo, N.; *et al.:* Idiopathic enlargement of the right atrium. *Am. J. Cardiol.,* **40:**620, 1977.

Bommer, W.; Weinert, L.; Neumann, A.; *et al.:* Determination of right atrial and right ventricular size by two-dimensional echocardiography. *Circulation,* **60:**91, 1979.

Desimone, A. R., and Kronzon, I.: Giant right atrium in Ebstein's anomaly. *Chest,* **79:**80, 1981.

Kushner, F. G.; Lam, W.; and Morganroth, J.: Apex sector echocardiography in evaluation of the right atrium in patients with mitral stenosis and atrial septal defect. *Am. J. Cardiol.,* **42:**733, 1978.

Pastor, B. H., and Forte, A. L.: Idiopathic enlargement of the right atrium. *Am. J. Cardiol.,* **8:**513, 1961.

Reeves, W. C.; Hallahan, W.; Schwiter, E. J.; *et al.:* Two-dimensional echocardiographic assessment of electrocardiographic criteria for right atrial enlargement. *Circulation,* **64:**387, 1981.

Seward, J. B.; Tajik, A. J.; Feist, D. J.; *et al.:* Ebstein's anomaly in an 88-year-old man. *Mayo Clin. Proc.* **54:**139, 1979.

INFERIOR VENA CAVA

Meltzer, R. S.; van Hoogenhuyze, D.; Serruys, P. W.; *et al.:* Diagnosis of tricuspid regurgitation by contrast echocardiography. *Circulation,* **63:**1093, 1981.

Meltzer, R. S.; McGhie, J.; and Roelandt, J.: Inferior vena cava echocardiography. *J. C. U.,* **10:**47, 1982.

Mintz, G. S.; Kotler, M. N.; Parry, W. R.; *et al.:* Real-time inferior vena caval ultrasonography: Normal and abnormal findings and its use in assessing right-heart function. *Circulation,* **64:**1018, 1981.

Reeves, W. C.; Leaman, D. M.; Buonocore, E.; *et al.:* Detection of tricuspid regurgitation and estimation of central venous pressure by two-dimensional contrast echocardiography of the right superior hepatic vein. *Am. Heart J.,* **102:**372, 1981.

Wise, N. K.; Myers, S.; Fraker, T. D.; *et al.:* Contrast M-mode ultrasonography of the inferior vena cava. *Circulation,* **63:**1100, 1981.

ATRIAL SEPTAL DEFECT

Bahler, A. S.; Moller, J.; Brik, H.; *et al.:* Paradoxical motion of the interventricular septum with right ventricular dilatation in the absence of shunting. *Am. J. Cardiol.,* **38:**654, 1976.

Bierman, F. Z., and Williams, R. G.: Subxiphoid two-dimensional imaging of the interatrial septum in infants and neonates with congenital heart disease. *Circulation,* **60:**80, 1979.

Botvinick, E. H., and Schiller, N. B.: The complementary roles of M-mode echocardiography and scintigraphy in the evaluation of adults with suspected left-to-right shunts. *Circulation,* **52:**1080, 1980.

Bourdillon, P. D. V.; Foale, R. A.; and Rickards, A. F.: Identification of atrial septal defects by cross-sectional contrast echocardiography. *Br. Heart J.,* **44:**401, 1980.

DeMaria, A. N.; Oliver, L. E.; Borgren, H. G.; *et al.:* Apparent reduction of aortic and left heart chamber size in atrial septal defect. *Am. J. Cardiol.,* **42:**545, 1978.

Diamond, M. A.; Dillon, J. C.; Haine, L. L.; *et al.:* Echocardiographic features of atrial septal defect. *Circulation,* **43:**129, 1971.

Dillon, J. C.; Weyman, A. E.; Feigenbaum, H.; *et al.:* Cross-sectional echocardiographic examination of the interatrial septum. *Circulation,* **55:**115, 1977.

Egeblad, H.; Berning, J.; Efsen, F.; *et al.:* Non-invasive diagnosis in clinically suspected atrial septal defect of secundum or sinus venosus type. Value of combining chest x-ray, phonocardiography and M-mode echocardiography. *Br. Heart J.,* **44:**317, 1980.

Fraker, T. D.; Harris, P. J.; Behar, V. S.; *et al.:* Detection and exclusion of interatrial shunts by two-dimensional echocardiography and peripheral venous injection. *Circulation,* **60:**327, 1979.

Hagan, A. D.; Francis, G. S.; and Sahn, D. J.: Ultrasound evaluation of systolic anterior septal motion in patients with and without right ventricular volume overload. *Circulation,* **59:**248, 1974.

Jardin, F.; Farcot, J. C.; Boisante, L.; *et al.:* Influence of positive end-expiratory pressure on left ventricular performance. *N. Engl. J. Med.,* **304:**387, 1981.

Kerber, R. E.; Dippel, W. F.; and Abboud, F. M.: Abnormal motion of the interventricular septum in right ventricular volume overload: Experimental and clinical echocardiographic studies. *Circulation,* **48:**86, 1973.

Lange, L. W.; Sahn, D. J.; Allen, H. D.; *et al.:* Subxiphoid cross-sectional echocardiography in infants and children with congenital heart disease. *Circulation,* **59:**513, 1979.

Lieppe, W.; Scallion, R.; Behar, V. S.; *et al.:* Two-dimensional echocardiographic findings in atrial septal defect. *Circulation,* **56:**447, 1977.

McCann, W. D.; Harbold, N. B.; and Giuliani, E. R.: The echocardiogram in right ventricular overload. *JAMA,* **221:**1243, 1972.

Meyer, R. A.; Schwartz, D. C.; Benzing, G.; *et al.:* Ventricular septum in right ventricular volume overload. An echocardiographic study. *Am. J. Cardiol.,* **30:**349, 1972.

Mirro, M. J.; Rogers, E. W.; Weyman, A. E.; *et al.:* Angular displacement of the papillary muscles during the cardiac cycle. *Circulation,* **60:**327, 1979.

Nanda, N. C., and Gramiak, R.: *Clinical Echocardiography.* C. V. Mosby, St. Louis, 1978.

Nasser, F. N.; Tajik, A. J.; Seward, J. B.; *et al.:* Diagnosis of sinus venosus atrial septal defect by two-dimensional echocardiography. *Mayo Clin Proc.,* **56:**568, 1981.

Pearlman, A. S.; Borer, J. S.; Clark, C. E.; *et al.:* Abnormal right ventricular size and ventricular septal motion after atrial septal defect closure: etiology and functional significance. *Am. J. Cardiol.,* **41:**295, 1978.

Radtke, W. E.; Tajik, A. J.; Gau, G. T.; *et al.:* Atrial septal defect: Echocardiographic observations. *Ann. Intern. Med.,* **84:**246, 1976.

St. John Sutton, M. G.; Tajik, A. J.; Mercier, L. A.; *et al.:* Assessment of left ventricular function in secundum atrial septal defect by computer analysis of the M-mode echocardiogram. *Circulation,* **60:**1082, 1979.

Schrieber, T. L.; Feigenbaum, H.; and Weyman, A. E.: Effect of atrial septal defect repair on left ventricular geometry and degree of mitral valve prolapse. *Circulation,* **61:**888, 1980.

Shub, C.; Dimopoulos, I.; Seward, J. B.; *et al.:* Imaging of sinus venosus atrial septal defect by two-dimensional echocardiography. *Am. J. Cardiol.,* **49:**974, 1982 (Abstr).

Tajik, A. J.; Gau, G. T.; and Ritter, D. G.: Echocardiographic patterns of right ventricular diastolic volume overload in children. *Circulation,* **46:**36, 1972a.

Tajik, A. J.; Gau, G. T.; and Schattenberg, T. T.: Echocardiogram in atrial septal defect. *Chest* **62:**213, 1972b.

Tajik, A. J.; Gau, G. T.; and Schattenberg, T. T.: Normal ventricular motion in atrial septal defect. *Mayo Clin. Proc.,* **47:**635, 1972c.

Wanderman, K. L.; Ovsyshcher, I.; and Gueron, M.: Left ventricular performance in patients with atrial septal defect. *Am. J. Cardiol.,* **41:**489, 1978.

Weyman, A. E.; Wann, S.; and Feigenbaum, H.; Mechanism of abnormal septal motion in patients with right ventricular volume overload. A cross-sectional echocardiography study. *Circulation,* **54:**179, 1976.

ANOMALOUS PULMONARY VENOUS DRAINAGE

Aziz, K. U.; Paul, M. H.; Bharati, S.; *et al.:* Echocardiographic features of total anomalous pulmonary venous drainage into the coronary sinus. *Am. J. Cardiol.,* **42:**108, 1978.

Bourdillon, P. D.; Foale, R. A.; and Somerville, J.: Persistent left superior vena cava with coronary sinus and left atrial connections. *Eur. J. Cardiol.,* **11:**227, 1980.

Danilowicz, D., and Kronzon, I.: Use of contrast echocardiography in the diagnosis of partial anomalous pulmonary venous connection. *Am. J. Cardiol.,* **43:**248, 1979.

Orsmond, G. S.; Ruttenberg, H. D.; Bessinger, F. B.; *et al.:* Echocardiographic features of total anomalous pulmonary venous connection to the coronary sinus. *Am. J. Cardiol.,* **41:**597, 1979.

Sahn, D. J.; Allen, H. D.; Lange, L. V.; *et al.:* Cross-sectional echocardiographic diagnosis of the sites of total anomalous venous drainage. *Circulation,* **60:**1317, 1979.

Tajik, A. J.; Gau, G. T.; and Schattenberg, G. G.: Echocardiogram in total anomalous pulmonary venous drainage. Report of case. *Mayo Clin. Proc.,* **47:**247, 1972.

ENDOCARDIAL CUSHION DEFECTS

Bass, J. L.; Bessinger, F. B.; and Lawrence, C.: Echocardiographic differentiation of partial and complete atrioventricular canal. *Circulation,* **57:**1144, 1978.

Beppu, S.; Nimura, Y.; Sakakibara, H.; *et al.:* Mitral cleft in ostium primum atrial septal defect assessed by cross-sectional echocardiography. *Circulation,* **62:**1099, 1980.

Hagler, D. J.; Tajik, A. J.; Seward, J. B.; *et al.:* Real-time wide-angle sector echocardiography: Atrioventricular canal defects. *Circulation,* **59:**149, 1979.

Hynes, J. K.; Tajik, A. J.; Seward, J. B.; *et al.:* Partial atrioventricular canal defect in elderly patients (Aged 60 years or older). *Am. J. Cardiol.,* **50:**59, 1982.

Pieroni, D. R.; Homcy, E.; and Freedom, R. M.: Echocardiography in atrioventricular canal defect. A clinical spectrum. *Am. J. Cardiol.,* **35:**54, 1975.

Williams, R. G., and Rudd, M.: Echocardiographic features of endocardial cushion defects. *Circulation,* **49:**418, 1974.

Yoshida, H.; Funabashi, T.; Nakaya, S.; *et al.:* Subxiphoid cross-sectional echocardiographic imaging of the "gooseneck" deformity in endocardial cushion defect. *Circulation,* **62:**1319, 1980.

EBSTEIN'S ANOMALY

Alipour, M.; Tarbiat, C.; and Nazarian, I.: Right ventricular endomyocardial fibrosis simulating Ebstein's anomaly. *Am. Heart J.,* **100:**859, 1980.

Farooki, Z. Q.; Henry, J. F.; and Green, E. W.: Echocardiographic spectrum of Ebstein's anomaly of the tricuspid valve. *Circulation,* **53:**63, 1976.

Henry, J. G.; Gordon, S.; and Timmis, G. C.: Corrected transposition of great vessels and Ebstein's anomaly of the tricuspid valve. Echocardiographic findings. *Br. Heart J.,* **41:**49, 1979.

Hirschklau, M. J.; Sahn, D. J.; Hagan, A. D.; *et al.:* Cross-sectional echocardiographic features of Ebstein's anomaly of the tricuspid valve. *Am. J. Cardiol.,* **40:**400, 1977.

Kambe, T.; Ichimiya, S.; Toguchi, M.; *et al.:* Apex and subxiphoid approaches to Ebstein's anomaly using cross-sectional echocardiography. *Am. Heart J.,* **100:**53, 1980.

Koiwaya, Y.; Narabayashi, H.; Koyanagi, S.; *et al.:* Early closure of the tricuspid valve in a case of Ebstein's anomaly with type B Wolff-Parkinson-White syndrome. *Circulation,* **49:**149, 1979.

Lundstrom, N. R.: Echocardiography in the diagnosis of Ebstein's anomaly of the tricuspid valve. *Circulation,* **47:**597, 1973.

Matsumato, M.; Matsuo, H.; Nagata, S.; *et al.:* Visualization of Ebstein's anomaly of the tricuspid valve by two-dimensional and standard echocardiography. *Circulation,* **53:**69, 1976.

Milner, S.; Meyer, R. A.; Venables, A. E.; *et al.:* Mitral and tricuspid valve closure in congenital heart disease. *Circulation,* **53:**513, 1976.

Monibi, A. A.; Neches, W. H.; Lenoz, C. C.; *et al.:* Left ventricular anomalies associated with Ebstein's malformation of the tricuspid valve. *Circulation,* **57:**303, 1978.

Ports, T. A.; Silverman, N. H.; and Schiller, N. B.: Two-dimensional echocardiographic assessment of Ebstein's anomaly. *Circulation,* **58:**336, 1978.

Tajik, A. J.; Gau, G. T.; and Giuliani, E. R.: Echocardiogram in Ebstein's anomaly with Wolff-Parkinson-White preexcitation syndrome, type B. *Circulation,* **47:**813, 1973.

Yuste, P.; Minguez, I.; Aza, V.; *et al.:* Echocardiography in the diagnosis of Ebstein's anomaly. *Chest,* **66:**3, 1974.

RV DYSPLASIA

Baran, A.; Nanda, N. C.; Falkoff, M.; *et al.:* Two-dimensional echocardiographic detection of arrhythmogenic right ventricular dysplasia. *Am. Heart J.,* **103:**1066, 1982.

Marcus, F. I.; Fontaine, G. H.; Guiraudon, G. *et al.:* Right ventricular dysplasia. *Circulation,* **65:**385, 1982.

Perrenoud, J. J.; Adamec, R.; Fournet, D. C.; *et al.:* Intérêt de l'échocardiographie dans le diagnostic de la maladie de Uhl. *Arch. Mal Coeur,* **75:**491, 1982.

Rossi, P.; Massumi, A.; Gillette, P.; *et al.:* Arrhythmogenic right ventricular dysplasia. *Am. Heart J.,* **103:**415, 1982.

RV SYSTOLIC OVERLOAD INCLUDING COR PULMONALE

Allen, H. D.; Taussig, L. M.; Gaines, J. A.; *et al.:* Echocardiographic profiles of the long-term cardiac changes in cystic fibrosis. *Chest,* **75:**428, 1979.

Alpert, J. S.; Francis, G. S.; Vieweg, W. V. T.; *et al.:* Left ventricular function in massive pulmonary embolism. *Chest,* **71:**108, 1977.

Gewitz, M.; Eshaghpour, E.; Holslaw, D. S.; *et al.:* Echocardiography in cystic fibrosis. *Am. J. Dis. Child.,* **131:**275, 1977.

Hirschfeld, S. S.; Fleming, D. G.; Doershuk, C.; *et al.:* Echocardiographic abnormalities in patients with cystic fibrosis. *Chest,* **75:**351, 1979.

Jacobstein, M. D.; Hirschfeld, S. S.; Winnie, G.; *et al.:* Ventricular interdependence in severe cystic fibrosis. A two-dimensional echocardiographic study. *Chest,* **80:**399, 1981.

Kasper, W.; Meinertz, T.; Kersting, F.; *et al.:* Echocardiography in assessing acute pulmonary hypertension due to pulmonary embolism. *Am. J. Cardiol.,* **45:**567, 1980.

Krayenbuehl, H. P.; Turina, J.; and Hess, O.: Left ventricular function in chronic pulmonary hypertension. *Am. J. Cardiol.,* **41:**1150, 1978.

Rosenthal, A.; Tucker, C. R.; Williams, R. G.; *et al.:* Echocardiographic assessment of cor pulmonale in cystic fibrosis. *Pediatr. Clin. North Am.,* **23:**327, 1976.

Ryssing, E.: Assessment of cor pulmonale in cystic fibrosis by echocardiography. *Acta Paediatr. Scand.,* **66:**753, 1977.

Tanaka, H.; Tei, C.; Nakao, S.; *et al.:* Diastolic bulging of the interventricular septum toward the left ventricle. An echocardiographic manifestation of negative interventricular gradient between left and right ventricles during diastole. *Circulation,* **62:**558, 1980.

RIGHT VENTRICULAR INFARCTION

Butman, S.; Olson, H. G.; Aronow, W. S.; *et al.:* Remote right ventricular myocardial infarction mimicking chronic pericardial constriction. *Am. Heart J.,* **103:**912, 1982.

Candell-Riera, J.; Figueras, J.; Valle, V.; *et al.:* Right ventricular infarction: relationships between ST segment elevation in V4R and hemodynamic, scintigraphic, and echocardiographic findings in patients with acute inferior myocardial infarction. *Am. Heart J.,* **101:**281, 1981.

D'Arcy, B., and Nanda, N. C.: Two-dimensional echocardiographic features of right ventricular infarction. *Circulation,* **65:**167, 1982.

Lorell, B.; Leinback, R. C.; Pohost, G. M.; *et al.:* Right ventricular infarction. Clinical diagnosis and differentiation from cardiac tamponade and pericardial constriction. *Am. J. Cardiol.,* **43:**465, 1979.

Miller, F. A.; Seward, J. B.; Gersh, B. J.; *et al.:* Two-dimensional echocardiographic findings in cardiac trauma. *Am. J. Cardiol.,* **50:**1022, 1982.

Sharpe, D. N.; Botvinick, E. H.; Shames, D. M.; *et al.:* The noninvasive diagnosis of right ventricular infarction. *Circulation,* **57:**483, 1978.

CYSTIC MASS SIMULATING DILATED RIGHT VENTRICLE

D'Cruz, I. A., and Pipit, C.: Echocardiographic diagnosis of an unusual anterior mediastinal mass. *Clin. Cardiol.,* **5:**464, 1982.

Farooki, Z. Q.; Adelman, S.; and Green, E. W.: Echocardiographic differentiation of a cystic and solid tumor of the heart. *Am. J. Cardiol.,* **39:**107, 1977.

MASSES IN THE RIGHT HEART CHAMBERS

Attar, S.; Lee, Y. C.; Singleton, R.; *et al.:* Cardiac myxoma. *Ann. Thorac. Surg.,* **29:**397, 1980.

Balk, A. H.; Wagenaar, S. S.; and Bruschke, A. V.: Bilateral cardiac myxomas and peripheral myxomas in a patient with recent myocardial infarction. *Am. J. Cardiol.,* **44:**767, 1979.

Battle-Diaz, J.; Stanley, P.; Kratz, V.; *et al.:* Echocardiographic manifestations of persistence of the right sinus venosus valve. *Am. J. Cardiol.,* **43:**850, 1979.

Caralis, D. G.; Kennedy, H. C.; Bailey, I.; *et al.:* Primary right cardiac tumor. Detection by echocardiographic and radioisotopic studies. *Chest,* **77:**100, 1980.

Chandaratna, P. A. N.; San Pedro, S.; Elkins, R. C.; *et al.:* Echocardiographic, angiocardiographic and surgical correlations in right ventricular myxoma simulating valvar pulmonary stenosis. *Circulation,* **55:**619, 1977.

Come, P. C.; Kurland, G. S.; and Vine, H. S.: Two-dimensional echocardiography in differentiating right atrial and tricuspid valve mass lesions. *Am. J. Cardiol.,* **44:**1207, 1979.

Covarrubias, E. A.; Sheikh, M. V.; and Fox, L. M.: Echocardiography and pulmonary embolism. *Ann. Intern. Med.,* **87:**720, 1977.

DeMaria, A.; Vismara, L. A.; and Miller, R. R.: Unusual echographic manifestations of right and left heart myxomas. *Am. J. Med.,* **59:**713, 1975.

Farooki, Z. Q.; Green, W. E.; and Arciniegas, E.: Echocardiographic pattern of right atrial tumor motion. *Br. Heart J.,* **38:**580, 1976.

Fitterer, D. J.; Spicer, M. J.; and Nelson, W. P.: Echocardiographic demonstration of bilateral atrial myxomas. *Chest,* **70:**282, 1976.

Frishman, W.; Factor, S.; Jordan, A.; *et al.:* Right atrial myxoma: Unusual clinical presentation and atypical glandular histology. *Circulation,* **59:**1070, 1979.

Fye, W. B., and Molina, J. E.: Right atrial angiosarcoma: Echocardiographic diagnosis and surgical correlation. *Johns Hopkins Med. J.,* **147:**111, 1980.

Goldschlager, A.; Popper, R.; Goldschlager, N.; *et al.:* Right atrial myxoma with right to left shunt and polycythemia presenting as congenital heart disease. *Am. J. Cardiol.,* **30:**82, 1972.

Gussenhoven, W. J.; Essed, C. E.; and Bos, E.: Persistent right sinus venosus valve. *Brit. Heart J.,* **47:**183, 1982.

Hada, Y.; Wolfe, C.; Murray, G. F.; *et al.:* Right ventricular myxoma. Case report and review of phonocardiographic and auscultatory manifestations. *Am. Heart J.,* **100:**871, 1980.

Hamer, J. P.; Nieveen, J.; Bergstra, A.; *et al.:* Left atrial myxoma moving from right atrium to left ventricle. Noninvasive and invasive techniques and surgical findings. *Acta Med. Scand.,* **205:**527, 1979.

Harbold, N. B., and Gau, S. T.: Echocardiographic diagnosis of right atrial myxoma. *Mayo Clin. Proc.,* **48:**284, 1973.

Henuzet, C.; Franken, P.; Polis, O.; *et al.:* Cardiac metastasis of rectal adenocarcinoma diagnosed by two-dimensional echocardiography. *Am. Heart J.,* **104:**637, 1982.

Jaffe, C. C.; Kelley, M. J.; and Taunt, K. A.: Two-dimensional echocardiographic identification of a right ventricle tumor. *Radiology,* **129:**471, 1978.

Lutz, J. F.; Hagan, A. D.; Vieweg, N. V. R.; *et al.:* "Pseudotumor" of the right ventricular outflow tract and congenital pulmonary valve regurgitation: A case report. *Am. Heart J.,* **100:**349, 1980.

Mahoney, L.; Schieken, R. M.; and Doty, D.: Cardiac rhabdomyoma simulating pulmonic stenosis. *Cathet. Cardiovasc. Diagn.,* **5:**385, 1979.

Malcolm, A. D.; Shiu, M. J.; and Jenkins, B. S.: Sarcoma obstructing right ventricular cavity: clinical, echocardiographic, hemodynamic and angiographic features. *Postgrad. Med. J.,* **55:**203, 1979.

Maurer, G., and Nanda, N. C.: Two-dimensional echocardiographic identification of intracardiac leiomyomatosis. *Am. Heart J.,* **103:**915, 1982.

Meyers, S. N.; Shapiro, J. E.; Barresi, V.; *et al.:* Right atrial myxoma with right to left shunting and mitral valve prolapse. *Am. J. Med.,* **62:**308, 1977.

Mills, P.; Wolfe, C.; Redwood, D.; *et al.:* Noninvasive diagnosis of sub-pulmonary outflow tract obstruction. *Br. Heart J.,* **43:**276, 1980.

Milner, S.; Abramowitz, J. A.; and Levin, S. E.: Rhabdomyoma of the heart in a newborn infant. Diagnosis by echocardiography. *Br. Heart J.,* **44:**244, 1980.

Mori, K.; Oonaka, M.; Tanaka, T.; *et al.:* Prolapsing right atrial myxoma. *Cardiology,* **64:**58, 1979.

Nanda, N. C.; Barold, S. S.; Gramiak, R.; *et al.:* Echocardiographic features of right ventricular outflow tumor prolapsing into the pulmonary artery. *Am. J. Cardiol.,* **40:**272, 1977.

Orita, Y.; Meno, H.; Kanaide, H.; *et al.:* Echocardiographic features of persistent right sinus venosus valve in an adult. *J. C. U.,* **10:**461, 1982.

Pernod, J.; Piwnica, A.; and Duret, J. C.: Right atrial myxoma: An echocardiographic study. *Br. Heart J.,* **40:**201, 1978.

Ports, T. Z.; Schiller, N. B.; and Strunk, B. L.: Echocardiography of right ventricular tumors. *Circulation,* **56:**439, 1977.

Powers, J. C.; Falkoff, M.; Heinle, R. A.; *et al.:* Familial cardiac myxoma: emphasis on unusual clinical manifestations. *J. Thorac. Cardiovasc. Surg.,* **77:**782, 1979.

Roelandt, J.; Bletter, W. B.; Leuftink, E. W.; *et al.:* Ultrasonic demonstration of right ventricular myxoma. *J.C.U.* **5:**191, 1977.

Rosenzweig, M. S., and Nanda, N. C.: Two-dimensional echocardiographic detection of circulating right atrial thrombi. *Am. Heart J.,* **103:**435, 1982.

Siltanen, P.; Tuuteri, L.; Noria, R.; *et al.:* Atrial myxoma in a family. *Am. J. Cardiol.,* **38:**252, 1976.

Snider, A. R.; Silverman, N. H.; Schiller, N. B.; *et al.:* Echocardiographic evaluation of ventricular septal aneurysms. *Circulation,* **59:**920, 1979.

Starkey, I. R., and deBono, D. P.: Echocardiographic identification of right-sided cardiac intracavitary thromboembolus in massive pulmonary embolism. *Circulation,* **66:**1322, 1982.

Steffens, T. G.; Mayer, H. S.; and Das, S. K.: Echocardiographic diagnosis of a right ventricular metastatic tumor. *Arch. Intern. Med.,* **140:**122, 1980.

Waxler, E. B.; Kawai, N.; and Kasparian, H.: Right atrial myxoma: Echocardiographic, phonocardiographic and hemodynamic signs. *Am. Heart J.,* **83:**251, 1972.

Werner, J. A.; Cheitlin, M. D.; Gross, B. W.; *et al.:* Echocardiographic appearance of the Chiari network: Differentiation from right heart pathology. *Circulation,* **63:**1104, 1981.

Yuste, P.; Asin, E.; Cerdan, F. J.; *et al.:* Illustrative echocardiogram: Echocardiogram in right atrial myxoma. *Chest,* **69:**94, 1976.

H
The Left Atrium

LEFT ATRIAL SIZE

The left atrial dimension is measured at end-systole (Fig. C-1) as the maximum distance between the anterior (leading) edge of the posterior aortic root echo and the anterior (leading) edge of the LA posterior wall echo. The LA dimension should be measured at an aortic root level at which the aortic valve can be clearly seen. In some difficult subjects, the aortic cusps cannot be visualized, in which case the identity of the aortic root may be ascertained by parallel motion of its anterior and posterior walls.

An element of uncertainty as to exactly which linear echo is the LA posterior wall is not uncommon. Often a "soft" fuzzy or indistinct echo, a few millimeters wide, is seen anterior to a subjacent "hard" well-defined linear echo. The latter should be considered the LA posterior wall for the purpose of LA dimension measurement.

It is also not rare to see a small echo-free space behind the LA posterior wall representing a pulmonary vein, or (near the atrioventricular function) the coronary sinus or descending thoracic aorta. In such cases, uncertainty as to the identity of the LV posterior wall echo can be avoided by scanning to a different LA area which usually eliminates the sonolucent retroatrial space.

In children, certain rare congenital anomalies—cor triatriatum, supramitral stenosing ring or membrane, or an intra-atrial baffle of Mustard operation—can present as a linear echo traversing the LA chamber, so that some uncertainty may exist as to the precise limits of the true LA cavity. Contrast echocardiography and hemodynamic studies may be required to make the diagnosis if the clinical presentation justifies it.

A mural thrombus adherent to the LA posterior wall likewise can produce abnormal linear echoes within the left atrium. The patient usually has a stenotic or prosthetic mitral valve, or else has a dilated left atrium associated with cardiomyopathy.

The normal LA dimension is between 20 and 40 mm. The upper limit of normal quoted by several authors is 22 mm/M^2 body surface area (Hirata et al., 1969; ten Cate et al., 1974; Brown et al., 1974; Feigenbaum, 1976). Angular deviation of the M-mode transducer from the perpendicular by 20° or even 10° can significantly alter the LA dimension recorded (Lester et al., 1979). LA dimensions obtained by the subcostal approach are not valid measures of LA diameter because the ultrasound beam, aimed more superiorly than posteriorly, transects the topmost part of the left atrium so that this chamber appears smaller than it does by the parasternal approach.

At Michael Reese Hospital, in patients of average size, LA dimensions between 40 and 50 mm are considered mild LA dilatation, between 50 and 60 moderate LA dilatation, between 60 and 70 marked dilatation; LA dimensions exceeding 70 mm deserve the appellation giant left atrium and in the most extreme examples attain the 90- to 100-mm range. These gradations of LA enlargement are arbitrary but convenient in daily practice. The actual values that classify the degree of LA dilatation could vary from one laboratory to another and should be decreased or increased when one is dealing with very small or very large patients, respectively.

The diameter of the aortic root is about the same as that of the left atrium in normal adults and older children (Brown et al., 1974), the average LA:AR ratio being 1.1 (range, 0.85 to 1.17). The patient's own aortic root can therefore be used as a convenient yardstick to assess the presence or absence of LA enlargement. For this purpose it must be assumed that the aortic root is of normal size. Thus, the LA:AR ratio cannot be used when the aortic root is dilated. Mild dilatation of the ascending aorta is common in aortic regurgitation or aortic valve stenosis (poststenotic); severe or aneurysmal dilatation is usually luetic or associated with Marfan's syndrome. In the latter type of case, the aneurysmal aortic root may compress the left atrium so that it appears abnormally narrow in the left parasternal scan.

Lewis and Takahashi (1976) found an excellent correlation between the pulmonary-systemic blood flow ratio and the echographic LA:AR ratio (r = 0.96) and a good correlation (r = 0.85) between the pulmonary-to-systemic flow ratio and the LA dimension corrected for body surface area. The LA:AR ratio seemed a very useful noninvasive means of assessing the extent of left-to-right shunts in children with ventricular septal defects when following such patients periodically. Rees et al. (1978) also found the LA:AR ratio useful in children with ventricular septal defects. They found that ratios exceeding 1.4:1 were associated with pulmonary-to-systolic flow ratios greater than 2:1. However, Lester et al. (1979) reported a far less satisfactory correlation between the LA:AR ratio and pulmonary-to-systemic blood flow ratio (r = 0.62). The value of echocardiography for this purpose thus remains controversial (Fuhrman et al., 1980).

In a series of children with various congenital cardiac defects, Yabek et al. (1976) found a good correlation between the M-mode echographic LA dimension and angiographically determined LA volume. These authors reported that the LA volume could be predicted by a regression equation; in normal subjects the factor used for multiplying the echographic LA dimension was 7.5 and in patients with large LA chambers it was 8.1.

When LA dilatation is marked, LA dimension exceeds LV dimension impressively (Fig. H-1).

On 2-D echocardiography, the LA diameter can be measured in long-axis and short-axis view (Schabelman et al., 1979), yielding essentially the same dimension that is measured in the conventional M-mode tracing. In addition, the LA dimension can also be measured in the apical four-chamber view, from the mitral ring (mitral valve attachment) to the posterosuperior atrial roof, at end-systole (Kushner et al., 1978). In normal subjects the upper limit by the latter method is 40 mm (mean, 35 ± 4 mm).

Two-D echocardiography is of real help in appreciating the presence and degree of LA enlargement (Gradin-Frimmer et al., 1982; Gehl et al., 1982) (Figs. H-2 to H-6). The disparity between a large left atrium and a normal aortic root is evident in long- and short-axis views. Dilatation of the left atrium is more evident in the apical four-chamber view than in the

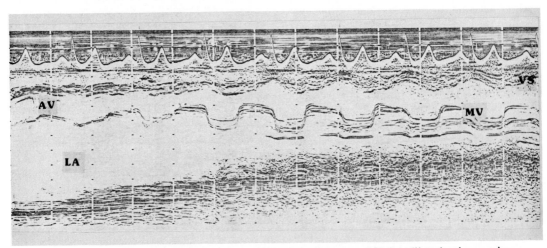

Fig. H-1. M-mode echographic scan from LA and aortic root to LV. LA dilatation is conspicuous (*left of figure*). The mitral valve shows changes typical of mitral stenosis.

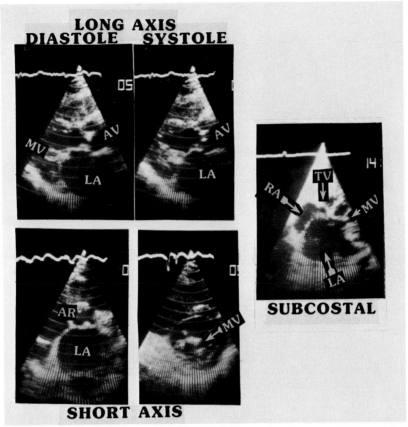

Fig. H-2. *Left.* 2-D echogram of an elderly woman admitted with atrial flutter. No diastolic murmur was heard but a history of rheumatic fever in childhood was forthcoming. The mitral valve appears stenotic in the long-axis view (*upper frames*) and short-axis view (*right lower frame*). The left atrium appears dilated to about 5 cm (*left upper and lower frames*).

Right. Subcostal 2-D echogram of another patient with marked LA enlargement secondary to rheumatic mitral valve disease. The atrial septum bulges into the right atrium, which appears dwarfed by the dilated LA.

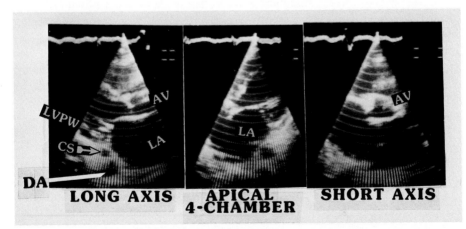

Fig. H-3. 2-D echogram of a patient with rheumatic mitral regurgitation. The left frame is in the long-axis view, the center frame in the apical 4-chamber view, and the right frame in the short-axis view. The left atrium is dilated (dimension about 6 cm). The anatomic relationships of the coronary sinus and descending aorta to each other, and to the LA and LV, are clearly visible in the left frame.

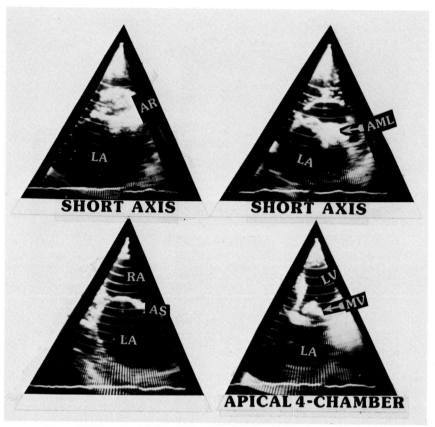

Fig. H-4. 2-D echogram of a man with calcific mitral stenosis. The left upper frame and right upper frame, in the short-axis view, show the dilated LA posterior to the aortic root and calcified anterior mitral leaflet, respectively. The calcified mitral valve and dilated LA are also evident in the right lower frame in the apical 4-chamber view. The left lower frame, in the *right* parasternal horizontal view, shows the dilated LA posterior to the smaller anterior RA.

long-axis view (Fig. H-5). Marked LA enlargement is associated with a striking alteration in its shape from ellipsoidal to spherical, a geometric attribute that can be appreciated in every view (Figs. H-4 and H-6). Rarely, a giant LA may extend or evaginate behind the LV to some extent (Fig. H-6).

Gehl *et al.* (1982) found that LA volume showed marked systolic increase in severe mitral regurgitation, whereas in mitral stenosis the LA volume was often excessively large, but showed little phasic change.

CLINICAL SIGNIFICANCE OF LEFT ATRIAL ENLARGEMENT

Left atrial size, as assessed radiographically, has long been an important diagnostic feature of mitral valve disease. Thus the clinician expects some LA dilatation in all patients with stenosis

or regurgitation (or both) of the mitral valve, except in some instances with only mild mitral valve lesions. The echocardiographic demonstration of LA dilatation likewise plays an important role in the evaluation of mitral valve disease, since considerable LA dilatation is the rule in patients with severe grades of mitral stenosis or regurgitation.

CORRELATION WITH ECG

Waggoner *et al.* (1976), Rubler *et al.* (1976), and Josephson *et al.* (1977) have examined the correlation between echocardiographic and electrocardiographic criteria of LA enlargement. Waggoner as well as Rubler found that P-wave morphology was reasonably specific but not very sensitive as an indicator of LA enlargement. In patients with atrial fibrillation, no correlation was found between LA size and the

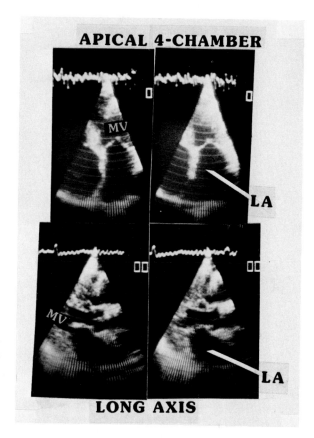

APICAL 4-CHAMBER

LONG AXIS

Fig. H-5. 2-D echogram of a 60-year-old hypertensive woman, in the long-axis view (*lower*) and apical 4-chamber view (*upper*). The LA dimension appears normal in the long-axis view, but definitely increased in the apical view. The latter view appears more sensitive in detecting LA dilatation.

type of atrial fibrillatory waves on the ECG. A lack of correlation between amplitude of fibrillatory atrial activity on the ECG and LA size was likewise described by Morganroth *et al.* (1979). Josephson *et al.* (1977) made the intriguing observation that LA dilatation on the echogram correlated with ECG manifestations of LA enlargement only in patients with mitral valve disease, but in those with coronary artery disease the electrocardiographic pattern was unrelated to LA size.

CORRELATION WITH ATRIAL FIBRILLATION

Another aspect of LA size that has deservedly aroused great interest is the relationship between LA dilatation and the occurrence or recurrence (after defibrillation) of atrial fibrillation. These considerations are pertinent to far-reaching decisions on prognosis, risk of thromboembolism, electrical conversion, cardiac surgery, anticoagulant therapy, antiarrhythmic drug therapy, and other aspects of clinical management.

DeMaria *et al.* (1975) measured LA dimension before and after cardioversion in 35 patients with ischemic heart disease or cardiomyopathy in atrial fibrillation. Conversion to sinus rhythm led to a prompt decrease in LA size. Effective atrial contraction (reflected in a normal "A" wave on the mitral valve) also reappeared immediately, as did a hemodynamic improvement as manifested by an increase in cardiac output. In two patients the conversion to sinus rhythm did not result in appearance of an "A" wave on the mitral valve (so-called electromechanical dissociation), and these patients soon reverted back to atrial fibrillation.

Henry *et al.* (1976) studied the incidence of atrial fibrillation in a large series of 85 patients with mitral valve disease, 50 with aortic valve disease, and 13 with hypertrophic cardiomyopathy. Several pertinent observations emerged from this important study: (1) Atrial fibrillation was rare in patients with LA dimension less than 40 mm, but was the rule in those with LA dimensions of 55 mm or more. Paroxysmal atrial fibrillation interrupting sinus rhythm was

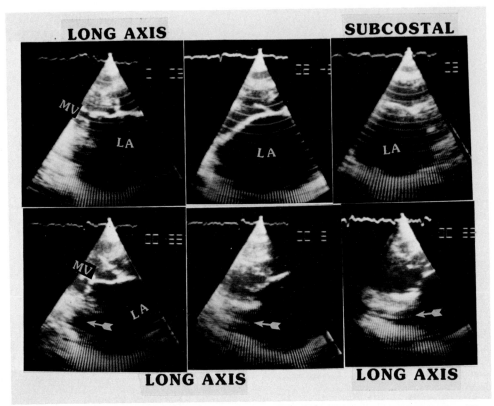

Fig. H-6. 2-D echogram of a 71-year-old woman with mitral stenosis and regurgitation. The LA is enormously dilated, to a maximum dimension of 9 cm, as in the long axis (*top, left*), subcostal (*top, right*), and partial short axis (*top, center*) views. In the lower frames, the long-axis view, note that the dilated LA extends behind the LV posterior wall (*arrows*). In the M-mode echogram, this manifested as an echo-free space posterior to the LV, simulating a pericardial or pleural effusion.

seen in patients with LA dimensions between 40 and 55 mm. (2) Cardioversion, while initially successful, was unlikely to result in sinus rhythm that did not revert back to atrial fibrillation within six months if the LA dimension exceeded 45 mm. (3) In patients with LA dimension of 45 mm or more, over 40 years of age, atrial fibrillation occurred in about 90 per cent of those with mitral valve disease and almost the same proportion of patients with hypertrophic cardiomyopathy. (4) Patients with hypertrophic cardiomyopathy, LA dimensions over 50 mm, and atrial fibrillation are especially prone to embolization following cardioversion.

In a subsequent paper the same group (Watson *et al.,* 1977) reported that no patients with ASH who had LA dimensions less than 45 mm had this arrhythmia. Most patients under 40 with LA dilatation before operation had 10 per cent or more reduction in LA dimension post-

operatively, whereas LA dilatation did not regress after surgery in those over 40. Thus prevention of atrial fibrillation and its attendant risks of embolization and congestive failure could be a possible indication for surgical therapy of IHSS in young patients.

To slightly modify a recommendation of Henry *et al.* (1976), it may be prudent to institute prophylactic anticoagulation in patients in sinus rhythm with mitral valve disease or hypertrophic cardiomyopathy if their LA dimension exceeds 40 mm and their age exceeds 40 years.

Sherrid *et al.* (1979) investigated the effect of mitral valve surgery on LA size, status of cardiac compensation, atrial fibrillation, and systemic embolization. Patients were evaluated an average of a year postoperatively: clinical improvement was usually associated with decrease in LA size (average decrease 20 per cent), whereas no diminution in LA size was noted

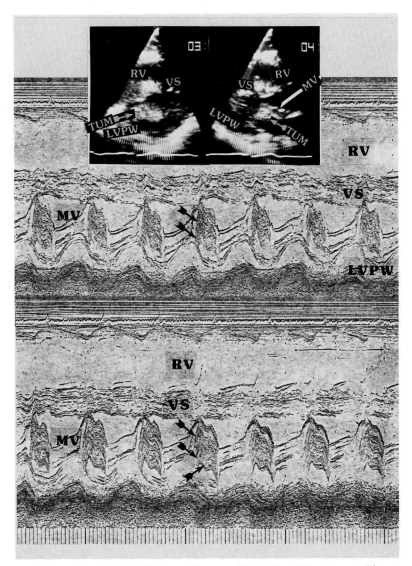

Fig. H-7. Echocardiogram of a 52-year-old man with a left atrial myxoma. The upper panel of the M-mode echogram is at a slightly lower LV level than the lower panel. The size, density, and motion of the tumor (*arrows*) is similar in the two segments, except that the posterior margin of the myxoma is better visualized in the lower panel. A small interval (clear space) can be discerned between anterior opening motion of the anterior mitral leaflet and anterior motion of the tumor mass.

Inset. 2-D echogram in the short-axis view (*left*) and long-axis view (*right*) in the same patient. Both frames are in diastole and show the LA myxoma as a mass protruding into the center of the LV.

in patients with persistent cardiac decompensation, whether caused by poor LV function or prosthetic valve dysfunction.

As expected, patients with chronic atrial fibrillation had larger LA chambers than those in sinus rhythm. Large left atria predispose to atrial fibrillation as well as to systemic emboli. In patients with established atrial fibrillation

the risk of embolization does not necessarily increase with increasing LA size. However, Sherrid *et al.* found that the combination of LA dilatation and low cardiac output is particularly ominous in this regard in patients with mitral valve disease. Prophylactic anticoagulation is therefore strongly recommended for this type of patient.

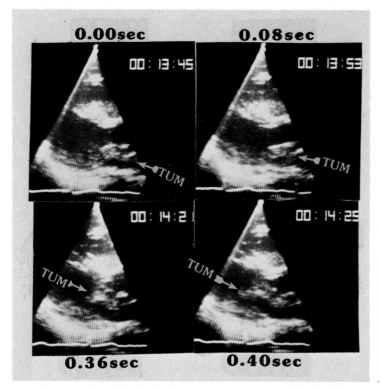

Fig. H-8. 2-D echogram of a patient with a left atrial myxoma (removed surgically), who had presented with recurrent strokes. The four frames, all in the long-axis view, are serial ones from the same cardiac cycle. The upper frames are in systole, the lower ones in diastole. In systole the LA myxoma manifests as an abnormal echo situated under the anterior mitral leaflet and aortic root. In diastole the tumor can be seen as an elongated fingerlike mass moving into the LV through the mitral valve.

PROLONGATION OR "PROLAPSE" OF DILATED LEFT ATRIUM BEHIND THE LEFT VENTRICLE

When the LA is markedly dilated, it occasionally may have a prolongation or extension that enlarges as a wedge-shaped continuation or "foot" of the LA chamber posterior to the basal LV posterior wall (Ratshin *et al.,* 1974; Reeves *et al.,* 1981; Foale *et al.,* 1982; Beppu *et al.,* 1982). An echo-free space is evident posterior to the LV posterior wall at mitral valve level, which could be mistaken for a pericardial or pleural effusion (Fig. N-36). Another condition it could mimic, even on the 2-D echogram, is pseudoaneurysm of the LV. Foale *et al.* (1982) described two instances of LA aneurysms arising from the LA appendages, which presented as large echo-free spaces *lateral* to the heart rather than behind it.

LEFT ATRIAL MYXOMA (Figs. H-7 and H-8)

In spite of the rarity of atrial myxomas in everyday practice, over a score of papers have been published in leading cardiology journals on their ultrasonic features (Schattenberg, 1968; Wolfe *et al.,* 1969; Popp and Harrison, 1969; Finegan and Harrison, 1970; Kostis and Moghadam, 1970; Spencer *et al.,* 1971; Nasser *et al.,* 1972; Pridie, 1972; Bass and Sharratt, 1973; Gustafson *et al.,* 1973; Johnson *et al.,* 1973; Kerber *et al.,* 1974; Martinez *et al.,* 1974; DeMaria *et al.,* 1975; Potts *et al.,* 1975; Fitterer *et al.,* 1976; Petsas *et al.,* 1976; Graham *et al.,* 1976; Huston *et al.,* 1978; Lappe *et al.,* 1978; Cosio *et al.,* 1978; Yoshikawa *et al.,* 1978; Hibi *et al.,* 1979; Stewart *et al.,* 1979; Kaminsky *et al.,* 1979; Ciraulo, 1979; Hamer *et al.,* 1979; Rajpal *et al.,* 1979; Sharratt *et al.,* 1979; Tanabe *et al.,* 1979; Hamada *et al.,* 1980; Paulsen *et al.,* 1980; Sandok *et al.,* 1980; Joseph *et al.,* 1980). Although uncommon, cardiac myxomas are potentially fatal yet permanently curable by surgery only if they are diagnosed in time, and echocardiography is foremost among the means by which the tumor is detected.

The usual echographic manifestations (Fig. H-4) are fortunately conspicuous and fairly specific:

1. An echo mass appearing just posterior to the anterior mitral leaflet in diastole. The den-

MASSES IN THE LEFT HEART CHAMBERS

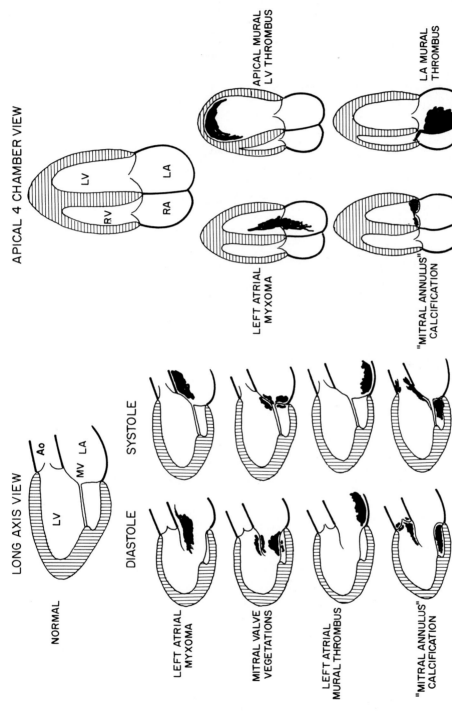

Fig. H-9. Diagram showing 2-D echographic appearances in the long-axis (*left*) and apical 4-chamber (*right*) views in patients with various types of masses in the LA or LV. The masses are depicted in solid black. Note that certain varieties of masses change position from systole to diastole, while others do so very little.

235

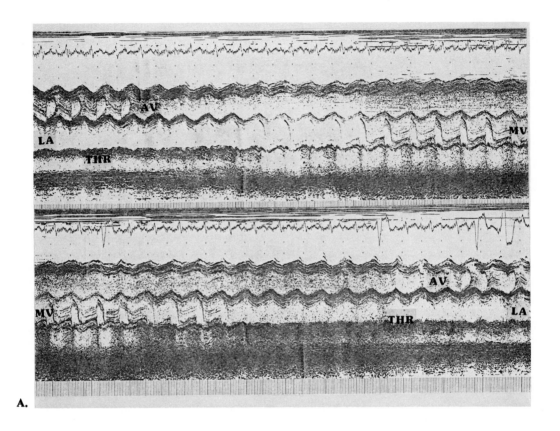

A.

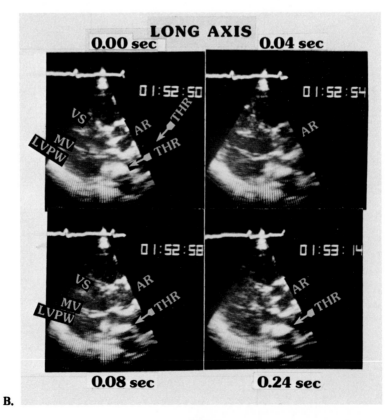

B.

236

LEFT ATRIAL MYXOMA 237

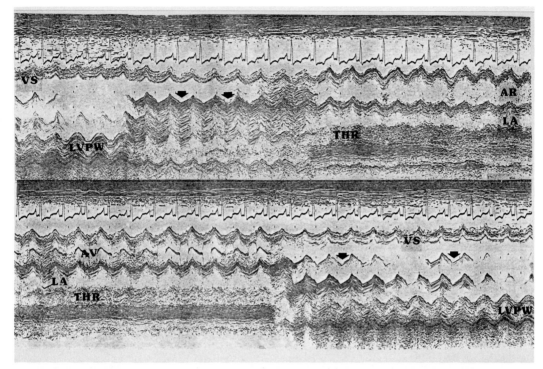

Fig. H-11. Segments from the M-mode echogram of a patient with a prosthetic porcine mitral valve (*arrows*). A thrombus (THR) is visible in the LA, adjacent to the LA posterior wall.

sity and texture of this echo mass can vary from "dense solid" or "dense stratified" to stippled or fluffy. It can usually be recognized as separate from the anterior mitral leaflet echo, especially in early diastole, i.e., the myxoma moves forward into the left ventricle an appreciable interval after the anterior mitral leaflet. Potts *et al.* (1975) pointed out that this echo-free margin adjacent to the DE segment of the anterior mitral echo was broad with small left atrial myxomas but minimal with large myxomas.

2. The anterior mitral leaflet echo may show a low or flat EF slope, thus resembling the diastolic motion of mitral stenosis. However, the leaflet does not appear thickened or calcified. The posterior mitral leaflet may be identified

just behind the tumor mass in diastole but more often is obscured by it.

3. In systole the myxoma disappears from the left ventricle but may be visible in the left atrium behind the aortic root. Sometimes the tumor mass is seen just behind the base of the mitral leaflet, as the ultrasound beam scans from mitral valve to aortic root.

Most published reports of left atrial myxomas describe tumors that are freely mobile, pedunculated, and attached to the left aspect of the interatrial septum and present echocardiographically as stated above. However, not all atrial neoplasms conform to this pattern. There are occasionally exceptions:

1. The left atrial myxoma may be confined

Fig. H-10. *A.* M-mode echogram of an elderly woman with an LA mural thrombus. The upper panel shows a scan from LA to LV; the lower panel a scan from LV to LA. The mural thrombus appears as a dense echo band within the LA, which appears separate from the LA posterior wall in the upper panel, but contiguous to the LA wall in the lower panel.

Fig. H-10. *B.* 2-D echogram of the same patient with an LA mural thrombus, showing 4 serial frames in the long-axis view. The first (*upper left*) and last (*lower right*) are at end-diastole; the other two are systolic, from the same cardiac cycle. The abnormal dense echo in the LA shows little or no change in position. An LA myxoma would have moved down into the LV in diastole and back up into the LA in systole.

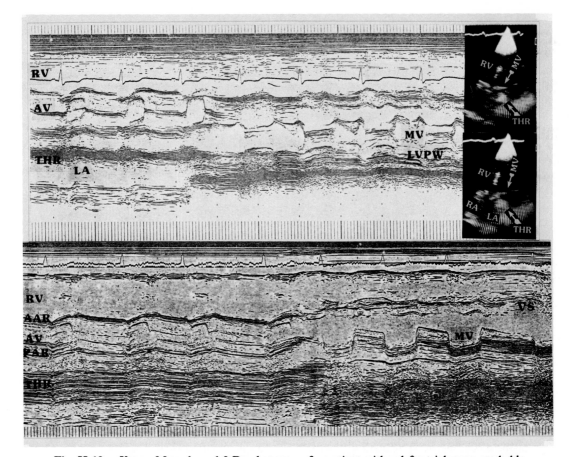

Fig. H-12. *Upper.* M-mode and 2-D echograms of a patient with a left atrial mass, probably a mural thrombus. The M-mode scan from LA to LV shows a dense echo band within the LA chamber, which meets the posterior wall at the atrioventricular junction. The 2-D echogram in the apical view in systole (*above*) and diastole (*below*) shows the LA mass as a dense echo between the mitral valve and LA wall.

Lower. M-mode echographic scan from LA to LV in a patient with mitral stenosis and a calcified mural thrombus adherent to the LA posterior wall. The thrombus presents echocardiographically as a dense mass about 2 cm wide, occupying the posterior half of the LA and causing the LA cavity to appear abnormally small.

to the left atrium in diastole as well as systole because it is sessile or has a short pedicle. Instances of this type have been reported by Johnson *et al.* (1973), Petsas *et al.* (1976), Lappe *et al.* (1978), Yoshikawa *et al.* (1978). Petsas *et al.* noted that visualization of the left atrial chamber by the suprasternal approach revealed abnormal echoes arising from the myxoma in all their three cases, two of which were not mobile enough to prolapse into the mitral valve orifice in the classic pattern.

2. Myxomas arising from the mitral valve itself can closely resemble a left atrial myxoma. An echo mass is seen just posterior to the anterior mitral leaflet.

3. Malignant sarcomatous left atrial tumors are extremely rare (Yasher *et al.,* 1979; Mahar *et al.,* 1979; Hamada *et al.,* 1980). Metastases from a malignant neurilemoma closely simulated a left atrial myxoma echographically (Ishikawa *et al.,* 1982). Such an invasive neoplasm can simulate a myxoma or even calcific mitral stenosis. Although the tumor protrudes into the mitral valve orifice in diastole like a myxoma, it may not retreat back into the left atrium in systole. Abnormal dense echoes thus persist in both systole and diastole, the pattern of mitral motion sometimes resembling that of mitral stenosis.

4. Rarely a left atrial myxoma of substantial

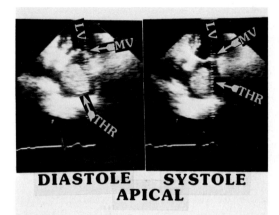

DIASTOLE   SYSTOLE
APICAL

Fig. H-13. 2-D echogram in the apical view of an elderly patient with mitral stenosis. In the left frame, in diastole, the mitral valve does not open normally, but presents a convex contour toward the LV. In the right frame, in systole, the mitral valve is closed. A large spherical echo mass within the LA is evident in both frames; it does not prolapse into the LV in diastole, as an LA myxoma usually would do. It represents a ball thrombus, a rare but notorious complication of mitral stenosis.

size is invisible to ultrasound (Stewart *et al.,* 1979). These authors ascribed the nonechogenic nature of the tumor in this patient to its great vascularity, the blood within the tumor rendering its acoustic properties similar to the blood in the LA. Fortunately, the vascularity caused an intense tumor "blush" on the angiocardio-gram. In another patient reported by Ciraulo (1979), coarse mitral flutter was evident, but the LA myxoma itself was not visualized on the echocardiogram. Another instance of mitral flutter in diastole, similar to that seen in patients with aortic regurgitation, recently has been reported by Baird (1981).

5. Large sonolucent areas within the mass of stippled echoes representing the atrial myxoma could be caused by hemorrhage within the tumor (Rahilly and Nanda, 1981) and, if present, possibly could help in differentiating myxomas from other masses (thrombi or large vegetations) in this region.

6. In a patient reported by Motro *et al.* (1982), the LA myxoma was adherent to the anterior mitral leaflet; the tumor stalk thus moved parallel to the anterior mitral leaflet and produced an "extra" mitral valve echo in the LA behind the aortic root.

TWO-D ECHOCARDIOGRAPHY

As pointed out by Feigenbaum (1976), 2-D echocardiography may not be more sensitive than the M-mode technique in detecting the presence of a left atrial myxoma, but it does permit an appreciation of certain aspects of the tumor that are difficult or impossible to ascertain by M-mode echography. These include its

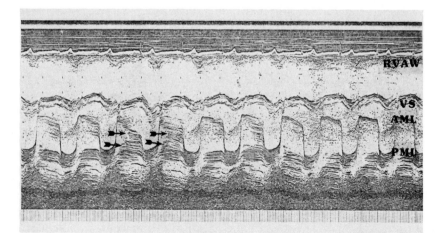

Fig. H-14. M-mode echogram of a patient with typical appearances of mitral stenosis: flat EF slope, marked sclerosis or calcification, and abnormal diastolic motion of the posterior mitral leaflet. In some beats (for example, the third and fourth) the space between the anterior and posterior leaflets appears to fill up with echoes simulating a pedunculated left atrial myxoma or clot. However, such an artifactual "mass" can be made to vanish by slight change in transducer direction and is probably attributable to the beam-width factor. 2-D echography would also help in excluding a mobile LA mass.

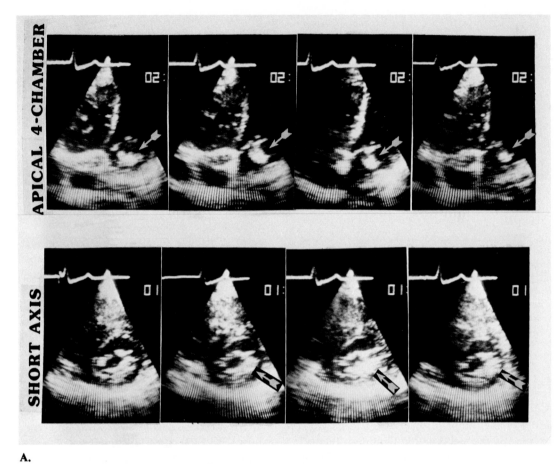

Fig. H-15. *A.* 2-D echogram of a patient with chronic renal failure and a large staphylococcal vegetation (infected mural thrombus) implanted directly on the mitral annulus (diagnosis established at autopsy).

Upper. Apical 4-chamber view. All four frames are in diastole, but the vegetation or thrombus shows considerable variation in size (appearing progressively smaller from left to right) with slight changes in direction of the 2-D probe.

Lower. Short-axis view. All four frames are in diastole, but the vegetation (*arrows*) appears progressively larger from left to right with slight alteration in the sector plane scanned.

shape, size, and motion characteristics (Figs. H-4 and H-5). The shape and size of LA myxomas viewed by cardiac ultrasound are quite variable (Lappe *et al.,* 1978; Yoshikawa *et al.,* 1978; Moses and Nanda, 1980). At times they are long, narrow, and fingerlike, penetrating deep into the LV in diastole; at the other end of the spectrum they may be large and massive, filling most of the LA chamber. Most cases fall between these two extremes.

LA myxomas exhibit a pattern of motion during the cardiac cycle that distinguishes them from most other intracardiac masses. They move abruptly back and forth between the LA

and LV through the mitral valve orifice. This differentiates them from (1) mitral valve vegetations, which are obviously attached to the leaflets and move along with them; (2) calcific masses in the "mitral annulus," region which appear fixed to the adjacent LV posterior wall and partake of its motion; (3) mural thrombi, which are likewise adherent to the subjacent LA or LV wall and move parallel to the underlying endocardium.

The amplitude of LA myxoma motion varies from one case to the other, probably depending on the length of the tumor pedicle, and the configuration and bulk of the tumor mass itself.

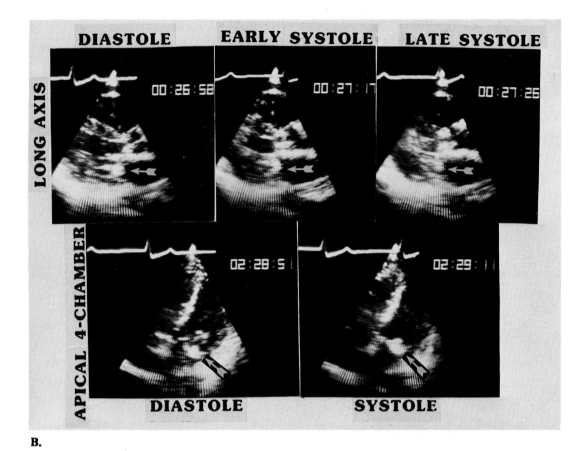

Fig. H-15. *B.* The 3 upper frames are from the same cardiac cycle: the first in diastole, the second in early systole, the third in late systole. The vegetation presents as a nodular echo on the atrial side of the base of the posterior mitral leaflet (*arrows*). The relationship of the vegetation to the mitral valve and LA is also demonstrated in the apical 4-chamber view, in diastole and systole (*lower frames*).

A small minority of documented LA myxomas have been sessile or almost so, with rather restricted mobility (Lappe *et al.,* 1978; Perry *et al.,* 1981); they are difficult to differentiate from LA mural thrombi.

Large, solid tumors occupying the LA cavity are associated with echo opacification of the LA space, i.e., the normally sonolucent area posterior to the aortic root is transformed to a mottled or cloudy or stratified, linear mass of echoes. Such an appearance can be produced by a large, nonmobile myxoma, a large ball thrombus (in mitral stenosis), a fibrosarcoma arising from the LA wall (Yoshikawa *et al.,* 1978), and by mediastinal malignant neoplasms invading the LA or compressing it from behind (Yoshikawa *et al.,* 1978).

In each of these situations, abnormal echoes suggestive of a solid mass within the LA and perhaps also posterior to the anterior mitral leaflet are seen in scans from LA to LV. When the tumor is intra-atrial with some (though limited) mobility, there tends to be a definite difference between systole and diastole as to the extent of abnormal echoes visualized behind the anterior mitral leaflet. When the tumor is extra-cardiac in the posterior mediastinum, the abnormal echo mass encroaching on the retro-aortic space and retromitral space (at the atrioventricular junction) shows no motion or variation during the cardiac cycle. Moreover, in the long-axis view it is evident that an external posterior mass is distorting the posterior cardiac contour, forming a large convex bulge that pushes the LA posterior wall anteriorly and reduces LA dimension.

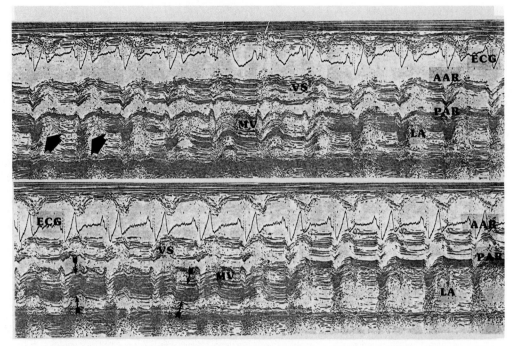

Fig. H-16. M-mode echographic scans in an elderly woman with heavy submitral (mitral annulus) calcification. In the upper panel, a scan is made from LA to LV and back to LA. In the lower panel, a scan is made from LV to LA. Dense echoes, apparently in the LA (*broad arrows*), arise from submitral calcification (*thin arrows*) but artefactually appear to extend into the LA because of the beam-width factor.

CONDITIONS SIMULATING LA MYXOMA (Fig. H-9, see page 235)

MITRAL VALVE VEGETATIONS

1. Large vegetations on the mitral leaflets, particularly the posterior leaflet, can closely resemble the M-mode echographic pattern of a left atrial myxoma. The brief delay between anterior motion of the anterior mitral leaflet and of the vegetation can cause a small, narrow space between anterior mitral echo and the echo mass of the large vegetation; this feature therefore is not entirely specific for a left atrial myxoma. Such large mitral vegetations are often fungal in nature (Pasternak *et al.,* 1976) but can also be bacterial, as in an instance of staphylococcal endocarditis reported by Nicholson *et al.* (1980).

To complicate the differential diagnosis further, about a dozen instances of infected myxomas have been reported, including a couple of cases with *Candida* as the causative organism (Joseph *et al.,* 1980). The echocardiographic picture is that of a noninfected myxoma (Gra-

ham *et al.,* 1976; Joseph *et al.,* 1980). However, the clinical presentation in the majority of reported patients was systemic embolization.

On 2-D echocardiography a mitral valve vegetation moves with and is clearly attached to the posterior mitral leaflet. Such motion is quite different from the to-and-fro motion of a pedunculated left atrial myxoma between left atrium and left ventricle.

2. *Left atrial thrombi* (Figs. H-10 to H-13, see pages 236–239) usually have very restricted mobility, being firmly adherent to the atrial endocardium. They are thus visualized, by M-mode and even better by 2-D echography, to remain fixed within the LA chamber throughout the cardiac cycle. LA myxomas are usually pedunculated and highly mobile so that in diastole they appear in the left ventricle and in systole retreat into the left atrium.

However, sessile myxomas or those with very short pedicles do occur and cannot be differentiated by ultrasound from left atrial thrombi. The distinction is important because the therapy for LA myxomas is surgical, whereas the manage-

[*Text continued on page 246.*]

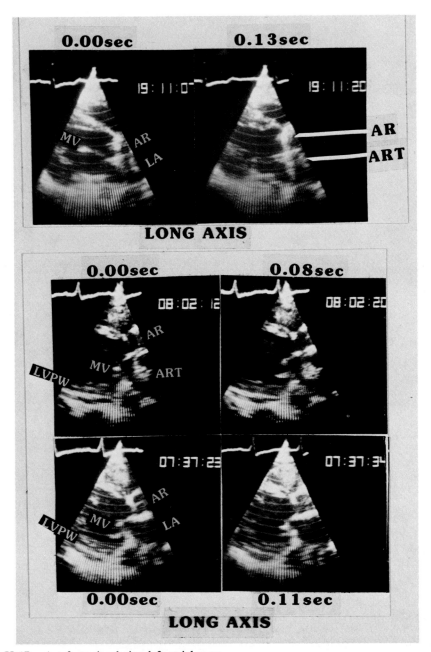

Fig. H-17. Artefacts simulating left atrial mass.

Upper. 2-D echogram in the long-axis view of a man with Bjork-Shiley aortic valve replacement. The left frame is in diastole; the right frame (0.13 sec later) is in systole. In the latter, reverberations from the prosthetic disk appear to come from the LA, and may therefore be mistaken from an LA mass. Such reverberations obviously emanate from the dense echo of the disk in the aortic root, and have no independent motion of their own.

Lower. 2-D echogram, in the long-axis view of an elderly woman with cardiomyopathy. The LV size shows little change from diastole to systole. The upper frames are serial ones from the same cardiac cycle. The lower frames are also serial, from a different cardiac cycle, in a slightly different plane. An apparently abnormal echo in the LA appears in the upper frames. It was thought to be a reverberatory artefact because (a) it disappeared with a minor change in probe direction (*lower frames*), and (b) it did not show motion from systole to diastole.

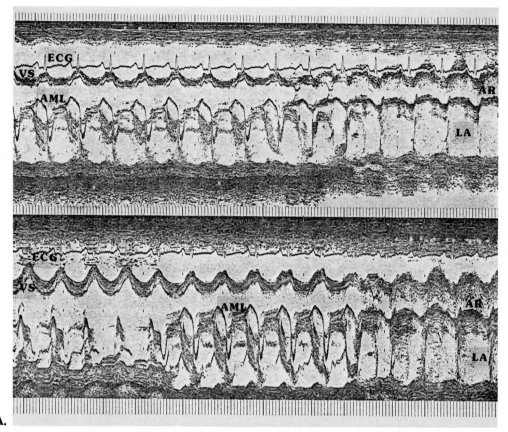

A.

Fig. H-18. *A.* Two scans from LV to LA, in a 5-year-old child, at slightly different transducer angulations. Abnormal echoes posterior to the anterior mitral leaflet are visible in both scans, but morphology of these echoes is different in the two panels because the beam traverses the peculiar structure at different levels. At surgery a thick diaphragm-like structure was removed from the left atrium; it was situated above the mitral valve and attached to the posterior leaflet by a thin band.

Fig. H-18. *B.* 2-D echogram in the same 5-year-old child demonstrating an abnormal structure within the LA. The four upper frames show how this structure undergoes striking changes in position and contour at different phases of the cardiac cycle. During diastole (*first two upper frames*) it tends to move through the mitral valve into the LV. During systole (*last upper frame*) it billows back into the LA like a sail. It thus appears like a sheet or membrane, attached to the LA posterior wall and connected to the posterior mitral leaflet but free of the anterior mitral leaflet.

The left lower frame, in the short-axis view, shows the abnormal structure, partly folded, below the anterior mitral leaflet. The next frame (*lower row center*), in the 4-chamber apical view, shows the abnormal structure divided into two parts, with a central clear area that leads into the mitral valve orifice. The right lower frame, in the subcostal 4-chamber view, shows the abnormal structure protruding into the LV inflow area.

At surgery a thick corrugated membrane was found spanning the LA chamber. It was attached to the posterior mitral leaflet but free of the anterior leaflet. Nonspecific inflammatory changes were found in this structure on histological examination, but no neoplastic tissue.

Fig. H-18. *C.* Serial frames from the same cardiac cycle in the same 5-year-old child with a thick membrane-like structure in the LA. The three frames, all in the apical 4-chamber view, show strikingly different echo patterns at different phases of the cardiac cycle. In late diastole (*left frame*) the abnormal structure appears to consist of two components that move apart to allow the passage of blood from LA to LV through the open mitral orifice. At the onset of systole (*center frame*) the abnormal LA structure appears to coil up and simulate an LA mass such as a myxoma. Later in systole the membrane seems to balloon out into a curved linear echo, presumably in response to the regurgitant mitral jet impinging upon it.

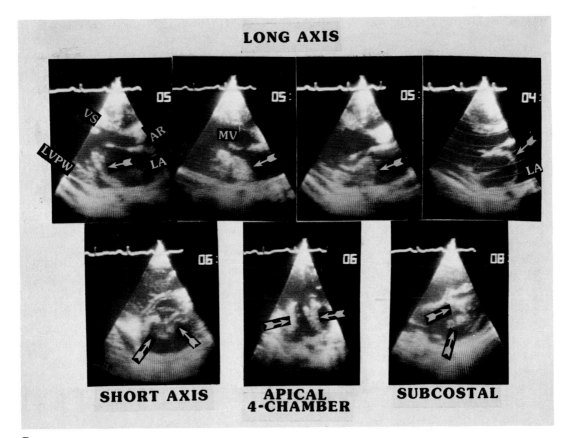

LONG AXIS

SHORT AXIS **APICAL 4-CHAMBER** **SUBCOSTAL**

B.

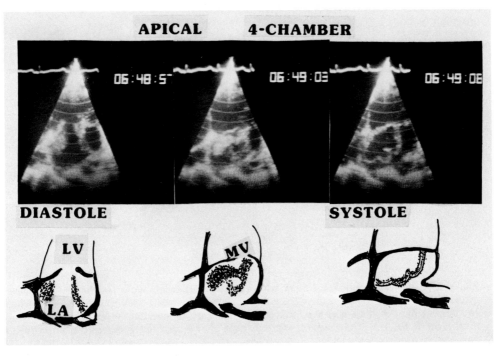

APICAL   4-CHAMBER

DIASTOLE   **SYSTOLE**

C.

ment of left atrial thrombi is medical (anticoagulant therapy).

Most reported instances of left atrial thrombi diagnosed by echocardiography have been in patients with mitral valve stenosis or mitral prostheses.

3. In mitral prolapse the posterior mitral leaflet is often very redundant and/or thickened due to myxomatous degeneration, so that it tends to gather into folds during diastole, simulating a vegetation or myxoma (see Fig. B-27). Two-D echocardiography helps in differentiating between the two diagnoses.

4. In mitral stenosis, the thickened anterior mitral leaflet can simulate an intramitral diastolic echo that could be mistaken for a myxoma (Fig. H-14, see page 239).

5. A vegetation on the mitral annulus does not show as much mobility as does one on a mitral leaflet but could simulate an LA thrombus or myxoma (Fig. H-15, see page 240- 241).

6. Reverberations from the aortic root, prosthetic aortic valves, or even the chest wall, also artefacts caused by the beam-width factor (from submitral calcification, Fig. H-16, page 242) or improper transducer angulation may produce "abnormal" echoes in the LA, on M-mode as well as 2-D echography (Fig. H-17, see page 243). Such artefactual echoes are often mistaken by neophytes for LA masses, which they can indeed resemble on isolated 2-D frames or short M-mode segments. In actual practice, the echocardiographer learns to avoid such pitfalls by technical adjustments including slight alterations in transducer location or angulation, gain setting, and so forth.

7. We have encountered recently a remarkable case of a thick supramitral membrane in the LA that simulated a myxoma on M-mode and 2-D echograms (Fig. H-18). However, during certain phases of the cardiac cycle the membrane or diaphragm ballooned into the LA, forming a band or linear echo that revealed its true nature.

Linear or band echoes in the LA are not usually mistaken for myxomas, but constitute a problem of differential diagnosis in themselves. They may represent the edge of a mural thrombus, various forms of congenital LA septa (cor triatriatum) or supramitral ring or diaphragm (Jacobstein and Hirschfeld, 1982), or mitral valve aneurysm (Lewis *et al.*, 1982). A

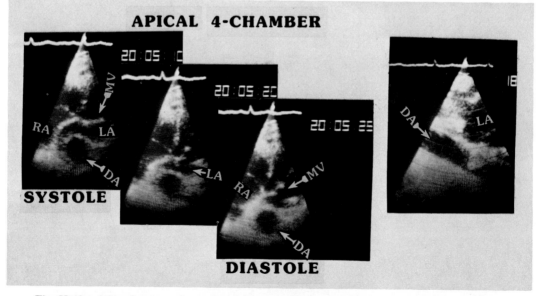

Fig. H-19. 2-D echogram of a patient with a dilated descending aorta. In the first 3 frames, in the apical 4-chamber view, the descending aorta (*DA*) appears as a round echo-free space just behind the LA, into which it protrudes. It appears to simulate an anomalous band or diaphragm in the LA. The frame at extreme right shows the dilated descending aorta in its long-axis view.

dilated descending aorta (Fig H-19) or coronary sinus can bulge into the LA and simulate such an LA structure.

LEFT ATRIAL THROMBI

Thrombotic masses within the LA are as frequent as neoplastic ones. However, unlike myxomas, LA thrombi occur almost exclusively in patients with mitral valve disease, including those with prosthetic mitral valves. Surgical and angiocardiographic observations indicate that 10 to 25 per cent of patients with mitral valve disease have LA thrombi. De Pace *et al.* (1981) reported a somewhat lower incidence (6 per cent) by 2-D echocardiography. One instance of an LA mural thrombus in association with IHSS has been described (D'Cruz *et al.*, 1982).

LA thrombi may be suspected in the M-mode echogram when abnormal linear or stratified echoes appear in the LA chamber posterior to the aortic root (Poehlmann *et al.*, 1975; Spangler and Okin, 1975; Graboys *et al.*, 1977). However, a linear echo in this area (probably arising from the atrial septum) is often seen in normal subjects. Reverberatory or beam-width artefacts from calcification in neighboring structures or prosthetic valves also can simulate LA thrombi.

Two-D echography, especially in the apical four-chamber view, is much superior to the M-mode technique for detecting LA thrombi (Mikell *et al.*, 1979; De Pace *et al.*, 1981). Such mural thrombi are usually not mobile and therefore do not prolapse into the LV during diastole as LA myxomas do. However, a small minority of cases of LA myxomas are sessile or are so enormous as to fill the LA almost completely; these have very little mobility and therefore resemble LA thrombi rather closely. Typically, a LA thrombus presents "as a mass of irregular nonmobile laminated echoes within an enlarged LA cavity, usually with broad base of attachment to the LA posterior wall" (De Pace *et al.*, 1981).

Cautions: (1) Come *et al.* (1981) have encountered two instances of LA thrombi (proven at surgery and autopsy, respectively, to be fairly large and located in the main LA cavity) which did not manifest at all on the 2-D echogram, possibly because the acoustic impedance characteristics of the thrombi did not differ sufficiently from those of the blood or LA wall to permit adequate reflection of ultrasound. (2) Clots in the LA appendage are common in patients with mitral stenosis but may be overlooked because this region is not clearly visualized by ultrasound. Consequently the failure to detect a mass in the LA by echography does not entirely exclude the presence of an LA thrombus.

REFERENCES

LEFT ATRIAL SIZE

Brown, O. R.; Harrison, D. C.; and Popp, R. L.: An improved method for echocardiographic detection of left atrial enlargement. *Circulation,* 50:58, 1974.

Feigenbaum, H.: *Echocardiography.* Lea & Febiger, Philadelphia, 1976.

Fuhrman, B. P.; Epstein, M. C.; Bass, J. L.; *et al.:* Predictive value of the echocardiographic left atrial dimension in isolated ventricular septal defect. *J.C.U.,* 8:347, 1980.

Gehl, L. G.; Mintz, G. S.; Kotler, N. M.; *et al.:* Left atrial volume overload in mitral regurgitation. *Am. J. Cardiol.,* 49:33, 1982.

Gradin-Frimmer, G.; Lassvik, C., Nylander, E.; *et al.:* Echocardiographic estimation of left atrial size from the apical view. *Eur. Heart J.,* 3:159, 1982.

Hirata, T.; Wolfe, S. B.; Popp, R. L.; *et al.:* Estimation of left atrial size using ultrasound. *Am. Heart J.,* 78:43, 1969.

Kushner, F. G.; Lam, W.; and Morganroth, J.: Apex sector echocardiography in evaluation of the right atrium in patients with mitral stenosis and atrial septal defect. *Am. J. Cardiol.,* 42:733, 1978.

Lester, L. A.; Vitullo, D.; Dodt, P.; *et al.:* An evaluation of left atrial/aortic root ratio in children with ventricular septal defect. *Circulation,* 60:364, 1979.

Lewis, A. B., and Takahashi, M.: Echocardiographic assessment of left-to-right shunt volume in children with ventricular septal defect. *Circulation,* 54:78, 1976.

Rees, A. H.; Rao, P. S.; Rigby, J. J.; *et al.:* Echocardiographic estimation of a left-to-right shunt in isolated ventricular septal defects. *Eur. J. Cardiol.,* 7:25, 1978.

Schabelman, S. E.; Schiller, N. B.; Auschentz, R. A.; *et al.:* Comparison of four two-dimensional echocardiographic views for measuring left atrial size. *Am. J. Cardiol.,* 41:391, 1979 (Abstr.).

ten Cate, F. J.; Kloster, F. E.; van Dorp, W. S.; *et al.:* Dimensions and volumes of left atrium and ventricle determined by single beam echocardiography. *Br. Heart J.,* 38:737, 1974.

Yabek, S. M.; Isabel-Jones, J.; and Bhatt, D. R.: Echocardiographic determination of left atrial volumes in children with congenital heart disease. *Circulation,* 53:268, 1976.

LEFT ATRIAL ENLARGEMENT

Beppu, S.; Kawazoe, K.; Nimura, Y.; *et al.:* Echocardiographic study of abnormal position and motion of the posterobasal wall of the left ventricle in cases of giant left atrium. *Am. J. Cardiol.,* 44:467, 1982.

DeMaria, A. N.; Lies, J. E.; King, J. K.; *et al.:* Echographic assessment of atrial transport, mitral movement and ventricular performance following electroversion of supraventricular arrhythmias. *Circulation,* 51:273, 1975.

Foale, R. A.; Gibson, T. C.; Guyer, D. E.; *et al.:* Congenital aneurysms of the left atrium: Recognition by cross-sectional echocardiography. *Circulation,* **66:**1065, 1982.

Henry, W. L.; Morganroth, J.; Pearlman, A. S.; *et al.:* Relation between echocardiographically determined left atrial size and atrial fibrillation. *Circulation,* **53:**273, 1976.

Josephson, M. E.; Kastor, J. A.; and Morganroth, J.: Electrocardiographic left atrial enlargement. Electrophysiologic, echocardiographic and hemodynamic correlates. *Am. J. Cardiol.,* **39:**967, 1977.

Morganroth, J.; Horowitz, L. N.; Josephson, M. E.; *et al.:* Relationship of atrial fibrillatory wave amplitude to left atrial size and etiology of heart disease. *Am. Heart J.,* **97:**184, 1979.

Ratshin, R. A.; Smith, M.; and Hood, W. P.: Possible false-positive diagnosis of pericardial effusion by echocardiography in presence of large left atrium. *Chest,* **65:**112, 1974.

Reeves, W. C.; Ciotola, T.; Babb, J. D.; *et al.:* Prolonged left atrium behind the left ventricular posterior wall: Two-dimensional echocardiographic and angiographic features. *Am. J. Cardiol.,* **47:**708, 1981.

Rubler, S.; Shah, N. N.; and Moallem, A.: Comparison of left atrial size and pulmonary capillary pressure with P wave of electrocardiogram. *Am. Heart J.,* **92:**93, 1976.

Sherrid, M. V.; Clark, R. D.; and Cohen, K.: Echocardiographic analysis of left atrial size before and after operation in mitral valve disease. *Am. J. Cardiol.,* **43:**171, 1979.

Waggoner, A. D.; Adyanthaya, A. V.; Quinones, M. A.; *et al.:* Left atrial enlargement: Echocardiographic assessment of electrocardiographic criteria. *Circulation,* **54:**553, 1976.

Watson, D. C.; Henry, W. L.; and Epstein, S. E.: Effects of operation on left atrial size and the occurrence of atrial fibrillation in patients with hypertrophic subaortic stenosis. *Circulation,* **55:**178, 1977.

LEFT ATRIAL TUMORS

Attay, S.; Lee, Y. C.; Singleton, R.; *et al.:* Cardiac myxoma. *Ann. Thorac. Surg.,* **29:**397, 1980.

Baird, M. G.: Left atrial myxoma causing fluttering of the posterior mitral leaflet. *Am. Heart J.,* **101:**851, 1981.

Bass, N. M., and Sharratt, G. P.: Left atrial myxoma diagnosed by echocardiography with observations on tumor movement. *Br. Heart J.,* **35:**1332, 1973.

Ciraulo, D. A.: Mitral valve fluttering: An echocardiographic feature of left atrial myxoma. *Chest,* **76:**95, 1979.

Cosio, F. G.; Maria, E.; Tascon, J.; *et al.:* Correlation of phono- and apexcardiographic findings with tumor motion in left atrial myxoma. *Chest,* **74:**686, 1978.

DeMaria, A. N.; Vismara, L. A.; and Miller, R. R.: Unusual manifestations of right and left atrial myxoma. *Am. J. Med.,* **59:**713, 1975.

Finegan, R. E., and Harrison, D. C.: Diagnosis of left atrial myxoma by echocardiography. *N. Engl. J. Med.,* **282:**1022, 1970.

Fitterer, J. D.; Spicer, M. J.; and Nelson, W. P.: Echocardiographic demonstration of bilateral atrial myxoma. *Chest,* **70:**282, 1976.

Graham, H. V.; von Hartitzsch, B.; and Medina, J. R.: Infected atrial myxoma. *Am. J. Cardiol.,* **38:**658, 1976.

Gustafson, A.; Eder, I.; Dahlback, O.; *et al.:* Left atrial myxoma diagnosed by ultrasound cardiography. *Angiology,* **24:**443, 1973.

Hamada, N.; Matsuzaki, M.; Kusukawa, R.; *et al.:* Malignant fibrous histiocytoma of the heart. *Jpn. Circ. J.,* **44:**361, 1980.

Hamer, J. P.; Nieveen, J.; Bergstra, A.; *et al.:* Left atrial myxoma moving from right atrium to left ventricle. *Acta Med. Scand.,* **204:**527, 1979.

Hibi, N.; Fukui, Y.; Nishimura, K.; *et al.:* Real-time observation of atrial myxoma with high speed B mode echocardiography. *J. C. U.,* **7:**34, 1979.

Huston, K. A.; Combs, J. J.; Lie, J. T.; *et al.:* Left atrial myxoma simulating peripheral vasculitis. *Mayo Clin. Proc.,* **53:**752, 1978.

Ishikawa, K.; Hirata, S.; and Fukuzumi, N.: Malignant neurilemmoma of left atrium. *Brit. Heart J.,* **47:**94, 1982.

Johnson, M. L.; Seiker, H. O.; Behar, V. S.; *et al.:* Echocardiographic diagnosis of a left atrial myxoma attached to the free left atrial wall. *J. C. U.,* **1:**75, 1973.

Joseph, P.; Himmelstein, D. U.; Mahowald, J. M.; *et al.:* Atrial myxoma infected with *Candida:* First survival. *Chest,* **78:**340, 1980.

Kaminsky, M. E.; Ehlers, K. H.; Engle, M. A.; *et al.:* Atrial myxoma mimicking a collagen disorder. *Chest,* **75:**93, 1979.

Kerber, R. E.; Kelly, D. H.; and Gutenkauf, C. H.: Left atrial myxoma. Demonstration by stop-action cardiac ultrasonography. *Am. J. Cardiol.,* **34:**838, 1974.

Kostis, J. B., and Moghadam, A. N.: Echocardiographic diagnosis of left atrial myxoma. *Chest,* **58:**550, 1970.

Lappe, D. C.; Bulkley, B. H.; and Weiss, J. L.: Two-dimensional echocardiographic diagnosis of left atrial myxoma. *Chest,* **74:**55, 1978.

Lee, Y. C., and Magram, M. Y.: Nonprolapsing left atrial tumor. *Chest,* **78:**332, 1980.

Mahar, L. J.; Lie, J. T.; Groover, R. V.; *et al.:* Primary cardiac myxosarcoma in a child. *Mayo Clin. Proc.,* **54:**261, 1979.

Martinez, E. C.; Giles, T. D.; and Burch, G. E.: Echocardiographic diagnosis of left atrial myxoma. *Am. J. Cardiol.,* **33:**281, 1974.

Morgan, D. L.; Palazola, J.; Reed, W.; *et al.:* Left heart myxomas. *Am. J. Cardiol.,* **40:**615, 1977.

Moses, H. W., and Nanda, N. C.: Real-time two-dimensional echocardiography in the diagnosis of left atrial myxoma. *Chest,* **78:**788, 1980.

Motro, M.; Schneeweiss, A.; Grenedier, E.; *et al.:* Mitral valve echocardiographic pattern within the left atrium. *Clin. Cardiol.,* **5:**136, 1982.

Nasser, W. K.; Davis, R. H.; Dillon, J. C.; *et al.:* Atrial myxoma. II. Phonocardiographic, echocardiographic, hemodynamic and angiographic features in nine cases. *Am. Heart J.,* **83:**810, 1972.

Nicholson, M. R.; Roche, A. H.; Keer, A. R.; *et al.:* Mitral valve vegetations in bacterial endocarditis resembling left atrial myxoma. *Aust. N. Z. J. Med.,* **10:**327, 1980.

Pasternak, R. C.; Cannom, D. S.; and Cohen, L. S.: Echocardiographic diagnosis of large fungal verruca attached to mitral valve. *Br. Heart J.,* **38:**1209, 1976.

Paulsen, W.; Wolewajka, A. J.; Boughner, D. R.; *et al.:* Left atrial myxoma: report of six cases and review of the literature. *Can. Med. Assoc. J.,* **123:**518, 1980.

Perry, L. S.; Ring, J. F.; Zeft, H. G.; *et al.:* Two-dimensional echocardiography in the diagnosis of left atrial myxoma. *Brit. Heart J.,* **45:**667, 1981.

Petsas, A. A.; Gottlieb, S.; Kingsley, B.; *et al.:* Echocardiography of left atrial myxoma. Usefulness of suprasternal approach. *Br. Heart J.,* **38:**627, 1976.

Popp, R. C., and Harrison, D. C.: Ultrasound for the diagnosis of atrial tumor. *Ann. Intern. Med.,* **71:**785, 1969.

Potts, J. L.; Johnson, L. W.; and Eich, R. H.: Varied manifestations of left atrial myxoma and the relationship of echocardiographic patterns to tumor size. *Chest,* **68:**781, 1975.

Pridie, R. B.: Left atrial myxomas in childhood: Presentation with emboli—diagnosis by ultrasonics. *Thora* **27:**759, 1972.

Rahilly, G. T., and Nanda, N. C.: Two-dimensional echographic identification of tumor hemorrhages in atrial myxomas. *Am. Heart J.,* **101:**237, 1981.

Rajpal, R. S.; Leibsohn, J. A.; Liekweg, W. G.; *et al.:* Infected left atrial myxoma with bacteremia simulating infective endocarditis. *Arch. Intern. Med.,* **139:**1176, 1979.

Sandok, B. A.; von Estorff, I.; and Giuliani, E. F.: CNS embolism due to atrial myxoma: Clinical features and diagnosis. *Arch. Neurol.,* **37:**485, 1980.

Schattenberg, T. T.: Echocardiographic diagnosis of left atrial myxoma. *Mayo Clin. Proc.,* **43:**620, 1968.

Sharratt, G. P.; Grover, M. L.; and Monro, J. L.: Calcified left atrial myxoma with floppy mitral valve. *Br. Heart J.,* **42:**608, 1979.

Spencer, W. H.; Peter, R. H.; and Orgain, E. S.: Detection of a left atrial myxoma by echocardiography. *Arch. Intern. Med.,* **128:**787, 1971.

Stewart, J. A.; Warnica, M. D.; Kirk, M. E.; *et al.:* Left atrial myxoma: False negative echocardiographic findings in a tumor demonstrated by coronary arteriography. *Am. Heart J.,* **98:**228, 1979.

Tanabe, J.; Williams, R. C.; and Diethrich, E. G.: Left atrial myxoma: Association with acute coronary embolization in an 11-year-old boy. *Pediatrics,* **63:**778, 1979.

Wolfe, S. B.; Popp, R. L.; and Feigenbaum, H.: Diagnosis of atrial tumors by ultrasound. *Circulation,* **39:**615, 1969.

Yasher, J.; Witoszka, M.; Savage, D. D.; *et al.:* Primary osteogenic sarcoma of the heart. *Ann. Thorac. Surg.,* **28:**594, 1979.

Yoshikawa, J.; Sabah, I.; Yanagibara, K.; *et al.:* Cross-sectional echocardiographic diagnosis of large left atrial tumor and extracardiac tumor compressing the left atrium. *Am. J. Cardiol.,* **42:**853, 1978.

LEFT ATRIAL LINEAR OR BAND ECHOES

Jacobstein, M. D., and Hirschfeld, S. S.: Concealed left atrial membrane: Pitfalls in the diagnosis of cor triatriatum and supravalve mitral ring. *Am. J. Cardiol.,* **49:**780, 1982.

Lewis, B. S.; Colsen, P. R.; Rosenfeld, T.; *et al.:* An unusual case of mitral valve aneurysm. *Am. J. Cardiol.,* **49:**1293, 1982.

LEFT ATRIAL THROMBI

Come, P. C.; Riley, M. F.; Markis, J. E.; *et al.:* Limitations of echocardiographic techniques in evaluation of left atrial masses. *Am. J. Cardiol.,* **48:**947, 1981.

D'Cruz, I. A.; Collison, H. K.; and Sreekanth, S.: Two-dimensional echocardiographic diagnosis of LA thrombus with hypertrophic cardiomyopathy. *Cardiovasc. Rev. and Rep.,* **3:**524, 1982.

De Pace, N. L.; Soulen, R. L.; Kotler, M. N.; *et al.:* Two-dimensional echocardiographic detection of intraatrial masses. *Am. J. Cardiol.,* **48:**954, 1981.

Graboys, T. B.; Sloss, L. J.; and Dokena, J. A.: Echocardiographic diagnosis of left atrial thrombus—a case report. *J. C. U.,* **5:**284, 1977.

Mikell, F. L.; Asinger, R. W.; Rourke, T.; *et al.:* Two-dimensional echocardiographic demonstration of left atrial thrombi in patients with prosthetic mitral valves. *Circulation,* **60:**1183, 1979.

Poehlmann, H. W.; Basta, L. L.; and Brown, R. E.: Left atrial thrombus detected by ultrasound—a case report. *J. C. U.,* **3:**65, 1975.

Spangler, R. D., and Okin, J. T.: Echocardiographic demonstration of a left atrial thrombus. *Chest,* **67:**716, 1975.

Yoshikawa, J.; Sabah, T.; Yanagihara, K.; *et al.:* Cross-sectional echocardiographic diagnosis of large left atrial tumor and extracardiac tumor compressing the left atrium. *Am. J. Cardiol.,* **42:**853, 1978.

I

The Left Ventricle

Various basic left ventricular (LV) M-mode patterns are depicted in Figure I-1. The manner of measuring LV dimensions and thicknesses of the LV wall and ventricular septum are shown in Figure A-5. Two-D echographic patterns of the LV are shown in Figure I-2.

LEFT VENTRICULAR WALL THICKNESS

Thickness of the left ventricular posterior wall is measured from the leading edge (anterior border) of its endocardial echo to the leading edge of its epicardial echo, at the level of the mitral chordae tendineae. In former years, this measurement was made by some at the peak of the R wave, by others just before the onset of atrial contraction. However, to standardize technique, the American Society of Echocardiography has required that all end-diastolic measurements, i.e., septal and left ventricular wall thickness as well as left ventricular internal diameter (LVID) and right ventricular internal diameter (RVID), be made at the onset of the QRS.

Pioneering measurements of LV wall thickness were made by Feigenbaum *et al.* (1968), Sjogren *et al.* (1970), Troy *et al.* (1972), and others. The importance of establishing the normal range of values gained emphasis when the diagnosis of LV hypertrophy by M-mode echocardiography was attempted (Abbasi *et al.,* 1973, Dunn *et al.,* 1977). The normal range of LV posterior wall thickness is 6 to 11 mm, according to Feigenbaum (1981). Other authors (Henry *et al.,* 1973; Browne *et al.,* 1977; Kleid and Arvan, 1978) agree on 11 mm as the upper normal limit, whereas some put the upper limit at 12 mm (Haft and Horowitz, 1978). The sex

and build of the subject should be taken into consideration; 12 mm may be normal for a hefty 6-ft, 200-lb man but is definitely abnormal for a slender 5-ft, 100-lb woman.

ABNORMALLY INCREASED LV POSTERIOR WALL THICKNESS

Under certain circumstances, the LV posterior wall can be thought erroneously to be abnormally thick:

1. *At papillary muscle* level, the thickness of the posterior papillary muscle is added to that of the LV posterior wall, so that the latter appears twice as thick as it really is. Scanning toward the basal LV, bringing into view the chordae tendineae and then the mitral cusps, reveals the true thickness of the LV posterior wall.

2. *Chordae tendineae* of the mitral valve, especially if thickened by old rheumatic inflammation, can be mistaken for LV posterior wall endocardium, so that the LV posterior wall appears twice as thick as it really is. Proper attention to gain and reject settings could identify the chordae and demonstrate a narrow space between them and the ventricular wall. A useful rule to follow is that, if several crowded linear echoes are to be identified, the fastest moving one is the LV posterior endocardium.

3. *Mitral annulus calcification* manifests as a dense, bandlike echo between the mitral valve and LV posterior wall. In some cases, a narrow space is seen between such calcification and the LV posterior wall. In others, the two are contiguous and the echo of mitral annulus calcification may be included mistakenly in the LV wall thickness. Close scrutiny of the fine echo pattern (D'Cruz *et al.,* 1976) reveals that the very dense, homogenous echo of a calcific deposit

M-MODE ECHOGRAPHY: VENTRICULAR PATTERNS

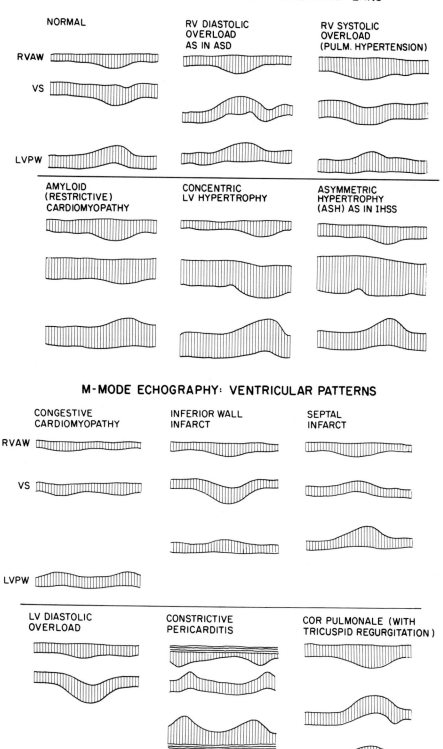

Fig. I-1. M-mode echographic patterns in a variety of conditions that affect LV or RV wall thickness and/or chamber size. Normal and abnormal systolic motion of the ventricular septum and/or LV posterior wall are also shown. The echocardiographer must become familiar with each of these patterns.

LEFT VENTRICULAR CONTOURS IN APICAL 4 CHAMBER VIEW

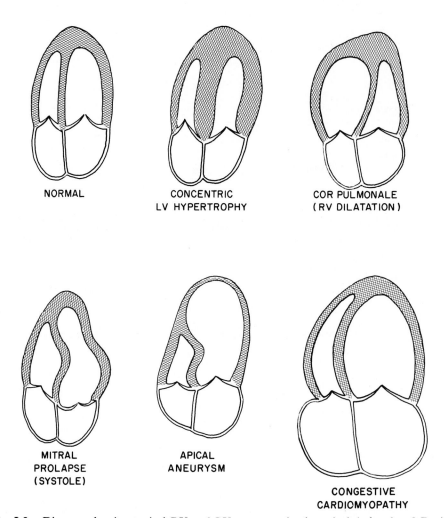

Fig. I-2. Diagram showing typical RV and LV contours, in the apical 4-chamber 2-D view, in various common cardiac conditions.

is distinguishable from the texture of the ventricular wall myocardium (Fig. I-3).

4. *Pericardium, thickened and sclerotic* by an old or chronic inflammatory process, is often adherent to the LV posterior wall epicardium; either the visceral pericardium or both visceral and parietal pericardial layers are fused together. As the LV posterior wall and pericardial echoes are fully contiguous and move together, their combined thickness easily may be mistaken echocardiographically for that of the ventricular wall alone (Fig. I-3). Again, identification of the thick pericardium and its visual separation from the LV posterior wall myocar-

dium is not difficult if the recording equipment has good resolution capability and aids such as gray-scale and switched-gain compensation are built into it.

Assuming that the fallacies mentioned above have been avoided, an abnormally thick LV posterior wall is usually caused by myocardial hypertrophy. Either an obvious cause for hypertrophy such as *aortic stenosis* or systemic *hypertension* is evident, in which case the hypertrophy is secondary to the enhanced afterload, or:

1. The individual has *hypertrophic cardiomyopathy* (obstructive or nonobstructive).

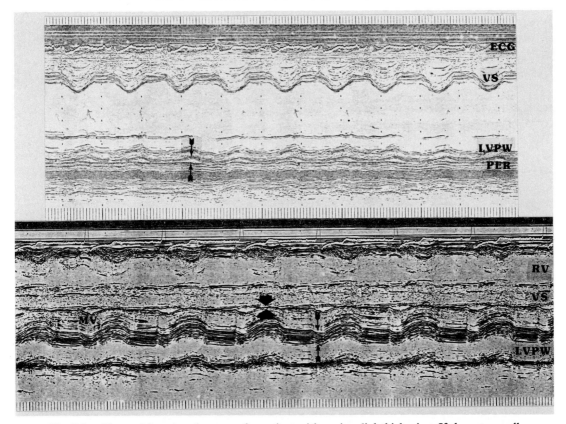

Fig. I-3. *Upper.* M-mode echogram of a patient with pericardial thickening. If the very small pericardial space (*arrows*) that appears between the LV posterior wall and thick pericardium in systole were overlooked, the combined LV wall and pericardial echoes could have been mistaken for a rather hypertrophied LV posterior wall.

Lower. M-mode echogram in a patient with concentric LV hypertrophy. The small LV chamber is further narrowed by posterior submitral annulus calcification (*thin arrows*). The mitral apparatus is thereby displaced anteriorly, attenuating the LV outflow tract to a slit (*broad arrows*). The submitral calcification can be easily distinguished from the subjacent LV posterior wall by the high density of its echo.

2. The individual is an *athlete*, especially a weight-lifter or wrestler, who has had prolonged training in heavy isometric exercise; the LV hypertrophy is a physiologic response to the increased stress.

3. Rarely, but importantly, abnormally thick ventricular walls may consist not entirely of myocardium but also of additional abnormal interstitial material such as amyloid, neoplastic or granulation, fibrous tissue (Borer *et al.*, 1977; Bass *et al.*, 1980). In such instances of *infiltrative* or *restrictive cardiomyopathy*, the echocardiographic triad of thick LV walls, normal-size LV cavity, and impaired LV contractility suggests the diagnosis in normotensive elderly patients presenting with congestive heart failure.

4. Very rarely, a *myocardial neoplasm*—rhabdomyoma (Farooki *et al.*, 1977), rhabdomyosarcoma (Orsmond *et al.*, 1976), fibroma (Etches *et al.*, 1980), or lymphomatous infiltration (Cabin *et al.*, 1981)—can simulate LV hypertrophy by producing gross thickening of the ventricular septum or LV wall. Farooki also described huge distention of the septum by a hydatid cyst within it, but the clear echo-free space representing the cystic fluid was morphologically different from the fine linear or stippled pattern associated with true hypertrophied myocardium.

5. A transient but striking increase in LV wall thickness has been reported in myocarditis (Hauser *et al.*, 1983).

The presence of abnormal systolic mitral anterior motion (SAM) and an excessive septal-

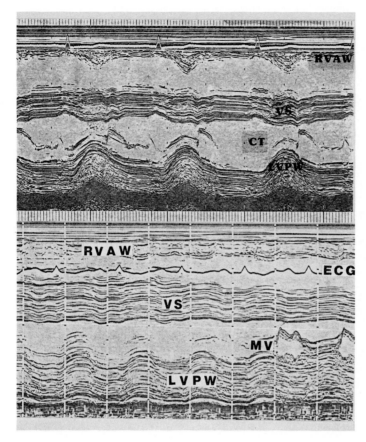

Fig. I-4. *Upper.* M-mode echogram showing concentric LV hypertrophy of mild to moderate degree. The LV chamber is of low normal size, and LV function appears normal.

Lower. M-mode echogram showing severe concentric LV hypertrophy. The ventricular septum and LV posterior wall are both over 2 cm thick. The LV end-diastolic interval dimension is unduly small (about 3 cm). The ventricular septum appears akinetic.

ventricular wall thickness ratio serves to identify IHSS, i.e., obstructive hypertrophic cardiomyopathy.

On the other hand, nonobstructive hypertrophic cardiomyopathy, especially the variety in which a transformation is occurring from a small-chambered hyperdynamic LV to the stage wherein chamber size increases and LV contractility decreases, may be difficult or even impossible to distinguish from infiltrative or "restrictive" cardiomyopathy. The latter includes amyloidosis, hypereosinophilia, sarcoidosis, and hemochromatosis. In both infiltrative and nonobstructive hypertrophic cardiomyopathy, (1) the LV wall is abnormally thick; (2) the LV chamber size is normal or mildly increased; and (3) LV function as measured by systolic fractional shortening of the LV internal dimension, or LV ejection fraction calculated from estimated end-diastolic and end-systolic volumes, may be normal.

Gross disparity between the thicknesses of the ventricular septum and LV posterior wall

favors hypertrophic cardiomyopathy, but its absence does not rule out this diagnosis.

Some examples of LV hypertrophy, as visualized by M-mode and 2-D echography, are shown in Figures I-4 to I-10.

LEFT VENTRICULAR HYPERTROPHY (Figs. I-3 to I-11)

The diagnosis of LV hypertrophy is an important part of the assessment of patients with hypertension, aortic valve disease, and other left heart conditions. Until recently, the electrocardiogram, sometimes supported by the vectorcardiogram, was the cardiologist's mainstay in determining the presence or absence of LV hypertrophy. During the 1970s, echocardiography has been shown to be as reliable or even more so than the ECG in this regard.

1. The M-mode echographic diagnosis of LV hypertrophy is based on increased thickness of the LV posterior wall and ventricular septum

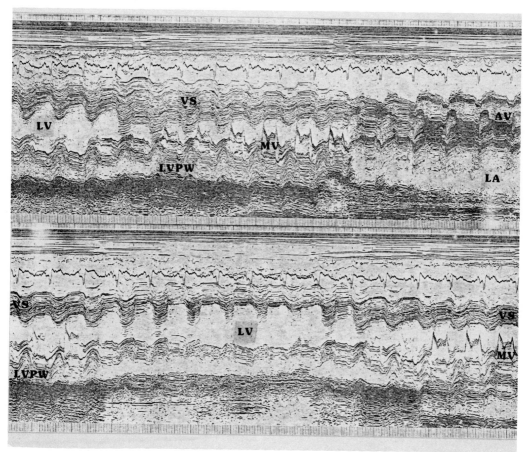

Fig. I-5. *Upper.* M-mode echocardiogram showing a scan from mid-LV to aortic root. There appears to be considerable concentric LV hypertrophy and diminution of LV internal dimension at mitral valve level, but these changes are less marked at mid-LV level.

Lower: A scan of the LV in the same patient, from mid-LV toward the apex and then back to mitral valve level, shows hypokinesis of the septum as well as of the LV posterior wall. The 2-D echogram revealed that the LV was narrow at its base but expanded into a huge apical aneurysm.

(12 mm or more). LV posterior wall thickness of 12 to 14 mm may be considered mild hypertrophy; 15 to 19 mm, moderate hypertrophy; and 20 mm or more, severe hypertrophy. Concentric LV hypertrophy, with equally thick LV posterior wall and septum, is the rule, so that the septal/LV wall ratio is close to 1 and does not exceed 1.3. However, 5 to 10 per cent of patients with LV hypertrophy secondary to hypertension, chronic renal failure, aortic stenosis, and so forth, have septal LV wall thickness ratios of the order of 1.3 or 1.4 (disproportionate septal hypertrophy). Massive hypertrophy of the ventricular septum, with normal or mildly increased LV posterior wall thickness and septal LV wall thickness ratios of 1.5 or more, is of course typical of hypertrophic cardiomyopathy

(including IHSS). The term "asymmetric septal hypertrophy" (ASH), if it is used at all, perhaps should be reserved for such cases. Bahler *et al.* (1977) correlated the electrocardiograms and vectorcardiograms with the echocardiograms of 30 normal volunteers. There was significant correlation between electrical potentials reflecting LV activation on ECG and VCG and thickness of the ventricular septum but not with thickness of the LV posterior wall. The authors favored the explanation that the LV posterior wall thickness did not accurately represent the thickness of the rest of the LV wall. Whether or not that is the reason for the discrepancy, it can be argued that data from this study of normal individuals do not negate the value of LV posterior wall thickness as a measure of

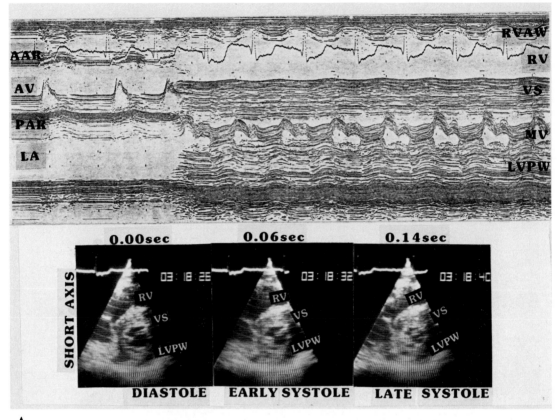

A.

Fig. I-6.   Concentric LV hypertrophy.

  A. Upper. M-mode echographic scan from aortic root to LV. The ventricular septum and LV posterior wall are equally hypertrophied, and the LV chamber is abnormally small. At first glance the aorta appears to override the hypertrophied septum. However, the continuity between the septum and anterior aortic root can be faintly discerned.

  Lower. 2-D echogram, in the short-axis view, showing serial frames from the same cardiac cycle. The LV is concentrically hypertrophied, with thick walls and a small cavity (about 3 cm in diameter), which narrows down to 2 cm in systole.

LV hypertrophy in abnormal hearts subject to LV pressure or volume overload.

  2. Gaasch (1979) called attention to his finding that the ratio of end-diastolic LV radius to LV wall thickness (R/Th ratio) has a constant relationship to LV systolic pressure in normal children and adults, as well as in the "physiologic hypertrophy" of athletes and patients with compensated chronic aortic regurgitation. He found the normal R/Th ratio to be 3.0 ± 0.7. Abnormally increased values of this ratio, signifying "inadequate hypertrophy," indicate a poor prognosis in patients with chronic aortic regurgitation or dilated cardiomyopathy. On the other hand, decreased R/Th ratios are the rule in patients with moderate to severe but compensated aortic stenosis, implying "appropriate hypertrophy," but also in patients with hypertrophic cardiomyopathy (including IHSS) in whom the hypertrophy may be considered inappropriate or inordinate.

  While the R/Th ratio has not yet found a place in the routine echocardiographic report, it is a useful concept in the sense that it suggests to the cardiologist that increased LV wall thickness is not synonymous with LV hypertrophy; it should be evaluated in the context of the LV internal dimension and volume.

LEFT VENTRICULAR MASS

The left ventricles of normal adult males weigh about 200 gm or less, and of normal adult females 140 gm or less (Reiner *et al.*, 1959). Theo-

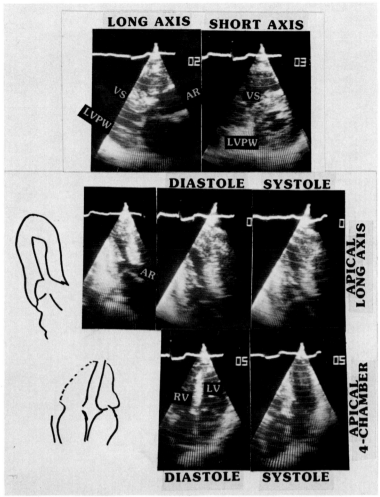

Fig. I-6. *B. Upper.* 2-D echogram in the long-axis (*left*) and short-axis (*right*) views, in the same patient with concentric LV hypertrophy. The septum is normally in about the same plane as the anterior aortic root. In this case, however, the hypertrophied septum seems to lie in a somewhat more posterior plane than the anterior aortic root (*left frame*) which explains why the M-mode echographic scan shows apparent overriding of the septum by the aortic root (*below*).

Center and Lower. 2-D echogram of the same patient in the apical long-axis view (*center*) and apical 4-chamber view (*lower*). In the center row, the LV image in the first frame has been expanded in the second and third frames. Concentric LV hypertrophy and the narrow LV chamber are well visualized.

retically, LV mass may be expected to represent a better measure of LV hypertrophy than LV wall thickness. Thus, patients with increased LV mass would include not only those with enhanced thickness of the LV wall and/or septum, but also those with dilated LV chambers with normal or only marginally thickened LV walls.

The LV posterior wall and septum are not necessarily of uniform thickness at all levels. The LV is sometimes much thicker toward the apex than at the base (Figs. I-10 and I-11).

Technical artefacts can cause fallacies in septal or LV wall thickness measurements (Fig. I-12).

Although LV mass estimations may not be made routinely in clinical echocardiographic practice, it well may be worth calculating the LV mass in patients for whom the presence or degree of LV hypertrophy has important clinical significance; systemic hypertension and aortic stenosis are common examples.

In a study correlating echocardiograms and electrocardiograms in 27 patients with LV hypertrophy by ECG criteria, increase in esti-

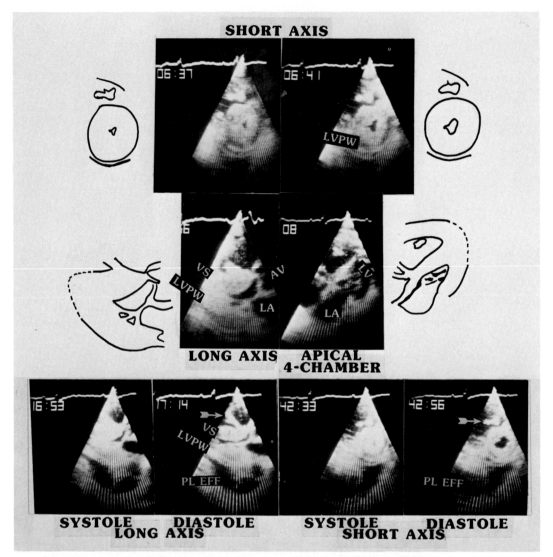

Fig. I-7. 2-D echogram of a patient with severe concentric LV hypertrophy.

Upper. In the short-axis view, the left at end-systole, the right in early diastole, systolic obliteration of the LV cavity is evident.

Center. In the long-axis view (*left*), and apical 4-chamber view (*right*) the narrow slitlike LV cavity is clearly depicted.

Lower. The 2 left frames are in the long-axis view, in systole and diastole; the 2 right frames are in the short-axis view, in systole and diastole. An unusual muscular band in the RV (*arrows*) is inserted on the thick ventricular septum. In the frame at extreme left, this band seems to merge with the septum, thus increasing its apparent thickness. A pleural effusion is present.

mated LV mass (more than 200 gm) was noted in 21, but increased thickness of the LV wall and septum in only 13 (McFarland *et al.*, 1978). Nine patients had normal thickness of the LV wall but dilated LV chambers and abnormally high LV mass.

LV mass can be calculated by the formula:

$$[(LVIDd + 2LVWT)^3 - LVIDd^3] \times 1.05$$

where LVIDd is the end-diastolic internal dimension of the left ventricle, LVWT is the end-diastolic LV wall thickness, and 1.05 is the specific gravity of myocardium (Feigenbaum, 1976; Bennett and Evans, 1974; Horton *et al.*, 1977). The formula is based on the assumption that the LV shape is perfectly ellipsoidal, that the LV wall thickness is uniform throughout the ventricle, and that the LV internal dimension

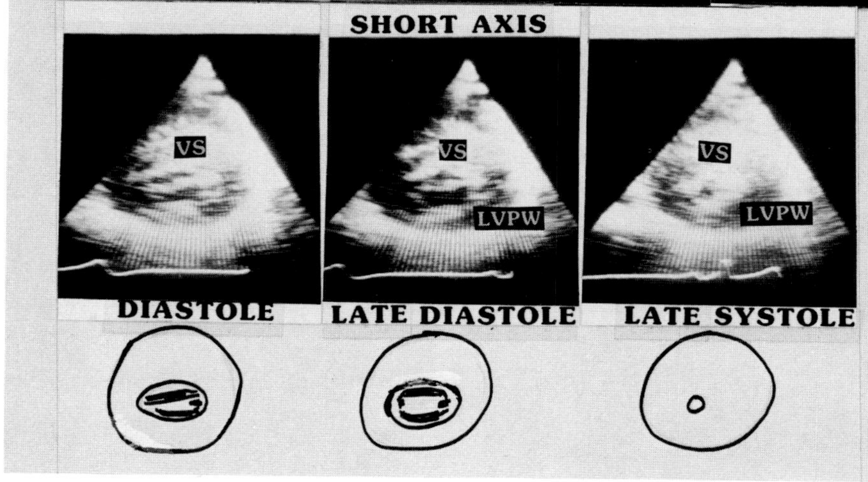

Fig. I-8. 2-D echogram of a patient with nonobstructive hypertrophic cardiomyopathy.

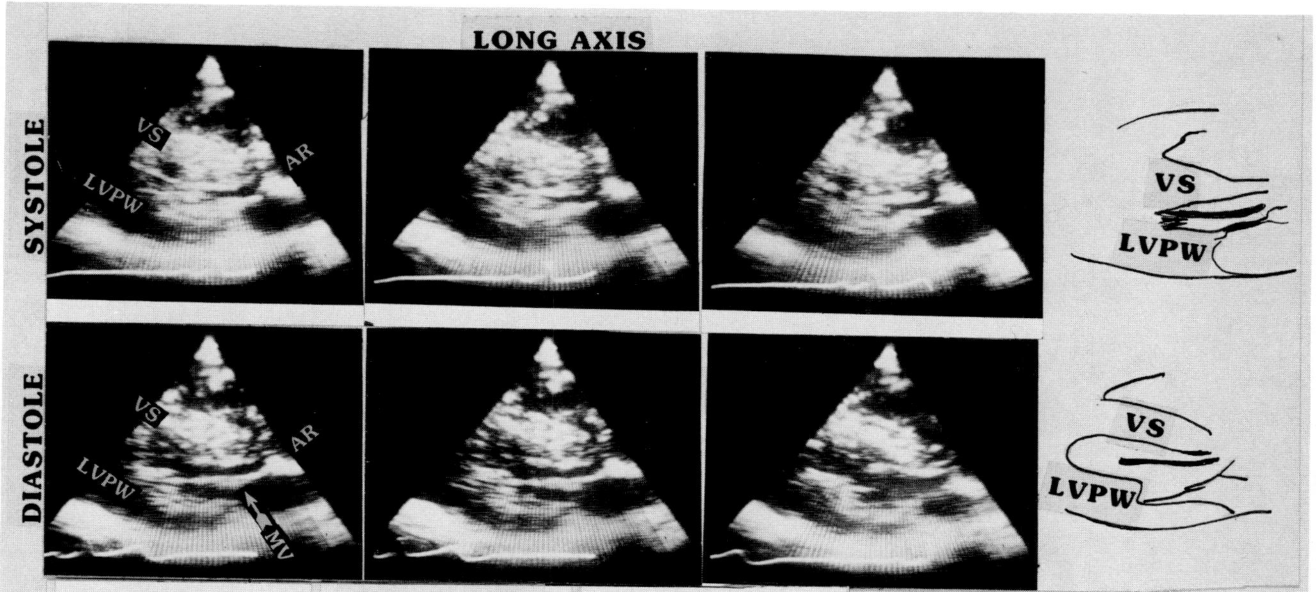

Fig. 1-8. *A.* Six serial frames, in the long-axis view, from the same cardiac cycle. The top 3 frames are systolic, the next 3 diastolic. The diastolic thickness of the ventricular septum is about twice that of the LV posterior wall. The LV cavity is narrowed to a slit, which almost obliterates during systole. It is traversed by a linear echo representing the anterior mitral leaflet and chordae tendineae.

Fig. I-8. *B.* Short-axis view, showing 3 successive frames from the same cardiac cycle. The second frame, in late diastole just after LA contraction, shows that the LV cavity is appreciably larger than in the first frame, reflecting the significant atrial contribution to LV filling. As in the long-axis view, conspicuous septal hypertrophy, small LV chamber size, and systolic LV cavity obliteration (third frame) are evident.

LONG AXIS

SHORT AXIS

SYSTOLE

DIASTOLE

DIASTOLE   LATE DIASTOLE   LATE SYSTOLE

A.

B.

259

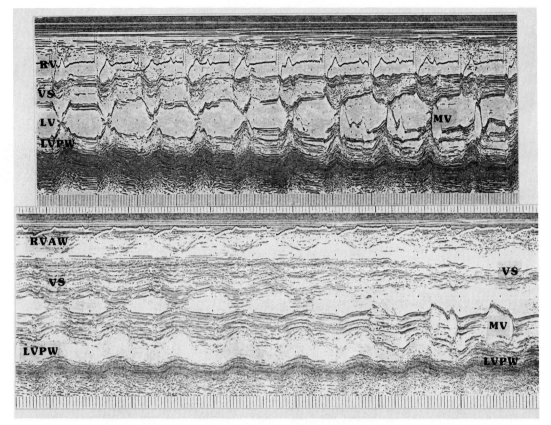

Fig. I-9. *Upper.* M-mode scan of the LV from apex to base, showing that the ventricular septum is much thicker toward the apex (*left*) than it is at mitral valve level (*right*). The varying pattern of mitral motion in diastole is attributable to A-V dissociation.

   Lower. M-mode echographic scan of the LV from its apex to its base (mitral valve level). There is concentric LV hypertrophy of considerable degree at papillary muscle level (*left*) but none at mitral valve level (*right*). Note also that the papillary muscle echo, in the left half of the figure, could simulate the LV posterior wall, in which case the actual LV posterior wall could be mistaken for a posterior pericardial effusion.

measured is the true minor LV axis; these assumptions are not entirely or invariably valid. The formula is based on the principle that the volume of LV myocardium can be obtained by subtracting the volume of the LV cavity from the external volume of the left ventricle, including its walls and the ventricular septum.

   Devereux *et al.* (1977) pointed out certain theoretical flaws in the formula for LV mass previously used by Troy *et al.* (1972), Bennett and Evans (1974), and others. In their version,

$$\text{LV mass} = 1.04\,[(\text{LVIDd} + \text{PWTd} + \text{IVSTd})^3 - (\text{LVID})^3] - 14\ \text{gm}$$

where LVIDd is the left ventricular internal diameter at end-diastole; PWTd is the LV posterior wall thickness at end-diastole; IVSTd is the interventricular septal thickness at end-dias-

tole. In making their measurements, these authors excluded the thickness of endocardial echo from the wall thickness measurements and included the thickness of the left septal and LV wall echo lines in the LV internal dimension measurement. The estimated LV mass by this method correlated well (r = 0.96) with actual anatomic LV mass measured at autopsy.

   Reichek and Devereux (1981) have recently compared the echocardiographic LV mass, ECG findings of LV hypertrophy (by the Romhilt-Estes score as well as the Sokolow-Lyon criteria), and the actual autopsy weight of the LV. They found that calculation of LV mass from the M-mode echogram was far superior to the ECG in sensitivity (93 per cent versus 50 and 21 per cent for the two ECG sets of criteria). The specificity of ECG and echo-

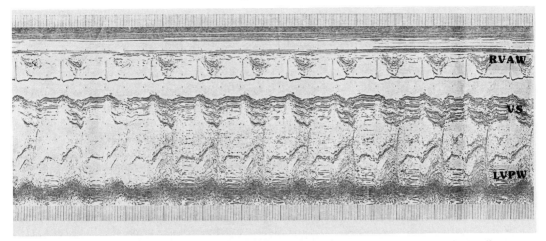

Fig. I-10. M-mode echogram of the LV. The ventricular septum and LV posterior wall are clearly depicted at the right of the figure, so that their thicknesses can be reliably measured. On the left side of the figure, the right (anterior) border of the septum is well defined, but its left (posterior) border has dropped out because the gain was set too low; the septum therefore appears thinner than it is.

graphic criteria was comparable (95 per cent). Helak and Reichek (1981) also tested the reliability of 2-D echographic quantification of LV mass in 13 patients with the LV weight as measured at autopsy. The formulae they used were the short-axis Simpson's rule and area-length ones; by both methods, a very good correlation was obtained between 2-D echographic and anatomic values (r = 0.93 and 0.92). Reichek *et al.* (1983) found that LV mass by 2-D echo during life correlated extremely well (r = 0.93) with actual LV weight in 21 autopsied subjects.

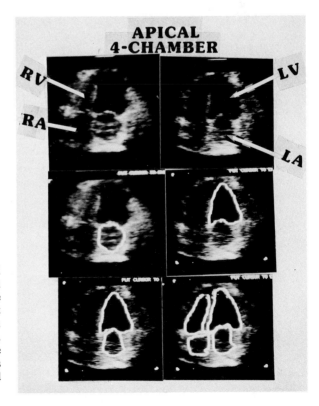

Fig. I-11. 2-D echogram in the apical 4-chamber view. In the center and bottom frames, a light-pen has been used to demarcate the individual cardiac chambers: the left atrium (*center, left*), the left ventricle (*center, right*), the left atrium and ventricle (*bottom, left*), all four chambers (*bottom, right*). The system was previously calibrated. The areas of the respective chambers can be measured electronically at the press of a button.

HYPERTENSIVE HEART DISEASE

Echocardiography has been used increasingly in the cardiac assessment of hypertensive patients (Dunn *et al.,* 1977; Browne *et al.,* 1977; Karliner *et al.,* 1977; Schlant *et al.,* 1977). Its diagnostic use in this setting falls into two categories:

1. To detect cardiovascular complications that hypertensive patients are more susceptible to than the general population, such as dissecting aortic aneurysm, impairment of LV performance, wall motion abnormalities due to ischemic heart disease and its complications.

2. To detect left ventricular hypertrophy. In patients with asymptomatic, uncomplicated hypertension, evidence of definite LV hypertrophy may influence the clinician in deciding whether or not to institute hypotensive drug therapy.

LV hypertrophy in hypertensives is usually

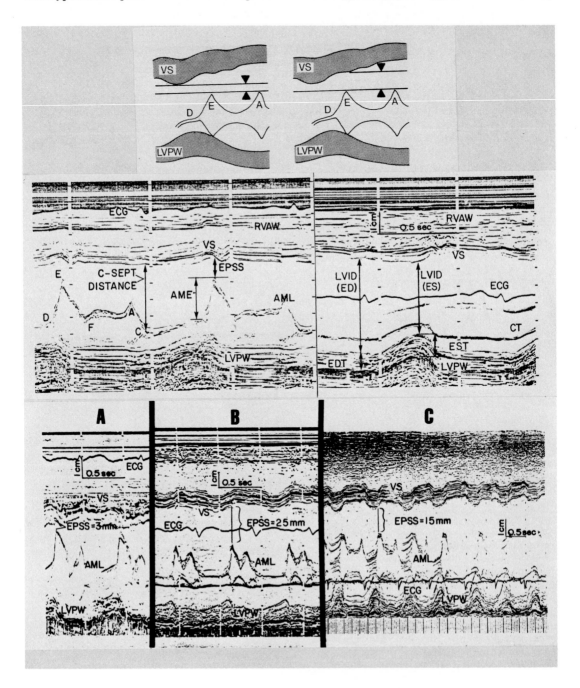

concentric, but occasionally the ventricular septum is hypertrophied to more than 1.3 times the thickness of the LV posterior wall. This was the case in 2 of 33 patients with chronic severe hypertension of Maron et al. (1978).

Safar et al. (1979) made the unexpected and intriguing observation that their patients with "borderline" hypertension tended to have abnormally thick septums but normal LV posterior wall thickness, but patients with "sustained" hypertension showed symmetric LV hypertrophy; the more severe the hypertension, the more likely the symmetry or equality of hypertrophy between septum and LV wall. These authors speculate that increased septal thickness represents the initial or earliest stage of LV hypertrophy. Of 79 hypertensives studied by Cohen et al. (1981), 29 had concentric LV hypertrophy; 8 had disproportionate septal thickening.

Estimation of LV mass (Dunn et al., 1977) is perhaps more sensitive and valuable for the purpose of detecting LV hypertrophy than measurement of LV wall thickness.

The importance of the echographic diagnosis of LV hypertrophy on the basis of increased LV wall thickness or LV mass lies in the accumulation of data suggesting that echocardiography is more sensitive in this respect than electrocardiography and chest x-ray (Dunn et al., 1977; Schlant et al., 1977; Savage et al., 1979). In other words, hypertensive heart disease probably can be identified at an earlier stage by ultrasound than by electrocardiography.

Several studies also suggest that serial echocardiography is useful in following patients with essential hypertension to detect regression or progression of hypertrophy or functional abnormalities (Schlant et al., 1982; Reichek et al., 1982; Fouad et al., 1982). These authors report improvement in LV function and regression of hypertrophy 12 to 24 months after successful control of hypertension by medical therapy.

Regarding LV function in uncomplicated asymptomatic cases of hypertension, it was found to be usually normal by Karliner et al. (1977) but often impaired by Dunn et al. (1977). Takahashi et al. (1980) found that LV contractile function was normal in hypertensive individuals with only mild increase in LV wall thickness, but subnormal in patients with more severe LV hypertrophy.

It is likely that large-scale, long-term studies will be done and their results published in the next few years to clarify the place of echocardiography in the *routine* assessment of hypertensive patients.

The echographic differentiation of hypertensive heart disease (concentric LV hypertrophy) from hypertrophic cardiomyopathy may not be easy. In both conditions, the septum and perhaps LV posterior wall are hypertrophied; the LV cavity, including its outflow tract, is abnor-

---

Fig. I-12. *Upper.* Diagram showing how mitral E point–septal separation (EPSS) is measured by the previous method (*left*) and our method (*right*). In the previous method, mitral-septal separation is the distance between the nadir of the left septal echo and the subsequent E peak. In our method, mitral-septal separation is measured at the instant of inscription of the E peak.

Center. Diagram showing how measurements are made: left ventricle at mitral valve level (*left*) and at chordae tendineae level (*right*) (ECG, electrocardiogram; RVAW, right ventricular anterior wall; VS, ventricular septum; LVPW, left ventricular posterior wall; AME, anterior mitral excursion; C-sept distance, mitral C point–septal separation; LVID, left ventricular internal diameter; ED, end-diastolic; ES, end-systolic; CT, chordae tendineae; EDT, end-diastolic thickness; EST, end-systolic thickness).

Lower. Echocardiograms showing mitral E point–septal separation in three individuals, each representing a different clinical situation: (a) a normal person (angio EF = 70%) showing normal EPSS (3 mm); (b) a patient with congestive cardiomyopathy (angio EF = 32%) showing considerably increased EPSS (25 mm); (c) a patient with coronary heart disease and aneurysm of the apical and anterior LV regions (angio EF = 40%). This patient had EPSS of 15 mm, suggesting impaired overall LV performance. Note that the LV internal diameter and systolic excursions of the LV posterior wall and septum appear normal at this LV level. Thus, EPSS proved a better indicator of LV performance than indices based on LV diameter or its systolic shortening fraction.

(Reproduced from D'Cruz, I. A., et al.: The superiority of mitral E point-ventricular septum separation to other echocardiographic indicators of left ventricular performance. *Clin. Cardiol.* **2:**140, 1979, with permission of the publishers.)

mally small. This topic was studied by Doi *et al.* (1980), who found that SAM and/or mid-systolic aortic valve closure was found in 82 per cent of patients with IHSS, 35 per cent of patients with nonobstructive hypertrophic cardiomyopathy, but not seen in patients with hypertension.

LEFT VENTRICULAR INTERNAL DIMENSION

Also known as the short or minor LV axis, the left ventricular internal dimension (LVID) is the distance between the left surface of the ventricular septum and the endocardial surface of the LV posterior wall. It is probably the most important measurement in echocardiographic practice and therefore worth considering in some detail.

Since the LV is of ellipsoidal and not cylindric shape, the width of the LV chamber varies depending on whether it is measured at the basal or mid- or near-apical level of the LV. Moreover, since the LV is contracting or filling during almost all of the cardiac cycle, its internal dimension is not a constant distance but is continually increasing or decreasing.

However, by convention and for standardization of procedure, the LVID refers to a specific dimension of the LV: the transverse or minor diameter or axis as visualized by ultrasound scanning from the left parasternal region, such that the ventricular septum and LV posterior wall are clearly defined at the level of the mitral chordae tendineae.

If it is not possible to visualize definite mitral chordae, bits and pieces ("remnants") of the tips of the mitral leaflets, or of the posterior leaflet alone, would probably be acceptable as indicating an LV level where the LVID could be measured. It must be emphasized that the LVID should be measured neither where the anterior and posterior mitral cusps or the anterior cusp alone is well seen, nor where the papillary muscles are in view.

As mentioned above, the LVID is constantly changing during each cardiac cycle, decreasing in systole and increasing in diastole. It thus could be represented by a continuum of cyclically variable values, but the only ones used for practical purposes are the end-diastolic (LVIDd) and end-systolic (LVIDs) dimensions.

The American Society of Echocardiography requires that the LVIDd be measured at the *onset* of the QRS complex and that the LVIDs is the smallest LV dimension, without reference to the ECG. The LVIDs is usually coincident, or almost so, with the most posterior systolic point of the left (posterior) septal contour and precedes the most anterior point of the LV posterior wall endocardial contour.

In practice, the measurement of the LVIDd and LVIDs is not always as simple and easy as would appear in diagrams or illustrations in textbooks or papers depicting how such dimensions are measured. Some of the difficulties encountered in everyday echocardiographic practice are as follows:

1. The LV posterior wall endocardium may be difficult to define in some cases. Other linear echoes that could possibly be mistaken for it include (a) the posterior mitral leaflet, (b) the posterior mitral chordae tendineae, (c) mitral annulus calcification (should the epicardial echo be weak or suppressed by inappropriate gain-setting, the following linear echoes could be mistaken for it), (d) intramyocardial linear echoes, (e) the LV posterior wall epicardium, (f) the inner layer of thickened stratified pericardium. A very helpful rule in differentiating LV posterior wall endocardium from other linear echoes in this region is that it is always the fastest moving (steepest) line in systole and early diastole.

2. The left border of the ventricular septum should be seen as a sharply defined, continuous linear echo, moving posteriorly in systole. It should be kept in mind that the septum is not necessarily of uniform thickness (Fig. I-9), also that it is not flat but curved along the minor as well as long axes of the LV. Moreover, it can happen that the ultrasound beam transects it obliquely rather than perpendicularly. It is not surprising, therefore, that the left septal border sometimes appears discontinuous, fuzzy, or even bizarre. The LVID should not be measured under such circumstances. The transducer or patient position should be altered until the ventricular septum is properly recorded.

Other linear echoes that could possibly be mistaken for the left septal border include (a) reverberations of the septum itself, of the right ventricular anterior wall of the chest wall, or of catheters or pacemaker wires in the right ventricle; (b) the right septal border; (c) right ventricular muscular bands; (d) portions of the tricuspid apparatus including the chordae; (e) artefacts caused by selective suppression of echoes near the septum, in which case the false "septal border" is a straight line perfectly parallel to the "main bang."

Painstaking attention to transducer position and direction, turning of the patient to the left lateral position, as well as adjustment of near-gain and damping controls, can overcome most technical problems relevant to proper septal visualization (Fig. I-10). As in other difficult applications of the echocardiographic art, there is no substitute for experience and patient endeavor.

EXTRACARDIAC FACTORS AFFECTING LVID MEASUREMENT

1. Large pericardial effusions cause excessive "swinging" motion of the ventricles. On the M-mode echogram, the anterior and posterior borders of the heart, particularly the former, are well defined in oscillatory motion, but individual cardiac structures such as the ventricular septum and valves may not be seen clearly because of the blurring caused by excessive rapid pendulous motion.

2. Normally, there are small cyclic respiratory variations in ventricular dimensions (Feigenbaum, 1976; Brenner *et al.,* 1978). During inspiration, the right ventricle enlarges while the left ventricle becomes slightly smaller. These changes are usually small, of the order of 1 to 3 mm at most, constituting 5 per cent or less of the LVID in adults.

In patients with tamponade caused by large pericardial effusions and certain other conditions associated with exaggerated respiratory effort such as pulmonary embolism and chronic obstructive lung disease (see Section N: Pericardial Disease, page 398), the inspiratory decrease and expiratory increase in LV dimension may be quite large.

THE UPPER LIMIT OF NORMAL RANGE FOR THE LVID

The normal upper limit of end-diastolic LV internal dimension is 56 mm, according to Feigenbaum (1981) and Nanda and Gramiak (1978). Haft and Horowitz (1978) and Kleid and Arvan

(1978) consider 53 mm as the maximum normal value. In my experience, normal persons, however large, very seldom if ever have LVID values over 56 mm.

On the other hand, the upper normal limit for LVID per square meter of both surface areas is quoted as 32 mm (Feigenbaum) or 31 mm (Kleid and Arvan). The upper normal limit would thus be 65 to 70 mm for very large individuals with body surface areas of 2.1 to 2.4 M^2. The upper limit of 31 or 32 mm per M^2 would yield false negatives in many cases in which the LV is actually dilated; it may be more applicable to persons of small to normal size.

Athletes trained in strenuous exertion of the "isotonic" type, such as long-distance running, basketball, boxing, and so forth, tend to have large left ventricles. Such dilatation is of course "physiologic," a response to the habitual large and prolonged increase in cardiac output they have to sustain (preload stress).

THE LV IN ATHLETES

Echocardiographic studies in numerous groups of athletes, including swimmers, runners, bicyclists, and Olympic competitors (Morganroth *et al.,* 1975; Roskoff *et al.,* 1976; Roeske *et al.,* 1976; Gilbert *et al.,* 1977; Allen *et al.,* 1977; Laurenceau *et al.,* 1977; DeMaria *et al.,* 1978; Ikäheimo *et al.,* 1979; Stein *et al.,* 1980; Nishimura *et al.,* 1980; Rost, 1982), have established that LV internal end-diastolic dimension and LV wall thickness show a statistically significant increase in comparison with control groups. It is of interest to note that Finnish long-distance runners tend to have thicker walls than sprinters (Ikäheimo *et al.,* 1979), or that middle-aged Japanese professional bicyclists tend to have more hypertrophy (but not more dilatation) than their younger counterparts (Nishimura *et al.,* 1980).

However, in all these instances, LV hypertrophy was of only mild degree. In most series, the majority of athletes did not have LV wall or septal thickness in excess of the upper limit of normal range (11 mm); in the remaining, it was at most 12 to 14 mm. It behooves the echocardiographer or cardiologist to inquire about athletic activities, especially when young individuals have LV wall thickness or LV dimensions slightly in excess of the normal range, to differentiate exercise-induced physiologic increases from abnormal pathologic ones.

LEFT VENTRICULAR DIASTOLIC OVERLOAD STATES

The echocardiographic assessment of LV function in patients with aortic or mitral valve regurgitation deserves special consideration for two main reasons: (1) the normal values for fractional shortening in systole of the LV internal dimension (FS) do not apply to these hemodynamic situations; when well compensated, patients with these valvular lesions have hyperdynamic left ventricles with increased stroke volumes; and (2) the preoperative LV internal dimension and FS have been shown to be valuable indicators of the prognosis after valve replacement surgery; these echocardiographic parameters have also proved useful in guiding the clinician assessing or following up asymptomatic patients with moderate to severe aortic regurgitation as to whether and when surgery is advisable.

The assessment of LV function in patients with chronic, severe aortic regurgitation has aroused the most interest (Danford et al., 1973; McDonald, 1976a; Johnson et al., 1976; Gaasch et al., 1978; Abdulla et al., 1980; McDonald and Jelinek, 1980). LV function in mitral regurgitation was studied by McDonald (1976b) and Saltissi et al. (1980). Some of the studies mentioned above were restricted to unoperated patients, whereas other investigators dealt with LV performance after aortic valve replacement (Venco et al., 1976; Gaasch et al., 1978; Schuler et al., 1979).

McDonald (1976a and b) found that compensated aortic regurgitation and mitral regurgitation were associated with increase in LV internal dimension (at end-diastole), LV stroke volume (LV end-diastolic volume minus LV end-systolic volume, both estimated echocardiographically), and increased thickness of the LV posterior wall. The increase in these parameters, in individual cases, was proportional to the severity of the regurgitation. McDonald observed that LV failure could coexist with an LV internal dimension FS that would be in the normal range for persons without diastolic overload.

Similar findings were reported by Rosenblatt

et al. (1976), who found that the commonly used indices of LV function (FS, echocardiographic ejection fraction, and V_{CF}) are increased in patients with compensated regurgitant lesions, normal in patients they categorized as "intermediately compensated," and decreased in those they designated "decompensated." In other words, the echocardiographer or clinician interpreting the echographic data of patients with significant aortic or mitral regurgitation must keep in mind that "normal" LV function in these situations will show values substantially higher than the usual normal range. Thus a patient with severe aortic or mitral regurgitation could be in obvious LV failure and yet have a FS of about 30 per cent.

Gaasch et al. (1978) showed that successful valve replacement surgery for aortic regurgitation results in the "normalization" of LV volume. In their series, the LV end-diastolic internal dimension fell from an average preoperative value of 69 mm to an average postoperative 55 mm within about a week. These authors found that a LV end-diastolic internal dimension to LV wall thickness ratio of more than 8 signified an unfavorable prognosis and persistence of LV dilatation after surgery.

Clark et al. (1980) demonstrated that serial M-mode echograms could provide valuable information in patients with valvular heart disease. They could divide their patients into three groups: (1) those with stable or improved LV size and function; (2) those who showed progressive LV dilatation but stable LV function (FS); and (3) those with obvious decompensation, with progressive decrease in FS and usually increase in LV size. They made the interesting observation that deterioration of LV function often occurred "silently" in patients who apparently did not experience a concomitant worsening of symptoms.

However, it must be mentioned that M-mode echographic estimations of LV volume and LV function are not always reliable and may not correlate well with the angiocardiographic estimations of LV size and function (Abdulla et al., 1980; Johnson et al., 1976) in patients with severe aortic regurgitation. The fallacies in LV internal dimension measurements are attributable to alterations in LV geometry in such patients and also perhaps to the possibility in very large hearts that the LV dimension measured may not correspond to the true minor LV axis.

Recent work by Henry *et al.* (1980) based on serial M-mode echocardiography in patients with moderate to severe aortic regurgitation, some of whom were subjected to surgery, has deservedly attracted wide attention. These authors showed that patients with preoperative LV end-systolic dimension exceeding 55 mm, or with FS less than 25 per cent, were at high risk of experiencing LV failure and dying after an otherwise successful operation, especially if they were positive for both of these adverse factors. Conversely, the outcome after surgery was excellent if the LV end-systolic dimension was less than 55 mm and FS more than 25 per cent, even if the regurgitation was severe.

Henry *et al.* followed up 37 patients with moderate to severe aortic regurgitation, 14 of whom developed symptoms while under observation and had valve replacement; 23 remained asymptomatic and continued under medical management and observation. They proposed the following guidelines on the basis of whether or not symptomatic or echocardiographic deterioration developed under observation:

1. An asymptomatic patient with aortic regurgitation whose LV end-systolic dimension is less than 50 mm is at low risk and can be followed safely by M-mode echocardiography at yearly intervals. Incidentally, the annual increments in LV end-systolic dimensions were nearly always less than 7 mm.

2. Asymptomatic patients with LV end-systolic dimensions of 50 to 54 mm may be followed by serial echocardiograms at four- to six-month intervals.

3. Patients with LV end-systolic dimensions of 55 mm or more are advised surgery, even if asymptomatic.

Other LV diastolic overload states include:
Anemia. M-mode echocardiographic studies have been done in patients with sickle cell anemia (Gerry *et al.*, 1976) and with β-thalassemia (Lewis *et al.*, 1978). The LV end-diastolic dimension is often increased in such chronic anemic states, but the indices of LV performance are usually normal, indicating the absence of a cardiomyopathic element.
Pregnancy. Stroke volume is increased in pregnancy, as are the V_{CF} and LV wall excursions. The LV size remains unchanged; a small increase in RV dimension may be noted (Rubler

et al., 1977). Laird-Meeter *et al.* (1979), who performed monthly echograms in 13 normal pregnant women as well as a postpartum echogram six weeks after delivery, concluded that the cardiac output in pregnancy increases at first by an increase in heart rate, but after the twentieth week by increase in stroke volume, accompanied by a mild increase in LV wall thickness.

LEFT VENTRICULAR FUNCTION

The noninvasive assessment of LV function has constituted one of the most important concerns of the modern clinical cardiologist. The measurement of the systolic time intervals from simultaneous recordings of the electrocardiogram, phonocardiogram, and external carotid pulse tracing introduced in the 1960s was a very useful achievement in this regard, but during the 1970s it has been increasingly overshadowed by echocardiographic and nuclear cardiology techniques.

Estimation of LV function by cardiac ultrasound has progressed through the following stages over the last decade:

1. Measuring the extent and velocity of the systolic excursion of the LV posterior wall.

2. Measuring the systolic thickening (increase in thickness during systole) of the LV posterior wall.

3. Measuring the fraction or percentage of systolic shortening of the LV internal dimension at end-diastole.

4. The LV end-diastolic volume and LV endosystolic volumes can be calculated from the corresponding LV internal dimensions by the application of a variety of formulae. The difference between the LV end-diastolic and end-systolic volumes thus estimated is the "M-mode echocardiographic stroke volume." The ratio of the stroke volume to LV end-diastolic volume is the "M-mode ejection fraction."

5. Measuring certain indirect indicators of overall LV function. Some of these, such as the ratio of the LV preejection to ejection period on the aortic valve echo or the mitral E point–septal separation, are fairly reliable, whereas other indices obtained from motion of the mitral valve, aortic valve, or aortic root are of equivocal or at least inadequately proven diagnostic value.

6. In addition to the preceding data taken from M-mode echocardiograms, 2-D echocardiograms in multiple views can display the entire length and breadth of the left ventricle. LV volumes and wall motion thus can be more completely visualized by this technique.

LV posterior wall motion can be taken as an indicator of LV function only if the entire left ventricle contracts uniformly. This is not the case in most patients with myocardial infarction as well as left bundle branch block, IHSS, and so forth. The normal systolic excursion of the LV posterior wall endocardial echo is 9 to 14 mm. Excursions less than 9 mm indicate hypokinesis; those over 14 mm indicate hyperdynamic LV contraction.

It is important to "normalize" systolic excursions of the LV wall by correcting for LV size in large ventricles, i.e., an excursion that would be normal for a normal or small ventricle would be subnormal for a dilated ventricle (Quinones et al., 1974). Thus, a systolic excursion of 9 or 10 mm would be normal for a LV internal dimension of 50 mm but not for one of 70 mm.

Although LV posterior wall systolic excursion and velocity are recorded routinely in many echocardiographic laboratories, few would use or quote these values as indicators of total LV function.

The percentage shortening of the LV internal dimension is

$$\frac{(LVIDd - LVIDs) \times 100}{LVIDd}$$

where LVIDd is the left ventricular internal diameter at end-diastole; LVIDs, the left ventricular internal diameter at end-systole. The normal range is 28 to 41 per cent. This index of LV function is commonly used and, together with the LVIDd itself, is the most important measurement in the echocardiographic report in most patients in adult cardiology practice.

The rate of LV circumferential fiber shortening (V_{CF}) is

$$\frac{LVIDd - LVIDs}{LVIDd \times LVET}$$

where LVET is the LV ejection time obtained by simultaneous external carotid pulse tracing. Normal values, expressed as circumferences per second, are in the range of 1.02 to 1.94 circumferences per sec (mean, 1.3). Values less than 1.0 are generally considered subnormal. Published reports indicate that the rate of LV circumferential shortening may be slightly better than the percentage of fractional shortening itself as a measure of LV contractility. However, neither of these indices would be valid for estimating *overall* LV function if:

1. The ventricular septum (or at least the part of it transected by the ultrasound beam) is hypokinetic or dyskinetic because of infarction, ischemia, or fibrosis;

2. The ventricular septum moves abnormally in systole, which can happen in a multitude of clinical situations—right ventricular overload as in atrial septal defect or tricuspid regurgitation, left bundle branch block, absent pericardium, constrictive pericarditis, previous open heart surgery, and so forth;

3. The LV posterior wall is hypokinetic, akinetic, or dyskinetic due to infarction or ischemia;

4. There are large areas of segmental hypokinesis, akinesis, or dyskinesis elsewhere in the left ventricle (commonly involving the LV apex and adjacent ventricular septum or anterolateral wall) so that there is compensatory hyperkinesis of the LV posterior wall and ventricular septum in the basal left ventricle, the part of the left ventricle scanned by the ultrasound beam in M-mode echocardiography. In such circumstances, the apparent LVID systolic shortening would be normal in spite of impaired overall LV performance.

All of these situations, affecting the validity of internal dimension shortening in systole, are frequently encountered in adult practice and, unfortunately, are particularly common in the type of patient who is sent to the echocardiographer for evaluation of LV function, i.e., middle-aged or elderly persons with symptoms suggestive of cardiac decompensation or ischemia.

LEFT VENTRICULAR VOLUME AND EJECTION FRACTION

During the early 1970s, echocardiography held out to clinicians the alluring prospect of being able to measure noninvasively the volume of the left ventricle; by estimating both end-diastolic and end-systolic volumes, it appeared that left ventricular ejection fraction would also be available (Popp and Harrison, 1969; Murray *et al.,* 1970; Pombo *et al.,* 1971; Gibson, 1972; Feigenbaum *et al.,* 1972; Betenkie *et al.,* 1973; Ludbrook *et al.,* 1973; Popp *et al.,* 1975).

Various formulae were devised, on the basis of certain geometric assumptions, which could be applied to the measured LVID so as to calculate the left ventricular volume. Some authors used the same formula for end-diastolic and end-systolic LV volumes, while others, assuming a systolic change in LV shape, used different formulae.

If Dd denotes the LV internal dimension at end-diastole, and Ds the LV internal dimension at end-systole, some formulae in common use are shown in the table below. The formula of Teichholz *et al.* (1976) is perhaps the most favored by echocardiographers at present. Yet other formulae have been proposed (Murray *et al.,* 1970; Gibson, 1972).

All the formulae mentioned above have been "validated" by their respective authors by comparing the LV volumes (calculated from the LVID values by the respective formulae) with the corresponding volumes obtained by angiocardiography; all reported a high degree of correlation between the two. However, a good correlation for a large group of patients as a whole should by no means be construed as proof that M-mode echocardiography is as accurate as angiocardiography or equivalent to it for the purpose of estimating LV volumes or LV ejection fractions in all patients.

Extrapolation of LVID on the M-mode tracing to LV volumes is dependent on several assumptions:

1. That the LV shape in all patients is a perfect prolate ellipse of revolution. This is true or almost so in normal hearts, but general LV dilatation is associated with a tendency to a more spherical shape. Ventricular aneurysms distort ventricular shape to a varying degree, depending on their size. In IHSS, the LV chamber may be attenuated to a narrow slit, encroached upon and distorted by a grossly hypertrophied and misshapen ventricular septum, not to mention hypertrophied papillary muscles.

2. That the minor (short) axis is exactly half the length of the long (major) axis. Very dilated left ventricles, which tend to a more spherical shape, have long-axis values of the order of 1.5 times the short-axis values.

3. That the LVID recorded on the M-mode tracing is the true geometric minor axis, passing through the true long axis and precisely perpendicular to it. In actual practice, it well can happen that the path of the ultrasound beam is somewhat eccentric rather than perfectly central (a chord rather than diameter of the LV circumference) and that it deviates by more than a few degrees from being exactly at right angles to the long axis.

4. That the above geometric assumptions prevail in systole as well as diastole. This postulate appears reasonable for normal hearts, and for those with generalized decrease (dilated cardiomyopathy) or increase (anemia, hyperthyroidism) in myocardial contractility. The presence of gross hypokinesis, akinesis, or dyskinesis (including aneurysm) in patients with ischemic heart disease, of course, will render the systolic LV shape very different from the diastolic LV shape.

5. That all segments of the LV chamber contract uniformly. Local akinesis of the ventricular septum or of the LV posterior wall transected by the ultrasound beam will give inappropriately high values for the LV internal systolic dimension, if the rest of the left ventricle is contracting well.

6. That the distance from the transducers to an object in the heart is precisely proportional to the time taken for the ultrasound beam to be reflected back from the object to the transducer. Because of the random error in trans-

AUTHOR	END-DIASTOLIC LV VOLUME	END-SYSTOLIC LV VOLUME
Pombo *et al.* (1971)	$0.962\ Dd^3 + 11.53$	$1.041\ Ds^3 + 6.25$
Feigenbaum (1971)	$0.922\ Dd^3 + 72.42$	$0.96\ Ds^3 + 42$
Fortuin (1971)	$59\ Dd - 153$	$47\ Ds - 120$
Teichholz *et al.* (1976)	$\left(\dfrac{7}{2.4 + Dd}\right) Dd^3$	$\left(\dfrac{7}{2.4 + Ds}\right) Ds^3$

mission velocity of ultrasound through non-homogeneous media, a small inaccuracy in measurement of intracardiac distances could creep in.

The following items are relevant to echocardiographic estimation of LV volume and ejection fraction:

1. It is worth emphasizing Feigenbaum's caveat (1976) that M-mode echocardiography does not *measure* the LV volume but only makes an *estimate* of it, a prediction that approximates the truth if the various geometric assumptions in a given patient are not far off the theoretical mark. This should be kept in mind by clinicians, who should not consider the calculated LV volumes in an echocardiographic report accurate to the last milliliter. In fact, some echocardiographic laboratories make no mention of LV volumes and base their statements of LV size only on the LVID values.

2. LV end-diastolic and end-systolic volumes, based on subcostal (subxiphoid) M-mode echographic measurements, correlated very well with the corresponding values on angiocardiography (Starlin *et al.,* 1980). The correlation of echographic and angiographic ejection fractions was not nearly as close; the echocardiographic estimation by both parasternal and subcostal approaches tended to give higher values than the angiocardiographic ejection fractions, the presumed "gold standard."

3. DeMaria *et al.* (1979) investigated the effect of heart rate (controlled by atrial pacing) on LV internal dimension and the indices of LV function calculated from echographic LV measurements in normal volunteers. They found that LV dimensions decreased considerably with increase in heart rate from 70 per min to 150 per min: the LV end-diastolic dimension decreased from a group mean of 48 to 30 mm, while the corresponding end-systolic dimension diminished from 30 to 23 mm; the velocity of circumferential fiber shortening (VCF) increased from a mean of 1.09 at 70 per min to 1.63 at 150 per min. However, the LV internal dimension systolic shortening fraction was *not* affected by heart rate.

4. In children, the LV internal dimension systolic shortening fraction (mean, 36 ± 4 per cent) and the ratio of LV preejection period to LV ejection time (mean, 0.31 ± 0.03) remain constant throughout childhood (Gutgesell *et*

al., 1977). On the other hand, mean VCF was higher and absolute values of LV preejection period and LV ejection time were shorter in younger children than in older children.

5. In children, Bhatt *et al.* (1978) found that LV volumes by M-mode echocardiography correlated well with cineangiography LV volumes if the LV was of normal size, but the correlation is much less satisfactory if the LV is dilated or the ventricular septal motion is abnormal.

6. In a study comparing the stroke volume calculated by eight different echocardiographic formulae with the stroke volume obtained by cineangiographic and thermodilution methods, the formulae based on characteristics of mitral and aortic valve motion emerged as failures. The formulae based on LV minor-axis measurements fared better, the one employing Teichholz's formula proving the best (Kronik *et al.,* 1979). Even these formulae were valid only if the LV contracted symmetrically or almost so; poor correlation between echographic and invasive methods was the rule in the presence of grossly asymmetric LV contraction patterns.

TWO-DIMENSIONAL ESTIMATION OF LV VOLUME (Fig. I-11)

Two-D echocardiography permits scanning of the whole LV chamber and therefore held out a promise of attaining a better picture of LV shape and quantification of LV volume than M-mode scan alone could provide. However, the 2-D views initially introduced (parasternal long-axis and short-axis views) could not image the LV apex very well, and the narrow (30°) sector angles then in use could not reveal more than a portion of the left ventricle at one time in the long-axis view. But the development of wide-angle sector scanners and the discovery that the entire left ventricle can be well visualized by placing the wide-angle probe at the apex and directing it toward the base of the left ventricle (i.e., aligning the probe along the LV long axis) made it possible to see clearly the entire LV chamber and to measure not only its long axis from base to apex but also its minor axis at various levels (Heng *et al.,* 1978; Chaudry *et al.,* 1978; Schiller *et al.,* 1979; Carr *et al.,* 1979; Folland *et al.,* 1979; Henry 1982).

Carr *et al.* (1979) demonstrated that the LV volume by the 2-D echo method consistently underestimated the LV volume when compared to the angiocardiographic LV volume estimation for reasons that are not entirely clear. However, the 2-D echo ejection fraction of the left ventricle correlated well with the angiocardiographic ejection fraction. Interobserver variability and variation between two studies performed within 24 hours and analyzed by the same observer were very small, not more than 1 to 3 per cent. Schiller et al. (1979) also found some discrepancy between angiographic and 2-D echocardiographic LV diastolic volumes ($r = 0.80$). However, the angioecho correlation in their patients was better for ejection fractions ($r = 0.87$) and systolic LV volumes ($r = 0.90$), which is noteworthy because 65 per cent of the patients had significant regional wall motion abnormalities. It is in such patients that M-mode echocardiography is notoriously inaccurate in assessing overall LV function.

Folland et al. (1979) in adults and Silverman et al. (1980) in a study of pediatric patients also reported that 2-D echocardiography was definitely superior to the M-mode technique in estimating LV volumes, and that the angioecho correlation was better for the ejection fraction than for actual LV volumes.

No standard method yet has been agreed upon for making 2-D measurements and calculations for LV volumes. The problem is which geometric model to choose that best represents LV shape (not only in normals but also in patients with abnormally small and abnormally dilated LV chambers). This in turn determines which 2-D views of the LV should be employed and which dimensions or measurements utilized for this purpose in each view.

Carr et al. (1979) recorded long-axis, short-axis, apical four-chamber (hemiaxial), and apical two-chamber (axial) views. They used varying combinations of pairs of orthogonal (perpendicular) views in different patients, depending upon which views provided the greatest clarity of endocardial definition in a given patient.

Schiller et al. (1979) used the parasternal short-axis view (an equivalent of the left anterior oblique angiocardiographic projection) and the apical long-axis two-chamber view (an equivalent of the right anterior oblique angiocardiographic projection). They used a modified Simpson's rule formula to calculate LV volume from measurements made in these two views.

Silverman et al. (1980) in their pediatric study used only apical views: the apical long-axis and apical four-chamber. Their calculations were made by the single-plane area-length method for each view, also by biplane area-length and Simpson's rule methods from the combined recorded outlines of two LV views.

Folland et al. (1979) compared five different algorithms for determining LV ejection fraction and volume and compared them with standard angiocardiographic and radionuclide methods. The five different geometric approaches (and respective formulae) were based on five correspondingly different assumptions as to the geometric shape of the LV. They found that the method based on modified Simpson's rule correlated best with the angiographic and radionuclide gold standard for ejection fraction estimation, with r values in the 0.75 to 0.80 range.

Recently, Quinones and associates (Quinones et al., 1981; Torteledo et al., 1983) devised a new 2-D echographic method for estimation of LV volumes and ejection fractions that involves measurements of the LV long axis and short axis at various levels in three views: the parasternal long-axis, apical long-axis, and apical four-chamber. This method has the advantage that area measurements are avoided, thus reducing the time expended and eliminating the difficult delineation of the entire LV endocardial contour (difficult because of dropout) on a single stop-frame. Quinones found a high correlation ($r > 0.90$) with the LV end-diastolic volumes, end-systolic volumes, and ejection fractions obtained by gated blood-pool imaging and by cineangiocardiography, even though the majority of his patients had coronary disease with LV dyssynergy.

It is hoped that a uniform 2-D echographic method for measuring and calculating LV volumes be agreed upon, combining practicality and convenience with reasonable accuracy and applicability to LV chambers of various sizes and shapes. Meanwhile, potential sources of error in recording technique, or limitations in scanning equipment, continue to be emphasized (Geiser et al., 1982; Stamm et al., 1982). On the other hand, Rich et al. (1982) claim that the LV ejection fraction, as estimated or guessed at by visual inspection, without measurement or calculations, correlated very well with the values obtained by invasive LV angiography and by gated nuclear angiography.

ESTIMATION OF LV FUNCTION ON THE BASIS OF THE MITRAL OR AORTIC ECHOGRAM

Because of the drawbacks of indices of LV function based on systolic shortening of the LVID in patients with segmental wall motion abnormalities, other indices that assess overall LV performance have aroused interest.

The LV preejection period (PEP) is the interval between the onset of inscription of the QRS complex and opening of the aortic valve. The LV ejection period (EP) is the interval between opening and closing of the aortic valve. Both PEP and EP can be measured directly from the aortic valve echogram, preferably run at a fast paper speed of 75 or 100 mm/sec (Stefadouros and Witham, 1975).

Fortunately, these systolic time intervals (as measured from the "mechanocardiogram"—simultaneous recording of the phonocardiogram, carotid pulse tracing, and electrocardiogram) were studied extensively a decade ago (Weissler *et al.*, 1968; Weissler *et al.*, 1969; Garrard *et al.*, 1970; Hodges *et al.*, 1972). The PEP/EP ratio was found to be a reliable index of LV performance, unaffected by heart rate. Stefadouros and Witham (1975) found a high degree (r = 0.98) of accord between the systolic time intervals measured by the previous method, utilizing phonocardiography and pulse tracing, and the echographic aortic-valve method. Differences between the two techniques were of negligible extent, never exceeding 15 msec for PEP or EP. The normal range for the PEP/EP ratio is 0.30 to 0.38. In hypercontractile states, such as hypertrophic cardiomyopathy, values in the region of 0.25 are common; on the other hand, in severe myocardial impairment, as in dilated cardiomyopathy with congestive failure, values of 0.40 to 0.60 or even more are often encountered.

This method does have certain shortcomings:

1. The apparent point of onset of the QRS complex in the ECG lead used may not be the true point of onset if the initial QRS inscription is isoelectric in that lead.

2. If left bundle branch block is present, pro-longation of the PEP could be due, at least in part, to delay in LV electrical activation rather than a slow rate of rise of LV pressure.

3. A very distinct and complete definition of the aortic valve, especially of its opening and closing, is necessary. Both cusps must be visualized; the exact moments of opening and closing cannot be pinpointed if only one cusp is delineated.

LV ISOVOLUMIC CONTRACTION TIME

The LV isovolumic contraction time forms part of the LV preejection period. It is the interval between mitral valve closure and aortic valve opening. Echocardiographically, these events are visualized easily on the mitral valve echogram and aortic valve echogram, respectively. Since the mitral and aortic valves cannot be visualized simultaneously by the same M-mode ultrasound transducer, the LV isovolumic contraction time can be obtained either by:

1. Simultaneous recording of the mitral and aortic valve echoes by different transducers but on the same tracing (dual echocardiography); or

2. Recording the mitral and aortic valve echoes successively, measuring the following intervals: (a) from QRS onset to mitral valve closing, and (b) from QRS onset to aortic valve opening; the LV isovolumic contraction time is the difference between the two (Hirschfeld *et al.*, 1976). These authors found that the interval varied with heart rate and age (in children). In their normal subjects, 1 to 19 years of age, the LV isovolumic contraction time varied between 20 and 50 msec. In children with myocardial disease, it was prolonged (40 to 100 msec). On the other hand, children with patent ductus arteriosus tended to have short intervals, less than 20 msec.

MITRAL VALVE E POINT–SEPTAL SEPARATION (Fig. I-12, see pages 262–63)

Massie *et al.* (1977) showed that the distance between the E peak of the anterior mitral leaflet and the left margin of the ventricular septum did not exceed 5 mm in individuals with normal LV function, but was usually greater than 5 mm in patients with decreased ejection fraction on angiocardiography. This index, sometimes abbreviated to EPSS (E point septal separation), correlated better with angiocardiographic ejection fraction than other commonly used indices of LV performance such as end-diastolic LVID, LVID systolic shortening fraction, ejection fraction based on LV volumes calculated from LVID measurements at end-systole and end-diastole, and LV posterior wall systolic thickening.

This superiority of the EPSS measurement to other indices of LV performance was confirmed in the studies of Lew et al. (1978), D'Cruz et al. (1979), and Child et al. (1981). D'Cruz et al. modified the method of measuring the mitral-septal separation: whereas Massie et al. (1977) measured the separation between the E point and the most posterior point on the left septal margin during the *preceding* systole, D'Cruz measured EPSS at the moment of inscription of the E peak. The normal upper limit by the latter method was 10 mm.

The recent study of Child et al. (1981) confirmed that the EPSS measurement accurately separated individuals with normal and abnormal LV function, irrespective of LV size. Increased LV internal dimension per se did not affect the EPSS unless depressed LV function coexisted.

The EPSS value is admittedly an arbitrary quantity that, on theoretical grounds, bears no obvious direct relationship to or dependence on LV contractility; moreover, as a diastolic observation, its ability to reflect accurately the quality of LV systolic contraction is not understood clearly. Nevertheless, EPSS is a valuable empiric indicator of overall LV performance. These are its advantages:

1. It is not affected by segmental wall abnormalities of the ventricular septum or LV posterior wall, but reflects overall LV function. An important practical consideration is that an abnormally large EPSS in a patient who has normal septal and LV posterior motion on the M-mode echocardiogram suggests that the patient has diminished overall LV performance due to a large akinetic or dyskinetic region involving the LV apex or adjacent myocardium.

2. It requires visualization of only the anterior mitral leaflet and left border of the ventricular septum, which can be recorded in almost all patients, even by relatively inexperienced echocardiographers. On the other hand, the indices of LV performance that depend on the LVID and its systolic shortening require simultaneous and clear recording of septal and LV posterior wall endocardium, sometimes a difficult task in emphysematous, obese, or elderly persons.

The disadvantages of EPSS as an index of LV function include:

1. It may not apply in patients with mitral stenosis, extensive mitral annulus calcification, or aortic regurgitation; these three entities have in common the frequent diminution of diastolic excursion of the anterior mitral leaflet, for mechanical reasons affecting diastolic motion of the mitral valve. Also, the EPSS cannot be measured, of course, in patients with prosthetic mitral valves.

2. In some patients with anteroseptal aneurysms, the ventricular shape may be so distorted by the anterior sharp septal bulge that mitral-septal separation is normal at basal LV level (just below the aortic root, a region of the septum that is usually spared by ischemic heart disease), but is considerably increased if the ultrasound beam, directed from a lower intercostal space, transects the aneurysmal, anteriorly bowed portion of the ventricular septum.

SYSTOLIC AORTIC ROOT MOTION

In the first detailed description of echocardiography of the aortic root, Gramiak and Shah (1970) noted that the aortic root moves anteriorly to an average distance of 10.4 mm in normal persons, but to a lesser extent in most patients with heart disease.

Subsequently, it was commonly observed by echocardiographers that patients with severe LV failure exhibited a marked diminution in aortic root systolic excursion. The relationship between aortic root excursion and LV function was examined quantitatively by Pratt et al. (1976) and Burggraf et al. (1978). Both groups found that the anterior excursion of the aortic root correlated well with stroke volume but did not correlate well with ejection fraction. In fact, it had been earlier claimed by Kleid and Schiller (1974) that the LV stroke volume (in milliliters) could be obtained by simply multiplying the systolic anterior excursion of the posterior aortic root (in millimeters) by the factor 6.4. Pratt as well as Burggraf found that the average anterior excursion of the posterior aortic wall (posterior aortic root, in echographic terminology) was about 9 mm. Burggraf et al. reported that the normal range was 7 to 12 mm, whereas ten patients with ischemic heart disease and heart failure as well as ten with congestive cardiomyopathy all had excursions of less than 7 mm.

Pratt et al. showed that aortic root systolic motion is sensitive to acute changes in stroke volume, such as those produced by the Valsalva maneuver and amyl nitrite inhalation. Thus it appears that systolic aortic root motion may have a role in investigating the effect of acute interventions of short duration on stroke volume, but has little place in the routine clinical assessment of LV function.

The atrial emptying index (AEI) was originally studied as an indirect method for diagnosing mitral stenosis. The AEI is the ratio of the posterior excursion of the posterior aortic root in the first third of diastole to the total posterior diastolic excursion (until onset of atrial contraction). Wasserman et al. (1980) recently have correlated the AEI with the pulmonary artery wedge pressure in 21 patients with no mitral stenosis. They found that a significant negative correlation existed between the AEI and the wedge pressure ($r = 0.91$). Patients with normal wedge pressure had an average AEI of 0.94 $\pm$ SD 0.06. Those with abnormally high wedge pressure had an average AEI of 0.61 $\pm$ 0.20. No patients with a normal wedge pressure had an AEI less than 0.80. No patient with a wedge pressure over 18 mm had an AEI more than 0.66.

There may in fact be a useful role for echocardiographic measurements such as systolic anterior aortic root excursion or velocity, LV preejection time ratio, mitral E point–septal separation, and other indirect indices of stroke volume or LV performance in the monitoring of acute or rapidly changing hemodynamic states. Thus, Kavey et al. (1980) used several such parameters serially to assess cardiac output and status in children during the 24 hours after open-heart surgery. It is possible that a similar application of echocardiography in adults suffering from acute LV failure may complement or partly replace the invasive monitoring methods now in use.

LV FUNCTION AS REFLECTED IN DIASTOLIC MITRAL VALVE MOTION

Abnormalities of mitral valve motion in patients with raised LV diastolic pressure or reduced compliance have long attracted attention because of their diagnostic importance. These patterns represent abnormalities of mitral echo morphology on the M-mode echogram due to abnormal diastolic behavior of the mitral leaflets resulting from abnormal LV physiology, in particular the rates of mitral flow during the various phases of LV filling. These changes are thus functional or pathophysiologic in origin (in contrast to changes attributable to intrinsic anatomic changes in the mitral cusps):

1. Low or flat EF slope secondary to stiff or noncompliant LV chambers (Layton et al., 1973; Quinones et al., 1974; DeMaria et al., 1976) and in patients with pulmonary hypertension (Duchak et al., 1972; Goodman et al., 1973; McLaurin et al., 1973).

2. Flutter of the anterior mitral leaflet, in most cases of aortic regurgitation. This may be accompanied in some instances by a flat or even negative (upsloping) EF segment of the anterior mitral echo because the anterior mitral leaflet is held down by the regurgitant aortic jet impinging on it.

3. Premature closure of the mitral valve in acute, severe aortic valve regurgitation (commonly due to aortic valve endocarditis); the LV diastolic pressure exceeds the LA pressure in late diastole, affecting mitral closure before onset of the QRS complex.

4. A notch or shoulder on the AC mitral slope (Konecke et al., 1973) is a useful sign of elevated LV diastolic pressure. Normally, the B point on the AC slope is barely perceptible as an abrupt increase in steepness of the slope. This echographic sign is an indication of significantly raised LV end-diastolic pressure; it also might be due to poor LV performance (Feigenbaum, 1976). In clinical practice, it is most often seen in patients with severe, diffuse LV dilatation and hypokinesis secondary to congestive cardiomyopathy or ischemic heart disease.

A similar interruption or prolongation of the AC slope can be seen in patients with abnormally long P-R intervals. The mitral valve attains a near-closure position during atrial relaxation, after the A peak, but the B and C points are delayed due to late onset of LV contraction. In order to avoid echographic false-positives due to prolonged P-R interval, the P-R minus AC interval was introduced as an index of raised LV end-diastolic pressure. Normally, the P-R interval is 0.06 sec or more greater than the AC interval. If the P-R exceeds the AC interval by less than 0.06 sec, it signifies a LV end-diastolic pressure of 20 mm or more, the atrial component of this pressure being 8 mm or more (Konecke et al., 1973).

Another caveat worth mentioning is that, in patients with fast heart rates, the "A" wave is sometimes diminutive and so almost "buried" in the EF slope. The EF and AC slopes are thus almost merged into one. The mitral cusp echogram should be scrutinized with special attention to the segment immediately following the P wave.

A recent study has confirmed the usefulness of the PR-AC interval (which was shown to be a fairly reliable indicator of raised pulmonary wedge pressure and decreased LV ejection fraction) in patients without valvular disease (Wilson et al., 1981). In this series, 90 per cent of patients with PR-AC intervals > 0.06 had pulmonary wedge pressures > 14 mmHg versus only 10 per cent of patients with wedge pressures less than this level.

5. The DE slope may be retarded in some patients with dilated LV chambers and gross LV failure (Konecke et al., 1973). In this mitral echographic pattern, it is the "E" peak that is delayed or attenuated, whereas the "A" peak is unduly prominent. In other words, the mitral valve opens fully only during the atrial contribution to LV filling, presumably due to powerful LA contraction. Some of the best examples of such mitral valve behavior are seen in patients with cor pulmonale and dilated RV chambers.

The clinical significance of this finding may be that LA contraction plays a crucial or predominant role in LV filling, so that arrhythmias such as atrial fibrillation or AV dissociation which deprive the LV of the atrial "kick" may well be particularly disastrous.

Caution: In aortic regurgitation, the DE excursion of the anterior mitral leaflet may be small or even absent because of the restraining effect of the jet emerging from the regurgitant aortic valve. The semiclosed or closed anterior mitral leaflet exhibits a rapid diastolic flutter.

MITRAL VALVE STROKE VOLUME

Rasmussen et al. (1978) from Feigenbaum's laboratory devised a formula for calculating mitral valve stroke volume using the rate of mitral valve opening (DE slope), separation between anterior and posterior mitral cusps at maximal opening (EE distance), P-R interval on the ECG, and heart rate. Thus, the mitral valve stroke volume (in ml) equals:

$$\left(\frac{EE \text{ (mm)}}{\text{Heart rate (beats/min)}} + \text{P-R (sec)}\right) \times 100$$
$$+ \frac{2 \times DE \text{ (mm/sec)}}{\text{Heart rate (beats/min)}}$$

This formula was tested prospectively in 80 consecutive patients, 54 of whom had coronary disease, by comparing the estimations obtained by it with those by Fick or thermodilution methods. The correlation was good (r = 0.90) for stroke volume and for cardiac output (r = 0.83). This method, which requires only a good mitral valve echogram, is worthy of wider trial in clinical practice.

LV POSTERIOR WALL MOTION

The earliest attempts to assess LV function by echocardiography included the measurement of the amplitude and velocity of the anterior systolic excursion of the LV posterior wall (Kraunz and Kennedy, 1970; McDonald et al., 1972). As an index of total LV performance, LV posterior wall motion has several limitations:

1. It is invalid if the entire LV does not contract uniformly, as in ischemic heart disease with local hypokinesis, akinesis, or dyskinesis; abnormal septal motion following cardiac surgery; IHSS; and so forth.

2. Excessive amplitude of LV wall motion accompanies pericardial effusions.

3. To be meaningful, LV wall excursions have to be related to the LV size in that patient (Quinones et al., 1974). Thus, an LV posterior wall excursion of 10 mm would be quite normal for a LV of 45 mm internal dimension but definitely subnormal for a dilated LV with internal dimension of 70 mm.

The normal anterior systolic excursion of the LV posterior wall was found to be 11.5 ± 1.7 mm by McDonald *et al.* (1972) and 13.9 ± 1.8 mm by Conetta *et al.* (1979). The mean velocity of the LV posterior wall endocardium during ejection, according to the latter authors, was 50.5 ± 8.0 mm.

For the purpose of calculating the LV posterior wall endocardial velocity, the duration of LV ejection is ascertained from a simultaneous external carotid pulse tracing (interval from onset of carotid upstroke to the dicrotic notch). Less preferably, if the arterial pulse tracing is not available, the onset of LV ejection is taken as 0.05 sec after the onset of the QRS complex and its completion the aortic component of the second heart sound or the smallest LV dimension.

Diastolic posterior motion of the LV posterior wall has been studied in detail by several investigators (Gibson and Brown, 1973; Fujii *et al.*, 1979; Conetta *et al.*, 1979). Thus, Conetta *et al.* found that the LV posterior wall endocardial echo moved posteriorly at 108 ± 28 mm per sec during rapid ventricular filling in early diastole, but at only 6.6 ± 1.8 mm per sec during slow ventricular filling. Although of much importance in the understanding of the pathophysiology of ventricular filling, abnormal values were documented in a wide variety of cardiac disease states and therefore were of little practical diagnostic value.

LEFT VENTRICULAR MASSES

Cardiac ultrasound probably surpasses all other diagnostic methods in the detection of abnormal masses within the left ventricle and demonstration of their anatomic relationship to various LV structures.

Radiography and fluoroscopy are useless for this purpose unless the intraventricular mass contains large amounts of calcium, and even so, precise localization of the calcification within the heart is not possible. Angiocardiography may reveal an LV mass only if it is so situated as to distort the normal LV contour in the particular projection or projections recorded, or is large enough to produce a filling defect within the opacified dye-shadow. Gated radioactive blood-pool scanning, while permitting noninvasive depiction of the LV chamber, can detect only gross distortion of LV shape; fine details of structure or motion are beyond its capabilities. Visualization of an LV mass by CAT scan is possible, if sufficiently large, but unlike 2-D echography, its motion characteristics cannot be appreciated.

Two-D echocardiography allows visualization of an LV mass in multiple views (long-axis, short-axis, apical four-chamber and two-chamber, subxiphoid), thus providing a more complete idea of its shape, anatomic location, and motion characteristics. Moreover, any number of repeat examinations is possible to elucidate diagnostic afterthoughts, to follow progress of a mass with passage of time (or with medical therapy), to detect possible recurrence after surgical removal, and so forth.

Left ventricular masses are of four main varieties:

1. Mural thrombi,
2. Neoplasms,
3. Extensive submitral (mitral annulus) calcific deposits,
4. Large vegetations of endocarditis.

It is only since the advent of 2-D echocardiography in the late 1970s that these various types of LV masses have been diagnosed during life and their frequency recognized. Of these, mural thrombi are by far the most commonly encountered in clinical echocardiographic practice.

MURAL THROMBI (Figs. I-13 to I-17)

Initial reports of detection of thrombi in the left ventricle by ultrasound were of solitary cases (Levisman *et al.*, 1975; Horgan *et al.*, 1976; DeJoseph *et al.*, 1977; Kramer *et al.*, 1978; van den Bos *et al.*, 1978; Kleid and Arvan, 1978). Later, several groups (Ports *et al.*, 1978; Meltzer *et al.*, 1979; DeMaria *et al.*, 1979; Quinones *et al.*, 1980; Drobac *et al.*, 1980; Come *et al.*, 1980; Nagri *et al.*, 1980) described series comprising 2 to 22 patients in whom wide-angle 2-D echocardiographic diagnosis of LV thrombi was substantiated by surgical, autopsy, or angiocardiographic data. Recent 2-D echocardiographic surveys of populations at

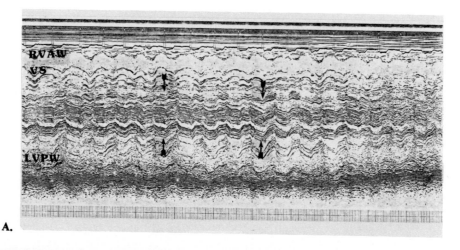

A.

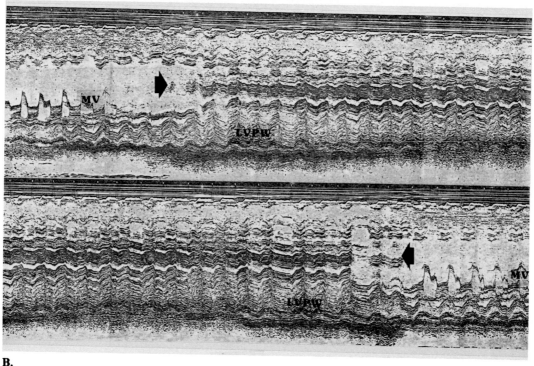

B.

Fig. I-13. *A.* M-mode echogram in a patient with a large apical mural thrombus, which manifests as dense echoes (*arrows*) that fill most of the LV chamber but are distinct from the ventricular septum and the LV posterior wall.

Fig. I-13. *B.* M-mode scans in the same patient of the LV from mitral valve level toward the apex (*upper*) and in the opposite direction (*lower*), showing the thrombus (*arrow*).

risk for LV mural thrombi formation have shown that such thrombi are by no means rare (Asinger *et al.,* 1980; Quinones *et al.,* 1980; Drobac *et al.,* 1980; Ezekowitz *et al.,* 1982; Stratton *et al.,* 1982; Gottdiener *et al.,* 1982).

Based on the data in these published reports

and personal experience, the following appear to be the echographic features of LV mural thrombi:

1. A definite mass, of variable size, adjacent to the LV endocardium. Either the surface of the thrombus or the whole of it produces rather

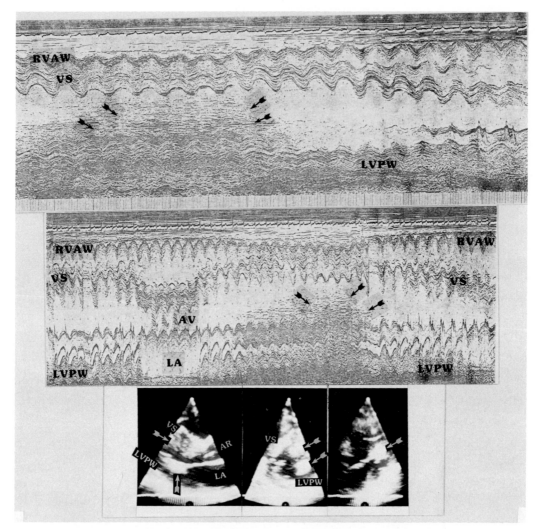

Fig. I-14. *Upper.* M-mode echogram of a patient with chronic renal failure and inferior wall myocardial infarction. A dense ill-defined echo fills most of the LV chamber at papillary muscle level, obscuring the normal LV wall pattern at this site. It probably represents a mural thrombus.

    Center. M-mode echogram at slow paper speed in the same patient, scanning from LV, to aortic root, to left atrium, then back to LV at papillary muscle level (showing the mural thrombus at this site), and finally once again to the mitral valve level.

    Lower. 2-D echogram of the same patient reveals an abnormally dense large mass at the site of the posterolateral papillary muscle, in long-axis (*left*), short-axis (*center*) and apical 4-chamber (*right*) views. The appearances are very suggestive of a long-standing mural thrombus. Another echo mass of lesser density anterior to it may represent another mural thrombus.

strong echoes, which may exceed the LV endocardial echo in density. Presumably such thrombi with strong reflecting qualities are long standing, containing dense fibrosis or even calcification. In other instances, the mural thrombi are of recent origin and probably possess acoustic properties not very different from those of blood; the abnormal echoes are therefore of a weak and indistinct nature. Such thrombi, of insubstantial density and nebulous outline, may be as important or even more important than the conspicuous, well-defined mural thrombi described above because they are more friable and apt to break off into the blood stream.

2. The LV apex is the most common site for mural thrombi; next in frequency comes the left aspect of the ventricular septum, then the lateral LV wall. The posterobasal and inferior LV walls are least affected.

3. Mural thrombi are seen almost exclusively

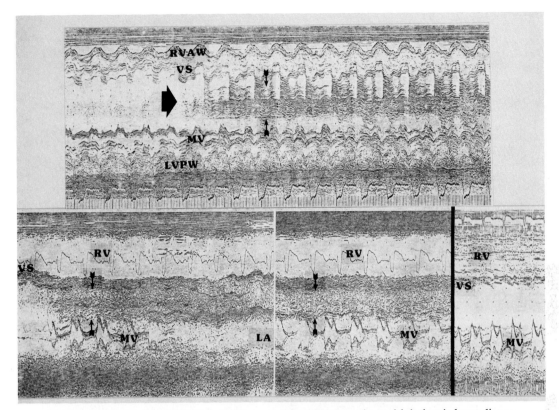

Fig. I-15. *Upper.* M-mode echographic scan of the LV in a patient with ischemic heart disease. An abnormal dense echo in the LV outflow region comes into view (*arrows*); it appears attached to be a mural thrombus attached to the ventricular septum.

Lower. M-mode echogram of a man with congestive cardiomyopathy. The left and middle panels revealed an abnormal echo-mass (*arrows*) in the LV outflow tract, between the mitral valve and ventricular septum. The echogram in the right panel, recorded four months earlier, showed no such abnormal LV mass, which was presumably a mural thrombus. Note that the erroneous diagnosis of abnormal septal hypertrophy (ASH) could easily have been made from the middle panel.

in left ventricles with segmental or diffuse dyssynergy (Quinones *et al.,* 1980; Asinger *et al.,* 1980), especially in proximity to akinetic or dyskinetic (perhaps aneurysmal) areas of the septum or ventricular wall (Lewin *et al.,* 1980). Thus, in clinical practice, it is in patients with myocardial infarction (recent or old) or with dilated congestive cardiomyopathy (Suzuki *et al.,* 1979; McManus *et al.,* 1983) that mural thrombi may be encountered, therefore a high index of suspicion on the part of the echocardiographer is warranted.

4. Mural thrombi show motion parallel and similar to that of the adjacent ventricular wall to which they adhere. This important characteristic makes it possible to differentiate them from artefacts caused by reverberations from the chest wall or anterior cardiac structures. Such

reverberations are sometimes quite prominent but are relatively stationary and do not participate in motion of the septum or other neighboring structures.

5. Pedunculated thrombi may have considerable mobility (van den Bos *et al.,* 1978; Come *et al.,* 1980) and may be indistinguishable preoperatively from a LV myxoma. Close examination of such pedunculated thrombi may reveal a rapid oscillatory or waving motion, like a flag fluttering in a strong wind. In one instance, a mobile LV mass was shown at operation to be a thrombus attached to a mitral chorda tendinea (Sabot *et al.,* 1979). In another example, the pedunculated thrombus, attached to the LV apex, partly broke off and caused a fatal cerebral embolism (Chen *et al.,* 1981). Strong evidence is accumulating that small, highly mobile LV

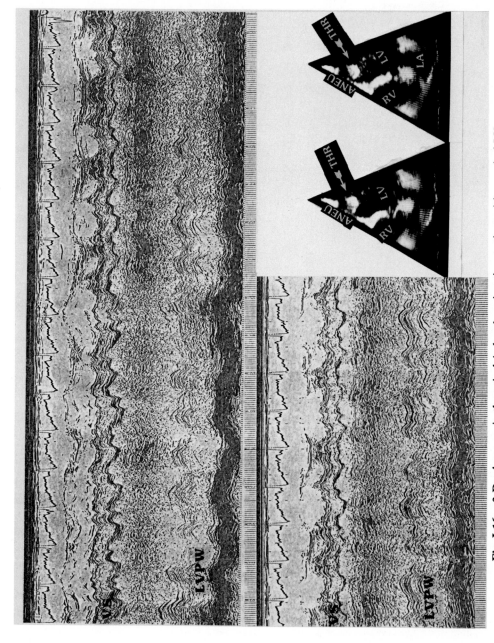

Fig. I-16. 2-D echogram, in the apical 4-chamber view, in a patient with an apical LV aneurysm following myocardial infarction. A mural thrombus is visible near the LV apex. M-mode echogram in the same patient showing extensive ill-defined echoes (dense in places) in the LV at papillary muscle level.

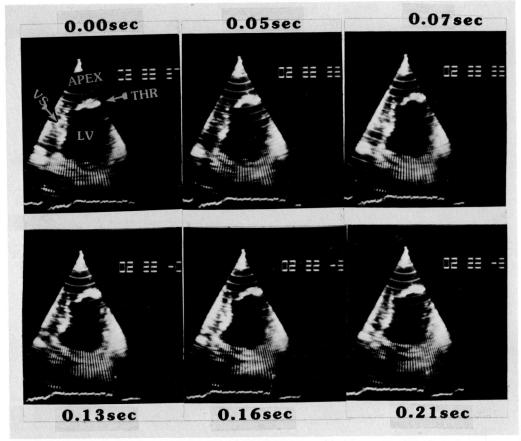

Fig. I-17. 2-D echogram, in the apical 4-chamber view, in a patient with LV apical dyskinesis secondary to myocardial infarction. Six serial frames from the same cardiac cycle are shown. The first frame is at end-diastole; the second to sixth frames are in progressively later phases of systole. An abnormal echo, representing the edge of an apical mural thrombus, changes contour during systole, distinguishing it from artefacts due to chest wall reverberation, which would be unchanged.

thrombi are far more ominous than large, flat, dense thrombi firmly adherent to the LV wall.

6. Mural thrombi have been found at surgery in patients whose 2-D echocardiograms before surgery were thought to reveal no thrombi (Meltzer *et al.*, 1979; DeMaria *et al.*, 1979). Perhaps some of these thrombi were overlooked because of their small size; in other instances, retrospective review of the echocardiograms showed faint, indefinite echoes at the affected sites, suggesting that some mural thrombi generate rather feeble echoes. It is also possible for a flat thrombus attached to the left septal endocardium to be mistaken for the septal surface itself, so that the septum appears falsely thick. On the other hand, 2-D echography may sometimes prove superior to angiocardiography in diagnosing apical LV thrombi (van Meurs-

van Woezik *et al.*, 1981). The sensitivity of 2-D echocardiography with regard to LV thrombi was 77 per cent, and specificity was 93 per cent in the series of Ezekowitz *et al.* (1982).

Because the diagnosis of mural thrombus within the LV chamber may be followed by far-reaching therapeutic decisions, such as the commencement of long-term anticoagulation, it is important to call attention to possible false-positive diagnoses that could easily ensnare the inexperienced:

1. The most common pitfall is an artefact caused by reverberation from the chest wall or the plastic casing of the sector-scanner probe. Such artefactual echoes are particularly likely to be mistaken for LV apical thrombi on the apical 2-D view; this is unfortunate because the

[*Text continued on page 284.*]

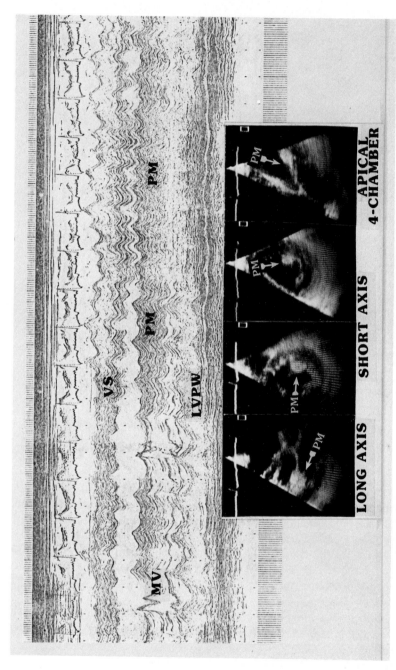

Fig. I-18. *Upper.* M-mode echogram of a normal patient with an unusually large posterior papillary muscle. When an LV scan is made from mitral valve level toward the LV apex, the mitral valve is seen to be continuous with a wide dense echo that moves parallel to the LV posterior wall and then merges with it.

Lower. 2-D echogram of the same patient, showing the prominent papillary muscle in long-axis view (*left*), short-axis view (*center*), and apical 4-chamber view (*right*). Thus, the 2-D echogram demonstrates that the large mass in the LV on the M-mode tracing is much more likely to be a normal variant (large papillary muscle) than a mural thrombus.

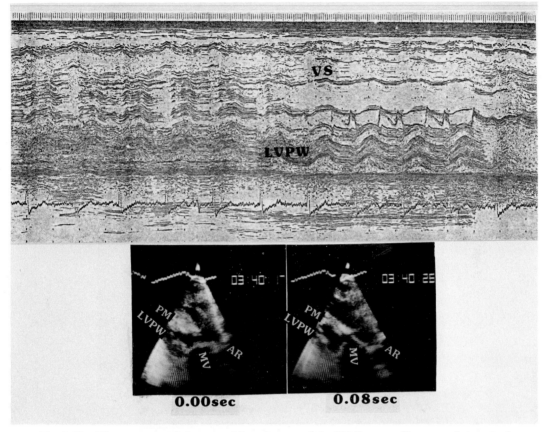

Fig. I-19. The upper panel shows an M-mode scan of the LV from papillary muscle to mitral valve level. Abnormal echoes within the LV chamber (*left half of figure*) raised the possibility of an LV thrombus. However, the 2-D echogram in the long-axis view showed that the apparent LV echo mass was in fact a large, prominent papillary muscle. This is clearly presented in the left frame, which is in systole; the right frame, in early diastole, demonstrates the changes in papillary muscle contour—elongation and thinning—that occur in diastole.

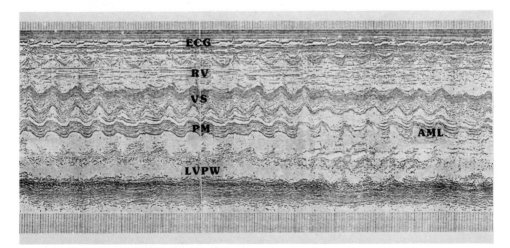

Fig. I-20. M-mode echogram showing a dense bandlike echo in the LV near the ventricular septum. Scanning toward the mitral valve reveals that this abnormal echo is continuous with the anterior mitral leaflet, thus identifying it as the apex of the anterior papillary muscle. It could simulate a mural thrombus.

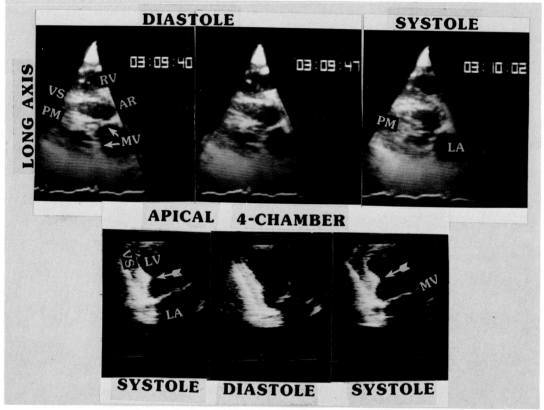

Fig. I-21. Normal variants of LV anatomy that simulate mural thrombi.

Upper. 2-D echogram in the long-axis view of a normal individual with prominent papillary muscle. The papillary muscle can be easily identified, in the left and center frames, because of its connection by chordae tendineae to the anterior and posterior mitral leaflets. However, in the right frame, which represents a slightly different plane, the connections between the papillary muscle and mitral leaflets are not as obvious, so that the papillary muscle could be mistaken for a mural thrombus. Such an error could be avoided by 2-D scanning: i.e., visualizing the abnormal echo in different planes by side-to-side rocking or rotation of the 2-D probe.

Lower. 2-D echogram in the apical 4-chamber view showing a local protuberance on the left margin of the ventricular septum (*arrows, left and right*) in systole, but not in diastole. It is perhaps attributable to a prominent or hypercontractile component of circular LV muscle. It should not be mistaken for a mural thrombus or tumor.

LV apex happens to be the most common site for clot formation. Reverberatory echoes can be distinguished from true thrombi by the fact that they are stationary and parallel to chest wall echoes; moreover, it may be possible to demonstrate, by slight changes in transducer direction, that the artefactual echo extends beyond the LV echo contour into the RV echo area, which would not happen with a true LV apical thrombus.

2. The posterior and anterior papillary muscles normally protrude into the LV cavity and therefore may be considered "normal" or "physiologic" masses. In older persons, the papillary muscle may appear unduly prominent because of sclerosis or calcification, or involvement in myocardial infarction. The echocardiographer must become familiar with the normal topography of the papillary muscles in all the various 2-D views so that they can be identified readily, and so that confusion with mural thrombi is minimized. For example, it may be difficult to distinguish a mural thrombus situated on the LV posterior wall from the posterior papillary muscle in the long-axis view, but it is likely to be a mural thrombus if, on the short-axis view, it is located at a site on the LV circumference other than those normally occupied. How-

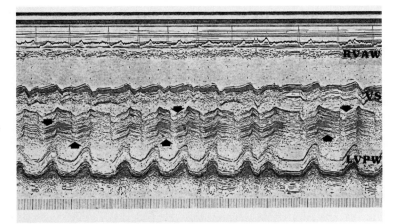

Fig. I-22. M-mode echogram of a patient with a Starr-Edwards mitral valve. The LV contains dense echoes arising from the prosthetic ball, which could possibly be mistaken for a myxoma or thrombus if the history of valve replacement is not available to the physician interpreting the echocardiogram. Scans to the aortic root and at different LV levels would permit recognition of typical motion of the ball and cage.

ever, mural thrombi can occur on the papillary muscle site. A blood cyst of a papillary muscle can present echocardiographically as a bizarre intra-LV mass (Hauser *et al.*, 1983).

3. In hypertrophied, small left ventricles, the endocardial echoes near the LV apex appear near the center of the LV chamber and on occa-

sion can simulate mural thrombi, especially when such endocardial echoes are fragmented due to partial dropout.

4. A prominence of the ventricular septum at its base is a common variant, attributable to undue hypertrophy or predominance of the circular muscle component of the LV at this

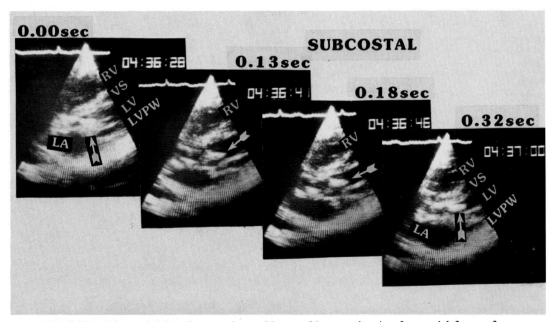

Fig. I-23. Subcostal 2-D echogram in an 85-year-old man, showing four serial frames from the same cardiac cycle. The first frame is in late diastole, the second in early systole, the third in midsystole, the fourth in late systole. In the first frame, there appears to be a large LV mass at its base. The subsequent systolic frames show that the mass becomes much smaller and occupies the region of the anterior mitral leaflet. This leaflet was very probably thickened by sclerotic degenerative changes. There was no evidence of old or recent endocarditis.

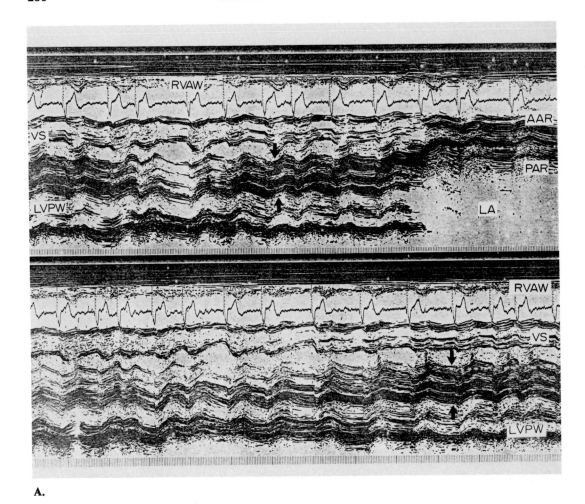

A.

Fig. I-24.   *A.* Segments of the M-mode echogram of an elderly patient with unusually extensive submitral calcification (*arrows*), which fills most of the LV chamber at this level and obscures the mitral valve. The aortic valve is also calcified, a commonly associated finding.

level. It becomes more prominent in systole (Fig. I-21) and may resemble a mural thrombus on a still-frame. When viewed in real time, it obviously moves and contracts with the rest of septal myocardium.

5. Prosthetic mitral valves, especially of long standing, can produce very dense echoes within the LV (Fig. I-22), but the history of valve replacement, typical motion of the disk or ball (in mechanical valves), and absence of mitral leaflet echoes should prevent any error.

6. Calcification in the mitral or submitral region, sometimes encountered in very elderly patients or those with chronic renal failure, can present on occasion as a dense LV mass, especially if of massive proportions (D'Cruz *et al.*,

1980). Figures I-23 and I-24 show such examples. Rarely, calcification in the region of the apex of a papillary muscle can be quite large and present as an impressive LV mass (I-25).

7. Recently an unusual, nebulous type of slow swinging echo in the LV near the apex was noted in patients with severe apical akinesis; this was attributed to echogenic regional blood stasis (Mikell *et al.*, 1982).

LEFT VENTRICULAR NEOPLASMS

Left ventricular tumors are of great rarity. Not more than twenty cases have been diagnosed by echocardiography. They may be located intramurally and present echographically as a tre-

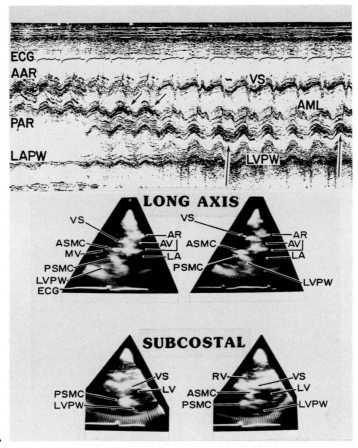

B.

Fig. I-24. *B.* The upper panel shows the M-mode echogram of a 50-year-old man with chronic renal failure and secondary hyperparathyroidism. There is calcification in the posterior submitral region (*upward arrows*), as well as in the base of the anterior mitral leaflet (*downward arrows*). The anterior submitral calcification (ASMC) and posterior submitral calcification (PSMC) are also identifiable on the 2-D echogram in the long-axis view (*above*) and subcostal view (*below*). Thus, careful analysis of the unusual, perplexing echo mass in the M-mode echogram, while a scan is made from aortic root to LV, reveals its true nature.

mendously thickened LV wall or ventricular septum. Such was the case in the patient of Farooki *et al.* (1977), a newborn infant with a septal rhabdomyoma; in a 32-year-old woman with a hemangioma distending the LV posterior wall reported by Ports *et al.* (1978); and in the cases of Biancaniello *et al.* (1982). Farooki *et al.* (1977) also described the ultrasound findings in a child with a hydatid cyst in the left ventricle that appeared partly embedded in the ventricular septum.

In other instances, the LV neoplasm was pedunculated, presenting echocardiographically as a mobile mass within the LV chamber. This was true of an intraventricular metastatic melanoma detected by Ports *et al.* (1978); a myxoma arising from an LV papillary muscle reported

by Morgan *et al.* (1977); and an LV papillary fibroelastoma reported by Ong *et al.* (1982).

LEFT ATRIAL MYXOMAS

Strictly speaking, left atrial myoxmas are not left ventricular masses since they arise in and are attached to the left atrial or atrial septal wall. However, left atrial myxomas often have long pedicles and fall deep into the left ventricle in diastole, even beyond the mitral valve leaflets into the mid- or apical left ventricle (Fig. I-26). The atrial origin of such a left ventricular mass can be suspected by visualizing its entry into the LV chamber between the mitral valve leaflets and its disappearance from the left ventricle during systole.

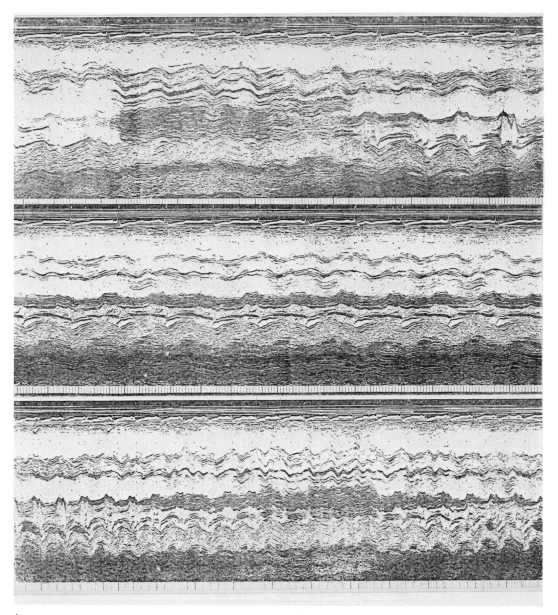

A.

Fig. I-25. *A. Upper.* M-mode echogram of an elderly patient showing a large dense echo occupying most of the left ventricle at mid-LV level, which disappears from view as a scan is made toward the mitral valve. LV thrombus or tumor were possible diagnoses.

Center and Lower. However, on further scans of the LV it was evident that the dense opacity extended to and moved with the anterior mitral leaflet echo. This finding, as well as the 2-D echographic appearances, indicate that the abnormal, dense echo was due to calcification in the anterior papillary muscle.

CALCIFIC LEFT VENTRICULAR MASSES (Figs. I-23 to I-25)

"Mitral annulus" calcification is easily recognized, in the vast majority of cases, as a dense, bandlike echo between the mitral valve and LV posterior wall. Occasionally, however, such calcification may attain large or even massive proportions and extend into the anterior as well as posterior submitral areas (so that the mitral

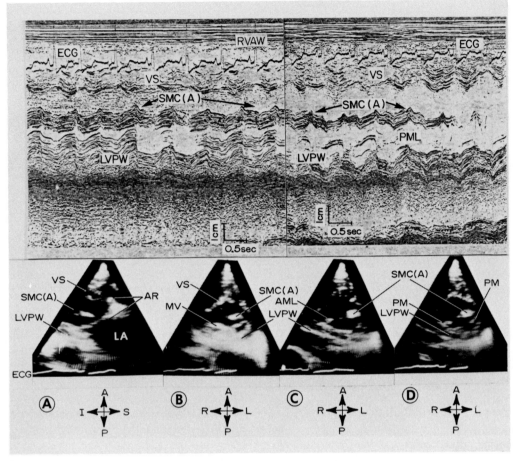

B.

Fig. I-25. *B.* Echocardiogram of another elderly patient with calcification in the region of the papillary muscle apex, which manifests as a dense mass in the anterior LV chamber on the M-mode echogram (*above*). This abnormal echo can be better localized on the 2-D echogram (*below*) on long-axis (*left frame*) and short-axis (*other 3 frames*) views.

leaflets are obscured, mostly or entirely, on the M-mode echogram) and present as a large, dense mass in the basal left ventricle (D'Cruz *et al.,* 1980). The true nature of the mass can be suspected if careful scanning from the mass upward to the aortic root and downward to the LV apex reveal:

1. Typical posterior mitral annulus calcification as a dense echo just anterior to the LV posterior wall.

2. Free edges of the mitral leaflets, of normal thickness; sometimes only the anterior mitral leaflet can be discerned, peeping over the dense bar of calcification.

3. Anterior submitral calcification superimposed on the anterior mitral leaflet; on scanning

to the aortic root, such calcification becomes continuous or contiguous to the posterior aortic root.

On 2-D echocardiography, submitral mitral annulus calcification is rather immobile, thus distinguishing it from other large LV masses in the mitral region, such as left atrial myxomas, large mitral (fungal or bacterial) valvular vegetations, and heavily calcified mitral cusps.

VEGETATIONS PRESENTING AS LV MASSES

Valvular vegetations in bacterial endocarditis usually present as shaggy or nodular thickening of valve cusps. They may be confused with LV

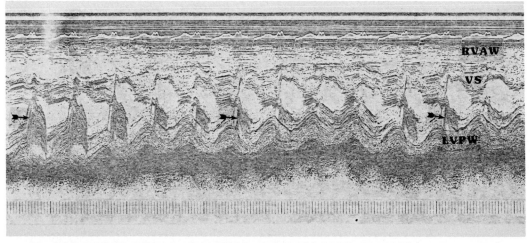

Fig. I-26. M-mode echogram of the LV in a patient with an LA myxoma (proven by surgical removal). The first 3 beats show the typical appearance of the myxoma (*arrows*) lying within the mitral valve in diastole, and retreating from view in systole. Thereafter the scan moves to the mid-LV level and the myxoma is still visible (*arrow*). The myxoma in this case was elongated and prolapsed into the LV almost to its apex in diastole.

masses of thrombotic or neoplastic nature only in exceptional instances when of very large size, which is common in fungal (*Candida*) vegetations but occasionally also in bacterial vegetations.

Aortic valve endocarditis can present as a "mass" in the LV outflow tract between the anterior mitral leaflet and ventricular septum just below the aortic valve. This mass, usually of small size, consists of a vegetation attached to a partly torn or detached aortic valve cusp that prolapses into the LV outflow tract in diastole but moves up into the aorta in systole. Fine diastolic flutter is evident on the prolapsing mass and on the anterior mitral leaflet as the regurgitant aortic jet sets them into vibratory motion.

ABNORMAL ECHOES IN THE LEFT VENTRICULAR OUTFLOW TRACT
(Figs. I-27 to I-30)

The term LV outflow tract refers to that part of the LV chamber that lies between the anterior mitral leaflet and the ventricular septum. It leads into the aortic root, and the aortic valve forms the upper boundary of the LV outflow area. This region is best seen echocardiographically in M-mode scans from LV to aortic root, and on 2-D echography in the long-axis view.

Abnormal echoes appearing in the LV outflow area may perplex the echocardiographer and in some instances could even be mistaken for the left septal border.

Such abnormal echoes include:

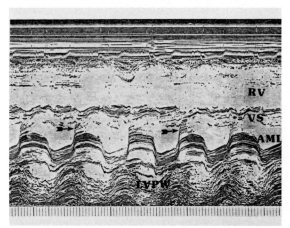

Fig. I-27. M-mode echogram of a patient with mitral stenosis. The mitral cusps are thickened and move abnormally in diastole. The most anterior part of the anterior mitral leaflet is seen only in early diastole (*arrows*), and drops out in the rest of diastole. This appearance could simulate a flail aortic valve leaflet. No aortic regurgitation was present in this patient.

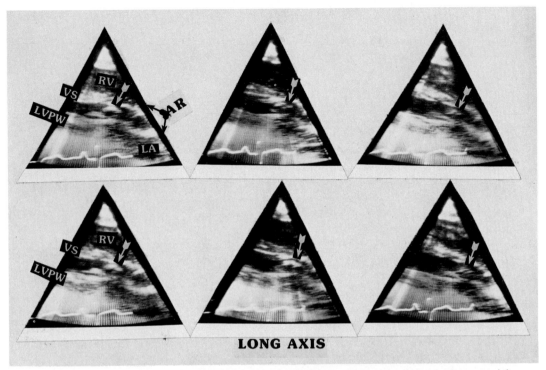

Fig. I-28. 2-D echogram of a 15-year-old boy with Down's syndrome, ostium primum atrial septal defect, and a cleft mitral valve. All 6 frames are diastolic and in the long-axis view. A pair of abnormal, short linear echoes appear between the septum and anterior mitral leaflet; they represent anomalous chordae tendineae connecting the anterior mitral leaflet to the crest of the ventricular septum.

1. Flail aortic cusp, usually secondary to bacterial endocarditis (Fig. D-10), occasionally to trauma (Gay *et al.,* 1983). The torn cusp prolapses into the LV outflow tract in diastole; in systole, it moves into the aortic root. The affected cusp may be rendered conspicuous by a vegetation adherent to it and by the diastolic flutter caused by the aortic regurgitant jet (Chandaratna *et al.,* 1977). On 2-D echography, in the long-axis view, the flail leaflet presents an unmistakable sight as it darts into the LV outflow area at the onset of diastole and back into the aortic root in early systole. Occasionally, the anterior mitral leaflet of a stenotic mitral valve may "drop out" in mid- to late diastole to simulate a flail aortic valve (Fig. I-27).

2. In patients with ostium primum atrial septal defects, anomalous chordae tendineae commonly connect the cleft anterior mitral leaflet to the upper rim of the ventricular septum. Such anomalous chordae are seen, on the long-axis view, as small, round or oval structures; they

tend to be somewhat thicker and denser in older patients (Fig. I-28).

3. False tendons in the LV have long been known to anatomists but have only recently been reported in the echographic literature (Nishimura *et al.,* 1981). Whereas normal chordae tendineae arise in one of the two papillary muscles and insert on the anterior or posterior mitral leaflet, false tendons pass from papillary muscle or LV wall to papillary muscle or LV wall. They present, on the M-mode echogram, as linear or band echoes near the ventricular septum. The 2-D echogram reveals the true situation by demonstrating not only the false tendon but also its ectopic origin or insertion (Fig. I-29). Other views, such as the short-axis and subcostal, also may show the anomalous structure as an abnormal echo in the anterior LV chamber.

4. Artefacts due to the beam-width effect can cause echoes arising from a calcified aortic valve to appear in the LV outflow tract. Scanning from LV to aortic root or in the reverse direc-

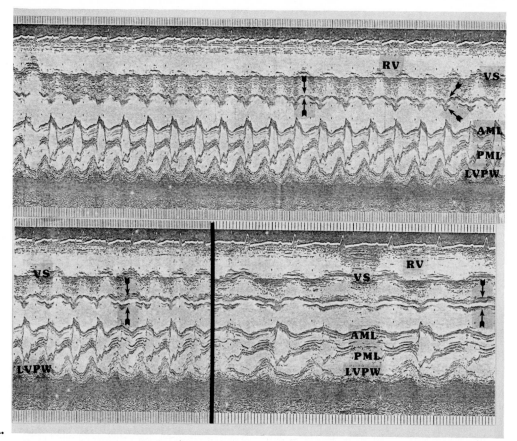

A.

Fig. I-29. *A. Upper.* M-mode echogram of a patient with what appeared on 2-D echography to be an anomalous chorda tendineae in the LV, inserting on the top of the ventricular septum rather than on the mitral valve. It appears as a thin echo just posterior to the septum (*arrows*). At a slightly different level (*left of figure*) the abnormal chordal echo merges with the septal echo at its site of insertion.

Lower. Echogram showing an anomalous chorda tendineae (*arrows*), about 1 cm posterior to the ventricular septum. If mistaken for the left septal border, the erroneous diagnosis of septal hypertrophy may have been made. The paper speed has been doubled in the right part of the panel.

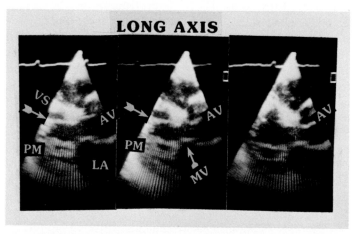

B.

Fig. I-29. *B.* 2-D echogram of the same patient with an anomalous band in the LV outflow tract. All 3 frames are in the long-axis view. The normal papillary muscle (PM) is attached to the anterior mitral leaflet. Just above it an accessory papillary muscle is attached to the ventricular septum by an anomalous chordal structure, apparent in the left and middle frames, but not in the right frame, which is in a slightly different plane.

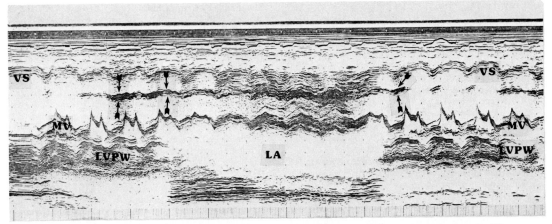

Fig. I-30. M-mode echogram showing a scan from LV to aortic root and back to LV. The aortic walls (anterior and posterior aortic root) are excessively sclerotic. An abnormal dense echo, apparently in the LV outflow tract, appears continuous with the dense anterior aortic root echo. It is attributable to the beam-width factor, producing the ultrasonic illusion of an abnormal structure in the LV outflow area.

tion (Fig. I-30) will reveal the continuity of the abnormal echo with dense aortic valve calcification.

5. Echoes arising from the anterior mitral leaflet or chordae can sometimes appear in the LV outflow area, but their connection with the anterior mitral leaflet is usually obvious. This applies to the linear echo in early systole attributable to anterior chordal buckling (in patients with mitral prolapse) or as a normal variant (Gardin *et al.,* 1981).

Ruptured mitral chordae tendineae can also cause abnormal echoes in the LV outflow area (Van Leeuwen *et al.,* 1982).

6. Membranes or bands situated below the aortic valve, and causing fixed discrete subvalvar stenosis, may cause bizarre LV outflow tract echoes. A unique case in which such a membrane was aneurysmal has been reported (Schneeweiss *et al.,* 1982).

7. Bulging of a ventricular septal aneurysm into the LV outflow tract has been reported (Barron *et al.,* 1982). The patient was a 41-year-old man with absent pulmonic valve and pulmonary hypertension.

REFERENCES

LV WALL THICKNESS, LVID, AND LV MASS

Abbasi, A. S.; MacAlpin, R. N.; Eber, L.; *et al.:* Left ventricular hypertrophy diagnosed by echocardiography. *N. Engl. J. Med.,* **289:**118, 1973.

Bahler, A. S.; Teichholz, L. E.; Gorlin, R.; *et al.:* Correlations of electrocardiography and echocardiography in de-termination of left ventricular wall thickness: Study of apparently normal subjects. *Am. J. Cardiol.,* **39:**189, 1977.

Bass, J. L.; Shrivastava, S.; Grabowski, G. A.; *et al.:* The M-mode echocardiogram in Fabry's disease. *Am. Heart J.,* **100:**807, 1980.

Bennett, D. H.; and Evans, D. W.: Correlation of left ventricular mass determined by echocardiography with vectorcardiographic and electrocardiographic voltage measurements. *Br. Heart J.,* **36:**981, 1974.

Bennett, D. H.; Evans, D. W.; and Raj, M. V. J.: Echocardiographic left ventricular dimensions in pressure and volume overload: Their use in assessing aortic stenosis. *Br. Heart J.,* **37:**971, 1975.

Borer, J. S.; Henry, W. L.; and Epstein, S. E.: Echocardiographic observation in patients with systemic infiltrative disease involving the heart. *Am. J. Cardiol.,* **39:**184, 1977.

Browne, P. F.; Desser, K. B.; Benchimol, A.; *et al.:* The echocardiographic correlates of left ventricular hypertrophy diagnosed by electrocardiography. *J. Electrocardiol.,* **10:**105, 1977.

Cabin, H. S.; Costello, R. M.; Vasudevan, G.; *et al.:* Cardiac lymphoma mimicking hypertrophic cardiomyopathy. *Am. Heart J.,* **102:**466, 1981.

D'Cruz, I.; Hirsch, L.; Prabhu, R.; *et al.:* Intramural myocardial echographic patterns during the cardiac cycle. *Circulation,* **54,** Suppl. II:84, 1976 (Abstr.).

Devereux, R. B.; Reichek, N.; Klunder, P. F.: Echocardiographic determination of left ventricular mass in man; anatomic validation of the method. *Circulation,* **55:**613, 1977.

Dunn, F. G.; Chandaratna, F.; deCarvalho, J. G. R.; *et al.:* Pathophysiologic assessment of hypertensive heart disease with echocardiography. *Am. J. Cardiol.,* **37:**789, 1977.

Etches, P. C.; Gribbin, B.; and Gunning, A. J.: Echocardiographic diagnosis and successful removal of cardiac fibroma in a 4-year-old child. *Br. Heart J.,* **43:**360, 1980.

Farooki, Z. Q.; Adelman, S.; and Green, E. W.: Echocardiographic differentiation of a cystic and a solid tumor of the heart. *Am. J. Cardiol.,* **39:**107, 1977.

Feigenbaum, H.: *Echocardiography.* Lea & Febiger, Philadelphia, 1981.

Feigenbaum, H.; Popp, R. C.; Chip, J. N.; et al.: Left ventricular wall thickness measured by ultrasound. *Arch. Intern. Med.*, **121**:391, 1968.

Gaasch, W. H.: Left ventricular radius to wall thickness ratio. *Am. J. Cardiol.*, **43**:1189, 1979.

Grossman, W.; McLaurin, L. P.; Moos, S. P.; et al.: Wall thickness and diastolic properties of the left ventricle. *Circulation*, **49**:129, 1974.

Haft, J. I.; and Horowitz, M. S.: *Clinical Echocardiography.* Futura Publishing Co., Mount Kisco, N.Y., 1978.

Hauser, A. M.; Gordon, S.; Cieszkoweski, M.; et al.: Severe transient left ventricular "hypertrophy" occurring during acute myocarditis. *Chest*, **83**:275, 1983.

Helak, J. W.; and Reichek, N.: Quantitation of human left ventricular mass and volume by two-dimensional echocardiography: in vitro anatomic validation. *Circulation*, **63**:1398, 1981.

Henry, W. L.; Clark, C. E.; and Epstein, S. E.: Asymmetric septal hypertrophy. Echocardiographic identification of the pathognomonic anatomic abnormality of IHSS. *Circulation*, **47**:225, 1973.

Horton, J. D.; Sherber, H. S.; and Lakatta, E. G.: Distance correction for precordial electrocardiographic voltage in estimating left ventricular mass, an echocardiographic study. *Circulation*, **55**:509, 1977.

Kleid, J. J.; and Arvan, S. B.: *Echocardiography: Interpretation and Diagnosis.* Appleton-Century-Crofts, New York, 1978.

McFarland, T. M.; Alam, M.; Goldstein, S.; et al.: Echocardiographic diagnosis of left ventricular hypertrophy. *Circulation*, **57**:1140, 1978.

Nanda, N. C., and Gramiak R.: *Clinical Echocardiography.* C. V. Mosby, St. Louis, 1977.

Ormsond, G. S.; Knight, L.; Debner, L. P.; et al.: Alveolar rhabdomyosarcoma involving the heart: An echocardiographic, angiocardiographic and pathologic study. *Circulation*, **54**:837, 1976.

Reichek, N., and Devereux, R. B.: Left ventricular hypertrophy: Relationship of anatomic, echocardiographic and electrocardiographic findings. *Circulation*, **64**:1139, 1981.

Reichek, N.; Helak, J.; Plappert, T.; et al.: Anatomic validation of left ventricular mass estimates from clinical two-dimensional echocardiography. *Circulation*, **67**:348, 1983.

Reiner, L.; Mazzoleni, A.; Rodriguez, F. L.; et al.: The weight of the human heart. I. Normal cases. *Arch. Pathol.*, **68**:68, 1959.

Sjogren, A. L.; Hytonen, I.; and Frick, M. H.: Ultrasonic measurements of left ventricular wall thickness. *Chest*, **57**:37, 1970.

Toshima, H.; Koga, Y.; and Kimura, N.: Correlations between electrocardiographic, vectorcardiographic, and echocardiographic findings in patients with left ventricular overload. *Am. Heart J.*, **93**:547, 1977.

Troy, B. L.; Pombo, J.; and Rackley, C. E.: Measurement of left ventricular wall thickness and mass by echocardiography. *Circulation*, **45**:602, 1972.

HYPERTENSIVE HEART DISEASE

Cohen, A.; Hagan, A. D.; Watkins, J.; et al.: Clinical correlates in hypertensive patients with left ventricular hypertrophy diagnosed with echocardiography. *Am. J. Cardiol.*, **47**:335, 1981.

Doi, Y. L.; Deanfield, J. E.; McKenna, W. J.; et al.: Echocardiographic differentiation of hypertensive heart disease and hypertrophic cardiomyopathy. *Br. Heart J.*, **44**:395, 1980.

Dunn, F. G.; Chandaratna, P.; deCarvalho, J. G. R.; et al.: Pathophysiologic assessment of hypertensive heart disease with echocardiography. *Am. J. Cardiol.*, **39**:789, 1977.

Fouad, F. M.; Nakashima, Y.; Tarazi, R. C.; et al.: Reversal of left ventricular hypertrophy in hypertensive patients treated with methyldopa. *Am. J. Cardiol.*, **49**:795, 1982.

Karliner, J. S.; Williams, D.; Gorwit, J.; et al.: Left ventricular performance in patients with left ventricular hypertrophy caused by systemic arterial hypertension. *Br. Heart J.*, **39**:1239, 1977.

Maron, B. J.; Edwards, J. E.; and Epstein, S. E.: Disproportionate septal thickening in patients with systemic hypertension. *Chest*, **73**:466, 1978.

Reichek, N.; Franklin, B. B.; Chandler, T.; et al.: Reversal of left ventricular hypertrophy by antihypertensive therapy. *Eur. Heart J.*, **3**, Suppl. A: 169, 1982.

Safar, M. E.; Lehner, J. P.; Vincent, M. I.; et al.: Echocardiographic dimensions in borderline and sustained hypertension. *Am. J. Cardiol.*, **44**:930, 1979.

Savage, D. D.; Drayer, J. I. M.; Henry, W. L.; et al.: Echocardiographic assessment of cardiac anatomy and function in hypertensive subjects. *Circulation*, **59**:623, 1979.

Schlant, R. V.; Felner, J. M.; Blumenstein, A.; et al.: Echocardiographic documentation of regression of left ventricular hypertrophy in patients treated for essential hypertension. *Eur. Heart J.*, **3**, Suppl. A: 171, 1982.

Takahashi, M.; Sasayama, S.; Kawai, C.; et al.: Contractile performance of the hypertrophied ventricle in patients with systemic hypertension. *Circulation*, **62**:116, 1980.

LV IN ATHLETES

Allen, H. D.; Goldberg, S. J.; Sahn, D. J.; et al.: A quantitative echocardiographic study of champion childhood swimmers. *Circulation*, **55**:142, 1977.

DeMaria, A. N.; Neumann, A.; Lee, G.; et al.: Alterations in ventricular mass and performance induced by exercise training in man evaluated by echocardiography. *Circulation*, **57**:237, 1978.

Gilbert, C. A.; Nutter, D. O.; Felner, J. M.; et al.: Echocardiographic study of cardiac dimensions and function in the endurance-trained athletes. *Am. J. Cardiol.*, **40**:528, 1977.

Ikäheimo, J. M.; Palatsi, I. J.; and Takkunen, J. T.: Noninvasive evaluation of the athletic heart-sprinters versus endurance runners. *Am. J. Cardiol.*, **44**:24, 1979.

Laurenceau, J. L.; Turcot, J.; and Dumesnil, J.: Echocardiographic findings in Olympic athletes. *Circulation*, **56**:III-25, 1977 (Abstr.).

Morganroth, J.; Maron, B. J.; Henry, W. L.; et al. Comparative left ventricular dimension in trained athletes. *Ann. Intern. Med.*, **82**:521, 1975.

Nishimura, T.; Yamada, Y.; and Kawai, C.: Echocardiographic evaluation of long-term effects of exercise on left ventricular hypertrophy and function in professional bicyclists. *Circulation*, **61**:832, 1980.

Roeske, W. R.; O'Rourke, R. A.; Klein, A.; et al.: Noninvasive evaluation of ventricular hypertrophy in professional athletes. *Circulation*, **53**:286, 1976.

Roskoff, W. J.; Goldman, S.; and Cohen, K.: The athletic heart: Prevalence and physiological significance of left ventricular enlargement in distance runners. *JAMA*, **236**:158, 1976.

Rost, R.: The athlete's heart. *Eur. Heart J.*, **3**, Suppl. A: 193, 1982.

Stein, R. A.; Michielli, D.; Diamond, J.; et al.: The cardiac response to exercise training: Echocardiographic analysis at rest and during exercise. *Am. J. Cardiol.*, **46**:219, 1980.

LV in Diastolic Overload States

Aortic and Mitral Valve Disease

Abdulla, A. M.; Frank, M. J.; Canedo, M. I.; *et al.:* Limitations of echocardiography in the assessment of left ventricular size and function in aortic regurgitation. *Circulation,* **61:**148, 1980.

Clark, R. D.; Korcuska, K.; and Cohn, K.: Serial echocardiographic evaluation of left ventricular function in valvular disease, including reproducibility guidelines for serial studies. *Circulation,* **62:**564, 1980.

Danford, H. G.; Danford, D. A.; Mielke, J. E.; *et al.:* Echocardiographic evaluation of the hemodynamic effects of chronic aortic insufficiency with observations on left ventricular performance. *Circulation,* **48:**253, 1973.

Gaasch, W. H.; Andrias, C. W.; and Levine, H. J.: Chronic aortic regurgitation: The effect of aortic valve replacement on left ventricular volume, mass and function. *Circulation,* **58:**825, 1978.

Henry, W. L.; Bonow, R. O.; Rosing, D. R.; *et al.:* Observations on the optimum time for operative intervention for aortic regurgitation. II. Serial echocardiographic evaluation of asymptomatic patients. *Circulation,* **61:**484, 1980.

Henry, W. L.; Bonow, R. O.; Borer, J. S.; *et al.:* Evaluation of aortic valve replacement in patients with valvular aortic stenosis. *Circulation,* **61:**814, 1980.

Johnson, A. D.; Alpert, J. S.; and Francis, G. S.: Assessment of left ventricular function in severe aortic regurgitation. *Circulation,* **54:**975, 1976.

McDonald, I. G.: Echocardiographic assessment of left ventricular function in aortic valve disease. *Circulation,* **53:**860, 1976a.

McDonald, I. G.: Echocardiographic assessment of left ventricular function in mitral valve disease. *Circulation,* **53:**865, 1976b.

McDonald, I. G.; and Jelinek, V. M.: Serial M-mode echocardiography in severe chronic aortic regurgitation. *Circulation,* **62:**1291, 1980.

Rosenblatt, A.; Clark, R.; Burgess, J.; *et al.:* Echocardiographic assessment of the level of cardiac compensation in valvular heart disease. *Circulation,* **54:**509, 1976.

Saltissi, S.; Crowther, A.; Byrne, C.; *et al.:* Assessment of prognostic factors in patients undergoing surgery for nonrheumatic mitral regurgitation. *Br. Heart J.,* **44:**369, 1980.

Schuler, G.; Peterson, K.; and Johnson, A. D.: Serial noninvasive assessment of left ventricular hypertrophy and function after surgical correction of aortic regurgitation. *Am. J. Cardiol.,* **44:**585, 1979.

Venco, A.; St. John Sutton, M. G.; Gibson, E. G.; *et al.:* Non-invasive assessment of left ventricular function after correction of severe aortic regurgitation. *Br. Heart J.,* **38:**1324, 1976.

Anemia

Gerry, J. L.; Baird, M. G.; and Fortuin, N. J.: Evaluation of left ventricular function in patients with sickle cell anemia. *Am. J. Med.,* **60:**1968, 1976.

Lewis, B. S.; Rachmilewitz, E. A.; Amitai, N.; *et al.:* Left ventricular function of B-thalassemia and the effect of multiple transfusions. *Am. Heart J.,* **96:**636, 1978.

Pregnancy

Laird-Meeter, K.; van de Ley, G.; Bom, T. H.; *et al.:* Cardiocirculatory adjustments during pregnancy—an echocardiographic study. *Clin. Cardiol.,* **2:**328, 1979.

Rubler, S.; Damani, P. M.; and Pinto, E. R.: Cardiac size and performance during pregnancy estimated with echocardiography. *Am. J. Cardiol.,* **40:**534, 1977.

LV Volume Estimation (M-Mode)

Betenkie, I.; Hutter, D. O.; Clark, D. W.; *et al.:* Assessment of left ventricular dimensions and function by echocardiography. *Am. J. Cardiol.,* **31:**755, 1973.

Bhatt, D. R.; Isabel-Jones, J. B.; Villoria, G. J.; *et al.:* Accuracy of echocardiography in assessing left ventricular dimensions and volume. *Circulation,* **57:**699, 1978.

Brenner, J. I.; Waugh, R. A.; and Harsh, R. D.: Effect of phasic respiration on left ventricular dimension and performance in a normal population: An echocardiographic study. *Circulation,* **57:**122, 1978.

DeMaria, A. N.; Neumann, A.; Schubart, P. J.; *et al.:* Systemic correlation of cardiac chamber size and ventricular performance determined with echocardiography and alterations in heart rate in normal persons. *Am. J. Cardiol.,* **43:**1, 1979.

Feigenbaum, H.; Popp, R. L.; Wolfe, S. B.; *et al.:* Ultrasonic measurement of left ventricle: A correlative study with angiocardiography. *Arch. Intern. Med.,* **129:**461, 1972.

Gibson, D. G.: Measurement of left ventricular volumes in man by echocardiography—comparison with biplane angiography. *Br. Heart J.,* **33:**614, 1972.

Gutgesell, H. P.; Paquet, M.; and Dunn, D. F.: Evaluation of left ventricular size and function by echocardiography: Results in normal children. *Circulation,* **56:**457, 1977.

Kronik, G.; Slany, J.; and Mosslacher, H.: Comparative value of eight M-mode echocardiographic formulas for determining left ventricular stroke volume. A correlative study with thermodilution and left ventricular single-plane cineangiography. *Circulation,* **60:**1308, 1979.

Ladipo, G. O. A.; Dunn, F. G.; and Pringle, T. H.: Serial measurements of left ventricular dimensions by echocardiography. Assessment of week-to-week inter- and intraobserver variability in normal subjects and patients with valvular heart disease. *Br. Heart J.,* **44:**284, 1980.

Linhart, J. W.; Mintz, G. S.; Segal, B. L.; *et al.:* Left ventricular volume measurements by echocardiography: Fact or fancy? *Am. J. Cardiol.,* **36:**114, 1975.

Ludbrook, P.; Karliner, J. S.; Peterson, K. L.; *et al.:* Comparison of ultrasound and cineangiographic assessment of left ventricular performance in patients with and without wall motion abnormalities. *Br. Heart J.,* **35:**1026, 1973.

Murray, J. A.; Johnston, W.; and Reid, J. M.: Echocardiographic determination of left ventricular performance. *Ann. Intern. Med.,* **72:**777, 1970.

Pombo, J. P.; Troy, B. L.; and Russell, R. O.: Left ventricular volumes and ejection fraction by echocardiography. *Circulation,* **43:**480, 1971.

Popp, R. L.; and Harrison, D. C.: An atraumatic method for stroke volume determination using ultrasound. *Clin. Res.,* **17:**258, 1969.

Popp, R. L.; Filly, K.; Brown, O. R.; *et al.:* Effect of transducer placement on echocardiographic measurement of left ventricular dimensions. *Am. J. Cardiol.,* **38:**537, 1975.

Quinones, M. A.; Pickering, E.; and Alexander, J. K.: Percentage of shortening of the echocardiographic left ventricular dimension: Its use in determining ejection fraction and stroke volume. *Chest,* **74:**59, 1978.

Starlin, M. R.; Crawford, M. H.; and O'Rourke, R. A.: Accuracy of subxiphoid echocardiography for assessing left ventricular size and performance. *Circulation,* **61:**367, 1980.

Teichholz, L. E.; Krevien, T.; and Herman, M. V.: Problems in echocardiographic volume determinations: Echocardiographic correlations in the presence or absence of asynergy. *Am. J. Cardiol.*, **37:**7, 1976.

LV VOLUME (2-D ECHO)

Carr, K. W.; Engler, R. L.; Forsythe, J. R.; *et al.:* Measurement of left ventricular ejection fraction by mechanical cross-sectional echocardiography. *Circulation,* **59:**1196, 1979.

Chaudry, K. R.; Ogawa, S.; Pauletto, J. F.; *et al.:* Biplane measurements of right and left ventricular volumes using wide-angle cross-sectional echocardiography. *Am. J. Cardiol.,* **41:**391, 1978.

Folland, E. F.; Parisi, A. F.; Moynihan, A. F.; *et al.:* Assessment of left ventricular ejection fraction and volumes by real-time, two-dimensional echocardiography. A comparison of cineangiographic and radionuclide techniques. *Circulation,* **60:**760, 1979.

Gehrke, J.; Leaman, S.; Raphael, M.; *et al.:* Noninvasive left ventricular volume determination by two-dimensional echocardiography. *Br. Heart J.,* **37:**911, 1975.

Geiser, E. A.; Skorton, D. J.; and Conetta, D. A.: Quantification of left ventricular function by two-dimensional echocardiography: Consideration of factors restricting image quality. *Am. Heart J.,* **103:**905, 1982.

Heng, M. K.; Wyatt, H. L.; Meerbaum, S.; *et al.:* An analysis of the reproducibility of two-dimensional echocardiographic measurements. *Am. J. Cardiol.,* **41:**390, 1978.

Henry, W. L.: Evaluation of ventricular function using two-dimensional echocardiography. *Am. J. Cardiol.,* **49:**1319, 1982.

Quinones, M. A.; Waggoner, A. D.; Reduto, L. A.; *et al.:* A new, simplified and accurate method for determining ejection fraction with two-dimensional echocardiography. *Circulation,* **64:**744, 1981.

Rich, S.; Sheikh, A.; Gallastegni, J.; *et al.:* Determination of left ventricular ejection fraction by visual estimation during real-time two-dimensional echocardiography. *Am. Heart J.,* **104:**603, 1982.

Schiller, N. B.; Aquatella, H.; Ports, T. A.; *et al.:* Left ventricular volume from paired biplane two-dimensional echocardiography. *Circulation,* **60:**547, 1979.

Silverman, N. H.; Ports, T. A.; Snider, A. R.; *et al.:* Determination of left ventricular volume in children: Echocardiographic and angiographic comparisons. *Circulation,* **62:**548, 1980.

Stamm, R. B.; Carabello, B. A.; Meyers, D. C.; *et al.:* Two-dimensional echocardiographic measurement of left ventricular ejection fraction. Prospective analysis of what constitutes an adequate determination. *Am. Heart J.;* **104:**136, 1982.

Teichholz, L. E.; Cohen, M. V.; Sonnenblick, E. H.; *et al.:* Study of left ventricular geometry and function by B-scan ultrasonography in patients with and without asynergy. *N. Engl. J. Med.,* **291:**1220, 1974.

Tortoledo, F. A.; Quinones, M. A.; Fernandez, G. L.; *et al.:* Quantification of left ventricular volumes by two-dimensional echocardiography: A simplified and accurate approach. *Circulation,* **67:**579, 1983.

LV FUNCTION ESTIMATION BY AORTIC AND MITRAL ECHOGRAMS

Burggraf, G. W.; Mathew, T.; and Parker, J. O.: Aortic root motion determined by ultrasound: Relation to cardiac performance in man. *Cathet. Cardiovasc. Diagn.* **4:**29, 1978.

Burrows, B.; Kettel, J. L.; Nideu, A. H.; *et al.:* Patterns of cardiovascular dysfunction in chronic obstructive lung disease. *N. Engl. J. Med.,* **286:**912, 1972.

Child, J. S.; Krivokapich, J.; Perloff, J. K.: Effect of left ventricular size on mitral E point to ventricular septal separation in assessment of cardiac performance. *Am. Heart J.,* **101:**797, 1981.

D'Cruz, I. A.; Lalmalani, G. G.; Sambasivan, V.; *et al.:* The superiority of mitral E point-ventricular separation to other echocardiographic indicators of left ventricular performance. *Clin. Cardiol.,* **2:**140, 1979.

DeMaria, A.; Miller, R. R.; Amsterdam, E. A.; *et al.:* Mitral valve early diastolic closing velocity on echogram: Relation to sequential diastolic flow and ventricular compliance. *Am. J. Cardiol.,* **37:**693, 1976.

Duchak, J. M.; Chang, S.; and Feigenbaum, H.: The posterior mitral valve echo and the echocardiographic diagnosis of mitral stenosis. *Am. J. Cardiol.,* **29:**628, 1972.

Garrard, C. L.; Weissler, A. M.; and Dodge, H. T.: The relationship of alterations in systolic time intervals to ejection fraction in patients with cardiac disease. *Circulation,* **42:**455, 1970.

Goodman, D. J.; Harrison, D. C.; and Popp, R. L.: Echocardiographic features of primary pulmonary hypertension. *Am. Heart J.,* **86:**847, 1973.

Gramiak, R., and Shah, P. M.: Echocardiography of the normal and diseased aortic valve. *Radiology,* **96:**1, 1970.

Hirschfeld, S.; Meyer, R.; Korfhagen, J.; *et al.:* The isovolumic contraction time of the left ventricle. An echographic study. *Circulation,* **54:**751, 1976.

Hodges, M.; Halpern, B. L.; Riesinger, G. C.; *et al.:* Left ventricular pre-ejection period and ejection time in patients with acute myocardial infarction. *Circulation,* **45:**933, 1972.

Kachel, R. G.: Left ventricular function in chronic obstructive pulmonary disease. *Chest,* **74:**286, 1978.

Kavey, R. E. W.; Krongrad, E.; and Gersony, W. M.: Perioperative echocardiographic evaluation of cardiovascular function: Assessment of changing hemodynamic state. *Circulation,* **62:**773, 1980.

Kleid, J. J., and Schiller, N. B.: *Echocardiographic Case Studies.* Medical Examination, New York, 1974, pp. 124–125.

Konecke, L. L.; Feigenbaum, H.; Chang, S.; *et al.:* Abnormal mitral valve motion in patients with elevated left ventricular diastolic pressures. *Circulation,* **47:**989, 1973.

Krayenbuhl, H. P.; Turine, J.; and Hess, O.: Left ventricular function in chronic pulmonary hypertension. *Am. J. Cardiol.,* **41:**1150, 1978.

Layton, C.; Gent, G.; Pridie, R.; *et al.:* Diastolic closure rate of normal mitral valve. *Br. Heart J.,* **35:**1066, 1973.

Lew, W.; Henning, H.; Schelbert, H.; *et al.:* Assessment of mitral valve E point–septal separation as an index of left ventricular performance in patients with acute and previous myocardial infarction. *Am. J. Cardiol.,* **41:**835, 1978.

Massie, B. M.; Schiller, N. B.; Ratshin, R. A.; *et al.:* Mitral-septal separation: New echocardiographic index of left ventricular function. *Am. J. Cardiol.,* **39:**1008, 1977.

McLaurin, L. P.; Gibson, T. C.; Waider, W.; *et al.:* An appraisal of mitral valve echocardiograms mimicking mitral stenosis in conditions with right ventricular pressure overload. *Circulation,* **48:**801, 1973.

Pratt, R. C.; Parisi, A. F.; Harrington, J. J.; *et al.:* The influence of left ventricular stroke volume on aortic root motion. An echocardiographic study. *Circulation,* **53:**947, 1976.

Quinones, M. A.; Gaasch, W. H.; and Waisser, E.: Reduction in the rate of diastolic descent of the mitral valve echogram in patients with altered left ventricular diastolic pressure-volume relations. *Circulation,* **49:**246, 1974.

Rasmussen, S.; Corya, B. C.; Feigenbaum, H.; *et al.:* Stroke volume calculated from the mitral valve echogram in patients with and without ventricular dyssynergy. *Circulation,* **58:**125, 1978.

Stefadouros, M. A., and Witham, A. C.: Systolic time intervals by echocardiography. *Circulation,* **51:**114, 1975.

Wasserman, A. G.; Meyer, J. F.; and Ross, A. M.: The relationship of pulmonary artery wedge pressure to the posterior aortic wall echocardiogram in patients free of mitral valve disease. *Am. Heart J.,* **100:**500, 1980.

Weissler, A. M.; Harris, W. S.; and Schoenfeld, D. C.: Systolic time intervals in heart failure in man. *Circulation,* **37:**149, 1968.

Weissler, A. M.; Harris, W. S.; and Schoenfeld, D. C.: Bedside techniques for the evaluation of ventricular function in man. *Am. J. Cardiol.,* **23:**577, 1969.

Wilson, J. R.; Robertson, J. F.; Halford, F.; *et al.:* Evaluation of M-mode echographic estimates of left ventricular function: Relationship of selected ultrasonic and hemodynamic parameters. *Am. Heart J.,* **101,** 249, 1981.

LV Posterior Wall Motion

Conetta, D. A.; Christie, L. G.; Wise, D. E.; *et al.:* Echocardiographic analysis of systolic and diastolic left ventricular wall motion in normal man. *Chest,* **76:**76, 1979.

Fujii, J.; Watanabe, H.; Koyama, S.; *et al.:* Echocardiographic study on diastolic posterior wall movement and left ventricular filling by disease category. *Am. Heart J.,* **98:**144, 1979.

Gibson, D., and Brown, D.: Measurement of instantaneous left ventricular dimension and filling rate in man, using echocardiography. *Br. Heart J.,* **35:**1141, 1973.

Kraunz, R., and Kennedy, J.: Ultrasonic determination of left ventricular wall motion in normal man: Studies at rest and after exercise. *Am. Heart J.,* **79:**36, 1970.

McDonald, I. G.; Feigenbaum, H.; and Chang, S.: Analysis of left ventricular wall motion by reflected ultrasound: Application to assessment of myocardial function. *Circulation,* **46:**14, 1972.

Quinones, M. A.; Gaasch, W. H.; and Alexander, J. K.: Echocardiographic assessment of left ventricular function: With special reference to normalized velocities. *Circulation,* **50:**42, 1974.

LV Tumors (Neoplasms)

Biancaniello, T. M.; Meyer, R. A.; and Gaum, W. E.: Primary benign intramural tumors in children. *Am. Heart J.,* **103:**852, 1982.

Farooki, Z. Q.; Adelman, S.; and Green, E. W.: Echocardiographic differentiation of a cystic and solid tumor of the heart. *Am. J. Cardiol.,* **39:**107, 1977.

Miller, J.; Teichholz, L. E.; Pickard, A. D.; *et al.:* Left ventricular myxoma. *Am. J. Med.,* **63:**816, 1977.

Morgan, D. L.; Palazola, J.; Reed, W.; *et al.:* Left heart myxomas. *Am. J. Cardiol.,* **40:**611, 1977.

Ong, L. S.; Nanda, N. C.; and Barold, S. S.: Two-dimensional echocardiographic detection and diagnostic features of left ventricular papillary fibroelastoma. *Am. Heart J.,* **103:**817, 1982.

Orsmond, G. S.; Knight, L.; Dehner, L. P.; *et al.:* Alveolar rhabdomyosarcoma involving the heart. An echocardiographic, angiographic and pathologic study. *Circulation,* **54:**837, 1976.

Ports, T. A.; Cogan, J.; Schiller, N. B.; *et al.:* Echocardiography of left ventricular masses. *Circulation,* **58:**528, 1978.

LV Thrombi

Asinger, R. W.; Mikell, F. L.; Francis, G.; *et al.:* Serial evaluation for left ventricular thrombus during acute transmural myocardial infarction using two-dimensional echocardiography. *Am. J. Cardiol.,* **45:**483, 1980.

Chen, C. C.; Webster, A. W.; and Morganroth, J.: Large mobile pedunculated left ventricular thrombus: Identification by two-dimensional echocardiography. *Clin. Cardiol.,* **4:**189, 1981.

Come, P. C.; Markis, J. E.; Vine, H. S.; *et al.:* Echocardiographic diagnosis of left ventricular thrombi. *Am. Heart J.,* **100:**523, 1980.

D'Cruz, I. A.; Devaraj, N.; Hirsch, L. J.; *et al.:* Unusual echocardiographic appearances attributable to submitral calcification simulating left ventricular masses. *Clin. Cardiol.,* **3:**260, 1980.

DeJoseph, R. L.; Shiroff, R. A.; Levinson, C. W.; *et al.:* Echocardiographic diagnosis of intraventricular clot. *Chest,* **71:**417, 1977.

DeMaria, A. N.; Bommer, W.; Newmann, A.; *et al.:* Left ventricular thrombi identified by cross-sectional echocardiography. *Ann. Intern. Med.,* **90:**14, 1979.

Drobac, M.; Rakowski, H.; Gilbert, B. W.; *et al.:* Two-dimensional echocardiographic recognition of mural thrombi: in-vivo and in-vitro studies. *Am. J. Cardiol.,* **45:**435, 1980 (Abstr.).

Ezekowitz, M. D.; Wilson, D. A.; and Smith, E. O.: Comparison of Indium 111 platelet scintigraphy and two-dimensional echocardiography in the diagnosis of left ventricular thrombi. *N. Engl. J. Med.,* **304:**1509, 1982.

Gottdiener, J.; VanVoorhees, L.; Gay, J.; *et al.:* Incidence and embolic potential of left ventricular thrombus in cardiomyopathy: Assessment by two-dimensional echocardiography. *Am. J. Cardiol.,* **49:**1029, 1982 (Abstr.).

Horgan, J. H.; O'M. Shiel, F.; and Goodman, A. C.: Demonstration of left ventricular thrombus by conventional echocardiography. *J. CU.,* **4:**287, 1976.

Kleid, J. J., and Arvan, S. B.: *Echocardiography: Interpretation and Diagnosis.* Appleton-Century-Crofts, New York, 1978, p. 246.

Kramer, N. E.; Rathod, R.; and Chawla, K. K.; *et al.:* Echocardiographic diagnosis of left ventricular mural thrombi occurring in cardiomyopathy. *Am. Heart J.,* **96:**381, 1978.

Levisman, J. A.; McAlpin, R. N.; Abbasi, A. S.; *et al.:* Echocardiographic diagnosis of a mobile pedunculated tumor in the left ventricular cavity. *Am. J. Cardiol.,* **36:**957, 1975.

Lewin, R. F.; Vidue, B.; Sclerovsky, G.; *et al.:* Two-dimensional real-time echocardiographic detection of a left ventricular aneurysm associated with mobile pedunculated thrombi. *Chest,* **77:**704, 1980.

McManus, B. M.; Goldberg, S. D.; Triche, T. J.; *et al.:* Elongate thrombus extending from left ventricular apex to outflow tract. *Am. Heart J.,* **105:**327, 1983.

Meltzer, R. S.; Guthaner, D.; Rakowski, H.; *et al.:* Diagnosis of left ventricular thrombi by two-dimensional echocardiography. *Br. Heart J.,* **42:**261, 1979.

Mikell, F. L.; Asinger, R. W.; Elsperger, K. J.; *et al.:* Regional stasis of blood in the dysfunctional left ventricle: Echocardiographic detection and differentiation from early thrombus. *Circulation,* **66:**755, 1982.

Nagri, N.; Popp, R. L.; and Coltart, D. J.: Diagnosis of

left ventricular thrombus by two-dimensional echocardiography. *Eur. J. Cardiol.,* **11:**235, 1980.

Ports, T. A.; Cogan, J.; Schiller, N. B.; and Rapaport, E.: Echocardiography of left ventricular masses. *Circulation,* **58:**528, 1978.

Quinones, M. A.; Nelson, J. C.; Winters, W. L.; *et al.:* Clinical spectrum of left ventricular mural thrombi in a large cardiac population: Assessment by two dimensional echocardiography. *Am. J. Cardiol.,* **45:**435, 1980 (Abstr.).

Sabot, G.; Fauvel, J. M.; and Bonnhoure, J. P.: Echocardiographic diagnosis of mobile left ventricular tumor. *Br. Heart J.,* **42:**112, 1979.

Stratton, J. R.; Light, G. W.; Pearlman, A. S.; *et al.:* Detection of left ventricular thrombus by two-dimensional echocardiography. *Circulation,* **66:**156, 1982.

Suzuki, S.; Yanagisawa, M.; Yano, S.; *et al.:* Cross-sectional echocardiographic findings of left ventricular thrombi in a ten-year-old patient with cardiomyopathy. *Jpn. Heart J.,* **20:**675, 1979.

van den Bos, A.; Vletter, B. B.; and Hagemeijer, F.: Progressive development of a left ventricular thrombus: Detection and evaluation studied with echocardiographic techniques. *Chest,* **74:**307, 1978.

van Meurs-Van Woezik, H.; Meltzer, R. S.; van den Brand, M.; *et al.:* Superiority of echocardiography over angiocardiography in diagnosing a left ventricular thrombus. *Chest,* **80:**321, 1981.

ABNORMAL ECHOES IN THE LV OUTFLOW TRACT

Barron, J. V.; Sahn, D. G.; Valdez-Cruz, L. M.; *et al.:* Two-dimensional echocardiographic features of ventricular septal aneurysm paradoxically bulging into the left ventricular outflow tract. *Am. Heart J.,* **104:**156, 1982.

Chandaratna, P. A. N.; Robinson, M. J.; Byrd, C.; *et al.:* Significance of abnormal echoes in the left ventricular outflow tract. *Br. Heart J.,* **39:**381, 1977.

Gardin, J. M.; Talano, J. V.; Stephanides, L.; *et al.:* Systolic anterior motion in the absence of asymmetric septal hypertrophy. A buckling phenomenon of the chordae tendineae. *Circulation,* **63:**181, 1981.

Gay, J. A.; Gottdiener, J. S.; Gomes, M. N.; *et al.:* Echocardiographic features of traumatic disruption of the aortic valve. *Chest,* **83:**150, 1983.

Nishimura, T.; Kondo, M.; Umadome, H.; *et al.:* Echocardiographic features of false tendons in the left ventricle. *Am. J. Cardiol.,* **48:**177, 1981.

Schneeweiss, A.; Motro, M.; Shem-Tor, A.; *et al.:* Echocardiographic diagnosis of a discrete membranous subaortic stenosis with aneurysm of the membrane. *Chest,* **82:**194, 1982.

Van Leeuwen, K.; Fast, J. H.; Deppenbrock, J. H. M.; *et al.:* Abnormal echoes in the left ventricular outflow tract caused by ruptured chordae tendineae of the mitral valve. *Chest,* **81:**103, 1982.

J

Hypertrophic Cardiomyopathy

Confirmation or exclusion of the diagnosis of hypertrophic cardiomyopathy constitutes one of the principal applications of ultrasound to cardiology. This important cardiac entity, unknown to medical science 25 years ago, was discovered by pathologists, cardiac surgeons, and "hemodynamic" cardiologists in the late 1950s and 1960s and came under intense study by echocardiographers all through the 1970s.

Fortunately, the ultrasound abnormalities characteristic of this disease are several and striking so that, in a classic case, the diagnosis can be made entirely on the basis of the echocardiographic findings with an extremely high degree of reliability.

On the other hand, each of these abnormalities on the M-mode echogram have been described individually in patients with various other cardiac conditions far removed from the entity of hypertrophic cardiomyopathy.

This has caused much confusion in clinical practice; it has become a semantic battleground where cardiologists misunderstand each other because they follow different schools of terminology.

The last decade has witnessed a regrettable tendency to introduce diagnostic labels, often not quite appropriate, to apply them to certain echographic signs, and then to use them as synonyms of clinical or pathologic disease entities.

A prime example is the acronym ASH (asymmetric septal hypertrophy). To some, it means asymmetry of a misshapen hypertrophied septum; to others, it is asymmetry of the left ventricle in the sense that in cut section a grossly thickened septum makes striking contrast with a relatively normal left ventricular free wall. To still others, it is synonymous with the whole clinicopathologic entity of hypertrophic cardiomyopathy.

Another important source of confusion in this field is lack of awareness of the wide spectrum of anatomic and functional variation with which hypertrophic cardiomyopathy can present:

1. More often than not, left ventricular outflow tract obstruction is present, but in a sizable minority—also known as nonobstructive ASH—there is no pressure gradient across the left ventricular outflow (Abbasi et al., 1972; Criley et al., 1975).

2. Not uncommonly, subaortic stenosis is slight or absent at rest but easily and consistently provoked by inotropic agents like digitalis or isoproterenol, or by maneuvers that decrease left ventricular size such as the Valsalva procedure or amyl nitrite inhalation. The LV outflow obstruction in such cases has been designated "latent," not to be confused with the "labile" variety wherein nonprovoked obstruction can be demonstrated on some occasions but not on others (Gilbert et al., 1980).

3. Usually the ventricular septum is much thicker than the left ventricular posterior wall, but uncommonly the two are of approximately equal thickness (concentric left ventricular hypertrophy), all other echographic and hemodynamic features being typical of IHSS.

4. The ventricular septum may not be of uniform thickness throughout its length. Sometimes it is the basal portion (near the mitral valve) that is inordinately thick, whereas in other instances septal hypertrophy is most prominent at mid-LV level, and in yet others it is at the LV apex that hypertrophy is most impressive (Yamaguchi et al., 1979).

5. The left ventricular chamber is typically narrow and attenuated, but some patients

evolve into a later stage wherein the ventricle dilates and loses its vigor of contraction so that features akin to congestive cardiomyopathy gradually appear.

All these aspects of controversy and confusion have their counterparts in clinical echocardiography, as is discussed below.

The ultrasound diagnosis of IHSS rests mainly on the demonstration of two cardinal abnormalities (Figs. J-1 to J-6):

1. An abnormally thick hypokinetic ventricular septum, much thicker than the left ventricular posterior wall, which contracts well and is of normal or only mildly increased thickness. In common usage, ASH is applied to this finding.

2. The acronym SAM is widely used to refer to abnormal systolic anterior motion of the anterior mitral leaflet of a distinctive type that consistently accompanies IHSS, the obstructive variety of hypertrophic cardiomyopathy.

Other echocardiographic findings, such as a small left ventricular chamber size, low mitral EF slope, and midsystolic partial closure of the aortic valve, are usually present but are less specific. They help or contribute to the diagnosis of IHSS only if ASH or SAM or both are evident.

Apart from the echocardiographic and hemodynamic considerations mentioned above, the diagnosis of hypertrophic cardiomyopathy has been rendered even more complex or ambiguous by entry into the arena of the histologist, who requires widespread appearances of myocardial fiber disarray, and the geneticist, who distinguishes between (1) a genetically transmitted disease found in first-degree relatives of the patients and (2) a nontransmitted variety. If at least five first-degree relatives of a patient have septal/LV wall ratios less than 1.3, the chances of the genetically transmitted true hypertrophic cardiomyopathy being present are 3 per cent or less (Maron *et al.,* 1978).

Wei *et al.* (1980) recognize even more categories of hypertrophic cardiomyopathy:

1. Wherein secondary LV hypertrophy oc-

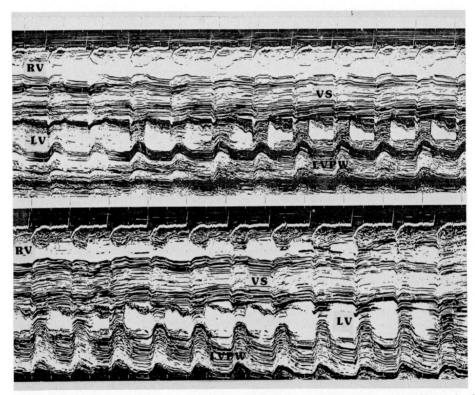

Fig. J-1. M-mode echocardiogram of a patient with classical IHSS, showing the LV at mitral valve level (*upper*) and at chordae level (*lower*). Abnormal systolic mitral motion (SAM) abutting the ventricular septum and associated mitral annulus calcification are evident in the upper panel. The ventricular septum is markedly hypertrophic, the LV posterior wall mildly hypertrophic. The LV chamber is abnormally small.

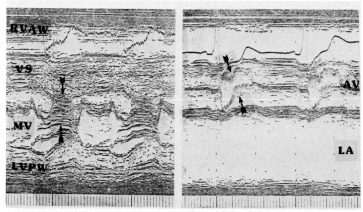

Fig. J-2. M-mode echogram of the LV at mitral valve level (*left*) and aortic root (*right*) in a patient with IHSS. The septum is markedly hypertrophied, more so than the LV posterior wall. SAM in this case consists of a conspicuous heap of multilayered echoes reaching from the normal mitral valve position up to the septum, during the latter two thirds of systole (*arrows*). In the right panel the aortic valve shows near-closure in midsystole (*arrows*). In the right panel the aortic valve shows near-closure in midsystole (*arrows*), with reopening of the anterior (right coronary) cusp but not of the posterior (noncoronary) cusp during the latter half of systole.

curs in response to severe aortic stenosis or severe long-standing hypertension, leading to a "permanent restructuring of the heart and a functional state similar to hypertrophic cardiomyopathy that may persist despite relief of the underlying causative lesion;

2. "A hypercontractile state in which hemodynamic features of hypertrophic cardiomyopathy may develop even in a normal heart under severe enough conditions of volume depletion or adrenergic stimulation," as reported earlier by the same group of investigators (Buckley and Fortuin, 1976).

Since echocardiography may reveal SAM or ASH superimposed on the original or primary cardiac pathology, it can well be imagined how complex or confused the diagnostic situation can become.

Since the echocardiographic recognition of IHSS 14 years ago (Moreya *et al.,* 1969; Shah *et al.,* 1969; Popp and Harrison, 1969; Pridie and Oakley, 1970), a sustained and intense interest in this entity has continued (Shah *et al.,* 1971, 1972; Henry *et al.,* 1974a, 1974b, 1975; Epstein *et al.,* 1974; Tajik and Giuliani, 1971; Rosen *et al.,* 1974; Morrow *et al.,* 1975; Rodger, 1976; Watson *et al.,* 1977; Chahine *et al.,* 1977; Schapira *et al.,* 1978; Maron *et al.,* 1978; ten Cate *et al.,* 1979; Doi *et al.,* 1980; Hanrath *et al.,* 1980; Wei *et al.,* 1980; Good-

win, 1980; Maron and Epstein, 1980; Gilbert *et al.,* 1980; Krajcer *et al.,* 1980).

ECHOCARDIOGRAPHIC ABNORMALITIES OF THE VENTRICULAR SEPTUM IN HYPERTROPHIC CARDIOMYOPATHY (Fig. J-7)

Normally the ventricular septum does not exceed 12 mm in end-diastolic thickness and is as thick as the left ventricular posterior wall (Henry *et al.,* 1974b). In hypertensive cardiomyopathy, the septum is 1.3 times or more as thick as the ventricular wall (Epstein *et al.,* 1974; Henry *et al.,* 1974b) and exceeds 1.3 cm in thickness. If the criteria for diagnosing ASH of hypertrophic cardiomyopathy are set at a minimum septal thickness of 1.5 cm and a minimum septal/ventricular wall ratio of 1.5, false positives are more effectively excluded (Abbasi *et al.,* 1972; Chandaratna *et al.,* 1978).

The usual ventricular level for measuring septal and left ventricular posterior wall thickness is that at which chordae tendineae are seen, below the mitral leaflet level. It has been pointed out that in some patients with IHSS (proven by catheterization and angiocardiography), an abnormally high septal/ventricular wall ratio

[*Text continued on page 304.*]

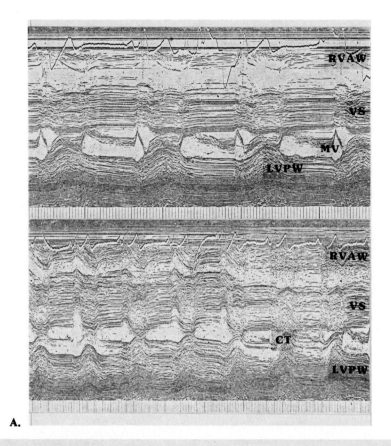

A.

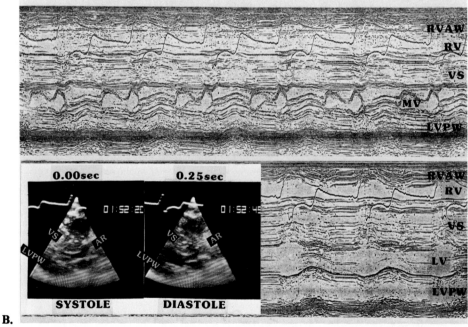

B.

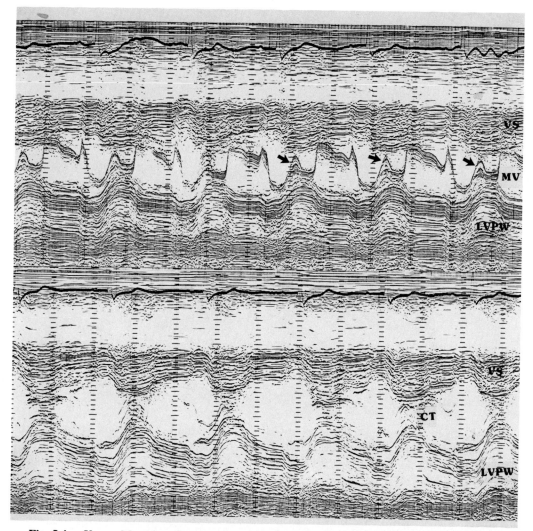

Fig. J-4. *Upper.* M-mode echogram of an elderly woman with a loud systolic ejection murmur. The upper panel shows concentric LV hypertrophy and posterior submitral mitral annulus calcification. The mitral valve exhibits abnormal systolic anterior motion (SAM) (*arrows*) of rather short duration (peak rather than plateau).

Lower. M-mode echogram of the same patient at the level of mitral chordae tendineae. At this level the LV posterior wall is actually thicker than the ventricular septum. Hypertrophy is marked in the former and mild in the latter.

Fig. J-3. *A. Opposite* M-mode echogram of a patient with findings typical of IHSS. The upper panel shows marked hypertrophy of the septum and mild hypertrophy of the LV posterior wall. Abnormal SAM of the mitral valve causes it to meet the left septal surface in midsystole. The lower panel shows even greater hypertrophy of the ventricular septum at chordae and papillary muscle level. The LV chamber is small. The posterior papillary muscle contacts the septum in midsystole.

Fig. J-3. *B. Opposite* The same patient a year later, on propranolol therapy. On M-mode as well as 2-D echography, the septal hypertrophy and diminutive LV chamber size appear unchanged, but typical SAM is no longer apparent.

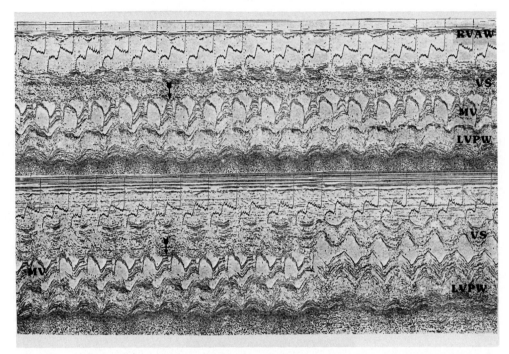

Fig. J-5.   M-mode echocardiogram of a patient with IHSS. Septal hypertrophy and SAM (*arrow*) are well visualized in the upper panel. The lower panel shows a LV scan from mitral level to chordae level (*right*), where septal thickness and motion appear normal, contrary to what is expected in IHSS.

is obtained only at the level of both mitral leaflets, whereas septal hypertrophy is less marked toward the apex, so that ASH is less prominent at that level.

Artefacts and other factors (Fig. J-7) can make the ventricular septum appear thicker on the M-mode echocardiogram than it really is for technical reasons such as:

1. Inadequate suppression of right ventricular echoes near the right septal border;

2. The ultrasound beam transecting the ventricular septum in an inappropriate direction, i.e., tangentially or obliquely (Fig. J-8) rather than perpendicularly (Fowles *et al.*, 1980).

Avoidance of fuzzy or discontinuous delineation of the endocardial echoes marking the right and left surfaces of the septum can be achieved by suitable adjustments of overall gain, near gain, transducer direction, patient positioning (left lateral), and repeated scanning of the septum from the aortic root level downward into the left ventricle as far as possible.

Even after artefacts due to technical reasons have been avoided, a reliable septal thickness may sometimes elude the echocardiographer because of uncertainty about:

1. The right septal echo. Unfortunately, it is common to encounter linear echoes in this region arising from right ventricular trabeculae or from some part of the tricuspid apparatus, which easily can be mistaken for the right septal border. Swan-Ganz catheters and pacemaker wires (Fig. J-9) in this location can likewise present as spurious septal echoes. Occasionally, a muscular band in the RV chamber can make the septum appear thicker than it actually is (Fig. J-10);

2. Identification of the left septal echo, less frequently a problem if care has been taken to record a sharp, continuous septal border. A mural thrombus adherent to the left septal surface can cause the septum to appear erroneously thick (Pollick *et al.*, 1982a); scanning to unaffected areas of the septum reveals true septal thickness and motion and identifies the mural thrombus. A neoplasm in the septal region could similarly simulate ASH (Isner *et al.*, 1979).

Reverberations from the chest wall echoes ("main bang"), right ventricular anterior wall, or catheters in the right ventricle may on occasion simulate the left septal border.

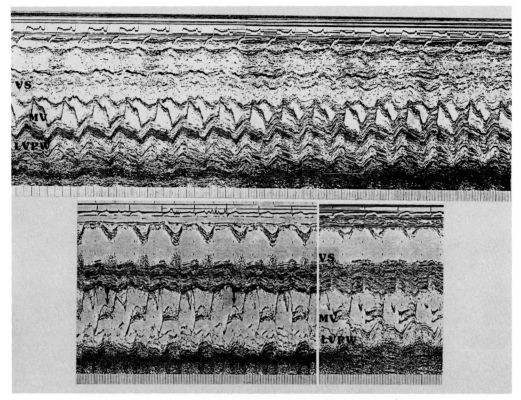

Fig. J-6. *Upper.* M-mode echogram of an elderly woman with hypertrophic cardiomyopathy and mild posterior submitral (mitral annulus) calcification. The ventricular septum and LV posterior wall are hypertrophied to about the same extent, and the LV chamber is abnormally small. Mitral systolic motion at first appears normal (*left*) but abnormal anterior motion (SAM) is revealed with only slight alteration in transducer direction (*right*).

Lower. M-mode echogram of a patient with hypertrophy of the ventricular septum but not of the LV posterior wall. Abnormal systolic anterior motion (*arrow*) of small amplitude is apparent in the left panel, but not with slight change in transducer direction (*right*). At cardiac catheterization, no LV outflow tract gradient was obtained at rest but a significant gradient could be provoked by norepinephrine.

SYSTOLIC SEPTAL MOTION AND THICKENING

The normal ventricular septum in systole moves posteriorly to an extent of at least 3 or 4 mm and undergoes an increase in thickness of at least 30 to 40 per cent. The very thick ventricular septum of IHSS, containing as it does a large mass of abnormal myocardium, presents the paradox of hypertrophy without enhanced power. Diminished septal contractility is reflected in poor posterior systolic excursions and subnormal systolic thickening—between 0 and 20 per cent (Rosen *et al.,* 1974).

In most cases of IHSS, the left ventricular posterior wall is of normal thickness and contracts vigorously, presumably to compensate for septal hypokinesis. However, it may be hypertrophied in patients with large subaortic pressure gradients or those with preexisting hypertension, but its end-diastolic thickness remains less than that of the ventricular septum.

When first described, a septal/left ventricular posterior wall thickness ratio of 1.3 or more was considered diagnostic of a long list of other cardiac conditions in which the septal thickness can equal or exceed 1.3 times the ventricular wall thickness. These conditions fall into three categories:

1. Those in which septal hypertrophy is merely part of RV hypertrophy, as the ventricular septum is as much a wall of the right ventricle as it is of the left. Thus it has been described in pulmonic stenosis (Maron *et al.,* 1977), trans-

SEPTAL HYPERTROPHY AND ITS SIMULATORS

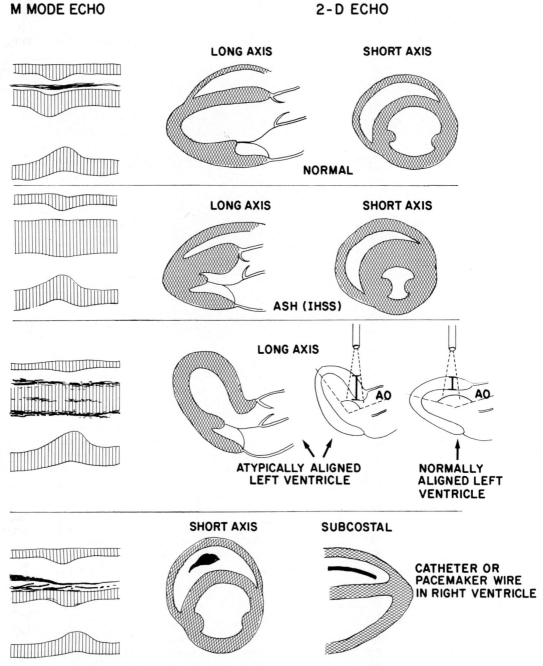

Fig. J-7. Diagram representing normal LV anatomy (*first row*) septal hypertrophy as in ASH (*second row*) and two common situations simulating septal hypertrophy (*third and fourth rows*). The M-mode appearance is shown in the left column; the 2-D appearances, in the center and right columns.

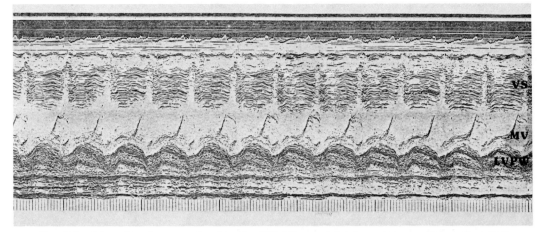

Fig. J-8. M-mode echogram showing the LV. The septal echo appears very broad at first sight, but on closer scrutiny it seems much thinner in diastole, which is rather brief in this patient because of tachycardia. In the septal hypertrophy of hypertrophic cardiomyopathy, there is little or no variation in septal thickness at different phases of the cardiac cycle. The LV posterior wall is of normal thickness. Apparent septal thickness was due to oblique or tangential orientation of the ultrasound beam through the septum.

position of great vessels (Nanda *et al.,* 1974), primary pulmonary hypertension (Goodman *et al.,* 1974; Maron *et al.,* 1977), Eisenmenger syndrome (Maron *et al.,* 1977), and normal infants (Larter *et al.,* 1976).

Maron *et al.* (1977) found a septal/LV wall ratio of 1.3 or more in 10 per cent of a large series of 304 patients (mainly adults), with both echographic and autopsy data, who had various types of congenital or acquired heart disease. Prevalence of disproportionate septal hypertrophy was more than 20 per cent in pulmonary stenosis and in primary pulmonary hypertension, but was less than 15 per cent in Eisenmenger syndrome, aortic and mitral valve disease, and did not occur in patients with atrial or ventricular septal defects. The absence of true hypertrophic cardiomyopathy in these patients with disproportionate septal hypertrophy was indicated by the absence of the histologic pattern of myocardial fiber disarray and the absence of ASH in first-degree relatives of these patients.

2. Abnormally thin left ventricular posterior wall due to infarction (Henning *et al.,* 1978). The septal/LV wall ratio is high not because of primary septal hypertrophy, but due to decrease in left ventricular posterior wall thickness secondary to replacement of myocardium by a varying degree of fibrous scar tissue. The septal thickness is normal, or in some cases

increased, due to compensatory hypertrophy or associated hypertension.

The following criteria were found useful in distinguishing hypertrophic cardiomyopathy from inferior myocardial infarction in patients with septal/LV posterior ratios of 1.3 or more (Stern *et al.,* 1978):

a. LV posterior wall *systolic* thickness less than 13 mm favors inferior wall infarction, because LV wall systolic thickening may be subnormal in infarction but would be high-normal or supranormal in hypertrophic cardiomyopathy.

b. An increase in septal/LV wall ratio during systole, as compared to diastole, favors inferior wall infarction, because septal contractility is normal or even supranormal while the inferior wall contraction is impaired. On the other hand, in hypertrophic cardiomyopathy, the LV wall is hypercontractile while the septum is hypocontractile.

c. Systolic excursion of the septum exceeding that of the LV posterior wall favors inferior wall infarction, for the same reasons.

d. Ratio of the septal thickness/systolic LV internal diameter less than 0.5 favors inferior wall infarction, because the combination of a very thick septum and an abnormally small LV results in this ratio exceeding 0.5 in patients with hypertrophic cardiomyopathy.

3. Those in whom left ventricular hypertro-

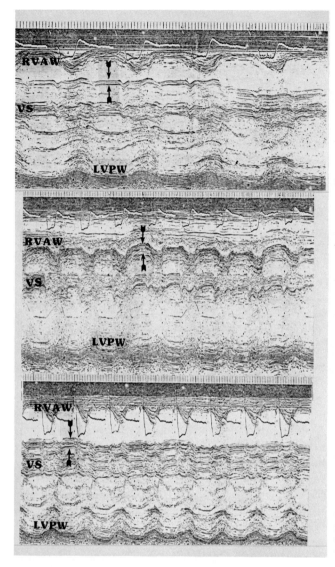

Fig. J-9. Pacemaker wire simulating abnormally thick ventricular septum.

Upper. M-mode echogram of a patient with a transvenous pacemaker. The pacemaker wire can be visualized in the RV chamber in a parasternal scan; the pacemaker echo is almost contiguous to the septal echo and tends to merge with it, at the right end of the figure. During the first 3 beats the wire can be seen (*arrows*) about 1.5 cm away from the septum and moving parallel to it. If the pacemaker echo were mistaken for the right septal border, mistaken diagnosis of a very thick septum could have been made.

Center and Lower. Subcostal (*center*) and parasternal (*lower*) echograms in a different patient with a pacemaker wire in the RV. In the center panel, the pacemaker (with perhaps surrounding endocardial fibrosis) presents as a dense echo (*arrows*) in the RV near the RV anterior wall, moving parallel to it. In fact, the pacemaker echo could be mistaken for the RV anterior wall, in which case the space between it and the true RV anterior wall could be mislabeled a small pericardial effusion. In the bottom panel in the same patient, the LV and RV are viewed in a different plane and the pacemaker echo (*arrows*) is very closely related to the septal echo and moves with it; this appearance could easily have been mistaken for marked septal hypertrophy, unless small areas of separation are detected.

phy is present, but instead of being concentric is atypically asymmetric in the sense that it affects the ventricular septum to a greater degree than the left ventricular free wall. The term "disproportionate septal thickening" (DST) proposed by Maron *et al.* (1977) seems an appropriate label for such cases; it serves to distinguish these patients from ASH associated with IHSS in the minds of clinicians, thus tending to prevent the error of confusing an innocuous anatomic variant with a myocardial disease of potentially grave prognosis. Into this category fall disproportionate septal hypertrophy in patients with hypertension (Criley *et al.*, 1975), aortic valve disease (Nanda *et al.*, 1974), coarc-

tation of the aorta (Scovil *et al.*, 1976), and chronic hemodialysis (Abbasi *et al.*, 1978).

Kansal *et al.* (1979) compared a group of 20 patients with IHSS to a group of 66 patients with LV hypertrophy due to aortic valve disease or chronic renal failure and a third group comprising 24 normal subjects. They found that a septal/LV wall ratio of 1.3 was of little value as a diagnostic criterion since it occurred often in patients with non-IHSS LV hypertrophy and even sometimes in normal individuals. They concluded that a septal/LV wall ratio ≥1.5 at mid-LV level will separate normal subjects from those with IHSS, but will fail to distinguish all or even most patients with non-IHSS

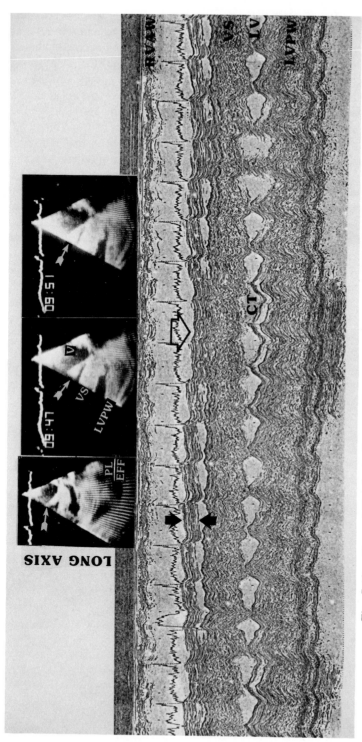

Fig. J-10. *Upper.* 2-D echocardiogram of a patient with concentric LV hypertrophy and a pleural effusion. The left frame is in the long-axis view. The center and right frames, on a larger scale, are in a plane intermediate between long- and short-axis views. An unusual echo in the RV (*arrows*) appears to be a muscular structure (probably the moderator band) inserted on the ventricular septum. It is not a papillary muscle because it has no connection with the tricuspid valve.

Lower. M-mode echogram of the same patient with extreme LV hypertrophy of concentric type. The LV chamber is very small. A muscular band about 8 mm thick is visible in the RV (*solid arrows*). At this site the band is quite separate from the right border of the ventricular septum. Elsewhere (*broad open arrow*) the band merges with the septum at its site of insertion, causing the apparent septal thickness to increase at this level.

309

LV hypertrophy from those with IHSS. A septal thickness of 15 mm or more will differentiate normal subjects from those with IHSS, but will not separate the latter from those with non-IHSS LV hypertrophy.

Gibson *et al.* (1979) found that as many as 40 of 100 patients with secondary LV hypertrophy of various etiologies had septum-to-LV posterior wall ratios of 1.3 or more.

ABNORMAL SYSTOLIC ANTERIOR MITRAL MOTION (SAM)

In IHSS the anterior mitral leaflet echo diverges in early systole into two linear components, one of which continues in its normal position, apposed to the posterior mitral leaflet; the other (abnormal) component moves rapidly forward to approach or touch the ventricular septum, remains in this abnormal position for a variable duration in midsystole, and finally moves rapidly back in the latter third of systole to rejoin the "normal" part of the mitral valve echo before the D point that signals mitral valve opening.

SAM thus consists of an abnormal hump or convexity atop the normal mitral echo. It is of variable amplitude and may be bluntly pointed, rounded, or flat-topped in contour. In its most classic form, the abnormal SAM echo appears as a dense line or band abutting against the posterior (left) border of the ventricular septum during the middle third of systole. The space between the SAM component and the normal component of the mitral valve echogram may be occupied by lesser horizontal linear echoes, which are presumed to arise from the anterior mitral leaflet or chordae tendineae. It has been demonstrated that a "pseudoejection" systolic sound can be recorded, 40 to 100 msec after onset of the upstroke of the external carotid pulse, which coincides with the abrupt halting anteriorly of SAM (Sze and Shah, 1976). Pollick *et al.* (1982b) found that the onset of the LV outflow pressure gradient was almost simultaneous with SAM–septal contact.

It is not uncommon for SAM to be of minor degree or even absent at rest but easily provoked by amyl nitrite inhalation, postextrasystolic potentiation, or the Valsalva maneuver (Fig. J-11). More often than not, the Valsalva maneuver does not yield satisfactory results because it is impossible for the echocardiographer to keep the mitral valve in full view during the thoracic exertions that accompany this procedure.

Postextrasystolic beats should be scrutinized for augmentation of SAM (Fig. J-12) when SAM is absent, minimal, or equivocal in the resting M-mode tracing. Angoff *et al.* (1978) have used an external mechanical cardiac stimulator to elicit ventricular premature beats for this purpose; however, this innovation has not entered routine echocardiographic practice.

When the ventricular rhythm is irregular (atrial fibrillation is not rare in patients with

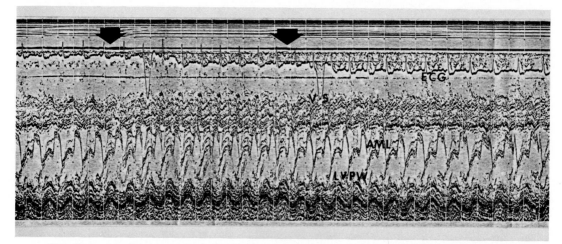

Fig. J-11. M-mode echogram at slow paper speed. At first, abnormal systolic anterior motion (SAM) of the mitral valve is not evident. It appears during the Valsalva maneuver (*interval between arrows*), and diminishes as the apneic phase ends.

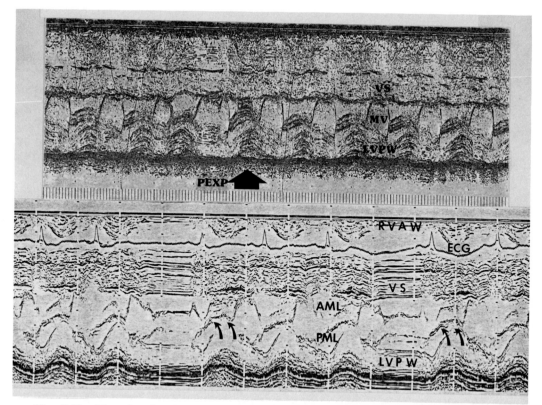

Fig. J-12. M-mode echograms of two different patients, both of whom show ASH (septum thicker than LV posterior wall) but no "classic" SAM on most leads. However, the beat following a long diastole (*arrows*) does show typical SAM, presumably because of the increased inotropy of such beats (PEXP, postextrasystolic pause). The ECG tracing is not clearly apparent in the upper panel because of baseline artefacts.

IHSS), SAM can vary in degree from beat to beat, presumably due to fluctuations in end-diastolic LV volume. Even in complete A-V block with regular ventricular rhythm in a patient with IHSS, a striking variation in the extent of SAM can be seen (Spilkin *et al.,* 1977). SAM decreased markedly when atrial systole preceded ventricular systole by an interval similar to the normal P-R interval; enhanced LV end-diastolic volume, in beats benefiting from an atrial contribution to ventricular filling, tended to diminish SAM and LV outflow obstruction.

When SAM is provokable on echocardiography, as above, a subaortic pressure gradient usually but not invariably can be elicited in the hemodynamic laboratory by acute inotropic drug intervention.

It is important to know whether the patient is or has recently been on digitalis if IHSS is being suspected. I have seen several patients

who had SAM when digitalized but not when off digitalis.

On the other hand, propranolol may suppress SAM in proven examples of IHSS, but this response is variable from one patient to another. A dose of propranolol that completely prevents SAM in one patient will be ineffective in another.

In clinical practice, the combination of ASH and SAM is a reliable predictor of dynamic LV outflow obstruction. Henry *et al.* (1974a) showed that the duration and degree of septal-mitral apposition correlate well with the severity of the subaortic pressure gradient found at cardiac catheterization. This has been confirmed recently by Gilbert *et al.* (1980), who found that systolic anterior motion of the anterior mitral leaflet such that it remains in contact with the ventricular septum during 30 per cent or more of echocardiographic systole (i.e., from C to D point) occurred in all 27 patients who demonstrated LV obstruction at rest, but in no patient with latent obstruction or no obstruction. These authors also found that aortic valve midsystolic notching (near-closure) was equally sensitive and almost as specific as an indicator of LV outflow obstruction. Surprisingly, left atrial enlargement was nearly as good a criterion of a dynamic LV outflow obstruction as SAM and aortic valve midclosure.

Others have observed that midsystolic near-closure of the aortic valve is not very sensitive as a criterion of LV outflow obstruction (normal aortic valve motion does not exclude a subaortic pressure gradient), but it may be useful diagnostically in the sense that it is perhaps more specific than ASH and SAM for this purpose (Chahine et al., 1977).

Chandaratna et al. (1978) pointed out that not only the aortic valve but also the aortic root exhibit abnormalities of systolic motion in patients with IHSS; when compared to normal subjects, anterior motion of the aortic root is steeper (more rapid) in early systole but flatter (slower) in the latter half of systole. In early diastole, the posterior motion of the aortic root is less steep (slower) than in normal subjects, but showed a more prominent late diastolic posterior motion—due to atrial contraction: the left atrium is hypertrophied in IHSS and capable of an unusually powerful atrial "kick."

Henry et al. (1974a) introduced an index of left ventricular outflow obstruction in IHSS based on measurements of the average distance between SAM and the ventricular septum and the duration of systole on the M-mode echogram. This index was shown to correlate well with the gradient at cardiac catheterization. Others have found that the predicted pressure gradient by Henry's index was often at variance with the actual gradient observed (Rosen et al., 1974).

In summary, well-marked SAM is consistently associated with a significant subaortic pressure gradient, but a quantitative echocardiographic prediction of pressure gradients is not necessarily reliable and not universally used in everyday clinical practice.

PSEUDO-SAM (Figs. J-13 and J-14)

The patterns of mitral motion that possibly can be mistaken for true SAM of IHSS are of different types, having been reported in a variety of cardiovascular situations. The term pseudo- or false SAM, if it is used at all, therefore should apply not to one specific pattern but to several different ones. These include:

1. Conditions associated with increased systolic anterior excursions of the left ventricular posterior wall as, for instance, in ventricular aneurysm elsewhere in the LV (Greenwald et al., 1975), pheochromocytoma (Cueto et al., 1979), aortic regurgitation, or mitral regurgitation. The mitral cusp echoes remain parallel to the left ventricular posterior wall endocardial echoes in systole. Systolic anterior motion of the mitral valve, though unduly large, is not suggestive of IHSS, because there is no separation of an anterior component that diverges from the main mitral echo to approach the ventricular septum. The occurrence of SAM in patients with atrial septal defects likewise has been attributed to vigorous systolic motion of the apical left ventricle. It should be added that true SAM has also been described in patients with pheochromocytoma (Shah et al., 1981).

2. Anterior mitral motion in patients with large pericardial effusions (Nanda et al., 1976), easily distinguished from true SAM because (a) swinging motion of the heart in a large pericardial effusion is evident; (b) such swinging or oscillation of the heart as a whole, and of the mitral valve and other structures along with it, disappears as soon as the effusion subsides or diminishes; and (c) on careful inspection, the mitral motion is different from true SAM: the mitral echo does not split into two components.

3. An early systolic anterior mitral motion seen in some instances of late systolic mitral prolapse. Although usually of brief duration and small amplitude, it exceptionally may be quite large, in which case it may closely resemble the *initial early systolic* phase of true SAM as seen in IHSS. However, in mitral prolapse, the mitral valve moves abruptly backward in midsystole to occupy an abnormally posterior position during the latter one half to one third of systole. Thus the late systolic phase of the mitral echo is inscribed anterior to the plane of the D point in true SAM, but posterior to it in pseudo-SAM of mitral prolapse.

4. A normal variant frequently encountered but rarely discussed in the literature, anterior

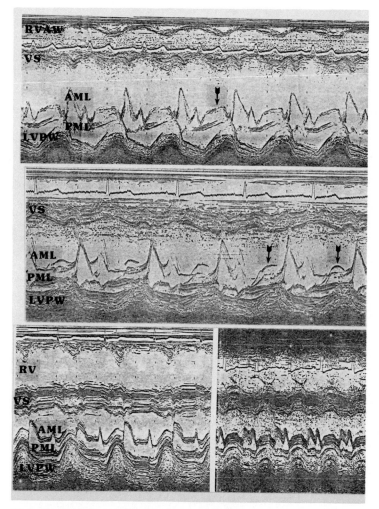

Fig. J-13.   Clinically insignificant SAM and pseudo-SAM.

Upper. M-mode echogram of a young woman with no abnormality on physical examination or ECG. The mitral valve shows systolic anterior motion as commonly seen with IHSS. However, the diagnosis of IHSS is very unlikely because of normal septal thickness and motion, and the fact that the LV size is top normal to mildly increased.

Center. M-mode echogram of a normal person showing linear echoes diverging from the main mitral valve echoes in early systole to move anteriorly; they are lost to view in late systole. This is a common normal variant, attributable to a rapid anterior buckling or whipping of one or more mitral chordae tendineae. No mitral prolapse was apparent in this patient.

Lower. M-mode echograms of two different patients with mild concentric LV hypertrophy secondary to hypertension. The linear echoes representing the mitral valve show large anterior excursions in systole. However, these excursions do not exceed in amplitude and velocity systolic anterior motion of the LV posterior wall. Mitral motion, in these patients is "physiologic" and does not constitute abnormal or pathologic SAM.

motion of the "anterior mitral echo" in early systole. This is a thin, linear echo that moves rapidly forward from the mitral echo just after the C point of mitral closure. It then "breaks off" and vanishes from view in midsystole or earlier, unlike true SAM, which completes the convexity of hump typical of SAM by returning

to the main mitral echo in late systole. Study of mitral motion by cross-sectional echocardiography in such patients suggests that a quick anterior whipping or buckling motion of anterior mitral chordae tendineae is responsible for this M-mode pattern.

5. An accessory "parachute" anterior mitral

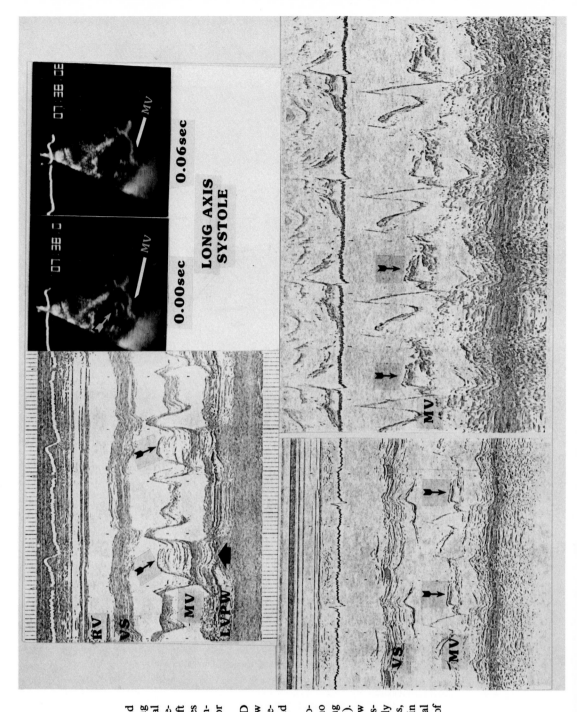

Fig. J-14. *Upper.* M-mode and 2-D echograms of a young woman with late systolic mitral prolapse and conspicuous anterior chordal buckling. In the left panel the upward arrow indicates mitral prolapse, and the downward arrows indicate the anterior buckling of the mitral chord.

The two frames of the 2-D echogram are systolic. The view shown here is intermediate between long axis (parasternal) and apical.

Lower. M-mode echocardiogram of an elderly man with no detectable heart disease, showing the LV at mitral valve level (*left*). On the right is an expanded view of the mitral valve. In early systole the mitral echo apparently splits into two components, which soon converge and meet in mid-systole. This is an unusual but "normal" buckling motion of a mitral chord.

leaflet producing an abnormal linear echo anterior to the mitral valve echo, with anterior convexity on the M-mode tracing very similar to true SAM (Cooperburg et al., 1976; Hatem et al., 1981). It differs from SAM in the finding that abnormal linear echoes persist also in diastole, partly superimposed on the anterior mitral leaflet but distinguishable from it.

SAM WITHOUT ASH AND WITHOUT HYPERTROPHIC CARDIOMYOPATHY (Figs. J-13 to J-15)

It has now been well established by several investigators (Buckley and Fortuin, 1976; Come et al., 1977; Mintz et al., 1978; Crawford et al., 1978; Maron et al., 1978; Udoshi et al., 1980; Gardin et al., 1981) that true SAM, indistinguishable from classic SAM as seen in IHSS, can occur in patients who have no ASH and may in fact have no other features of hypertrophic cardiomyopathy.

Maron et al. (1978) reported five patients with concentric LV hypertrophy and SAM who had large systolic pressure gradients between LV and aorta. Two of them had genetically transmitted true hypertrophic cardiomyopathy (documented by myocardial fiber disarray in the septum and ASH in first-degree relatives), whereas the other three did not. Maron et al. thus showed that SAM can occur in patients who have concentric LV hypertrophy not related to familial hypertrophic cardiomyopathy, and also that patients with familial hypertrophic cardiomyopathy occasionally can have concentric rather than asymmetric hypertrophy. They emphasized, however, that these are exceptional instances and should not distract the clinician from the really close association between SAM and IHSS in the vast majority of patients encountered in practice.

In patients with IHSS, the phenomenon known to echocardiographers as SAM has been attributed to various anatomic alterations in this disease; the LV shape, mitral leaflets, chordae, papillary muscles, and septal deformity have all been incriminated. How, then, can SAM be explained when it occurs in the absence of such anatomic abnormalities as in the four patients of Buckley and Fortuin (1976)? The factor common to these unusual cases of SAM seems to be an abnormal hypercontractile LV

producing LV ejection dynamics like those typical of IHSS. In other words, the cardiac physiology, but not its anatomy, resembles that of IHSS. Mintz et al. (1978) believed that the small LV size and reduced width of the LV outflow tract in their patients may have contributed to causation of SAM. Buckley and Fortuin also thought that SAM in their patients was somehow related to vigorous contraction of a small LV, in the setting of hypovolemia and the intravenous administration of norepinephrine.

Gardin et al. (1981) reported SAM in 15 patients, 5 of whom had mitral prolapse; the other 10 had no organic heart disease. These authors made the important 2-D echographic observation that SAM in their patients represented anterior "buckling" of mitral chordae tendineae, rather than movement of the entire anterior mitral leaflet into the LV outflow tract.

OTHER ECHOCARDIOGRAPHIC SIGNS OF IHSS

Small left ventricular chamber size. The left ventricular end-diastolic dimension is abnormally small or, at most, at the lower limit of normal range in nearly all patients with IHSS. Since the ventricle contracts vigorously, left ventricular end-systolic dimension is even more impressively reduced in IHSS (Tajik and Giuliani, 1971; Sanderson et al., 1978).

The left atrium is often dilated secondary to mitral regurgitation or reduced left ventricular compliance. Exceptionally, with severe mitral regurgitation, the left atrium reaches huge proportions. Increased left atrial size in patients with IHSS is associated with the appearance of atrial fibrillation. Following resection of myocardium in the left ventricular outflow tract, or mitral valve replacement, the dilated left atrium may return to normal size (Watson et al., 1977).

Mitral EF slope. A low or flat EF slope of the anterior mitral leaflet, attributable to low compliance of a hypertrophied, small-chambered left ventricle, is now known to be a very nonspecific echographic finding. However, during the early years of cardiac ultrasound, its similarity to the anterior mitral leaflet pattern of mitral stenosis was confusing. It, therefore, was referred to as a "pseudostenosis" pattern,

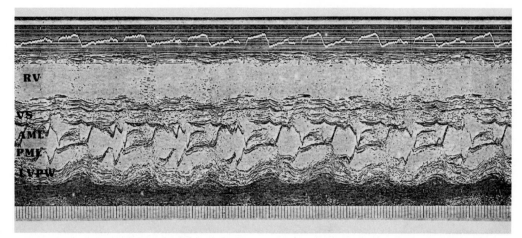

Fig. J-15. M-mode echocardiogram showing abnormal systolic anterior motion (SAM) of the mitral valve. The appearances are not typical of IHSS, inasmuch as the ventricular septum is only mildly hypertrophied and only mildly thicker than the LV posterior wall.

to be distinguished from true mitral stenosis by normal (posterior) diastolic motion of the posterior mitral leaflet.

Midsystolic closure of the aortic valve in a patient with hypertrophic cardiomyopathy signifies a substantial subaortic pressure gradient. It is discussed elsewhere (pp. 148–51).

In actual practice, perhaps the most common cardiac condition requiring differentiation from IHSS is the concentrically hypertrophied left ventricle of hypertensive heart disease. In both entities, the left ventricle has thick walls and an abnormally small chamber; the mitral valve EF slope tends to be low or flat.

In hypertensive elderly patients, the aortic valve is often sclerotic or calcified, resulting in a systolic murmur at the aortic area which also may be heard at the apex. A septal/posterior wall ratio of over 1.3 and SAM are typical of IHSS but not hypertensive heart disease. However, in an occasional hypertensive patient, the ventricular septum does hypertrophy to a greater extent than the left ventricular posterior wall (disproportionate septal hypertrophy). It is also not very unusual in patients with very small, cramped left ventricular chambers for the anterior mitral leaflet to lie quite close to the ventricular septum in systole; at a particular transducer angulation, an appearance resembling SAM can sometimes be recorded, but not with other transducer directions or positions. If a real uncertainty persists in symptomatic

patients with such perplexing echographic patterns, hemodynamic studies may be necessary to clarify the diagnosis.

Septal–mitral valve separation at the onset of systole. This refers to the distance between the mitral C point and the left border of the ventricular septum. Doi *et al.* (1980) found that if this criterion was set at 27 mm, maximum sensitivity and specificity were achieved for separating patients with hypertrophic cardiomyopathy from normal subjects, i.e., mitral C point–septal distance less than 27 mm made hypertrophic cardiomyopathy a likely diagnosis. Patients with left ventricular outflow obstruction (IHSS) tend to have smaller values than those without obstruction—less than 25 mm in the Hammersmith series (Doi *et al.,* 1980). Henry *et al.* (1975) found that only 6 per cent of patients without obstruction had a mitral C point–septal separation less than 20 mm, while 66 per cent of those with obstruction (IHSS) satisfied this criterion.

The mitral C point–septal distance may be abnormally small also in (1) posterior submitral (mitral annulus) calcification, which tends to displace the mitral leaflets anteriorly (D'Cruz *et al.,* 1977). (2) Very small-chambered, thick-walled left ventricles are sometimes seen in patients with severe hypertension. Since submitral calcification is more frequent in hypertensives, both factors act together to narrow the left ventricular outflow tract.

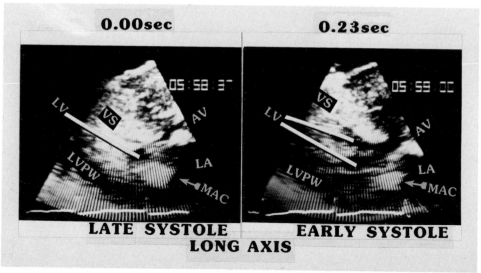

0.00sec   **0.23sec**

LATE SYSTOLE   EARLY SYSTOLE
LONG AXIS

Fig. J-16. 2-D echocardiogram showing an end-systolic frame (*left*) and an end-diastolic frame, 0.23 sec later (*right*), from the same cardiac cycle. The ventricular septum is greatly hypertrophied and the LV chamber unduly small. Posterior submitral (mitral annulus) calcification tends to displace the mitral valve anteriorly. In systole the mitral valve abuts against the ventricular septum (*left*).

TWO-DIMENSIONAL ECHOCARDIOGRAPHY (Figs. J-16 to J-18)

Ultrasound studies of hypertrophic cardiomyopathy using the 2-D technique have been reported by several authors (Henry *et al.*, 1975; Rodger, 1976; Cohen *et al.*, 1976; Schiller and Silverman, 1978; Martin *et al.*, 1979; Yamaguchi *et al.*, 1979). The principal features of IHSS on M-mode echography—

1. Abnormal increase in thickness and abnormal decrease in contractility of the ventricular septum,

2. Septal thickness strikingly greater than that of the LV posterior wall,

3. Abnormal systolic anterior motion of the anterior mitral leaflet, and

4. Hyperkinetic LV posterior wall motion—can all be recognized and thus confirmed on the 2-D recording, both in long-axis and short-axis views.

Certain additional features have been described on 2-D echocardiography:

1. A peculiar "ground-glass" appearance, characterized by multiple small, speckled echoes, affects the ventricular septum to a variable extent—20 to 100 per cent of septal length

(mean, 50 per cent), and 16 to 40 per cent of LV circumference (mean, 25 per cent)—and involves the left rather than right portion of this structure (Martin *et al.*, 1979). These authors ascribe this distinctive ultrasound pattern to the presence of multiple closely spaced reflecting interfaces of materials with markedly different densities or acoustic impedence, which might be due to the altered orientation of myocardial fibers and fibrosis in the abnormal septum of IHSS. The only other condition associated with a similar appearance is cardiac amyloidosis (Martin *et al.*, 1979).

2. The shape of the LV chamber in the long-axis view is often recognizably different in IHSS. Instead of the normal ellipsoidal shape in diastole, the LV cavity becomes slitlike. The hypertrophied papillary muscles and blunted LV apex also contribute to the altered contour of the chamber. On the other hand, concentric hypertrophy of the LV as seen in hypertension or aortic valve stenosis tends to produce a wedge-shaped or triangular chamber, tapering from its base to a narrow apex. Although the LV cavity can become extremely narrow in systole, in IHSS a small but appreciable space can be seen posterior to the papillary muscles in the short-axis view, so that complete oblitera-

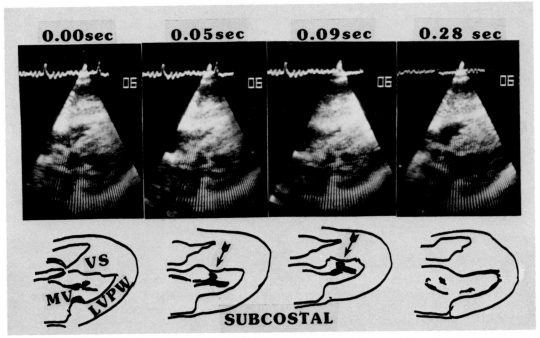

Fig. J-17. Serial frames, in the subcostal view, from the echocardiogram of a patient with IHSS. The second frame is 0.05 sec, the third 0.09 sec, and the fourth 0.28 sec after the first frame. The first 3 frames are in systole, the fourth in the ensuing diastole. The excessively thick, wedge-shaped ventricular septum, tapering to its attachment with the anterior aortic root, is clearest in the fourth frame. The anterior mitral leaflet moves anteriorly in systole (SAM) in the second and third frames to abut against the septum.

tion of the LV cavity (suggested by some hemodynamic studies) does not occur (Martin *et al.*, 1979). The shape of the ventricular septum in IHSS has been described as *catenoid* (Silverman *et al.*, 1982), i.e. concave to the left in the transverse plane and convex to the left in the sagittal plane. This shape is believed to cause septal akinesis and to play a crucial role in abnormal LV mechanics of IHSS.

3. In the short-axis view, the papillary muscles and mitral cusps and chordae are displaced anteriorly, so that the LV outflow tract is rendered abnormally small.

4. Two-D echography permits recognition of patients with pseudothickening of the basal septum on M-mode echocardiography (Fowles *et al.*, 1980). In these patients, the long axis of the LV and ventricular septum is unusually angulated with respect to the chest wall, such that the basal septum (adjacent to the aortic root) is oblique or even almost tangential to the M-mode ultrasound beam rather than perpendicular to it. Typically, the septum appears ill defined but fallaciously thickened at mitral

valve level; at mid-LV level, the septum, if it can be visualized at all, is of normal thickness. Two-D echography in the long axis reveals the abnormal ventricular angulation and normal septal thickness.

5. An abnormal pattern of coaptation in IHSS has been noted recently (Shah *et al.*, 1981) in the apical four-chamber view; the posterior mitral leaflet coapts with the middle third of the anterior leaflet. In normal subjects, the two leaflets coapt at their tips.

Much of the impetus to the 2-D study of patients with IHSS has arisen from attempts to resolve the controversy surrounding the precise anatomic site of obstruction of LV outflow and that bearing on the mechanism of production of SAM, controversies that date back almost to the description of IHSS itself. Martin *et al.* (1979) interpret their 2-D findings as in favor of the theory that SAM results from a Venturi effect causing the mitral valve apparatus to be drawn up anteriorly into the high-velocity blood stream flowing through the narrow LV outflow tract.

However, it must be added that previous investigators using 2-D echography to study the same problem arrived at different conclusions. Thus Rodger (1976) believed that "displacement of posterior papillary muscle above and in front of the mitral leaflets produces chordal slackening, and that it is displacement of the chordae tendineae by the blood flowing to the aortic root during LV ejection which is responsible for SAM of the mitral leaflets." Cohen *et al.* (1976) suggested that LV "outflow tract narrowing is probably caused by hypertrophy of the ventricular septum which in itself contributes to the narrowing, but which also displaces the papillary muscles and thus produces abnormal traction of the mitral valve and striking anterior displacement of the valve apparatus." Henry *et al.* (1975) did not think SAM could be attributed to contraction of malaligned papillary muscles.

Tajik *et al.* (1979) recognized three possible sites of LV obstruction in their 20 patients with IHSS studied by 2-D echocardiography:

1. High, caused by apposition of septum and anterior mitral leaflet;

2. Upper third of the LV outflow tract, caused by apposition of a "lemon-shaped" septum hypertrophied in its upper two thirds and the free edge (and chordal attachments) of the anterior mitral leaflet;

3. Mid-LV, caused by apposition of the ventricular septum and hypertrophied, malpositioned papillary muscles.

Tajik also pointed out that excessive hypertrophy often extends into the anterolateral LV wall. He emphasized that septal hypertrophy is frequently not uniform; it can involve only the upper third, lower third, or upper two thirds of the septal length.

Yet another anatomic variant of hypertrophic

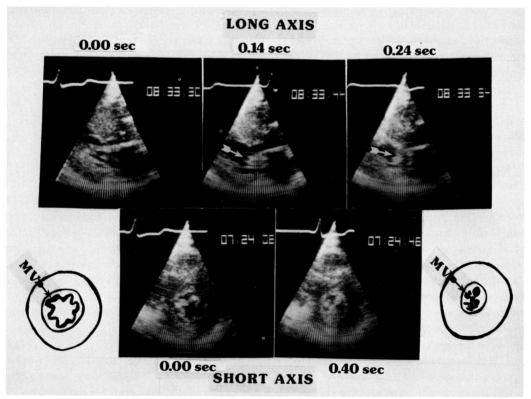

Fig. J-18. 2-D echogram of a patient with IHSS. Of the 3 upper frames, in the long-axis view, the first is in diastole, the second in early systole and the third in midsystole. Of the 2 lower frames, in the short-axis view, the left is in diastole and the right in end-systole. Note SAM of the anterior mitral leaflet, at its junction with its chordae tendineae, as it moves toward the thick ventricular septum (*top center and right frames*) and also that the mitral chordae leaflet junction appears to gather into folds in systole, accounting for the SAM effect and the multiple layered appearance of the mitral echoes in systole on M-mode.

cardiomyopathy was recently reported from Japan (Yamaguchi *et al.,* 1979) and South Africa (Stengo *et al.,* 1982). Marked concentric hypertrophy of the apical and near-apical LV was demonstrated on M-mode and 2-D echocardiography in a series of no less than 30 patients who showed LV hypertrophy by voltage criteria and very deep, "giant" T-wave inversions in left chest leads. Hypertension and coronary artery disease were excluded as a cause of the LV hypertrophy. On 2-D echography (long axis) and on angiocardiography (RAO projection), the LV chamber exhibited a characteristic spadelike contour caused by symmetric encroachment of the hypertrophied septum and LV wall in the vicinity of the LV apex. This unusual apical variant of hypertrophic cardiomyopathy occasionally does occur in the United States (Maron *et al.,* 1982) and differs in minor details from the Japanese type.

A bizarre variant of IHSS has been described (Tecklenberg *et al.,* 1978) in which the LV was constricted at midlevel by a ring of local hypertrophy; the obstructed LV apex was elongated into a diverticulum-like structure; mitral prolapse and regurgitation were also present.

The spectrum of hypertrophic cardiomyopathy has now expanded to include not only patients with no LV obstruction, but also some with no septal or LV wall hypertrophy on the M-mode echogram (Maron *et al.,* 1981). These authors described an interesting series of 16 patients in whom hypertrophic cardiomyopathy was suspected because of ECG abnormalities and either symptoms or belonging to a family with definite instances of the entity in one or more members. The M-mode echogram was normal, but 2-D echography revealed regional LV hypertrophy in unusual locations: the ventricular septum posteriorly (7 cases) or near the apex (2 cases), the anterior or lateral LV wall (7 cases). Short-axis views of the LV at successive LV levels from mitral valve level toward and beyond the papillary muscle level ("short-axis sweep") were particularly useful in demonstrating the hypertrophied segments. Such unduly thickened segments made a striking contrast with the normal thickness of LV wall or septum elsewhere on the LV circumference.

In the latest of a series of authoritative papers on the entity, Maron *et al.* (1981) have classified

hypertrophic cardiomyopathy into four categories on the basis of the 2-D echographic appearances in 125 patients:

Type I. Hypertrophy confined to the anterior portion of the ventricular septum.

Type II. Hypertrophy of the entire septum but not of the LV free wall.

Type III. Hypertrophy of "substantial portions" of the septum as well as anterolateral LV free wall. This was the most common variety (52 per cent of cases), worse than the others because these patients experienced (1) more severe functional limitation and (2) a higher incidence of LV outflow obstruction.

Type IV. Hypertrophy affecting regions of the LV other than the basal anterior septum: the apical septum, the posterior septum, or the anterolateral LV free wall.

Finally, 2-D echocardiography has a role in the postoperative assessment of patients with IHSS subjected to septal myomectomy. The M-mode technique can demonstrate diminished septal thickness, but the site and extent of myocardial resection are well appreciated only by 2-D echocardiography (Krajcer *et al.,* 1980).

CRITERIA FOR IHSS: CURRENT STATUS

Every pathologic and echocardiographic abnormality reported in hypertrophic cardiomyopathy, originally hailed as highly diagnostic or even pathognomonic, was reported eventually in several other conditions. Recently, the shortcomings and inadequacies of ultrasound in the diagnosis of IHSS have received much attention (Wei *et al.,* 1980; Goodwin, 1980), and there is general agreement that no diagnostic criterion, echocardiographic or even angiocardiographic, achieves an ideal 100 per cent specificity and 100 per cent sensitivity.

However, the disappointment and frustration that the clinical cardiologist feels on being informed that echocardiography is not as reliable a test for diagnosing or excluding IHSS as was once thought should by no means lead to abandonment of echocardiography for this purpose.

Notwithstanding the wide spectrum of anatomic and hemodynamic variations encountered (Fig. J-19), and the many echocardiographic faces of hypertrophic cardiomyopathy, it is the opinion of those who have studied the problem most extensively that hypertrophic cardiomyopathy—defined as "a hypertrophied nondilated left ventricle in the absence of cardiac or systemic disease that itself could produce left ventricular hypertrophy" (Maron and Epstein, 1980)—should continue to be regarded as a distinct disease entity (Maron and Epstein, 1980; Goodwin, 1980). In an analysis of the findings in a series of 1,600 patients, about one third of whom had hypertrophic cardiomyopathy, the specificity of ASH was 98 per cent and of SAM 97 per cent. Although not perfect, these two criteria, especially in combination, remain extremely useful in the clinical diagnosis of hypertrophic cardiomyopathy, especially IHSS.

OTHER CARDIAC CONDITIONS COMPLICATING OR ASSOCIATED WITH IHSS

The considerable body of echocardiographic literature that has accumulated on the topic of IHSS has extended to include a variety of other entities which have been observed in patients with IHSS. In some of these, as with associated fixed aortic stenosis, it is possible that this was the primary lesion that somehow predisposed to IHSS.

Bacterial endocarditis, on the other hand, is clearly a complication of IHSS (Wang *et al.*, 1975; LeJemtel *et al.*, 1979). In yet other instances, the association with another cardiac disease was merely fortuitous. Finally, there are some conditions that seem to have a relationship with IHSS that is as intriguing as it is unexplainable.

The combination of dynamic muscular subvalvular stenosis (IHSS) with *fixed stenosis of valvular or subvalvular* (discrete membrane) type has aroused much interest among echocardiologists (Nanda *et al.*, 1974; Chung *et al.*, 1974; Bloom *et al.*, 1975; Feizi *et al.*, 1978; Krajcer *et al.*, 1978; Hagaman *et al.*, 1980). The echographic findings include features of both the fixed site of stenosis and the dynamic component (such as SAM). It is important that those responsible for the ultrasound study as well as those involved in the hemodynamic procedure are alert to the possible coexistence of both lesions, lest the patient go to surgery with an incomplete diagnosis.

Mitral annulus calcification is not uncommon in elderly patients with IHSS (Kronzon and Glassman, 1978), perhaps because hypertension predisposes to both. Echocardiographic depiction of the LV anatomy in such cases suggests that large calcific masses in the posterior mitral annulus region can displace the mitral annulus anteriorly and thus aggravate an already diminished mitral-septal distance. The surprisingly high prevalence of IHSS in the elderly population also has been emphasized by Whiting *et al.* (1971), Krasnow and Stein (1978), and Albin *et al.* (1977). It suggests that (1) these elderly individuals suffer from a benign form of the disease that was no obstacle to longevity, or (2) IHSS, in some unknown manner, has developed *de novo* late in life (implying a very different origin from the genetically transmitted form commonly seen in younger individuals).

Bacterial endocarditis has been described in patients with IHSS (Wang *et al.*, 1975; LeJemtel *et al.*, 1979). Vegetations have been seen on the mitral valve and chordae as well as on the thickened plaque on the left septal surface against which the anterior mitral leaflet and attached chordae tendineae abut. The affected septal surface and the anterior mitral leaflet showed thickening and multilayered linear echoes on M-mode echography, presumably originating from the vegetations or inflammatory endocardial thickening. However, such changes must be considered nonspecific since they are not rare in other patients with IHSS who have no endocarditis.

Progression to LV dilatation in serial echographic examinations has been described in two patients in congestive heart failure who had had surgery a few years earlier for relief of LV outflow obstruction (IHSS) (ten Cate and Roelandt, 1979). LV dilatation and impaired LV function were also noted in four patients with IHSS who had sustained *myocardial infarction* (Maron *et al.*, 1979). Small to normal LV chamber size and enhanced LV contractility are so uniformly seen in hypertrophic cardiomyopathy that the development of LV dilatation and hypokinesis is most unusual and should suggest these complications. Come and Riley (1982) have reported the disappearance of dynamic LV outflow obstruction (as well as SAM) in three patients with IHSS after myocardial infarction,

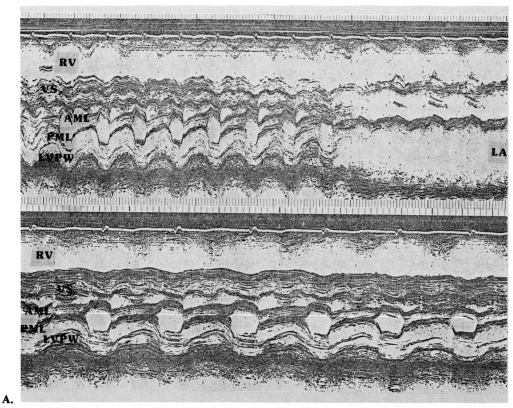

Fig. J-19. *A.* M-mode echogram of an elderly normotensive woman with a loud ejection systolic murmur as well as apical systolic murmur. The ECG showed LV hypertrophy. Abnormal SAM is absent, but the LV outflow tract appears quite narrow in systole. The septum shows regional hypertrophy and the LV is hypercontractile (see Fig. J-19B). This patient may have a variant of hypertrophic cardiomyopathy.

even though the site of infarction was remote from the ventricular septum.

Pericardial effusions associated with IHSS were described by Alimurung *et al.* (1979). Smith *et al.* (1977) showed that hypertrophic cardiomyopathy was the principal type of heart disease complicating *Friedrich's ataxia.* Thompson *et al.* (1980) reported the appearance of hypertrophic cardiomyopathy in six patients three to five years after *aortic valve replacement,* none of whom had evidence of the disease preoperatively. Chandaratna *et al.* (1978) encountered 16 patients with ASH in a series of 190 patients with *mitral valve prolapse.* Septum-to-LV posterior wall ratios in these 16 patients ranged from 1.5 to 2.5 (mean, 1.9); however, it seems uncertain as to whether all or even most of these patients had real hypertrophic cardiomyopathy.

An unexpected and intriguing association between *hypothyroidism* and ASH was reported in no less than 17 patients by Santos *et al.* (1980); 5 of them also had SAM. Ten of these patients reverted to a euthyroid state with L-thyroxine therapy, and the echographic abnormalities regressed. The hypertrophic cardiomyopathy in these patients was thus reversible, although its pathogenesis remains quite obscure.

Riggs *et al.* (1980) emphasized the heterogeneous nature of IHSS in pediatric practice. Whereas the entity in older children resembles that seen in adults, in neonates IHSS is transient and related to hypertension or to diabetes in the mother. In infants with transposition of great vessels, the LV outflow tract obstruction is really subpulmonic and therefore of quite a different hemodynamic significance.

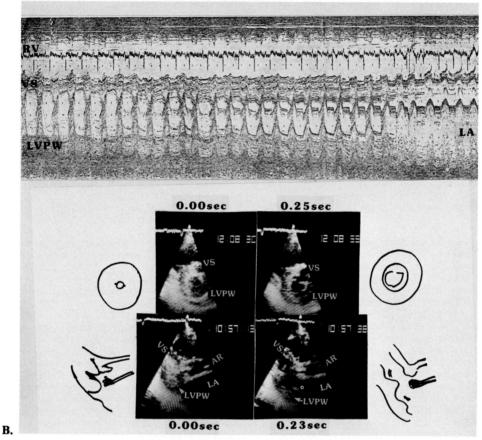

Fig. J-19. *B. Upper.* M-mode scan in the same patient, at slow paper speed, of the LV from apex to base and to LA. The ventricular septum is much thicker at mitral valve level (*center*) than it is near the apex (*left*).

Lower. 2-D echogram of the same patient. The two upper frames are in the short axis, the second 0.25 sec after the first. The two lower frames are in the long axis, the second 0.23 sec after the first. The systolic frames, on the left, show almost complete obliteration of the LV cavity. The diastolic frames, on the right, demonstrate the extent of the LV chamber; the ventricular septum is thick at mitral level but of normal thickness at mid-LV level.

REFERENCES

HYPERTROPHIC CARDIOMYOPATHY

Abbasi, A. S.; MacAlpin, R. N.; Eber, L. M.; *et al.:* Echocardiographic diagnosis of idiopathic hypertrophic cardiomyopathy without left ventricular obstruction. *Circulation,* **46:**897, 1972.

Angoff, G. H.; Wistran, D.; Sloss, L. J.; *et al.:* Value of a noninvasively induced ventricular extrasystole during echocardiographic and phonocardiographic assessment of patients with idiopathic hypertrophic subaortic stenosis. *Am. J. Cardiol.,* **42:**919, 1978.

Chahine, R. A.; Raizner, A. E.; Ishimori, T.; *et al.:* Echocardiographic, hemodynamic and angiocardiographic correlations in hypertrophic cardiomyopathy. *Br. Heart J.,* **39:**945, 1977.

Chahine, R. A.; Raizner, A. E.; Nelson, J.; *et al.:* Midsystolic closure of aortic valve in hypertrophic cardiomyopathy. Echocardiographic and angiographic correlation. *Am. J. Cardiol.,* **43:**17, 1979.

Chandaratna, P. A. N.; Chu, W.; Schecter, E.; *et al.:* Hemodynamic correlates of echocardiographic aortic root motion. Observation on normal subjects and patients with idiopathic hypertrophic subaortic stenosis. *Chest,* **74:**183, 1978.

Cohen, M. V.; Teichholz, L. E.; and Gorlin, R.: B-scan ultrasonography in idiopathic hypertrophic subaortic stenosis. Study of left ventricular outflow tract and mechanism of obstruction. *Br. Heart J.,* **38:**595, 1976.

Criley, J. M.; Blaufuss, A. H.; and Abbasi, A. S.: Nonobstructive idiopathic hypertrophic subaortic stenosis. *Circulation,* **52:**963, 1975.

D'Cruz, I. A.; Cohen, H. C.; Prabhu, R.; *et al.:* Clinical manifestations of mitral annulus calcification, with emphasis on its echocardiographic features. *Am. Heart J.,* **94:**367, 1977.

Doi, Y. L.; McKenna, W. J.; Chetty, S.; *et al.:* Prediction of mortality and serious ventricular arrhythmia in hypertrophic cardiomyopathy. An echocardiographic study. *Br. Heart J.,* **44:**150, 1980.

Doi, Y. L.; McKenna, W. J.; Gehrke, J.; *et al.:* M-mode echocardiography in hypertrophic cardiomyopathy: Diagnostic criteria and prediction of obstruction. *Am. J. Cardiol.,* **45:**6, 1980.

Epstein, S. E.; Henry, W. L.; Clark, C. E.; *et al.:* Asymmetric septal hypertrophy. *Ann. Intern. Med.,* **81:**650, 1974.

Gibson, D. G.; Traill, T. A.; Hall, R. J. F.; *et al.:* Echocardiographic features of secondary left ventricular hypertrophy. *Br. Heart J.,* **41:**54, 1979.

Gilbert, B. W.; Pollick, C.; Adelman, A. G.; *et al.:* Hypertrophic cardiomyopathy: Subclassification by M-mode echocardiography. *Am. J. Cardiol.,* **45:**861, 1980.

Goodwin, J. F.: Hypertrophic cardiomyopathy: A disease in search of its own identity. *Am. J. Cardiol.,* **45:**177, 1980.

Hanrath, P.; Mothey, D. G.; Siegert, R.; *et al.:* Left ventricular relaxation and filling pattern in different forms of left ventricular hypertrophy. An echocardiographic study. *Am. J. Cardiol.,* **45:**15, 1980.

Henry, W. L.; Clark, C. E.; Glancy, D. L.; *et al.:* Echocardiographic measurement of the left ventricular outflow gradient in idiopathic hypertrophic subaortic stenosis. *N. Engl. J. Med.,* **288:**989, 1974a.

Henry, W. L.; Clark, C. E.; Roberts, W. C.; *et al.:* Differences in distribution of myocardial abnormalities in patients with obstructive and nonobstructive asymmetric septal hypertrophy. *Circulation,* **50:**447, 1974b.

Henry, W. L.; Clark, C. E.; Griffith, J. M.; *et al.:* Mechanism of left ventricular outflow obstruction in patients with obstructive asymmetric septal hypertrophy. *Am. J. Cardiol.,* **35:**337, 1975.

Krajcer, Z.; Lufschanowski, R.; and Angelini, P.: Septal myomectomy and mitral valve replacement for idiopathic hypertrophic subaortic stenosis. An echocardiographic and hemodynamic study. *Circulation,* **62** (Suppl. I):158, 1980.

Maron, B. J.; Henry, W. L.; and Roberts, W. C.: Comparison of echocardiographic and necropsy measurements of ventricular wall thickness in patients with and without disproportionate septal thickening. *Circulation,* **55:**341, 1977.

Maron, B. J.; Gottdiener, J. S.; Goldstein, R. E.; *et al.:* Hypertrophic cardiomyopathy: The great masquerader. *Chest,* **74:**659, 1978.

Maron, B. J., and Epstein, S. E. Hypertrophic cardiomyopathy: Recent observations regarding the specificity of three hallmarks of the disease. Asymmetric septal hypertrophy, septal disorganization, and systolic anterior motion of the anterior mitral leaflet. *Am. J. Cardiol.,* **45:**141, 1980.

Maron, B. J.; Gottdiener, J. S.; and Epstein, S. E.: Patterns and significance of distribution of left ventricular hypertrophy in hypertrophic cardiomyopathy. *Am. J. Cardiol.,* **48:**418, 1981.

Maron, B. J.; Bonow, R. O.; Seshagiri, T. N. R.; *et al.:* Hypertrophic cardiomyopathy with ventricular septal hypertrophy localized to the apical region of the left ventricle. *Am. J. Cardiol.,* **49:**1838, 1982.

Martin, R. P.; Rakowski, H.; French, J.; *et al.:* Idiopathic hypertrophic subaortic stenosis viewed by wide-angle, phased-array echocardiography. *Circulation,* **59:**1206, 1979.

Moreya, E.; Kleid, J. J.; Shimada, H.; *et al.:* Idiopathic hypertrophic subaortic stenosis diagnosed by reflected ultrasound. *Am. J. Cardiol.,* **23:**32, 1969.

Morrow, A. G.; Reitz, B. A.; Epstein, S. E.; *et al.:* Operative treatment in hypertrophic subaortic stenosis: Techniques and results of pre- and post-operative assessments in 83 patients. *Circulation,* **52:**88, 1975.

Pollick, C.; Koilpillai, C.; and Howard, R.: Left ventricular thrombus demonstrating canalization and mimicking asymmetric septal hypertrophy on echocardiographic study. *Am. Heart J.,* **104:**641, 1982a.

Pollick, C.; Morgan, C. D.; Gilbert, B. W.; *et al.:* Muscular subaortic stenosis: The temporal relationship between systolic anterior motion of the anterior mitral leaflet and the pressure gradient. *Circulation,* **66:**1087, 1982b.

Popp, R. L., and Harrison, D. C.: Ultrasound in the diagnosis and evaluation of therapy of idiopathic hypertrophic subaortic stenosis. *Circulation,* **40:**905, 1969.

Pridie, R. B., and Oakley, C. M.: Mechanism of mitral regurgitation in hypertrophic obstructive cardiomyopathy. *Br. Heart J.,* **32:**203, 1970.

Rodger, J. C.: Motion of mitral apparatus in hypertrophic cardiomyopathy with obstruction. *Br. Heart J.,* **38:**732, 1976.

Rosen, R. M.; Goodman, D. J.; Ingham, R. E.; *et al.:* Hypertrophic subaortic stenosis: ventricular septal thickening and excursion. *N. Engl. J. Med.,* **291:**1317, 1974.

Sanderson, J. E.; Traill, T. A.; St. John Sutton, M. G.; *et al.:* Left ventricular relaxation and filling in hypertrophic cardiomyopathy. *Br. Heart J.,* **40:**596, 1978.

Schapira, J. N.; Stemple, D. R.; and Martin, R. P.: Single and two-dimensional echocardiographic visualization of the effects of septal myectomy in idiopathic hypertrophic subaortic stenosis. *Circulation,* **58:**850, 1978.

Schiller, N. B., and Silverman, N. H.: Two-dimensional ultrasonic cardiac imaging. In: Kleid, J. J., and Arvan, S. B. (eds.): *Echocardiography: Interpretation and Diagnosis.* Appleton-Century-Crofts, New York, 1978, p. 392.

Shah, P. M.; Gramiak, R.; and Kramer, D. H.: Ultrasound localization of left ventricular outflow obstruction in hypertrophic obstructive cardiomyopathy. *Circulation,* **40:**3, 1969.

Shah, P. M.; Gramiak, R.; Adelman, A. G.; *et al.:* Role of echocardiography in diagnostic and hemodynamic assessment of hypertrophic subaortic stenosis. *Circulation,* **44:**891, 1971.

Shah, P. M.; Gramiak, R.; Adelman, A. G.; *et al.:* Echocardiographic assessment of the effects of surgery and propranolol on the dynamics of outflow obstruction and hypertrophic subaortic stenosis. *Circulation,* **45:**516, 1972.

Shah, P. M.; Taylor, R. D.; and Wong, M.: Abnormal mitral valve coaptation in hypertrophic obstructive cardiomyopathy: Proposed role in systolic anterior motion of mitral valve. *Am. J. Cardiol.,* **48:**258, 1981.

Silverman, K.G.; Hutchins, G. M.; Weiss, J. C.; *et al.:* Catenoidal shape of the interventricular septum in idiopathic hypertrophic subaortic stenosis: Two-dimensional echocardiographic confirmation. *Am. J. Cardiol.,* **49:**27, 1982.

Spilkin, S.; Mitha, A. S.; Matisonn, R. E.; *et al.:* Complete heart block in a case of idiopathic hypertrophic subaortic stenosis. *Circulation,* **55:**418, 1977.

Stengo, L.; Dansky, R.; Pocock, W. A.; *et al.:* Apical hypertrophic nonobstructive cardiomyopathy. *Am. Heart J.,* **104:**635, 1982.

Sze, K. C., and Shah, P. M.: Pseudoejection sound in hypertrophic subaortic stenosis: An echocardiographic correlative study. *Circulation,* **54:**504, 1976.

Tajik, A. J., and Giuliani, E. R.: Echocardiographic observations in idiopathic hypertrophic subaortic stenosis. *Mayo Clin. Proc.,* **49:**89, 1971.

Tajik, A. J.; Seward, J. B.; and Hagler, D. G.: Detailed

analysis of hypertrophic obstructive cardiomyopathy by wide-angle two-dimensional sector echocardiography. *Am. J. Cardiol.,* **43:**348, 1979 (Abstr.).

Tecklenberg, P. L.; Alderman, E. L.; Billingham, M. E.; *et al.:* Diverticulum of the left ventricle in hypertrophic cardiomyopathy. *Am. J. Med.,* **64:**707, 1978.

ten Cate, F. J.; Hugenholtz, P. G.; VanDorp, W. G.; *et al.:* Prevalence of diagnostic abnormalities in patients with genetically transmitted asymmetric septal hypertrophy. *Am. J. Cardiol.,* **43:**731, 1979.

Watson, D. C.; Henry, W. L.; and Epstein, S. E.: Effects of operation on left atrial size and the occurrence of atrial fibrillation in patients with hypertrophic subaortic stenosis. *Circulation,* **55:**178, 1977.

Wei, J. Y.; Weiss, J. L.; and Bulkley, B. H.: The heterogeneity of hypertrophic cardiomyopathy: An autopsy and one-dimensional study. *Am. J. Cardiol.,* **45:**25, 1980.

Yamaguchi, H.; Ishimura, T.; Nishiyama, S.; *et al.:* Hypertrophic nonobstructive cardiomyopathy with giant negative T waves (apical hypertrophy): Ventriculographic and echocardiographic features in 30 patients. *Am. J. Cardiol.,* **44:**401, 1979.

ASH OR DST OTHER THAN IHSS

Abbasi, A. S.; MacAlpin, R. M.; Eber, L. M.; *et al.:* Left ventricular hypertrophy diagnosed by echocardiography. *N. Engl. J. Med.,* **289:**118, 1973.

Abbasi, A. S.; Slaughter, J. C.; and Allen, M. W.: Asymmetric septal hypertrophy in patients on long-term hemodialysis. *Chest,* **74:**548, 1978.

Fowles, R. E.; Martin, R. P.; and Popp, R. L.: Apparent asymmetric septal hypertrophy due to angled interventricular septum. *Am. J. Cardiol.,* **46:**386, 1980.

Goodman, D. J.; Rossen, R. M.; and Popp, R. L.: Echocardiographic pseudo idiopathic hypertrophic aortic stenosis. *Chest,* **66:**573, 1974.

Henning, H.; O'Rourke, R. A.; Crawford, M. H.; *et al.:* Inferior myocardial infarction as a cause of asymmetrical septal hypertrophy. An echocardiographic study. *Am. J. Cardiol.,* **41,** 817, 1978.

Isner, J. M.; Falcone, M. W.; Virmani, R.; *et al.:* Cardiac sarcoma causing "ASH" and simulating coronary heart disease. *Am. J. Med.,* **66:**1025, 1979.

Kansal, S.; Roitman, D.; and Sheffield, L. T.: Interventricular septal thickness and left ventricular hypertrophy. An echocardiographic study. *Circulation,* **60:**1058, 1979.

Larter, W. E.; Allen, H. D.; Sahn, D. J.; *et al.:* The asymmetrically hypertrophied septum: Further differentiation of its causes. *Circulation,* **53:**19, 1976.

Maron, B. J.; Clark, C. E.; Henry, W. L.; *et al.:* Prevalence and characteristics of disproportionate ventricular septal thickening in patients with acquired or congenital heart disease. *Circulation,* **55:**489, 1977.

Maron, B. J.; Savage, D. D.; Clark, C. E.; *et al.:* Prevalence and characteristics of disproportionate ventricular septal thickening in patients with coronary artery disease. *Circulation,* **57:**250, 1978.

Scovil, J. A.; Nanda, N. C.; Gross, C. M.; *et al.:* Echocardiographic studies of abnormalities associated with coarctation of the aorta. *Circulation,* **52:**953, 1976.

Stern, A.; Kessler, K. M.; Hammer, W. J.; *et al.:* Septal-free wall disproportion in inferior infarction: The echocardiographic differentiation from hypertrophic cardiomyopathy. *Circulation,* **58:**700, 1978.

Tajik, A. J.; Gau, G. T.; and Schattenberg, T. T.: Echocardiographic "pseudo-IHSS" pattern in atrial septal defect. *Chest,* **62:**324, 1972.

SAM WITHOUT ASH AND PSEUDO-SAM

Bulkley, B. H., and Fortuin, N. J.: Systolic anterior motion of the mitral valve without asymmetric septal hypertrophy. *Chest,* **69:**694, 1976.

Come, P. C.; Bulkley, B. H.; Goodman, A. D.; *et al.:* Hypercontractile cardiac states simulating hypertrophic cardiomyopathy. *Circulation,* **55:**901, 1977.

Cooperberg, P.; Hazell, S.; and Ashmore, P. G.: Parachute accessory anterior mitral valve leaflet causing left ventricular outflow tract obstruction. Report of a case with emphasis on the echocardiographic findings. *Circulation,* **53:**908, 1976.

Crawford, M. H.; Groves, B. M.; and Horwitz, L. D.: Dynamic left ventricular outflow tract obstruction and systolic anterior motion of the mitral valve in the absence of asymmetric septal hypertrophy. *Am. J. Med.,* **65:**703, 1978.

Cueto, L.; Arriaga, J.; and Zinser, J.: Echocardiographic changes in phaeochromocytoma. *Chest,* **76:**600, 1979.

Gardin, J. M.; Talano, J. V.; Stephanides, L.; *et al.:* Systolic anterior motion in the absence of asymmetric septal hypertrophy. *Circulation,* **63:**181, 1981.

Greenwald, Y.; Yap, J. F.; Franklin, M.; *et al.:* Echocardiographic mitral systolic motion in left ventricular aneurysm. *Br. Heart J.,* **37:**684, 1975.

Hatem, J.; Sade, R. M.; and Taylor, A.: Supernumerary mitral valve producing subaortic stenosis. *Chest,* **79:**483, 1981.

King, J. F.; DeMaria, A. N.; Miller, R. R.; *et al.:* Markedly abnormal mitral valve motion without simultaneous intraventricular pressure gradient due to uneven mitral-septal contact in idiopathic hypertrophic subaortic stenosis. *Am. J. Cardiol.,* **34:**360, 1974.

Levisman, J. A.: Systolic anterior motion of the mitral valve due to hypovolemia and anemia. *Chest,* **70:**687, 1976.

Maron, B. J.; Gottdiener, J. S.; Roberts, W. C.; *et al.:* Left ventricular outflow tract obstruction due to systolic anterior motion of the anterior mitral leaflet in patients with concentric left ventricular hypertrophy. *Circulation,* **57:**527, 1978.

Mintz, G. S.; Kotler, M. N.; Segal, B. L.; *et al.:* Systolic anterior motion of the mitral valve in the absence of asymmetric septal hypertrophy. *Circulation,* **57:**256, 1978.

Nanda, N. C.; Gramiak, R.; and Gross, C. M.: Echocardiography of cardiac valves in pericardial effusion. *Circulation,* **54:**500, 1976.

Oakley, C. M.: Surgical correction of IHSS. *Circulation,* **51:**951, 1975.

Popp, R. L.; Owen, R. B.; Silverman, J. F.; and Harrison, D. C.: Echocardiographic abnormalities in the mitral valve prolapse syndrome. *Circulation,* **49:**428, 1974.

Shub, C.; Williamson, M. C., and Tajik, A. J.: Dynamic left ventricular outflow tract obstruction associated with pheochromocytoma. *Am. Heart J.,* **102:**286, 1981.

Udoshi, M.; Shah, A.; Fisher, V. J.; *et al.:* Systolic anterior motion of the mitral valve with and without asymmetric septal hypertrophy. *Cardiology,* **66:**147, 1980.

IHSS ASSOCIATED WITH OTHER CONDITIONS

With Fixed Aortic Stenosis

Bloom, K. R.; Meyer, R. A.; Bove, K. E.; *et al.:* The association of fixed and dynamic left ventricular outflow obstruction. *Am. Heart J.,* **89:**586, 1975.

Chung, K. J.; Manning, J. A.; and Gramiak, R.: Echocardiography in coexisting hypertrophic subaortic stenosis and fixed left ventricular outflow obstruction. *Circulation,* **49:**673, 1974.

Feizi, O.; Farber-Brown, G.; and Emanuel, R.: Familial study of hypertrophic cardiomyopathy and congenital aortic valve disease. *Am. J. Cardiol.,* **41:**956, 1978.

Hagaman, J. F.; Wolfe, C.; and Craige, E.: Early aortic valve closure in combined idiopathic hypertrophic subaortic stenosis and discrete subaortic stenosis. *Am. J. Cardiol.,* **45:**1083, 1980.

Harrison, E. E.; Shar, S. S.; Martin, H.; *et al.:* Co-existing right and left hypertrophic subvalvular stenosis and fixed left ventricular obstruction due to aortic valve stenosis. *Am. J. Cardiol.,* **40:**133, 1977.

Krajcer, Z.; Orzan, F.; Pechacek, L. W.; *et al.:* Early systolic closure of the aortic valve in patients with hypertrophic subaortic stenosis and discrete subaortic stenosis: Correlation with pre-operative and post-operative hemodynamics. *Am. J. Cardiol.,* **41:**823, 1978.

Nanda, N. C.; Gramiak, R.; Shah, P. M.; *et al.:* Echocardiography in the diagnosis of idiopathic hypertrophic subaortic stenosis coexisting with aortic valve disease. *Circulation,* **50:**752, 1974.

In Childhood

Maron, B. J.; Henry, W. L.; Clark, C. E.; *et al.:* Asymmetric septal hypertrophy in childhood. *Circulation,* **53:**9, 1976.

Pitcher, D.; Wainwright, R.; Brennand-Roper, D.; *et al.:* Cardiac tumors: Noninvasive detection and assessment by gated cardiac blood pool radionuclide imaging. *Br. Heart J.,* **44:**143, 1980.

Riggs, T.; Hirschfeld, S.; and Rajai, H.: The pediatric spectrum of dynamic left ventricular obstruction. *Am. Heart J.,* **99:**300, 1980.

In Old Age

Albin, E. L.; Chandaratna, P. A.; Littman, B. B.; *et al.:* Idiopathic hypertrophic subaortic stenosis in the elderly. *Am. J. Med. Sci.,* **274:**163, 1977.

Berger, M.; Rethy, C.; and Goldberg, E.: Unsuspected hypertrophic subaortic stenosis in the elderly diagnosed by echocardiography. *J. Am. Geriatr. Soc.,* **27:**178, 1979.

Habibzadeh, M. A.: Idiopathic hypertrophic subaortic stenosis and aortic regurgitation in an 84-year-old man. *J. Am. Geriatr. Soc.,* **28:**515, 1980.

Krasnow, N., and Stein, R. A.: Hypertrophic cardiomyopathy in the aged. *Am. Heart J.,* **96:**326, 1978.

Kronzon, I., and Glassman, E.: Mitral ring calcification in idiopathic hypertrophic subaortic stenosis. *Am. J. Cardiol.,* **42:**60, 1978.

Whiting, R. B.; Powell, W. J.; and Dinsmore, R. E.: Idiopathic hypertrophic subaortic stenosis in the elderly. *N. Engl. J. Med.,* **285:**196, 1971.

With Bacterial Endocarditis

LeJemtel, T. H.; Factor, S. M.; Koenigsberg, M.; *et al.:* Mural vegetations at the site of endocardial trauma in infective endocarditis complicating idiopathic subaortic stenosis. *Am. J. Cardiol.,* **44:**569, 1979.

Wang, K. Gobel, F. L.; and Gleason, D. F.: Bacterial endocarditis in IHSS. *Am. Heart J.,* **89:**359, 1975.

With Pericardial Effusion

Alimurung, B. N.; Felner, J. M.; and Schlant, R. C.: Echocardiography in the diagnosis of idiopathic subaortic stenosis co-existing with pericardial effusion. *Chest,* **76:**187, 1979.

With Myocardial Infarction

Come, P. C., and Riley, M. F.: Hypertrophic cardiomyopathy: Disappearance of auscultatory, carotid pulse and echocardiographic manifestations of obstruction following myocardial infarction. *Chest,* **82:**451, 1982.

Maron, B. J.; Epstein, S. E.; and Roberts, W. C.: Hypertrophic cardiomyopathy and transmural myocardial infarction without significant atherosclerosis of the extramural coronary arteries. *Am. J. Cardiol.,* **43:**1086, 1979.

With LV Dilatation

ten Cate, R. J., and Roelandt, J.: Progression to left ventricular dilatation in patients with hypertrophic obstructive cardiomyopathy. *Am. Heart J.,* **97:**762, 1979.

With RV Outflow Obstruction

Cardiel, E. A.; Alonso, M.; Delcan, J. L.; *et al.:* Echocardiographic sign of right-sided hypertrophic obstructive cardiomyopathy. *Br. Heart J.,* **40:**1321, 1978.

With Friedrich's Ataxia

Smith, E. R.; Saugalang, V. E.; and Hefferman, C. P.: Hypertrophic cardiomyopathy: The heart disease of Friedrich's ataxia. *Am. Heart J.,* **93:**478, 1977.

With Aortic Valve Replacement

Thompson, R.; Ahmed, M.; Pridie, R.; and Yacoub, M.: Hypertrophic cardiomyopathy after aortic valve replacement. *Am. J. Cardiol.,* **45:**33, 1980.

With LV Fibromuscular Bands

Hall, R. R.; Baum, R. S.; Bryson, A. L.; *et al.:* Obstructive hypertrophic cardiomyopathy and apical mid diastolic murmur. Association with left ventricular fibromuscular bands. *Chest,* **73:**866, 1978.

K

Coronary Heart Disease

M-MODE ECHOCARDIOGRAPHY

Recognition of the normal pattern of motion of the LV posterior wall and ventricular septum during the early 1970s was followed by a spate of papers on abnormal motion of these structures in patients with coronary disease as recorded on the M-mode echogram. However, only a limited portion of the LV posterior wall, between the mitral annulus and posterior papillary muscle, can be explored adequately by M-mode echography. Even less of the ventricular septum can be visualized in this mode, amounting to only a small fraction of the total septal expanse. Observations on systolic thickening and motion of the LV wall were therefore restricted to these areas. All other parts of the LV, including the LV apex as well as the anterior and inferior walls and septum adjacent to the apex, are usually invisible by the M-mode technique since they lie beyond the reach of the ultrasound beam.

The ability to image the entire LV, and to visualize abnormalities of shape and contraction affecting all of its segments, has not only vastly expanded the scope of cardiac ultrasound but also exposed the serious limitations of M-mode echocardiography in the assessment of ischemic heart disease. At present, the diagnostic role of the M-mode technique in coronary disease is merely that of a preliminary survey of the basal and mid-LV, which should be followed by imaging and real-time recording of the LV chamber in the long-axis, short-axis, and apical views.

Therefore, a rather brief account of the M-mode findings in ischemic heart disease will appear here, in spite of the considerable body of literature on the topic that accumulated during the early and mid-1970s (Inoue et al., 1971;

Wharton, et al., 1971; Fogelman et al., 1972; Ratshin et al., 1972; Jacobs et al., 1973; Kerber and Abboud, 1973; Corya et al., 1974a and b, 1975; Goldstein and deJong, 1974; Heikkila and Nieminen, 1975; Kerber et al., 1975; Wildlansky et al., 1975; Nieminen and Heikkila, 1976a and b; Dortimer et al., 1976; Feigenbaum et al., 1976).

During the late 1970s, further observations were made on wall motion abnormalities in coronary disease, including their reversibility under certain circumstances, the identification of myocardial scarring, and the prediction of prognosis on the basis of echocardiographic findings (Corya et al., 1977; DeMaria et al., 1977; Morrison et al., 1977, 1978; Massie et al., 1978; Rasmussen et al., 1978; Wiener et al., 1979).

At about the same time, the great potential of 2-D echocardiography in detection of local LV asynergy was amply demonstrated (Kisslo et al., 1977; Heger et al., 1979, 1980; Eaton et al., 1979; Nixon et al., 1980). The 1980s might well witness the establishment of 2-D echocardiography as a routine procedure in the assessment of both acute and chronic phases of ischemic heart disease.

SEGMENTAL ABNORMALITIES OF SYSTOLIC LV WALL MOTION AND THICKENING

Local segmental impairment of LV wall motion, as distinguished from diffuse or generalized diminution of LV contractility, commonly is caused by coronary heart disease. In general, the detection of regional hypokinesis, akinesis, or dyskinesis of the LV wall is presumptive evidence of ischemic heart disease unless proven otherwise.

LOCAL ABNORMALITIES OF LV POSTERIOR WALL MOTION (Figs. K-1 to K-3)

The normal systolic excursion of the LV posterior wall endocardium is 9 to 14 mm in amplitude. Infarction or ischemia of this LV region may manifest as hypokinesis with abnormally small systolic anterior excursions. Less commonly, the LV posterior wall is akinetic, showing no systolic excursions at all. Paradoxic (posterior) systolic motion is rather rare and usually signifies a ventricular aneurysm.

Three distinct segments of the LV posterior wall can be identified by M-mode scanning:

1. Basal LV level, where the mitral valve leaflets are well visualized;

2. Mid-LV level, where mitral chordae tendineae are well visualized;

3. Papillary muscle level, where the LV wall abruptly doubles in thickness because of the presence of the posterior papillary muscle at this site.

The basal segment of the LV posterior wall is commonly spared by ischemic heart disease, and it is the mid-LV portion at chordae level, also perhaps at papillary muscle level, which shows diminished or absent systolic excursions. Very exceptionally, an infarcted LV posterior wall will actually move paradoxically (posteriorly) on the M-mode echogram (Fig. K-3). Posterior systolic motion of the LV posterior wall may be seen in patients with very large pericardial effusions associated with pendulous or "swinging" cardiac motion. Such abnormal mobility of the ventricles is recognized easily on M-mode and 2-D echography; LV wall motion promptly returns to normal as the pericardial effusion subsides or is tapped.

Abnormal posterior motion of the LV posterior wall in patients with swinging hearts in large pericardial effusions (Fig. N-12) should not therefore be mistaken for true LV wall akinesis or dyskinesis.

Repeated scans of the LV chamber along its long axis, from the left atrium to basal LV and then to mid-LV and papillary muscle levels as far toward the apex as possible, are desirable to record disparities in systolic excursions at different sites (Figs. K-1 and K-2).

Two important technical fallacies can simulate hypokinesis of the LV posterior wall:

1. Inability to record the true endocardial echo due to inappropriate setting of the gain or reject. The epicardial echo, an intramural echo within the LV wall itself, or chordal echoes, all of which have a lesser amplitude of systolic excursion, could be mistaken for the endocardial echo.

2. The ultrasound beam is tangential or oblique to the direction of LV posterior wall motion, as may happen when the transducer is tilted toward the LV apex. The amplitude of LV posterior wall excursion appears smaller than it would if the beam was parallel to the direction of motion, i.e., perpendicular to the wall itself (Feigenbaum, 1976).

Compensatory hyperkinesis of the septum, opposite the region of hypokinesis or akinesis

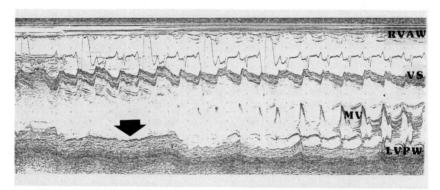

Fig. K-1. M-mode echographic scan of the LV from mid-LV to mitral valve level, in a patient with alcoholic cardiomyopathy, but normal coronary arteries. The LV posterior wall is akinetic at mid-LV level (*arrow*) and hypokinetic at mitral valve level. The ventricular septum shows normal systolic motion. The LV is dilated.

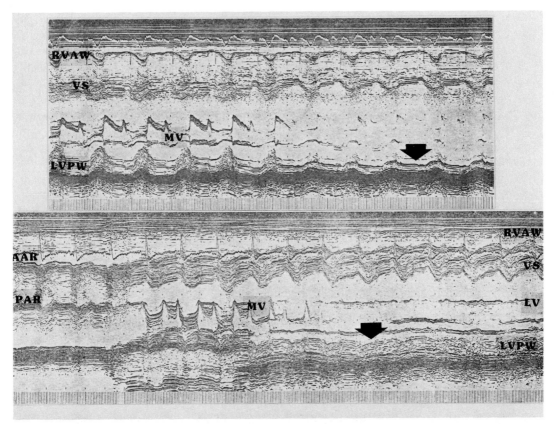

Fig. K-2. *Upper.* M-mode echographic scan of the LV from mitral to chordae level in a patient with inferior wall infarction. The LV posterior wall motion and thickness are normal at mitral valve level, but at mid-LV level the LV posterior wall is abnormally thin and hypokinetic (*arrow*). Septal motion appears normal.

Lower. M-mode echographic scan from LA to LV at mitral and then chordae level, in a patient with posteroinferior wall infarction. The ventricular septum moves normally. The LV posterior wall is akinetic (*arrow*). A slightly different pattern of LV posterior wall motion at mitral valve level could possibly be due to transmitted pulsations from the thoracic descending aorta (echo-free space) just behind it.

in the LV posterior wall, is very characteristic of ischemic heart disease. Striking contrast between vigorous contraction of the ventricular septum and feeble systolic motion of the LV posterior wall at the same LV level is very persuasive evidence of posteroinferior wall ischemia or infarction.

Similarly, attenuation or lack of septal contraction is often compensated for by vigorous systolic excursions of the LV posterior wall. Contraction of the LV posterior wall causes it to thicken in systole. Systolic increase in thickness in normal subjects has been quoted as ranging from 36 to 95 per cent (Nanda and Gramiak, 1978), and from 21 to 92 per cent (Corya *et al.,* 1977). Acute as well as old healed

infarctions of the LV posterior wall may present with diminished or even absent systolic thickening of this structure on the M-mode tracing. However, the echographic finding of normal LV posterior wall thickening by no means excludes the presence of infarction, which has presumably spared the area visualized on the echogram. Diminished systolic thickening and systolic anterior excursions of the LV posterior wall are also the rule in congestive (dilated) cardiomyopathy but are accompanied by diminished septal systolic thickening and excursions. In ischemia or infarction of the LV posterior wall, on the other hand, the ventricular septum opposite the hypokinetic LV wall shows normal or vigorous contraction.

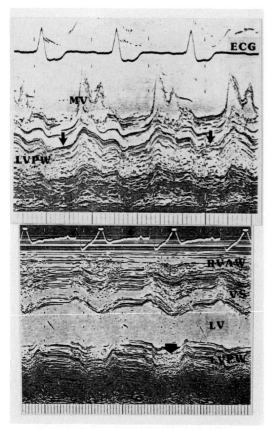

Fig. K-3. Paradoxic systolic motion of the LV posterior wall in myocardial infarction.

Upper. M-mode echogram of a patient with an inferior wall aneurysm following myocardial infarction. LV posterior wall motion is the reverse of normal, i.e., it moves posteriorly in systole and anteriorly in early diastole. Note that the contour of the LV posterior wall echo appears almost normal, until its relationship to the ECG, and therefore to the cardiac cycle, is noticed. Also note that the apposed mitral leaflets passively follow the LV posterior wall motion, simulating mitral prolapse (a form of pseudo-prolapse).

Lower. M-mode echogram of a patient with an inferior wall LV aneurysm following myocardial infarction. During systole the LV posterior wall moves dyskinetically, i.e., posteriorly in systole (*arrow*). The septum is hypertrophied and moves normally.

ABNORMALITIES OF MOTION AND THICKENING OF THE VENTRICULAR SEPTUM (Figs. K-4, K-5, and K-6)

Considerable attention has been paid to systolic behavior of the ventricular septum in ischemic heart disease, in particular to septal hypokinesis

or akinesis as evidence of obstruction in the left anterior descending artery (Gordon and Kerber, 1977; Corya *et al.,* 1977; Joffe *et al.,* 1977; Kolibash *et al.,* 1977; Cody *et al.,* 1980). Whereas some of these authors found a close correlation between significant stenosis of this coronary artery and abnormal septal motion (systolic posterior excursion less than 3 mm, or systolic anterior motion), others reported that abnormal septal motion is a relatively insensitive marker of severe left anterior descending artery stenosis, i.e., many patients with narrowing or even occlusion of this artery manifest septal excursions within the normal range (at least 3 to 4 mm).

The weight of published evidence on this topic seems to permit the general statement that abnormal septal motion indicates significant stenosis of the left anterior descending artery, probably proximal to the septal "perforator" branches of this artery (Gordon and Kerber, 1977). Studying septal perfusion by intracoronary injections of radio-labeled macroaggregated albumin, Kolibash *et al.* (1977) reported that the presence of abnormal septal motion on echocardiography strongly suggests absent septal perfusion and most likely infarction in patients with jeopardized left anterior descending artery stenosis. Normally, the ventricular septum at mid-LV (mitral chordae) level thickens in systole to the extent of 30 to 65 per cent of its end-diastolic thickness (Nanda and Gramiak, 1978); 14 to 57 per cent in the series of Corya *et al.* (1977).

Lack or diminution of systolic septal thickening at mid-LV level suggests infarction or ischemia of this region and is therefore usually accompanied by diminished, absent, or paradoxic excursions. There is some evidence that patients with acute anteroseptal infarction (transmural anteroseptal infarct on the ECG) have a better prognosis if they exhibit normal septal motion and systolic thickening than if either or both of these features are abnormal (Wiener *et al.,* 1979). Absence or decrease in systolic septal thickening, combined with absent or decreased systolic excursions, is frequently encountered in hypertrophic cardiomyopathy (including IHSS) as well as in congestive cardiomyopathy. In the former, the septum is very thick, the LV posterior wall contracts vigorously, and the LV chamber is small; in the latter, septal thick-

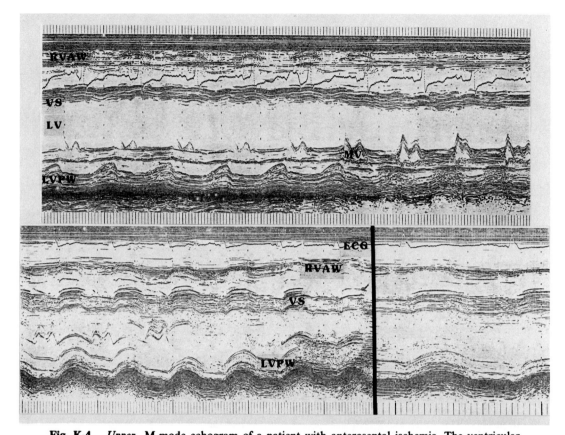

Fig. K-4.   *Upper.* M-mode echogram of a patient with anteroseptal ischemia. The ventricular septum appears akinetic at chordae tendineae level and the LV chamber is wider at this level than it is at mitral valve level. Angiocardiography revealed a large anteroseptal LV aneurysm.

Lower. M-mode echogram of a patient with recent aortic valve replacement. The ventricular septum shows abnormal systolic anterior motion at the level of mitral chordae. The right panel was recorded at faster paper speed, the better to show temporal relationships between motion of the septum, LV posterior wall, and ECG.

ness is normal, the LV wall is hypokinetic, and the LV is dilated.

Paradoxic anterior septal motion or lack of normal posterior motion in systole has been reported in a large number of cardiac conditions of very diverse pathology. The more common among these include left bundle branch block, right ventricular diastolic overload, recent open-heart surgery, right ventricular pacing, and constrictive pericarditis (Fig. K-5).

The abnormal septal motion of left bundle branch block is distinctive in that a rapid brief posterior "dip" very early in systole precedes the slower anterior motion. Abnormal systolic sepal motion is often (but not always) seen after coronary bypass and other cardiac surgery, on M-mode as well as 2-D echography (Rubenson *et al.,* 1982; Kerber *et al.,* 1982). Its mechanism

(i.e., whether it is due to septal myocardial damage or to altered cardiac motion secondary to sternal-cardiac adhesions) remains controversial. A characteristic feature of right ventricular diastolic overload is that the ventricular septum shows considerable systolic thickening, in contrast to absent or minimal systolic thickening typical of ischemic involvement.

Rasmussen *et al.* (1978) further extended the potential diagnostic scope of echocardiography in coronary heart disease by demonstrating that regional fibrotic (scar) replacement of myocardium manifested echocardiographically as abnormal thinness (less than 7 mm, or less than 30 per cent of adjacent healthy ventricular wall) and abnormally high density of echoes reflected from the affected area. The latter can be explained on the assumption that dense fibrous

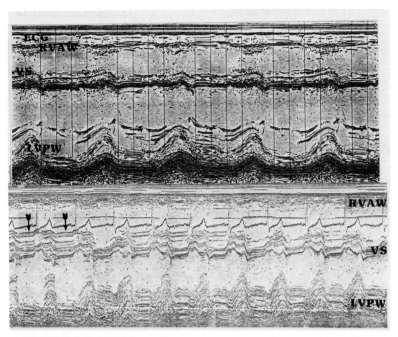

Fig. K-5. Abnormal septal motion.

Upper. M-mode echogram of a patient who had had recent coronary bypass graft surgery. The LV is visualized at chordae tendineae level. It shows normal contraction of the LV posterior wall but abnormal motion (of so-called type B) of the ventricular septum.

Lower. M-mode echogram of the LV at chordae tendineae and papillary muscle level; the ventricular septum is thinner than the LV posterior wall, and at first glance may appear to exhibit abnormal paradoxic systolic motion. However, closer scrutiny shows that anterior septal motion begins before inscription of the QRS complex and is therefore due to atrial contraction. After the QRS is inscribed, the septum moves posteriorly in normal manner. This figure also illustrates another possible pitfall in interpretation: at left (first 3 beats) the septum appears unduly thick because of linear echoes in the RV moving (*arrows*) parallel to the septum. The echoes probably originate from the tricuspid apparatus.

scar tissue in the infarcted septum is a better reflector of ultrasound than normal myocardium. Fibrous replacement in a LV posterior wall infarct can likewise manifest with abnormal thinness and density of the affected area on the echographic tracing.

"LINEAR" M-MODE SCANNING OF THE LV ANTERIOR WALL

The anterior LV wall is beyond the range of scanning from the conventional M-mode site—the left sternal edge. However, in some patients it is possible to obtain adequate echoes from the LV anterior wall by linear scanning, as follows: With the patient in the left lateral position, the left ventricle approaches the left anterior chest wall more closely. The transducer is first placed near the left margin of the septum,

as usual, to visualize the septum and LV posterior wall at chordae level. The transducer is then moved laterally along the chest wall, in contact with it, so as to be directly over the LV rather than RV. At this point, the ventricular septum is no longer seen, while the LV anterior wall lies just under the chest wall. Infarction of this area of the LV wall will manifest as marked hypokinesis or akinesis.

In practice, good quality echoes of the anterior LV are seldom obtained by this method because of intervening lung tissue.

In conclusion, M-mode echography reliably depicts wall motion abnormalities in ischemic heart disease *if* the affected myocardial region lies within the area visualized in this mode. Moreover, it may be possible to diagnose myocardial scarring on the basis of an abnormal, thinned, and dense LV wall or septum. How-

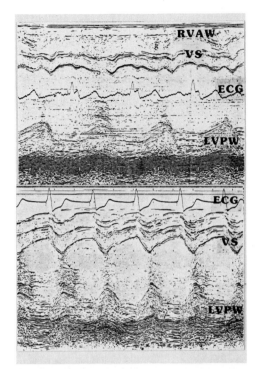

Fig. K-6. Atypical septal systolic motion in patients with left bundle branch block.

Upper. M-mode echogram in a patient with left bundle branch block. The septum exhibits a brief posterior motion early in systole, as in left bundle branch block, but then moves posteriorly (i.e., no paradoxic anterior motion is visible).

Lower. M-mode echogram in a patient with a transvenous pacemaker. The ventricular septum shows normal systolic motion.

ever, in spite of claims that M-mode echography from multiple left parasternal sites (Heikkila and Nieminen, 1980) can diagnose wall motion abnormalities in all cases of myocardial infarction, it is the experience of most echocardiologists that a considerable proportion of infarcts involving the apex and adjacent septum and/or anterolateral wall are visualized only by 2-D echography.

TWO-DIMENSIONAL ECHOCARDIOGRAPHY

Using multiple views, 2-D echocardiography permits visualization of the entire LV, except in a small percentage of patients in whom technically satisfactory recordings cannot be obtained because of emphysema, obesity, unfavorable thoracic shape, and so forth. Since most areas of the heart can be imaged in two or even

three of the various views (parasternal long- and short-axes, apical four-chamber and long-axis, and when possible subcostal), the detection of a local wall motion abnormality in one view can be corroborated by abnormal contour or behavior of the same segment in another view.

A good correlation between 2-D echographic recognition of LV wall motion abnormalities and autopsy findings of infarction was established in a series of 20 autopsied patients (Weiss *et al.*, 1981). These authors found that echography tended to overestimate the area of infarction, either because myocardium adjacent to infarcted areas was reversibly ischemic or because normal myocardium showed abnormal motion when in close proximity to scar tissue of infarction.

Kisslo *et al.* (1977) compared abnormalities of LV wall motion on 2-D echography in long- and short-axis views to those detected by biplane cineangiocardiography in a series of 105 patients. They divided the LV into five regions: anterolateral, posterolateral, apical, septal, and inferior. In about 80 per cent of LV segments that were seen adequately by the 2-D technique, the angiographic and echographic findings were in accord. Discrepancies between the two techniques in the other 20 per cent of LV segments examined were analyzed and attributed to inadequacy of the 2-D endocardial image, motion of the heart as a whole distorting the imaging plane, errors in angiogram interpretation, and so forth.

Heger *et al.* (1979, 1980) correlated the 2-D echogram with the electrocardiogram in 44 patients with myocardial infarction. They divided the LV into nine segments, as follows: the circumference of the basal LV as viewed in short axis was divided into four segments: anterior, lateral, posterior, and medial (septal); the mid-LV likewise was divided into a similar set of four segments; the ninth segment was the LV apex. They noted a very close correlation between the ECG localization of myocardial infarction and the 2-D echographic detection of LV wall motion abnormalities.

A close correlation of 2-D echographic and electrographic localization of acute myocardial infarction studied 2 to 12 hours after onset of symptoms was reported by Visser *et al.* (1981). They found 2-D echography a reliable method not only for early localization but also quantification of extent of the acute infarct, which correlated with the peak CPK-MB value. Several recent studies have focused attention on the role of 2-D echocardiography, in patients admitted with chest pain and suspected myocardial infarction or unstable angina, in detecting the presence and extent of LV wall motion abnormality and in assessing prognosis (Gibson *et al.*, 1982; Horowitz *et al.*, 1982; Horowitz and Morganroth, 1982; Loh *et al.*, 1982; Nixon *et al.*, 1982).

The American Society of Echocardiography Committee on Nomenclature and Standards has recently recommended a standard nomenclature for identifying myocardial wall segments. The committee first divides the myocardium into (1) LV free wall, (2) ventricular septum, and (3) RV free wall. The LV free wall and ventricular septum are subdivided along the long axis into basal, mid-, and apical regions of equal length. The committee's recommendation about subdivision in the short-axis views is more complex and based on an elaborate radial coordinate system.

Apical views are most helpful in detecting abnormalities of apical and septal motion and in appreciating overall LV geometry (Fig. K-7).

In everyday clinical practice, it is probably sufficient to view the LV in as many views as possible, make a qualitative description of LV shape, and mention the site and degree of wall motion abnormality. A few still frames may be photographed to document the LV abnormalities for the medical record or teaching purposes. The cardiologist responsible for the patient or for making therapeutic decisions should be encouraged to view the videotape in real time. The few minutes thus spent may be worth more than an elaborate echocardiographic report laden with a multitude of numerical data and computerized calculations.

TRANSIENT OR PROVOKED CHANGES IN LV CONTRACTION

M-mode as well as 2-D echography has been used to record acute minute-to-minute changes in LV wall motion, either spontaneous as in

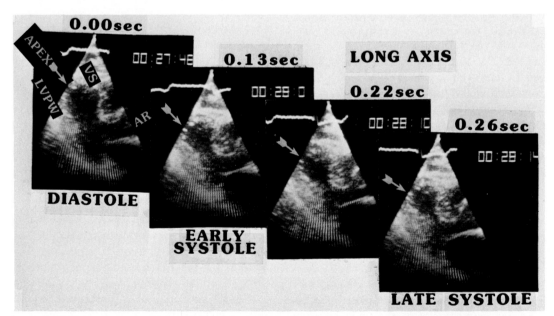

Fig. K-7. 2-D echogram showing four serial frames, in the long-axis view, of a patient with ECG evidence of anteroseptal and apical infarction. The first frame is in end-diastole, the next three are in progressively later phases of systole. The base of the LV contracts vigorously but the LV apex (*arrow*) appears relatively hypokinetic.

Prinzmetal's variant of angina (Gerson *et al.*, 1979) or provoked by various means:

1. By mechanical production of a ventricular premature beat; postextrasystolic potentiation results in enhanced contraction of normal as well as previously hypokinetic LV segments (Cohn *et al.*, 1979).

2. Morrison *et al.* (1977) demonstrated very good correlation between reversibility of wall motion abnormality as seen on echography and the same segments visualized on ventriculography by sublingual nitroglycerin administration.

3. Exercise echocardiography, using supine bicycle exercise, has been developed to unmask areas of hypokinesis during transitory, exertion-induced ischemia (Mason *et al.*, 1979; Wann *et al.*, 1979). There are obvious technical difficulties in obtaining satisfactory echocardiograms during exercise, but those who have pioneered this approach claim it is feasible as well as diagnostically useful. Wann used sublingual nitroglycerin immediately after exercise to demonstrate reversibility of exercise-provoked LV wall motion impairment.

Recently, Mitamura *et al.* (1981) found handgrip exercise highly specific in unmasking LV wall motion abnormalities and thereby predicting the presence of severe or multivessel stenosis of coronary arteries. However, the sensitivity of this method was relatively low, i.e., only 65 per cent of patients with proven coronary stenosis whose resting 2-D echogram revealed normal wall motion showed abnormal LV wall motion during handgrip exercise.

Maurer and Nanda (1981) obtained 2-D echograms before and immediately after gradual treadmill exercise; findings were correlated with angiocardiography and thallium perfusion scans performed five to ten minutes and also three hours after the exercise test. Exercise-induced wall motion abnormalities were detected in 19 of 23 patients with significant coronary artery disease and no prior myocardial infarction as well as in five with known previous infarction.

Quantitation of LV performance during upright bicycle exercise was studied in patients with severe angina by 2-D echography in apical views (Crawford *et al.*, 1983). In normal subjects the LV ejection fraction increased from 57 per cent at rest to 71 per cent at peak exercise (mean), but remained unchanged in the angina patients.

In conclusion, it may be stated that at present exercise echography is still in the investigative phase and has not yet been incorporated into the routine workup of patients with ischemic heart disease. It is to be hoped that a standardized, practicable, and reliable procedure eventually will be established for this purpose.

LEFT VENTRICULAR ANEURYSMS

M-mode echocardiography has a limited role in the diagnosis of LV aneurysms because the basal LV chamber (near the mitral annulus), which is the part of the ventricle best seen by this technique, is seldom the location for aneurysmal change.

Aneurysms of the LV *inferior wall* manifest as akinesis, or in some instances dyskinesis (posterior systolic motion) of the LV posterior wall, usually at chordae tendineae LV level. Patients with aneurysms of the *ventricular septum* exhibit lack of motion or paradoxic (anterior) motion of this structure during systole, also commonly at chordae level. In a few cases of aneurysm of the LV anterior wall, it may be possible to visualize directly the akinetic or paradoxic motion of the *LV anterior wall* by the linear scan technique, sliding the transducer laterally along the chest wall with the patient lying in a left lateral position. In the subcostal view, the "LV posterior wall" recorded is actually the posterolateral rather than inferior (diaphragmatic) LV wall, so that *posterolateral aneurysms* are seen best by this approach, which is especially suitable for thin patients with low diaphragms and lax epigastric muscles.

In all of these situations, however, it would be difficult to make a definite diagnosis of a ventricular aneurysm on the M-mode findings done. Whereas LV aneurysms are always associated with wall motion abnormalities of the affected region, the reverse is not necessarily true; akinesis or dyskinesis on M-mode echocardiography is not synonymous with aneurysm formation.

Visualization of distortion of ventricular shape in diastole is essential for diagnosing an aneurysm [an "anatomical aneurysm," according to Cabin and Roberts (1980)]; the deformation of contour, of course, is even more pronounced in systole because the aneurysmal area expands while the rest of the LV chamber decreases in size. On the other hand, if wall motion abnormalities are present without aneurysmal bulging, the left ventricle retains its normal diastolic shape; only in systole does the LV configuration look abnormal, preferably when viewing the video image in real time or slow motion ["functional aneurysm" in the terminology of Cabin and Roberts (1980)].

Nevertheless, M-mode echographic appearances suggestive of ventricular aneurysm can be recognized in some patients with large aneurysms involving the LV apex and adjacent myocardium (Figs. K-8 and K-9):

1. Normally the width of the LV chamber gradually narrows as a scan is made from the basal left ventricle (at mitral valve level) toward the mid-left ventricle (at chordae level) and then on toward the LV apex. Thus, the LV posterior wall and septum approach each other at papillary muscle level and may almost come in contact in systole at near-apical level. This appreciation of the normal conical or tapering LV shape is recorded best at a slow paper speed (10 mm/sec) during such LV scans (Fig. A-9). It is important to keep in mind that this tapering LV effect is seen best with the ultra-

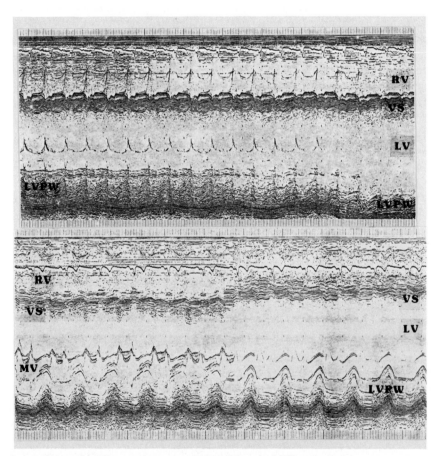

Fig. K-8. Abnormal LV scans in two patients with apical LV aneurysms.

Upper. M-mode echographic scan of the LV from chordae level toward the LV apex, in a patient with a large apical aneurysm. The LV dimension progressively increased, whereas normally the LV tapers toward its apex. The ventricular septum is akinetic, and the LV posterior wall at this level is hypokinetic.

Lower. M-mode echographic scan of the LV from mitral valve level to chordae tendineae level, in a patient with a postinfarction aneurysm of the anteroseptal and apical LA wall. The diagnosis can be suspected on this M-mode tracing because of septal akinesis and widening of the LV dimension toward the apex.

sound transducer placed as low as possible on the left parasternal area. It may not be evident when the left ventricle is scanned from higher left intercostal spaces.

In patients with large LV aneurysms at or near its apex, the LV chamber width actually *increases* as a scan is made from LV base toward its apex (Figs. K-8 and K-9), as was well demonstrated in the publications of Feigenbaum and associates (Feigenbaum *et al.,* 1976; Dillon *et al.,* 1976). Dillon *et al.* found that if the LVID measured at mid-LV (chordae) level was less than 33 mm/M² body surface area, and at low LV (nearer LV apex) level less than 38 mm/M², the prognosis after surgical excision of the aneurysm was excellent; all their 11 patients in this group survived surgery. On the other hand, all but one of their seven patients who did not survive operation had mid-LV dimensions over 33 mm/M² and low LV dimensions exceeding 38 mm/M².

Thus, although the LV apex itself is hidden to view by M-mode examination, careful scanning of the left ventricle from base to apex can reveal useful information about LV shape that can lead to at least the suspicion of a large apical LV aneurysm. Confirmation of this diagnosis by cross-sectional echocardiography, radionuclide studies, and angiocardiography then may lead to successful aneurysmectomy. M-mode echocardiography, therefore, can help in screening patients with ischemic heart disease to select possible candidates with this potentially lethal, yet correctable, complication of myocardial infarction.

If the "apical" LV aneurysm is large enough to involve also a considerable extent of the ventricular septum or of the inferior wall, akinesis or hypokinesis of the affected myocardium may be visualized at mid- or low LV levels.

Caution: M-mode recordings of the LV posterior wall and ventricular septum at basal or even mid-LV levels can be very misleading if these regions show vigorous contraction as a compensatory mechanism in response to the adverse hemodynamic effect of a large apical aneurysm. This is especially apt to occur if the patient had concentric LV hypertrophy and a

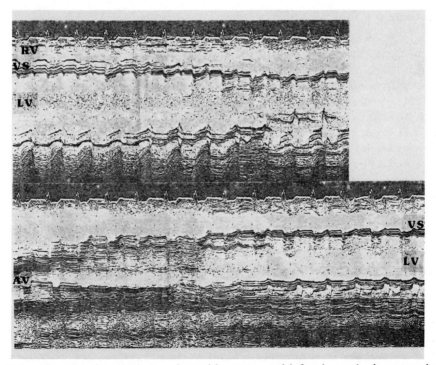

Fig. K-9. M-mode echogram in a patient with anteroseptal infarction and a large ventricular aneurysm involving the septum and apex. The upper panel shows a scan from chordae level toward the mitral valve, by the parasternal approach. The lower panel shows a scan from aortic root to LV, by the subcostal approach. The infarcted septum is thin and shows abnormal systolic motion. Left bundle branch block could also account for abnormal septal motion. The LV is considerably dilated, more so toward the apex than the base.

small LV chamber previous to the myocardial infarction and aneurysm formation. M-mode echography then may reveal normal LV width and normal contraction at mitral valve level. Two-D echocardiography demonstrates that the normal basal LV myocardium leads to a large ballooning of the remainder of the LV chamber (Fig. K-12).

2. Whereas most ventricular aneurysms merge gradually with surrounding healthy myocardium, in some instances the aneurysm tends to be saccular—an abrupt outpouching of the ventricular wall with relatively sharp edges demarcating healthy from dyskinetic infarcted myocardium. In such cases, M-mode scanning from basal LV (mitral valve) level toward the apex may demonstrate an abrupt and considerable (2 cm or more) posterior displacement as the sweep moves from normal to aneurysmal wall (Petersen et al., 1972; Kreamer et al., 1973).

A similar finding is seen also in some patients with large ballooning aneurysms of the ventricular septum. In such cases, the septum adjacent to the aortic root (basal level) appears normal, but at mid-LV level the septal echo tends to drop out, i.e., it can be recorded only incompletely on M-mode echocardiography because this abnormal part of the septum is tangential rather than perpendicular to the ultrasound beam. The aneurysmal configuration of the septal contour is recognized readily on long-axis and apical 2-D views.

3. It is worth looking carefully at the pattern of anterior mitral leaflet motion in patients with suspected aneurysms or dyskinesis at or near the LV apex. If the aneurysm or abnormality of LV wall motion is large enough to seriously impair overall LV performance, the anterior mitral leaflet might exhibit a notch on the AC slope, or the mitral E point–septal separation (EPSS) is abnormally large.

In a patient who shows apparently satisfactory motion of the septum and LV posterior wall at mitral valve level, such mitral valve motion abnormalities alert the cardiologist to the possibility of an aneurysm or gross impairment of contractility elsewhere in the LV chamber. Further investigative procedures to explore this possibility are then in order.

4. Ogawa et al. (1978) found that the peak LV wall systolic motion was delayed in patients with inferior wall aneurysms. Thus, the ratio R-to-LVPW peak/LV ejection time was 1.35 or more in 16 of 18 patients with inferior wall aneurysms but not in normals.

2-D ECHOCARDIOGRAPHY OF VENTRICULAR ANEURYSM (Figs. K-10 to K-14)

Distortion of LV shape due to aneurysm formation was recognized on B-scans by Yoshikawa et al. (1974). However, real-time 2-D echocardiography, using a mechanical oscillating sector-scanner, soon proved to have obvious technical and diagnostic advantages over B-scanning. Weyman et al. (1976) found it capable of visualizing aneurysms of virtually every part of the LV in a series of 31 patients with angiographically proven LV aneurysms. These authors found 2-D echography vastly superior to the previously used indicators of LV aneurysm: M-mode echography, chest x-rays, physical examination, and electrocardiograms (persistent ST elevations).

Weyman et al. (1976) defined a LV aneurysm as an "interruption in the normal contour of the LV wall occurring during both diastole and systole." They distinguished three types of LV aneurysm: apical, anterior, and posterior, which often occurred in combination.

Weyman visualized apical aneurysms by moving the 2-D probe over laterally from the left parasternum toward the apex, though still keeping its plane of oscillation oriented in the LV long axis.

By experience and comparison with LV angiograms, the echocardiographer comes to recognize certain basic LV patterns (Fig. K-15), including those of LV aneurysms; it must be kept in mind that variation in severity of abnormal contour and various combinations of lesions often occur in practice.

The advent of the apical four-chamber and apical long-axis views greatly improved the echocardiographer's appreciation of LV shape. Aneurysms of the LV apex were recognizable as akinetic or dyskinetic bulbous expansions of the LV apex, easily distinguishable from its normal tapering, conical contour. Exceptionally, a small slender protrusion of the LV chamber may be detected (Estevez et al., 1976)—a congenital diverticulum quite different in shape,

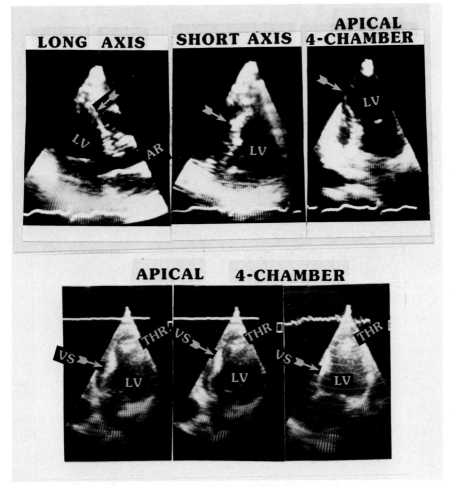

Fig. K-10. 2-D echogram in two different patients with LV aneurysms.

Upper. 2-D echogram of a patient with an anteroseptal aneurysm. The left frame is in the long-axis view, the center frame in the short-axis view, and the right frame in the apical 4-chamber view. The septal aneurysm (*arrows*) can be seen as a bulge anteriorly and to the right.

Lower. 2-D echogram of a patient with an apical aneurysm, which appears as a bulbous round dilatation of the LV apex. The aneurysm contains a mural thrombus, which is better defined in the left and center frames than in the right frame.

size, and pathogenesis from the more usual postinfarction aneurysm. Aneurysms involving the ventricular septum, as well as anterior, anteroseptal, and anteroapical aneurysms, can be seen well in the apical four-chamber and/or apical long-axis views (Chiaramida *et al.*, 1980; Rogers *et al.*, 1980; Sorensen *et al.*, 1982; Baur *et al.*, 1982).

The short-axis view is suitable for imaging the distortion of LV shape and motion caused by posteroinferior aneurysms affecting the lower half of the circular LV contour in this view. Septal, anteroseptal, or anterolateral aneurysms cause similar contour and motion

changes of the affected segment of the upper half of the LV circle that contrast strikingly with the normal motion of the unaffected myocardium.

Even more important than the location and size of the LV aneurysm to the patient's prognosis and to the clinician are the extent and contractility of the nonaneurysmal LV. This is crucial to the decision as to whether the patient is a suitable surgical candidate and, therefore, whether a hemodynamic study is in order or not.

LV aneurysms frequently have sessile or pedunculated thrombi adherent to their walls. The

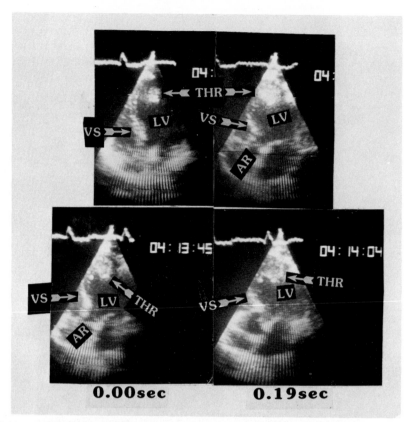

Fig. K-11. 2-D echogram (apical 4-chamber views) of a patient with a huge LV aneurysm involving most of the LV except its basal portion. A mural thrombus can be seen at the LV apex within the aneurysm.

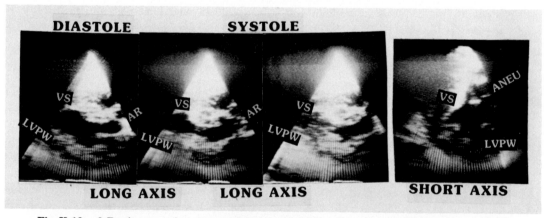

Fig. K-12. 2-D echogram of a patient with concentric LV hypertrophy secondary to hypertension and an LV aneurysm involving the apex and adjacent ventricular septum. The first three frames are in the long-axis view: the first in diastole, the second at midsystole, the third at end-systole. The base of the LV contracts well, so that the septum and LV posterior wall almost meet (*third frame*). However, nearer the apex the LV does not contract as well. In the right frame, in the short-axis view, an aneurysmal area, containing a mural thrombus, is visible in the anteroseptal area.

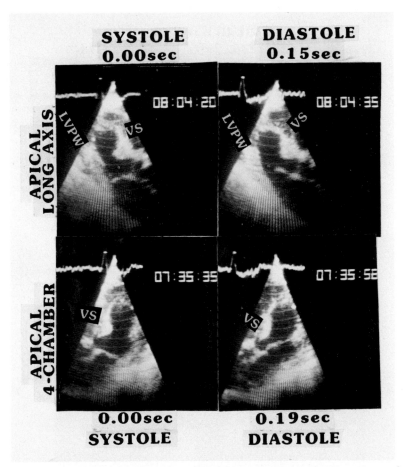

Fig. K-13. 2-D echogram of an elderly woman with a small apical LV aneurysm following myocardial infarction. The two upper frames, in the apical long-axis view, are from the same cardiac cycle; the two lower frames, in the apical 4-chamber view, are from another cardiac cycle. The frames on the left are at about end-diastole; the frames on the right are near end-diastole. The LV contracts well at its base but not at its apex. The LV as a whole is not dilated.

shape of an aneurysm—whether a shallow protrusion or a deep sac—may have some bearing on the likelihood of mural thrombi within it being swept away into the blood stream (Cabin and Roberts, 1980). By providing reliable information about the shape and size of an LV aneurysm and the presence or absence of clot within it, 2-D echography is of great help to the clinician in making decisions about anticoagulant therapy (Lewin *et al.,* 1980).

DIFFERENTIATION BETWEEN TRUE AND FALSE ANEURYSMS OF THE LEFT VENTRICLE

True LV aneurysms are produced by bulging or ballooning of the weakened infarcted LV wall; the wall of the aneurysm is thus the LV wall itself, albeit thinned or scarred by fibrous replacement of myocardium. *Pseudoaneurysms* are caused by rupture of the LV wall with escape of blood into a large false sac, the walls of which are formed by pericardium and surrounding mediastinal structures. Whereas true aneurysms are by far the more common of the two, pseudoaneurysms are important because they carry a grave prognosis but are correctable surgically if diagnosed in time. Until 2-D echography and radionuclide angiography became available, the noninvasive diagnosis of both true and false LV aneurysms was difficult or impossible in most cases. The onset of LV pseudoaneurysms may be accompanied by severe, prolonged chest pain, hypotension, and

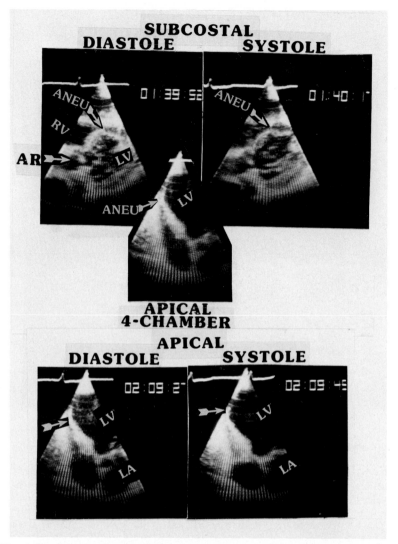

Fig. K-14. 2-D echogram of a patient with an aneurysm (ANEU) of the ventricular septum. The upper frames are in the subcostal view, the left in diastole and the right in systole, 0.25 sec later. The center frame is in the apical 4-chamber view. The aneurysmal segment of the septum bulges toward the RV.

The lower two frames are also in the apical view, the left in diastole, the right frame in systole, 0.22 sec later. Note that the ventricular septum bulges toward the right (*arrow*) in diastole as well as in systole, but more so in systole.

abrupt deterioration of cardial compensation; it can thus resemble extension of acute myocardial infarction. Two-D echocardiography provides the clinician with a rapid bedside means of distinguishing between these two catastrophes.

On the M-mode echogram, LV pseudoaneurysms present as a large, echo-free space posterior to the LV, which could be mistaken for a pericardial or left pleural effusion (Roelandt *et al.*, 1975; Morcerf *et al.*, 1976; Mills *et al.*,

1977; Aintablian *et al.*, 1979; Davidson *et al.*, 1977). An anatomically similar example secondary to staphylococcal endocarditis of the mitral valve has been described (Saksena *et al.*, 1978).

The 2-D echocardiographic visualization of a pseudoaneurysm was first reported by Roelandt *et al.* (1975) using a linear array system, but technically better depiction of the anatomy of the false aneurysm, its relation to the LV chamber, and the break in the LV wall leading

LEFT VENTRICULAR PROFILES IN PARASTERNAL LONG-AXIS VIEW

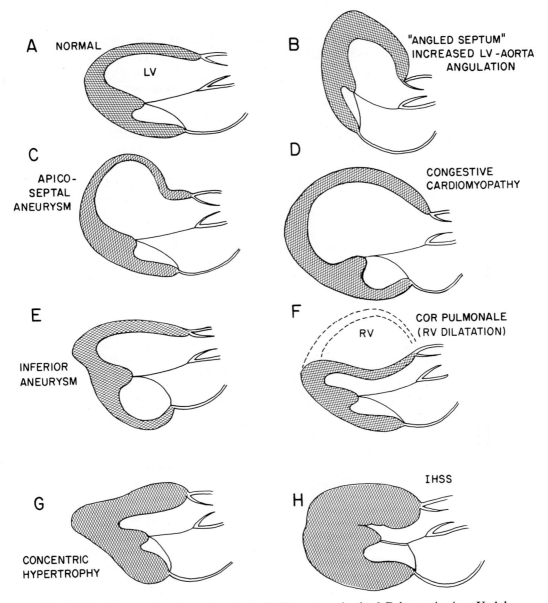

Fig. K-15. Diagram showing various typical LV contours in the 2-D long-axis view. Unduly thick LV walls and small LV chambers are characteristic of *G* and *H*. A small LV chamber (but not hypertrophy) may be seen in *F*. Ventricular aneurysms (*C* and *E*) must be differentiated from diffuse LV dilatation (*D*). Note the abnormal LV alignment (*B*) compared to normal alignment (*A*). *A* also shows normal LV shape.

into the aneurysmal sac was presented by Sears *et al.* (1977), Katz *et al.* (1979), and Gatewood and Nanda (1980).

Katz *et al.* (1979) recognized that the main difference between true and false LV aneurysms, discernible on 2-D echography, was that true aneurysms opened into the LV through large mouths as wide as the aneurysm itself. On the other hand, pseudoaneurysms communicate with the main LV chamber through a narrow neck much smaller than the largest width of the aneurysm.

Gatewood and Nanda (1980) confirmed this in a series of four patients with pseudoaneurysm in all of whom the neck of the false aneurysm was less than half as wide as the dilated sac itself. In seven other patients with true LV aneurysms, these authors found that the mouth of the aneurysm was 0.9 to 1.0 times the maximum width of the aneurysm. Another diagnostic feature was that the aneurysmal space could be seen extending behind the LV wall in pseudoaneurysms but not in true aneurysms.

Catherwood *et al.* (1980) recently described the 2-D echographic findings of five patients with LV pseudoaneurysms. They reemphasized the narrowness of the orifice or neck by which the aneurysmal sac communicates with the LV as a valuable diagnostic means of distinguishing false from true aneurysms; they also called attention to two other diagnostic criteria: sharp discontinuity of the endocardial image at the site of the ventricular rupture (orifice into pseudoaneurysm) and the saccular or globular contour of the aneurysmal chamber.

A large pseudoaneurysm at the LV apex recently was described by Alter *et al.* (1981).

A diverticulum of the LV is a rare anomaly that also can communicate with the LV chamber through a narrow neck, usually at the LV apex; however, such diverticula tend to be slender protrusions (Estevez *et al.,* 1976), very unlike the large, round or oval cavernous paracardiac spaces representing pseudoaneurysms on the 2-D echocardiogram.

RUPTURE OF LV WALL

This dreaded complication of acute myocardial infarction commonly is believed to be immediately fatal. However, Hagemeijer *et al.* (1980) reported four cases in whom the diagnosis was made at the bedside by 2-D echography. Weak LV contractions were observed following each QRS on the ECG. This is relevant because "electromechanical" dissociation is believed typical of this complication. Echocardiography was crucial to a successful outcome after surgery in another case of cardiac rupture 13 hours after onset of myocardial infarction. Echography demonstrated a pericardial effusion and immediate paracentesis improved the hemodynamic state sufficiently to permit emergency reconstructive surgery (Eisenmann *et al.,* 1978).

POSTINFARCTION RUPTURE OF THE VENTRICULAR SEPTUM

No specific M-mode findings have been reported in this complication of myocardial infarction. DeJoseph *et al.* (1975) described a case in which the ventricular septum appeared akinetic before rupture but after rupture showed a prominent early diastolic posterior "dip" during the phase of rapid early ventricular filling.

Chandaratna *et al.* (1975) reported three patients, all of whom had right ventricular dilatation with normal (not paradoxic) septal motion. One patient exhibited an unusual mitral diastolic echo pattern characterized by transient middiastolic closure with prompt reopening. Rosenthal *et al.* (1979) described diastolic fluttering of the posterior mitral leaflet in a patient who had no flail leaflet at surgery.

Kerin *et al.* (1976) described a patient with acute anterior myocardial infarction in whom discontinuity of the ventricular septum was demonstrated on repeated scans from LV to aortic root. In this case, the septal tear was shown (at surgery) to be at the topmost part of the muscular ventricular septum. Much more commonly, the septal rupture occurs lower in the septum at a level that cannot be visualized by M-mode echography.

It must be kept in mind, however, that septal dropout can be produced artefactually in LV-to-LA scans, especially if the heart is so aligned in the thorax that the septal plane is oblique rather than parallel to the chest wall.

Recently, 2-D echocardiography in the four-chamber apical view has been used successfully to confirm the diagnosis of ventricular septal rupture and even to locate its site in patients who developed a loud systolic murmur in the setting of acute myocardial infarction (Scanlan *et al.,* 1979; Egeblad and Hauns, 1979; Farcot *et al.,* 1980; Mintz *et al.,* 1981; Drobac *et al.,* 1983).

1. It may be possible to visualize the actual rupture as an oblique or transverse, narrow, echo-free hiatus interrupting the continuity of the septal myocardium. Such a gap may be more conspicuous in systole than in diastole. Viewing the videotape in slow motion and in frame-by-frame sequence is necessary for optimal appreciation of this sign.

2. The area of septum containing the rupture is usually dyskinetic and bulges toward the right ventricle. This septal aneurysmlike deformity may be accompanied by an apparent convexity of the upper septum in the opposite direction, i.e., toward the LV outflow tract.

3. Farcot *et al.* (1980) used contrast 2-D echography (microbubbles produced by right atrial injection of the patient's own blood) to opacify the RV chamber. The jet of unopacified blood coming across the rupture in the septum could be identified by its negative "washout" contrast effect. This sign was detected in 5 of Drobac's 12 patients; however, right-to-left passage of microbubbles through the defect was noted in 11.

In an important recent paper, Rogers *et al.*

(1980) described the 2-D echographic findings in six consecutive patients with acute inferior myocardial infarction complicated by rupture of the ventricular septum. All had aneurysms of the septum at the site of rupture. Septal dyskinesis produced conspicuous bulging of the septum into the RV in the parasternal short-axis view. Aneurysms of this type may be seen well in the subcostal four-chamber view (Fig. K-16). The association of septal aneurysm formation with septal rupture is important because (1) the aneurysm contributes to the deterioration of LV function, and (2) 2-D echographic visualization of the septal aneurysm would strengthen the suspicion of septal rupture in a patient with an inferior myocardial infarction

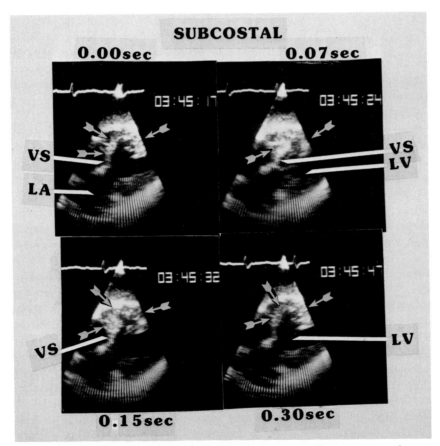

Fig. K-16. 2-D echogram in the subcostal view of a patient with aneurysm and rupture of the ventricular septum following acute myocardial infarction. The four frames are serial ones from the same cardiac cycle. The arrows indicate the aneurysmal area of the septum, which expands in the systolic frames (*top left and bottom right*) as compared to the diastolic frames (*top right and bottom left*). The septal rupture cannot be distinctly visualized; it was proven by cardiac catheterization and angiocardiography, and at surgery. On follow-up, two years later, the patient is well.

who develops a systolic murmur and lapses rapidly into cardiac failure.

The development of a new, loud systolic murmur and abrupt worsening in cardiac status in a patient with acute myocardial infarction also could be due to acute, severe mitral regurgitation secondary to papillary muscle rupture. Echocardiography may reveal LV posterior wall akinesis or hypokinesis and vigorous septal contractions with conspicuous diastolic flutter of the untethered posterior mitral leaflet (Bareiss *et al.*, 1977; Ahmad *et al.*, 1978). Thus the ventricular septum appears hyperdynamic in papillary muscle rupture or dysfunction but aneurysmal and dyskinetic in septal rupture, constituting a valuable diagnostic clue to clinicians coping with this type of cardiac emergency.

PAPILLARY MUSCLE RUPTURE

A few echocardiographic reports of this grave complication of acute myocardial infarction have appeared (Bareiss *et al.*, 1977; Ahmad *et al.*, 1978; Erbel *et al.*, 1981; Nishimura *et al.*, 1983). A combination of some of the following echographic findings in a patient with a recent inferior wall infarction and a loud systolic murmur should suggest the diagnosis. On *M-mode* echography:

1. Decreased systolic excursions of the LV posterior wall, with compensatory septal hyperkinesis,
2. Coarse rapid fluttering of the posterior mitral leaflet,
3. LV dilatation,
4. Mitral prolapse.

On *2-D* echography:

5. A mobile mass of echoes attached to mitral chordae tendineae moving erratically in the LV chamber,
6. Loss of the papillary muscle's normal contour in the long-axis view; its base is discernible but the tip seems "amputated" (Mintz *et al.*, 1981).

These authors pointed out that only 2-D echography could distinguish between papillary muscle rupture and papillary muscle fibrosis or dysfunction without rupture, the clinical presentations being very similar.

ASSESSMENT OF LV FUNCTION IN PATIENTS WITH CORONARY HEART DISEASE

Overall LV performance is an important consideration in the prognosis and management decisions for patients with acute as well as old myocardial infarction.

It has been shown by many authors that the correlation between angiocardiographic ejection fractions and the M-mode echocardiographic equivalent parameters such as the LVID systolic shortening fraction, velocity of circumferential fiber shortening (VCF), and ejection fraction based on LV end-diastolic and end-systolic volumes (calculated by various formulas from the LVID measurements) is often unsatisfactory in patients with regional LV dyssynergy. All too often these patients are precisely the ones for whom decisions are to be made about coronary angiography, coronary bypass surgery, fitness for rehabilitation programs, and return to work, and so forth—decisions that are based mainly or at least partly on overall LV function.

One approach to the noninvasive assessment of LV performance is the measurement of systolic time intervals by phonocardiography and external carotid pulse tracing. Stack *et al.* (1976) showed that the LV PEP/EP ratio and the LVID systolic shortening fraction correlated well with each other in a series that included a large number of patients with ischemic heart disease.

Moreover, these authors found that these two indices of LV performance were more sensitive measures of LV dysfunction in patients with previous transmural infarction than third or fourth heart sound gallops (documented by phonocardiography) and abnormal cardiothoracic ratios by chest roentgenogram.

Another valuable noninvasive method of assessing LV function, much in use in recent years, is the application of radionuclide blood pool scanning procedures. Several studies have now been done, documenting a good correlation of ejection fractions by this technique with ejection fractions in the same patients by invasive angiocardiography and recently by echocardiography.

Although reliable, such nuclear cardiology

techniques are limited to some degree by considerations of cost and availability of equipment and isotopic material. Moreover, because of the specialized personnel and nature of materials used, the procedure cannot be done at any time and in any place. On the other hand, echocardiography can be done at the patient's bedside at very short notice, provided a person with the necessary skill is available.

Because of the potential fallacies in estimating LV function by formulas based on M-mode LVID measurements in patients with regional abnormalities of LV wall shape or motion, echocardiographers turned to the mitral and aortic valves, the motion of which is known to reflect LV performance (Fig. K-17) because valve motion is affected by changes in LV pressures and stroke volume. This topic is discussed in the chapter on LV function.

CORONARY ARTERIES (Figs. K-18 to K-22)

LEFT MAIN CORONARY ARTERY

Since Weyman *et al.* (1976) showed that the left main coronary artery could be imaged adequately and stenosis of its lumen recognized

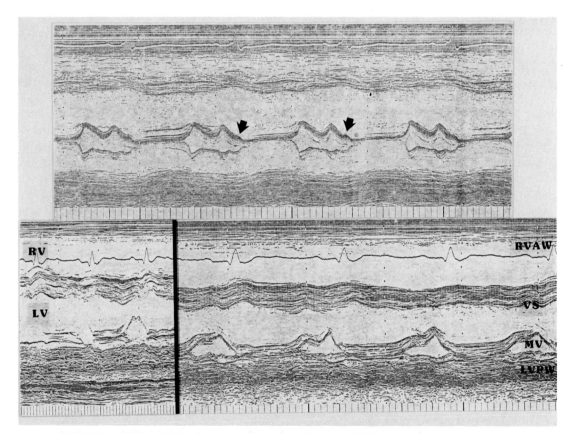

Fig. K-17. Abnormal mitral valve motion as a reflection of LV dysfunction.
Upper. M-mode echogram in a man with a large apical aneurysm. The LV is extremely dilated. The mitral valve shows a notch or bump on its AC slope (*arrows*), indicating a significantly elevated LV end-diastolic pressure. The LV end-diastolic pressure was 36 mm and ejection fraction 26 per cent.
Lower. M-mode echocardiogram of a patient with inferior myocardial infarction and concentric LV hypertrophy. The LV posterior wall is akinetic. The LV is not dilated. The mitral valve opens slowly in early diastole (low DE slope) and opens more fully with atrial contraction, as is well visualized in the right panel. Cardiac catheterization showed impaired LV performance and raised LV diastolic pressure.

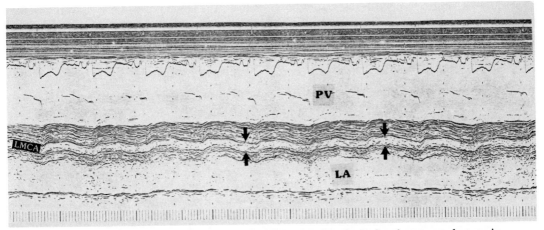

Fig. K-18. M-mode echogram of a normal person, showing the atriopulmonary sulcus region, which is situated between the pulmonary artery and valve anteriorly, and the LA posteriorly. The left main coronary artery is visualized as a narrow echo-free space about 5 mm wide, within the dense echoes of the atriopulmonary sulcus (*arrows*).

by 2-D echography, the application of cardiac ultrasound has aroused great interest among cardiologists. Although the left main coronary artery forms but a small segment of the coronary arterial tree, critical stenosis of this vessel is a strong indication for bypass-graft surgery. A noninvasive means of diagnosing left main coronary artery stenosis would enable the clinician to proceed promptly to angiographic confirmation and then to surgical correction. On the other hand, a reliable noninvasive method of excluding left main coronary stenosis would perhaps be reassuring to those clinicians who favor a conservative policy in investigating and managing their patients with suspected coronary disease.

The left main coronary artery may be visualized sometimes by M-mode echography as a narrow, echo-free space a few millimeters wide within the dense echoes of the "atriopulmonary sulcus," just posterior to the pulmonic valve (Fig. K-18).

The left main coronary artery is visualized by first bringing the aortic root into view in the short-axis view and then making slight changes in transducer direction until the left main coronary artery is seen as a pair of parallel linear echoes issuing from the left margin of the aortic root at about the three- or four-o'clock position and running directly leftward. The pulmonic valve and left main coronary artery are in about the same short-axis plane so that maneuvering the pulmonic valve into view

helps in finding the artery. The origin of the right coronary artery may be seen at about the 11-o'clock position in a slightly different plane (Fig. K-21).

Fortunately, the left main coronary artery courses through a region at the base of the heart called the atriopulmonary sulcus posterior to the main pulmonary artery that provides a background of dense echoes [attributable to pericardial fat (Rogers *et al.,* 1980)], against which the coronary artery is imaged as a narrow, echo-free band (Figs. K-19 to K-21).

In some individuals, only the ostium of the artery and its proximal few millimeters can be recorded; in others, the whole length of the artery can be seen; in yet others, its bifurcation and proximal segments of the anterior descending and circumflex arteries can be discerned. Frame-by-frame scrutiny of the videotape is necessary because the left main coronary echo moves in and out of view during the cardiac cycle, revealing itself fully for only tantalizingly brief fractions of a second.

When the left main coronary artery is stenotic, the linear echoes representing its walls appear thickened and show an "inward bending" at the site of stenosis (Weyman *et al.,* 1976). Feigenbaum and his group have continued to pioneer improvements in 2-D technique for this purpose, studying the left main coronary artery and its branches in vitro in cadaver hearts (Rogers *et al.,* 1980) and using digital processing of acoustic signals to detect athero-

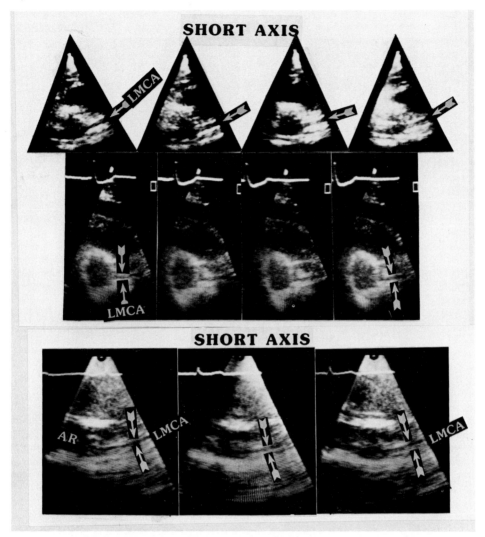

Fig. K-19. 2-D echograms, in the short-axis view, of the aortic root and left main coronary artery in three patients who had patent coronary arteries on coronary angiography. The left main coronary artery emerges from the aortic root at about the four- or 5-o'clock position.

sclerotic coronary calcification. In a prospective study of 100 patients, this technique was highly sensitive (99 per cent) but less specific (65 per cent) as an indicator of significant atherosclerotic obstruction of the left coronary system (Rogers *et al.,* 1980).

Chandaratna *et al.* (1980) confirmed that the presence or absence of significant stenosis of the left main coronary artery could be ascertained reliably by short-axis 2-D visualization of the artery as described above. These authors remarked that it was sometimes difficult to distinguish stenosis of the left anterior descending artery from that of the left main coronary artery. However, the left main coronary could

be visualized adequately in only about 60 per cent of their series of 123 patients. Technically excellent imaging of the artery may not be difficult in young persons but is often impossible in the elderly, obese, and emphysematous; unfortunately, the old, the corpulent, and heavy smokers are very well represented among candidates for coronary disease.

One group of investigators (Ogawa *et al.,* 1980; Chen *et al.,* 1980) has visualized the left main coronary artery by employing a different 2-D echographic approach. They visualize the heart in the apical four-chamber view and then angle the probe slightly to bring the aortic root into view; the probe is then rotated clockwise

SHORT AXIS

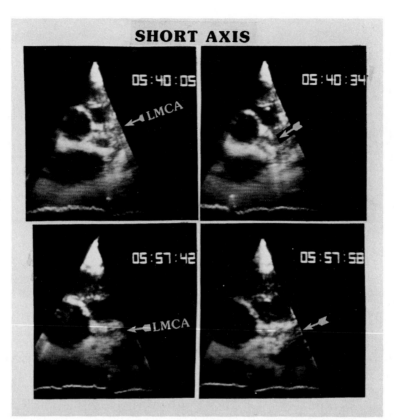

Fig. K-20. 2-D echogram in the short-axis view of a patient with probable calcification of the left main coronary artery. The upper two frames are from the same cardiac cycle; the lower two frames are from another cardiac cycle. The two left frames are systolic; the two right ones are diastolic. The image has been expanded in the lower two frames. The lumen of the left main coronary artery can be seen in all four frames. Dense areas on either side of the artery lumen may represent coronary artery calcification or dense sclerosis.

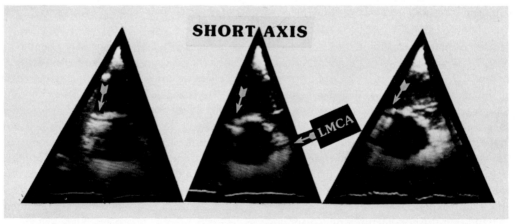

Fig. K-21. 2-D echogram, in the short axis-view, of a patient with normal coronary arteries. The right coronary artery can be seen to emerge from the aortic root at about the 11-o'clock position in all three frames. The origin of the left main coronary artery is also apparent in the center frame, at about the three- or four-o'clock position.

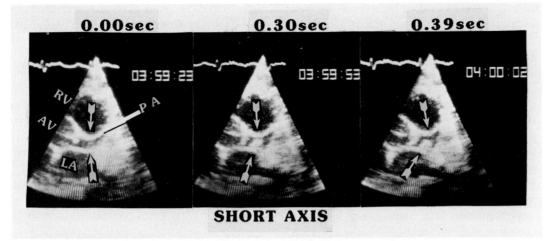

Fig. K-22. 2-D echogram in the short-axis view of a patient with a small to moderate pericardial effusion. Unusual echographic appearances (*arrows*) are evident in the region of the atriopulmonary sulcus, i.e., to the left of the aortic root, between the pulmonary artery (PA) anteriorly and the left atrium (LA) posteriorly. A small echo-free space, which fluctuates in width and contour during the cardiac cycle, is visible. The space appears to be an extension of the pericardial fluid into this recess, the anterior boundary of which is the posterior wall of the main pulmonary artery, while the shifting posterior boundary is the LA appendage. Still frames of such appearances could possibly be mistaken for dilatation or aneurysm of the left main coronary artery.

until the left main coronary artery comes into view. This technique was successful in imaging the left main coronary in 70 per cent of patients. Patency of the artery was identified correctly in 34 of 36 patients, stenosis in 12 of 16 patients.

It must be stated that at the present time the 2-D echocardiographic diagnosis of left main coronary artery patency or stenosis appears promising but by no means an established procedure. It remains to be shown that echocardiographers in general can reproduce the good results of the groups who recently have published their encouraging reports (Rink *et al.*, 1982; Friedman *et al.*, 1982).

ANOMALOUS ORIGIN OF THE LEFT CORONARY ARTERY FROM THE PULMONARY ARTERY

This important congenital anomaly can be visualized by 2-D echography (Yoshikawa *et al.*, 1978; Fisher *et al.*, 1981). The left coronary artery can be seen emerging from the posterior aspect of the pulmonary artery. The root of the pulmonary artery is visualized by first viewing the aortic root in the short axis and then tilting the probe slightly to obtain a slightly higher plane (Fisher *et al.*, 1981).

CORONARY ARTERY ANEURYSMS

In 2-D echography the left main coronary artery can be visualized as a narrow, echo-free band emerging from the left margin of the aortic root in the short-axis view. Aneurysmal dilatation of this artery manifests as a round widening or lacuna of the echo-free space (Weyman *et al.*, 1976; Moses *et al.*, 1979) against the contrasting background of the echo-dense area left of the aortic root, posterior to the pulmonary artery and anterior to the upper left pole of the left atrium. Aneurysms of the proximal right coronary artery have also been seen on 2-D echography (Karlsberg *et al.*, 1980).

Whereas large aneurysms of the proximal main coronary arteries are quite rare in adults, they are common in Kawasaki's disease, a peculiar mucocutaneous lymph node syndrome prevalent in Japanese children but also occasionally encountered in the United States. Yoshikawa *et al.* (1979) and Yoshida *et al.* (1979) could demonstrate large saccular aneurysms of the left or right coronary artery (confirmed by coronary angiography) in children or young adults afflicted with Kawasaki's disease. Two-D echographic appearances of this nature were seen in none of eight other children with Kawasaki's disease but normal coronary angiograms, nor in a group of normal controls.

Hiraishi *et al.* (1979) performed 2-D echographic studies in 58 children with Kawasaki's disease and found abnormal "fusiform" or "spherical" left main coronary artery patterns in seven. Five of these had coronary angiograms which confirmed the diagnosis in all. No such patterns were encountered in 30 normal subjects, who exhibited the normal "linear" pattern wherein the artery is represented by two parallel lines enclosing a narrow clear space. The use of 2-D echography in diagnosis of coronary artery aneurysms was documented further by Chung *et al.* (1982) and Yoshida *et al.* (1982). The latter authors used the subcostal approach to visualize right coronary artery aneurysms.

The echocardiographer may have to distinguish aneurysms of the coronary arteries from circumscribed echo-free spaces representing other structures adjacent to the aortic root (in the short-axis view). These include the pulmonary artery and its main branches, the left atrial appendage, and pericardial fluid around the latter structure (Fig. K-22). Congenital aneurysms of the sinuses of Valsalva and dilated coronary arteries feeding coronary arteriovenous fistulas (Yoshikawa *et al.,* 1982) could also simulate aneurysms of the proximal right or left coronary artery on the 2-D echocardiogram.

Gnepp *et al.* (1979) reported a remarkable instance of a huge aneurysm arising from the origin of the right coronary artery in a 62-year-old man. Its location between the aortic root and RV outflow tract permitted it to encroach on the pulmonary valve orifice and cause pulmonic valve stenosis and regurgitation. In the M-mode echogram, the thrombus-filled aneurysm, adjacent to the crest of the ventricular septum, simulated marked septal hypertrophy; the large aneurysmal mass was interposed between the aortic root and RV outflow tract, compressing the latter.

CORONARY EMBOLISM

Acute coronary embolization, resulting in myocardial infarction in an 11-year-old boy, occurred as a complication of a left atrial myxoma. The latter was diagnosed on echocardiography (Tanabe *et al.,* 1979). Myocardial

infarction or ischemia at an unexpectedly early age thus may constitute an indication for 2-D echography, not only for assessing LV function but also because of the possibility of revealing a coronary artery aneurysm, anomalous coronary artery origin (Yoshikawa *et al.,* 1978), or a source of emboli in the left heart chambers.

REFERENCES

Cody, R. J.; Salcedo, E. E.; Phillips, D. F.; *et al.:* M-mode echocardiography in anteroseptal myocardial infarction. *Chest,* **77**:781, 1980.

Corya, B. C.; Feigenbaum, H.; Rasmussen, S.; *et al.:* Anterior left ventricular wall echoes in coronary artery disease, linear scanning with a single element transducer. *Am. J. Cardiol.,* **34**:652, 1974a.

Corya, B. C.; Feigenbaum, H.; Rasmussen, S.; *et al.:* Echocardiographic features of congestive cardiomyopathy compared with normal subjects and patients with coronary artery disease. *Circulation,* **49**:1153, 1974b.

Corya, B. C.; Rasmussen, S.; Knoebel, S. B.; *et al.:* Echocardiography in acute myocardial infarction. *Am. J. Cardiol.,* **36**:1, 1975.

Corya, B. C.; Rasmussen, S.; Feigenbaum, H., *et al.:* Systolic thickening and thinning of the septum and posterior wall in patients with coronary artery disease, congestive cardiomyopathy and atrial septal defect. *Circulation,* **55**:109, 1977.

DeMaria, A. N.; Angel, J.; Amsterdam, E. A.; *et al.:* Applications of echocardiography in acute myocardial infarction: Development of a prognostic index and estimation of left ventricular filling pressure. In: Mason, D. T. (ed.): *Advances in Heart Disease,* Vol 1. Grune & Stratton, New York, 1977, pp. 367–376.

Dortimer, A. C.; DeJoseph, R. L.; Shiroff, R. A.; *et al.:* Distribution of coronary artery disease: prediction by echocardiography. *Circulation,* **54**:724, 1976.

Eaton, L. W.; Weiss, J. L.; Buckley, B. H.; *et al.:* Regional cardiac dilatation after acute myocardial infarction. Recognition by two-dimensional echocardiography. *N. Engl. J. Med.,* **300**:57, 1979.

Feigenbaum, H.; Corya, B. C.; Dillon, J. C.; *et al.:* Role of echocardiography in patients with coronary artery disease. *Am. J. Cardiol.,* **37**:775, 1976.

Fogelman, A. M.; Abbasi, A. S.; Pearce, M. L.; *et al.:* Echocardiographic study of the abnormal motion of the posterior left ventricular wall during angina pectoris. *Circulation,* **46**:905, 1972.

Gibson, R. S.; Bishop, H. L.; Stamm, R. B.; *et al.:* Value of early two-dimensional echocardiography in patients with acute myocardial infarction. *Am. J. Cardiol.,* **49**:110, 1982.

Goldstein, S., and deJong, W. J.: Changes in left ventricular wall dimension during regional myocardial ischemia. *Am. J. Cardiol.,* **34**:56, 1974.

Gordon, M. J., and Kerber, R. E.: Interventricular septal motion in patients with proximal and distal left anterior descending coronary artery lesions. *Circulation,* **55**:338, 1977.

Heger, J. J.; Weyman, A. E.; Wann, L. S.; *et al.:* Cross-sectional echocardiography in acute myocardial infarction: detection and localization of regional left ventricular asynergy. *Circulation,* **60**:531, 1979.

Heger, J. J.; Weyman, A. E.; Wann, L. S.; *et al.:* Cross-sectional echocardiographic analysis of the extent of left ventricular asynergy in acute myocardial infarction. *Circulation,* **61**:1113, 1980.

Heikkila, J., and Nieminen, M. S.: Echoventriculographic detection, localization, and quantification of left ventricular asynergy in acute myocardial infarction: a correlative echo and electrocardiographic study. *Br. Heart J.,* **37**:46, 1975.

Heikkila, J., and Nieminen, M. S.: Echoventriculography in acute myocardial infarction. *Clin. Cardiol.,* **3**:26, 1980.

Horowitz, R. S., and Morganroth, J.: Immediate detection of early high-risk patients with acute myocardial infarction using two-dimensional echocardiographic evaluation of left ventricular regional wall motion abnormalities. *Am. Heart J.,* **103**:814, 1982.

Horowitz, R. S.; Morganroth, J.; Parretto, C.; *et al.:* Immediate diagnosis of acute myocardial infarction by two-dimensional echocardiography. *Circulation,* **65**:323, 1982.

Inoue, K.; Smulyan, H.; Mookherjee, S.; *et al.:* Ultrasonic measurement of left ventricular wall motion in acute myocardial infarction. *Circulation,* **43**:778, 1971.

Jacobs, J. J.; Feigenbaum, H.; Corya, B. C.; *et al.:* Detection of left ventricular asynergy by echocardiography. *Circulation,* **48**:263, 1973.

Joffe, C. D.; Brik, H.; Teichholz, L. E.; *et al.:* Echocardiographic diagnosis of left anterior descending coronary artery. *Am. J. Cardiol.,* **40**:11, 1977.

Kerber, R. E., and Abboud, F. M.: Echocardiographic detection of regional myocardial infarction. *Circulation,* **47**:997, 1973.

Kerber, R. F.; Marcus, M. L.; Ehrhard, J.; *et al.:* Correlation between echocardiographically demonstrated segmental dyskinesis and regional myocardial perfusion. *Circulation,* **52**:1097, 1975.

Kerber R. E., and Litchfield R.: Postoperative abnormalities of interventricular septal motion. *Am. Heart J.,* **104**:263, 1982.

Kisslo, J. A.; Robertson, D.; Gilbert, B. W.; *et al.:* A comparison of real-time, two-dimensional echocardiography and cineangiography in detecting left ventricular asynergy. *Circulation,* **55**:134, 1977.

Kolibash, A. J.; Beaver, B. M.; Fulkerson, P. K.; *et al.:* The relationship between abnormal echocardiographic septal motion and myocardial perfusion in patients with significant obstruction of the left anterior descending artery. *Circulation,* **56**:780, 1977.

Loh, I. K.; Charuzi, Y.; Beeder, C.; *et al.:* Early diagnosis of nontransmural myocardial infarction by two-dimensional echocardiography. *Am. Heart J.,* **104**:963, 1982.

Massie, B.; Kleid, J. J.; and Schiller, N.: Echocardiography in ischemic heart disease. Present status and future perspectives. *Am. Heart J.,* **96**:543, 1978.

Maurer, G., and Nanda, N. C.: Two-dimensional echocardiographic evaluation of exercise-induced left and right ventricular asynergy: Correlation with thallium scanning. *Am. J. Cardiol.,* **48**:720, 1981.

Mitamura, H.; Ogawa, S.; Hori, S.; *et al.:* Two-dimensional echocardiographic analysis of wall motion abnormalities during handgrip exercise in patients with coronary artery disease. *Am. J. Cardiol.,* **48**:711, 1981.

Morrison, C. A.; Bodenheimer, M. M.; Feldman, M. S.; *et al.:* Ventriculographic-echocardiographic correlation in patients with asynergy. *JAMA,* **239**:1855, 1978.

Nanda, N. C., and Gramiak, R.: *Clinical Echocardiography.* C. V. Mosby, St. Louis, 1978.

Nieminen, M. S., and Heikkila, J.: Echoventriculography in acute myocardial infarction. II. Monitoring of left ventricular performance. *Br. Heart J.,* **38**:271, 1976a.

Nieminen, M., and Heikkila, J.: Echoventriculography in acute myocardial infarction. III. Clinical correlations and implications of the noninfarcted myocardium. *Am. J. Cardiol.,* **38**:1, 1976b.

Nixon, J. V.; Narahara, K. A.; and Smitherman, T. C.: Estimation of myocardial infarction in patients with acute myocardial infarction by two-dimensional echocardiography. *Circulation,* **62**:1248, 1980.

Nixon, J. V.; Brown, C. N.; and Smitherman, T. C.: Identification of transient and persistent segmental wall motion abnormalities in patients with unstable angina by two-dimensional echocardiography. *Circulation,* **65**:1497, 1982.

Prakash, R., and Aronow, W. S.: Spontaneous changes in hemodynamics in uncomplicated acute myocardial infarction: A prospective echocardiographic study. *Angiology,* **28**:677, 1977.

Rasmussen, S.; Corya, B. C.; and Feigenbaum, H.: Detection of myocardial scar tissue by M-mode echocardiography. *Circulation,* **57**:230, 1978.

Ratshin, R. A.; Rackley, C. E.; and Russell, R. O.: Serial evaluation of left ventricular volumes and posterior wall movement in the acute phase of myocardial infarction using diagnostic ultrasound. *Am. J. Cardiol.,* **29**:286, 1972.

Rubenson, D. S.; Tucker, C. R.; London, E., *et al.:* Two-dimensional echocardiographic analysis of segmental left ventricular wall motion before and after coronary artery bypass surgery. *Circulation,* **66**:1025, 1982.

Stack, R. S.; Lee, C. C.; Reddy, B. P.; *et al.:* Left ventricular performance in coronary artery disease evaluated with systolic time intervals and echocardiography. *Am. J. Cardiol.,* **37**:331, 1976.

Visser, C. A.; Lie, K. I.; Kan, G.; *et al.:* Detection and quantification of acute, isolated myocardial infarction by two-dimensional echocardiography. *Am. J. Cardiol.,* **47**:1020, 1981.

Weiss, J. L.; Bulkley, B. H.; Hutchins, G. M.; *et al.:* Two-dimensional echocardiographic recognition of myocardial injury in man: Comparison with postmortem studies. *Circulation,* **63**:401, 1981.

Wharton, C. F.; Smithers, C. S.; and Sowton, E.: Changes in left ventricular movement after acute myocardial infarction measured by reflected ultrasound. *Br. Med. J.,* **4**:75, 1971.

Widlansky, S.; McHenry, P. L.; Corya, B. C.; *et al.:* Coronary angiography, echocardiographic and electrocardiographic studies on a patient with variant angina due to coronary artery spasm. *Am. Heart J.,* **90**:631, 1975.

Wiener, I.; Meller, J.; Packer, M.; *et al.:* Prognostic value of echocardiographic evaluation of septal function in acute anteroseptal myocardial infarction. *Am. Heart J.,* **97**:726, 1979.

TRANSIENT CHANGES IN LV CONTRACTION

Cohn, P. F.; Angoff, G. H.; and Sloss, L. J.: Noninvasively-induced postextrasystolic potentiation of ischemic and infarcted myocardium in patients with coronary artery disease. *Am. Heart J.,* **97**:187, 1979.

Crawford, M. H.; Arron, K. W.; and Vance, W. S.: Exercise 2-dimensional echocardiography. Quantitation of left ventricular performance in patients with severe angina pectoris. *Am. J. Cardiol.,* **51**: 1983.

Gerson, M. C.; Noble, R. J.; Wann, L. S.; *et al.:* Noninvasive documentation of Prinzmetal's angina. *Am. J. Cardiol.,* **43**:329, 1979.

Mason, S. J.; Weiss, J. L.; Weisfeldt, M. L.; *et al.:* Exercise echocardiography: detection of wall motion abnormalities during ischemia. *Circulation,* **59:**50, 1979.

Morrison, C. A.; Bodenheimer, M. M.; Feldman, M. S.; et al.: The use of echocardiography of determination of reversible posterior wall asynergy. *Am. Heart J.,* **94:**140, 1977.

Wann, L. S.; Faris, J. V.; Childress, R. H.; et al.: Exercise cross-sectional echocardiography in ischemic heart disease. *Circulation,* **60:**1300, 1979.

LV Aneurysms

Baur, H. R.; Daniel, J. A.; and Nelson, R. R.: Detection of left ventricular aneurysm on two-dimensional echocardiography. *Am. J. Cardiol.,* **50:**191, 1982.

Cabin, H. S., and Roberts, W. C.: Left ventricular aneurysm, intra-aneurysmal thrombus and systemic embolus in coronary heart disease. *Chest,* **77:**586, 1980.

Chiaramida, S. A.; Goldman, M. A.; and Zema, M. J.: Cross-sectional echocardiographic diagnosis of acquired aneurysm of the interventricular septum. *J. C. U.,* **8:**356, 1980.

Dillon, J. C.; Feigenbaum, H.; Weyman, A. E.; et al.: M-mode echocardiography in the evaluation of patients for aneurysmectomy. *Circulation,* **53:**657, 1976.

Estevez, C. M.; Weyman, A. E.; Feigenbaum, H.: Detection of a left ventricular diverticulum by cross-sectional echocardiography. *Chest,* **69:**544, 1976.

Kambe, T.; Nishimura, K.; Hibi, N.; et al.: Real time observation of left ventricular aneurysm by B mode echocardiography. *J. C. U.,* **6:**405, 1978.

Kreamer, R.; Kerber, R. E.; and Abboud, F. M.: Ventricular aneurysm: Use of echocardiography. *J. C. U.,* **1:**60, 1973.

Lewin, R. F.; Vidne, B.; Sclarovsky, S.; et al.: Two-dimensional real-time echocardiographic detection of a left ventricular aneurysm associated with mobile pedunculated thrombi. *Chest,* **77:**704, 1980.

Ogawa, S.; Panletto, F. J.; Moghadam, A. M.; et al.: Delayed peak of the posterior wall. A new echocardiographic index of posterior wall aneurysm. *Chest,* **73:**382, 1978.

Petersen, J. L.; Johnston, W.; Hessel, E. A.; et al.: Echocardiographic recognition of left ventricular aneurysm. *Am. Heart J.,* **83:**244, 1972.

Rogers, E. W.; Glassman, R. D.; Feigenbaum, H.; et al.: Aneurysms of the posterior interventricular septum with postinfarction ventricular septal defect. *Chest,* **78:**741, 1980.

Weyman, A. E.; Peskoe, S. M.; Williams, E. S.; et al.: Detection of left ventricular aneurysms by cross-sectional echocardiography. *Circulation,* **54:**936, 1976.

Yoshikawa, J.; Owaki, T.; Kato, H.; et al.: Ultrasonic diagnosis of ventricular aneurysm. *Circulation,* **49:**30, 1974.

LV Pseudoaneurysm

Aintablian, A.; Hamby, R. I.; and Jaffe, J. R.: Left ventricular pseudoaneurysm identified by cross-sectional echocardiography. *Ann. Intern. Med.,* **90:**935, 1979.

Alter, B. R.; Lewis, M. E.; Vargas, A.; et al.: Noninvasive diagnosis of left ventricular pseudoaneurysm by radioangiography and echography. *Am. Heart J.,* **101:**236, 1981.

Catherwood, E.; Mintz, G. S.; Kotler, M. N.; et al.: Two-dimensional echocardiography recognition of left ventricular aneurysm. *Circulation,* **62:**294, 1980.

Davidson, K. H.; Parisi, A. F.; Harrington, J. J.; et al.: Pseudoaneurysm of the left ventricle: an unusual echocardiographic presentation. *Ann. Intern. Med.,* **86:**430, 1977.

Gatewood, R. P., and Nanda, N. C.: Differentiation of left ventricular pseudoaneurysm from true aneurysm with two-dimensional echocardiography. *Am. J. Cardiol.,* **46:**869, 1980.

Katz, R. J.; Simpson, A.; DiBianco, R.; et al.: Noninvasive diagnosis of left ventricular pseudoaneurysm. Role of two-dimensional echocardiography and radionuclide gated pool imaging. *Am. J. Cardiol.,* **44:**372, 1979.

Mills, P. G.; Ross, J. D.; Delaney, D. J.; et al.: Echophonographic diagnosis of left ventricular pseudoaneurysm. *Chest,* **72:**365, 1977.

Morcerf, S. P.; Duarte, E.; Salcedo, E. E.; et al.: Echocardiographic findings in false aneurysm of the left ventricle. *Cleve. Clin. Q.,* **43:**711, 1976.

Roelandt, J.; Brand, M.; Vletter, W. B.; et al.: Echocardiographic diagnosis of pseudoaneurysm of the left ventricle. *Circulation,* **52:**466, 1975.

Saksena, F. B.; Kramer, N. E.; Towne, W. D.; et al.: Infective aneurysm of the left ventricle: angiographic and echocardiographic features. *Am. Heart J.,* **96:**384, 1978.

Sears, T. C.; Ong, Y. S.; Starke, H.; et al.: Left ventricular pseudoaneurysm identified by cross-sectional echocardiography. *Ann. Intern. Med.,* **90:**935, 1977.

Sorenson, S. S.; Crawford, M. H.; Richards, K. L.; et. al.: Noninvasive detection of ventricular aneurysm by combined two-dimensional echocardiography and equilibrium radionuclide angiography. *Am. Heart J.,* **104:**145, 1982.

Rupture of the LV Wall

Eisenmann, B.; Bareiss, P.; Pacifico, A. D.; et al.: Anatomic, clinical and therapeutic features of acute cardiac rupture. Successful surgical management fourteen hours after myocardial infarction. *J. Thorac. Cardiovasc. Surg.,* **70:**78, 1978.

Hagemeijer, F.; Verbaan, C. J.; Souke, P. C.; et al.: Echocardiography and rupture of the heart. *Br. Heart J.,* **43:**45, 1980.

Postinfarction Rupture of the Ventricular Septum

Chandaratna, P. A. N.; Balachandran, P. K.; Shah, P.; et al.: Echocardiographic observations on ventricular septal rupture complicating acute myocardial infarction. *Circulation,* **51:**506, 1975.

DeJoseph, R. L.; Seides, S. F.; Lindner, A.; et al.: Echocardiographic findings in ventricular septal rupture in acute myocardial infarction. *Am. J. Cardiol.,* **36:**346, 1975.

Drobac, M.; Gilbert, B.; Howard, R.; et al.: Ventricular septal defect after myocardial infarction: Diagnosis by two-dimensional contrast echocardiography. *Circulation,* **67:**335, 1983.

Egeblad, H., and Hauns, S.: Echocardiographic findings in ventricular septal rupture and anterior wall aneurysm complicating myocardial infarction. *Acta Med. Scand. (Suppl.),* **627:**164, 1979.

Farcot, J. C.; Boisante, L.; Rigaud, M.; et al.: Two-dimensional echocardiographic visualization of ventricular septal rupture after acute anterior myocardial infarction. *Am. J. Cardiol.,* **45:**370, 1980.

Kerin, N. Z.; Edelstein, J.; and DeRue, R. G.: Ventricular septal defect complicating acute myocardial infarction: Echocardiographic demonstration confirmed by angiocardiograms and surgery. *Chest,* **70:**560, 1976.

Mintz, G. S.; Victor, M. F.; and Kotler, M. N.: Two-dimensional echocardiographic identification of surgically correctable complications of acute myocardial infarction. *Circulation,* **64:**91, 1981.

Rogers, E. W.; Glassman, R. D.; Feigenbaum, H.; *et al.:* Aneurysms of the posterior interventricular septum with postinfarction ventricular septal defect. *Chest,* **78:**741, 1980.

Rosenthal, R.; Kleid, J. J.; and Cohen, M. V.: Abnormal mitral valve motion associated with ventricular septal defect following acute myocardial infarction. *Am. Heart J.,* **98:**638, 1979.

Scanlan, J. G.; Seward, J. B.; and Tajik, A. J.: Visualization of ventricular septal rupture utilizing wide-angle two-dimensional echocardiography. *Mayo Clin. Proc.,* **54:**381, 1979.

Silverman, B.; Kozma, G.; Silverman, M.; *et al.:* Echocardiographic manifestations of post infarction ventricular septal rupture. *Chest,* **68:**778, 1975.

Van Mechelen, R.; van Hemel, N. M.; and van Rijk, P. P.: Noninvasive diagnosis of pseudoaneurysm of the left ventricle. *Br. Heart J.,* **40:**812, 1978.

POSTINFARCTION RUPTURE OF A PAPILLARY MUSCLE

Ahmad, S.; Kleiger, R. E.; Connors, J.; *et al.:* The echocardiographic diagnosis of rupture of a papillary muscle. *Chest,* **73:**232, 1978.

Bareiss, P.; Eisenmann, B.; Geitner, S.; *et al.:* Massive mitral insufficiency due to spontaneous and isolated rupture of a posterior papillary muscle. Echocardiographic study, treatment by assisted circulation and prosthetic valve replacement. *Arch. Mal. Coeur,* **70:**1213, 1977.

Erbel, R.; Schweizer, P.; Bardos, P.; *et al.:* Two-dimensional echocardiographic diagnosis of papillary muscle rupture. *Chest,* **79:**595, 1981.

Mintz, G. S.; Victor, M. F.; Kotler, M. N.; *et al.:* Two-dimensional echocardiographic identification of surgically correctable complications of acute myocardial infarction. *Circulation,* **64:**91, 1981.

Nishimura, R. A.; Schaff, H. V.; Shub, C.; *et al.:* Papillary muscle rupture complicating acute myocardial infarction: Analysis of 17 patients. *Am. J. Cardiol.,* **51:**373, 1983.

CORONARY ARTERIES

Chandaratna, P. A. N.; Aronow, W. S.; Murdock, K.; *et al.:* Left main coronary arterial patency assessed with cross-sectional echocardiography. *Am. J. Cardiol.,* **46:**91, 1980.

Chen, C. C.; Morganroth, J.; Ogawa, S.; *et al.:* Detecting left main coronary artery disease by apical, cross-sectional echocardiography. *Circulation,* **62:**288, 1980.

Chung, K. J.; Brand, T. L.; Fulton, D. R.; *et al.:* Cardiac and coronary arterial involvement in infants and children from New England with mucocutaneous lymph node syndrome (Kawasaki disease). *Am. J. Cardiol.,* **50:**137, 1982.

Fisher, E.; Sepehri, B.; Lendrum, B.; *et al.:* Two-dimensional echocardiographic visualization of the left coronary artery in anomalous origin of the left coronary artery from the pulmonary artery. *Circulation,* **63:**698, 1981.

Friedman, M. J.; Sahn, D. J.; Goldman, S.; *et al.:* High predictive accuracy for detection of left main coronary artery disease by antilog signal processing of two-dimensional echocardiographic images. *Am. Heart J.,* **103:**194, 1982.

Gnepp, D. R.; Deglin, S. M.; and Bekheit, J.: Massive coronary arterial aneurysm. *Am. J. Cardiol.,* **44:**184, 1979.

Hiraishi, S.; Yashiro, K.; and Kusano, S.: Noninvasive visualization of coronary arterial aneurysm in infants and young children with mucocutaneous lymph node syndrome with two-dimensional echocardiography. *Am. J. Cardiol.,* **43:**1225, 1979.

Karlsberg, R. P.; Eisenstein, I.; Aronow, W. S.; *et al.:* Noninvasive visualization of right coronary artery aneurysms. *Cardiology,* **66:**18, 1980.

Moses, H. W.; Huddle, R. A.; Nanda, N. C.; *et al.:* Surgical management of an aneurysm of the left main coronary artery. *Ann. Thorac. Surg.,* **27:**569, 1979.

Ogawa, S.; Chen, C. C.; Hubbard, F. E.; *et al.:* A new approach to visualize the left main coronary artery using apical cross-sectional echocardiography. *Am. J. Cardiol.,* **45:**301, 1980.

Rink, L. D.; Feigenbaum, H.; Goldberg, R. W.; *et al.:* Echocardiographic detection of left main coronary artery obstruction. *Circulation,* **65:**719, 1982.

Rogers, E. W.; Feigenbaum, H.; Weyman, A. E.; *et al.:* Evaluation of left coronary artery anatomy in vitro by cross-sectional echocardiography. *Circulation,* **62:**782, 1980a.

Rogers, E. W.; Feigenbaum, H.; Weyman, A. E.; *et al.:* Possible detection of atherosclerotic coronary calcification by two-dimensional echocardiography. *Circulation,* **62:**1046, 1980b.

Weyman, A. E.; Feigenbaum, H.; Dillon, J. C.; *et al.:* Noninvasive visualization of the left main coronary artery by cross-sectional echocardiography. *Circulation,* **54:**169, 1976.

Yoshida, H.; Funahashi, T.; Nakaya, S.; *et al.:* Mucocutaneous lymph node syndrome. A cross-sectional echocardiographic diagnosis of coronary aneurysms. *Am. J. Dis. Child.,* **133:**1244, 1979.

Yoshida, H.; Maeda, T.; Funabashi, T.; *et al.:* Subcostal two-dimensional echocardiographic imaging of peripheral right coronary artery in Kawasaki disease. *Circulation,* **65:**956, 1982.

Yoshikawa, J.; Owaki, T.; Kato, H.; *et al.:* Ultrasonic features of anomalous origin of the left coronary artery from the pulmonary artery. *Jpn. Heart J.,* **19:**46, 1978.

Yoshikawa, J.; Yanagihara, K.; Owaki, T.; *et al.:* Cross-sectional echocardiographic diagnosis of coronary artery aneurysms in patients with the mucocutaneous lymph node syndrome. *Circulation,* **59:**133, 1979.

Yoshikawa, J.; Katao, H.; Yanagibara, K.; *et al.:* Noninvasive visualization of the dilated main coronary arteries in coronary artery fistulas by cross-sectional echocardiography. *Circulation,* **65:**600, 1982.

CORONARY EMBOLIZATION

Tanabe, J.; Williams, R. L.; Diethrich, E. B.; Left atrial myxoma: association with acute coronary embolization in an 11-year-old boy. *Pediatrics,* **63:**778, 1979.

L

Dilated Cardiomyopathy

For two decades, primary myocardial disease has been classified into three categories: hypertrophic, congestive or dilated, and restrictive. This clinicopathologic classification can be applied equally well to the echocardiographic appearances of myocardial disease (Morganroth and Chen, 1980).

Hypertrophic cardiomyopathy, either with idiopathic subaortic stenosis (IHSS) or without LV outflow obstruction, is dealt with in a separate chapter.

CONGESTIVE (DILATED) CARDIOMYOPATHY

Twenty years ago, this diagnosis was acceptable only after all other forms of heart disease had been excluded by exhaustive investigation and often only at autopsy. During the 1950s and 1960s, it gradually became apparent that the entity had a typical profile on the bases of symptoms, physical signs, x-ray silhouette, and electrocardiogram. The definitive diagnosis required the angiocardiographic demonstration of patent coronary arteries and of diffuse LV dilatation and hypokinesis. Echocardiography certainly facilitates the noninvasive diagnosis of congestive cardiomyopathy (Abbasi *et al.,* 1973; Kotler *et al.,* 1973) by providing a constellation of consistent echographic characteristics. The risk and expense of hemodynamic studies thus may be avoided except in a few cases with atypical or special features.

M-Mode Echocardiography (Figs. L-1 to L-8)

LV dilatation and functional impairment are cardinal features. The LV internal dimension in both diastole and systole are abnormally in-creased; the LV systolic shortening fraction and echographic ejection fraction are decreased. The most extreme LV dilatation and impairment of function in clinical practice are seen in patients with advanced or end-stage cardiomyopathy of this type. Thus it is not rare to record an LV internal dimension of about 80 mm, a systolic shortening faction of about 12 per cent, and an ejection fraction of about 20 per cent.

Some authors (Roberts and Ferrans, 1975; Isner *et al.,* 1980) believe that the adjective "dilated" is more appropriate than "congestive" to describe this type of myocardial disease because of the vague connotation of the latter term. From the echocardiographer's viewpoint, it is true that significant LV dilatation and lack of significant increase in septal or LV wall end-diastolic thickness are the rule in congestive cardiomyopathy, while the reverse is almost invariably true of hypertrophic cardiomyopathy.

In a series of 37 children with congestive cardiomyopathy (Ghafour and Gutgesell, 1979), LA and LV diameters were approximately 1.5 times that predicted by body weight; systolic decrease in LV diameter (fractional shortening) was half that of normal children, but higher in the asymptomatic patients than in those with symptoms of cardiac decompensation. One third of patients improved after digitalis and diuretics, and these showed improvement of LV function by echographic parameters in serial echocardiograms. However, one or more indices remained abnormal in all, even when symptoms disappeared and the chest x-ray returned to normal.

Packer *et al.* (1980) have shown that LV size is of prognostic and therapeutic as well as diagnostic importance in patients with refractory LV failure. When the LV end-diastolic

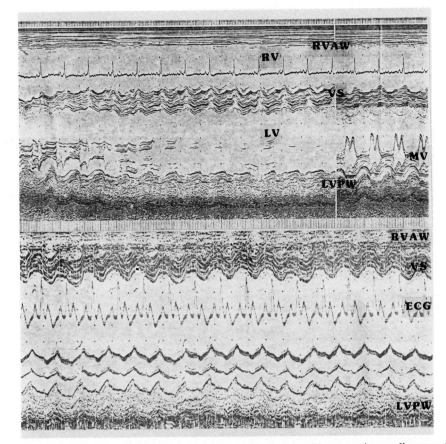

Fig. L-1. *Upper.* M-mode echogram of a 50-year-old woman with congestive cardiomyopathy. The coronary arteries were normal by coronary arteriography. The LV posterior wall is akinetic, more so at mitral valve level than at chordae tendineae level.

    Lower. M-mode echogram of a young man with congestive cardiomyopathy of idiopathic type; the diagnosis was confirmed at autopsy a year later. The LV is markedly dilated, but the RV is abnormally small. The LV posterior wall is mildly hypertrophied. It and the ventricular septum are both hypokinetic. The ECG shows atrial tachycardia with 2:1 A-V conduction.

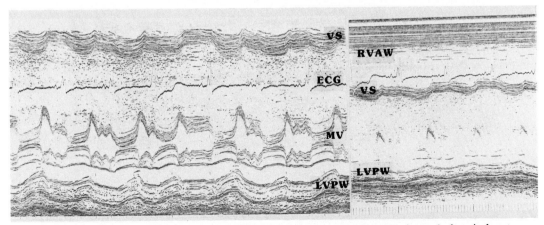

Fig. L-2. M-mode echogram in a patient with congestive cardiomyopathy and chronic heart failure. The LV is dilated, with hypokinesis of septum as well as LV posterior wall (*right panel*). In the left panel, at mitral valve level, the mitral-septal separation is very much increased, indicating poor overall LV function. Following the premature beat, alternation in excursions of the LV posterior wall and septum can be seen.

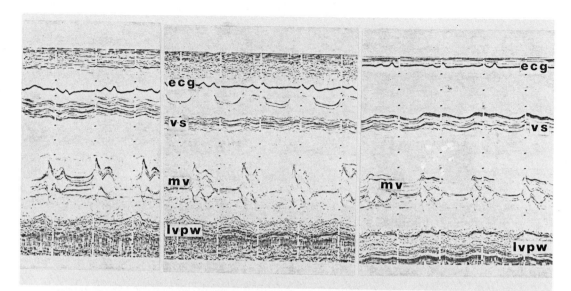

Fig. L-3. Segments from the M-mode echogram of a 38-year-old man with alcoholic cardiomy-opathy. The LV is dilated and large mitral-septal separation indicates poor overall LV performance. Motion of the LV posterior wall is small but qualitatively normal in the left and middle panels, but at a different transducer direction (*right panel*) the LV posterior wall shows dyskinetic motion.

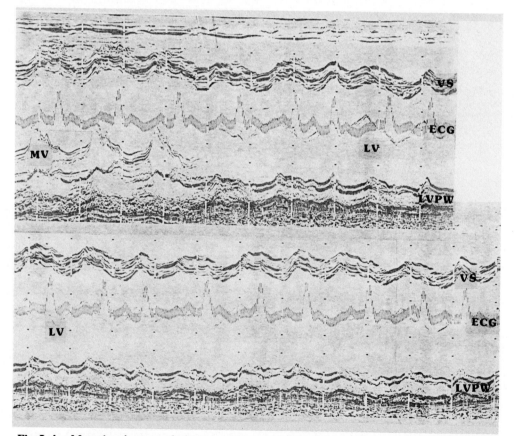

Fig. L-4. M-mode echogram of a 15-year-old boy with congestive cardiomyopathy, documented at autopsy. The LV is dilated. An unusual finding is dyskinetic systolic motion of the LV posterior wall at this level.

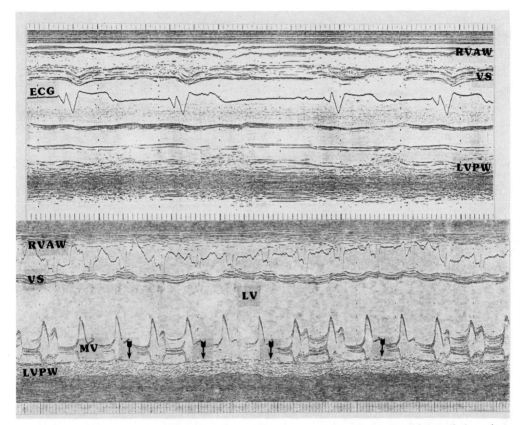

Fig. L-5. *Upper.* M-mode echogram of a patient with cardiomyopathy and left bundle branch block. The LV is markedly dilated (75 mm). The LV posterior wall is hypokinetic. The ventricular septum is hypokinetic but systolic motion typical of left bundle branch block can be detected: brief early systolic posterior motion, followed by a slower anterior motion.

Lower: M-mode echogram of a 20-year-old man with the Duchenne type of muscular dystrophy. The LV posterior wall is akinetic (*arrows*). Increased mitral E point–septal separation suggests that overall LV performance is poor.

dimension exceeded 60 mm, 60 per cent of patients were improved by vasodilator (hydralazine) therapy; of those with smaller LV size (less than 60 mm), only 2 of 16 improved, whereas 10 deteriorated.

VENTRICULAR WALL MOTION IN CONGESTIVE (DILATED) CARDIOMYOPATHY

Whatever its etiology, primary myocardial disease is typically a diffuse process with involvement of the whole myocardium. Thus the LV posterior wall as well as the ventricular septum may be expected to show diminished systolic excursions at all levels. This is indeed true as a general rule and is what distinguishes congestive cardiomyopathy echographically and angiocardiographically from coronary heart disease, which is characterized by poor contraction of one region accompanied by unduly vigorous or at least normal contraction of nonischemic myocardium elsewhere in the left ventricle. Corya *et al.* (1974) found that the sum of the excursions of the LV posterior wall and ventricular septum is usually 12 mm or less in congestive cardiomyopathy, but usually more than 12 mm in patients with ischemic heart disease. This cutoff value of 12 mm is a convenient yardstick to separate the two entities, both very commonly encountered in routine clinical echocardiographic practice.

However, certain important exceptions to this general rule do exist:

1. A small percentage of patients with severe multivessel coronary disease have diffuse LV dilatation and hypokinesis on angiocardiography as well as on echocardiography. Their ven-

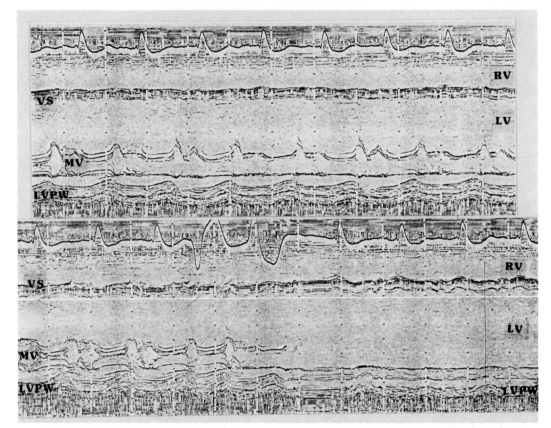

Fig. L-6. *Upper.* M-mode echogram of a 55-year-old woman with congestive cardiomyopathy. The coronary arteries were normal on coronary arteriography. The septum appears akinetic and the LV posterior wall hypokinetic.

Lower. LV scan in the same patient from mitral valve level to chordae level. At this level the LV posterior wall is thinner and more hypokinetic than it is at mitral valve level.

tricular wall motion thus is indistinguishable from that of cardiomyopathy; to such cases the controversial term "ischemic cardiomyopathy" is sometimes applied.

2. Patients with acute myocardial infarction in cardiogenic shock show hypokinesis not only of the infarcted area but also of the remaining LV myocardium.

3. An occasional patient with typical clinical and pathologic findings of cardiomyopathy exhibits local areas of akinesis (Figs. L-3, L-4, and L-6) in the septum or the LV posterior wall (Burch *et al.*, 1974; Laurenceau *et al.*, 1979; D'Cruz *et al.*, 1980). One may suppose that, although the entire LV is involved by the disease process, some areas are more affected than others, and rarely large areas of fibrotic scarring occur (D'Cruz *et al.*, 1980). Thus there is no area of the LV that shows normal or increased systolic motion, which helps in differen-

tiating such patients from those with coronary disease.

4. Mitral regurgitation is not uncommon in patients with marked LV dilatation and congestive cardiomyopathy. The LV diastolic overloading in this situation provokes an increased stroke output and thus an enhanced ventricular wall and septal motion, as compared to the same heart without (or before) mitral regurgitation. The amplitude of systolic excursion may approach the normal range, deceiving the echocardiographer into the erroneous conclusion that LV function is normal.

5. Whereas paradoxic septal motion is in some cases attributable to left bundle branch block (Fig. L-5), in others it could be due to tricuspid regurgitation (Fig. L-7).

Levisman (1977) called attention to the fact that some patients with dilated cardiomyopathy and mitral regurgitation show normal to in-

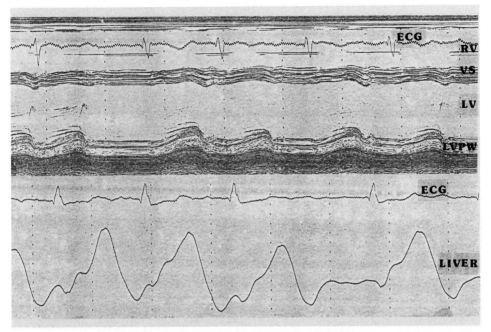

Fig. L-7. M-mode echogram showing dilatation of both ventricles (*upper panel*) in a patient with congestive cardiomyopathy. Abnormal systolic motion of the ventricular septum in this patient was attributable to tricuspid regurgitation. The lower panel shows systolic hepatic pulsations of florid tricuspid regurgitation.

creased systolic motion (but no systolic thickening) of the ventricular septum, the LV posterior wall appearing very hypokinetic by contrast. He postulated that large systolic septal excursions were not attributable to preservation of normal septal contraction, but were due to passive septal displacement caused by its anterior displacement by diastolic LV overload.

The mitral echogram in congestive cardiomyopathy presents typical features:

1. Both mitral leaflets are visualized together in the so-called double-diamond configuration. Normally, in LV scans it is easy to record the anterior mitral leaflet without the posterior leaflet and vice versa, but in dilated cardiomyopathy it may be impossible to do so.

2. During systole, the apposed mitral leaflets may appear as multiple horizontal lines rather than as one or two linear echoes. Such systolic mitral echoes may show a slight "sag" (posterior convexity) which should not be mistaken for prolapse; deeper or more pronounced posterior loops are needed to make the latter diagnosis. Features **1** and **2** above are not attributable to intrinsic pathology of the mitral leaflets, but rather to an alteration of LV geometry such

that the mitral ring (and with it the leaflets) changes its alignment with the chest wall (and therefore the ultrasound beam).

3. The anterior (DE) diastolic opening excursion of the anterior mitral leaflet may be diminished. The separation between anterior and posterior mitral cusps may seem even smaller than it really is because the valve cusps appear suspended within the wide expanse of the dilated LV chamber. This appearance should not be mistaken for mitral stenosis because the mitral leaflets retain their normal M- and W-shaped motion patterns.

4. The EF slope is normal. This, too, helps in excluding true mitral stenosis.

5. The separation between the anterior mitral leaflet E point and the left border of the ventricular septum (EPSS) is abnormally wide; values of 25 to 40 mm are common in severe dilated cardiomyopathy. The upper limit of normal is 5 mm by the method of Massie *et al.* (1977) and 10 mm by that of D'Cruz *et al.* (1979).

6. LV mural thrombi are very commonly found at autopsy in patients with idiopathic dilated cardiomyopathy (Isner *et al.*, 1980). Such

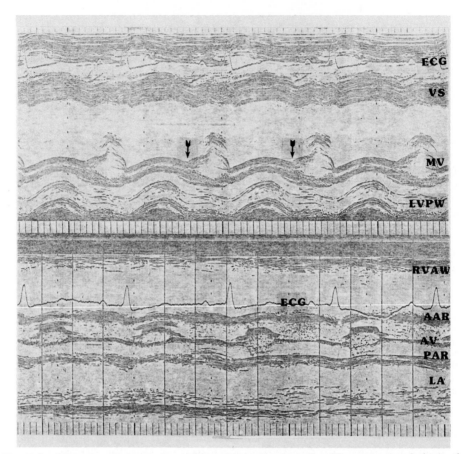

Fig. L-8. M-mode echogram of a patient with cardiomyopathy. The upper panel shows that mitral valve opening (D point) is very delayed (*arrows*) and the DE slope unduly small. Mitral opening occurs long after the peak of LV posterior systolic motion. The lower panel demonstrates aortic valve motion. Using the ECG as a reference point for measuring time intervals, it is evident that the mitral valve opens long after end-systole (aortic valve closure); that is, the isovolumic relaxation period is abnormally prolonged.

thrombi may be detected on M-mode echocardiography, should the clot be situated in or near the basal LV within the ambit of the ultrasound beam (Kramer *et al.,* 1978; D'Cruz *et al.,* 1980).

2-D Echocardiography (Fig. L-9)

Good visualization of all the cardiac chambers and valves is the rule, as the very dilated heart approaches the precordium more closely and so enlarges the ultrasound "window" available to the echocardiographer.

The 2-D appearance is as typical as the M-mode one. The LV is diffusely dilated and diffusely hypokinetic. Usually, all four cardiac chambers are enlarged, although LV dilatation is the most conspicuous. A change in LV shape

from the ellipsoid toward the spheroid is to be expected with very dilated ventricles and is best appreciated in the long-axis and apical four-chamber views. In real-time viewing, the mitral valve cusps move briskly and freely, although their diastolic excursions are of small amplitude.

Another interesting 2-D echographic finding, in the short-axis view, is that the ratio of diastolic mitral valve orifice area to LV cross-section area is markedly reduced in patients with dilated cardiomyopathy, compared with normal subjects (Pollick *et al.,* 1982). A similar reduction of the ratio of aortic valve orifice to aortic root area was also noted by these authors.

Chandaratna and Aronow (1981) studied LV geometry in the 2-D long-axis view in 11 patients with congestive cardiomyopathy and mi-

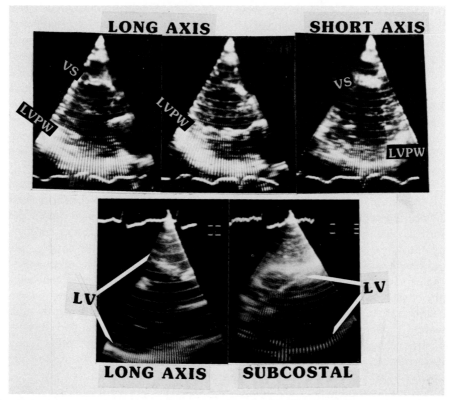

Fig. L-9. 2-D echogram of a patient with alcoholic cardiomyopathy of severe degree. The left and middle frames are in the long-axis view, the right frame is in the short-axis view. The LV is dilated, and there is little decrease in LV size from end-diastole (*left*) to systole (*middle*).

2-D echogram of a patient with dilated cardiomyopathy. The LV internal diameter is markedly increased (about 8 cm), as can be seen in long axis (*left*) and subcostal (*right*) views. The calibration marks are 1 cm apart. The left ventricle was diffusely hypokinetic when viewed in real time.

tral regurgitation. They compared them to 11 others with cardiomyopathy but no mitral regurgitation and 23 normal controls. All those with cardiomyopathy had LV dilatation, but the mitral annulus in some patients was not dilated or at least not dilated in proportion to the degree of LV dilatation. Thus mitral ring dilatation is not the only explanation for mitral regurgitation in such patients; other mechanisms such as malalignment of papillary muscles or loss of sphincteric action of the annulus region may have a role.

ECHOCARDIOGRAPHY IN SPECIFIC FORMS OF MYOCARDIAL DISEASE

Serial M-mode echograms were done in 14 children, aged 8 to 17 years, with *acute rheumatic fever* (Shieken and Kerber, 1976). In patients with mitral or aortic valve regurgitation but

without cardiac failure, LV contractility appeared normal. However, those with valve regurgitation and congestive failure had subnormal LV function. Serial tracings in the latter group showed progressive improvement, confirming the impression that myocardial inflammation had depressed LV function in the acute phase. Moreover, rebound rheumatic activity during steroid withdrawal was associated with transient decrease in LV contractility. Lewis *et al.* (1979) described four patients, "critically ill" with severe cardiac failure and valve incompetence, who had acute rheumatic carditis. Echocardiography showed that LV function was "relatively well-preserved." Valve replacement was successfully performed, as medical treatment had been found ineffective.

Aquatella *et al.* (1980) performed M-mode as well as 2-D echographic studies in 64 patients with *Chagas' disease* in Venezuela. They found that 11 had the classic echocardiographic features of dilated or congestive cardiomyopathy, but 18 others demonstrated a distinctive picture characterized by marked hypokinesis of the posteroinferior LV wall and apex but relative sparing of the ventricular septum. Two-D echography in the apical view was very helpful in detecting early cardiac involvement by identifying a peculiar aneurysmal dilatation or pouch at the LV apex.

Chronic *alcoholics* comprise a large proportion of patients with congestive cardiomyopathy in hospital practice in most American urban centers. Echocardiography in these individuals shows diffuse LV dilatation and hypokinesis, with normal thickness of LV wall and septum. However, alcoholic cardiomyopathy may be revealed at an early asymptomatic stage as mild hypertrophy of the ventricular septum and LV wall, and an increase in LV mass. At this stage of the disease, LV dimension and LV function on the M-mode echogram may appear almost normal (Akanas *et al.*, 1980).

Mathews *et al.* (1981) also found echographic abnormalities in asymptomatic alcoholics, which they divided into two subgroups: (1) Those with LV diastolic dimension less than 10 per cent above predicted value, normal fractional shortening, and mildly increased LV wall thickness. In my experience, such patients often present with atrial tachyarrhythmias and belong to a mid- to upper socioeconomic stratum. (2) Those with a LV diastolic dimension 10 to 24 per cent above predicted value and a borderline low fractional shortening. This type of patient tends to belong to a lower socioeconomic level and represents an early stage of the classic type of symptomatic alcoholic cardiomyopathy with very dilated and diffusely hypokinetic left ventricles.

LV function has been evaluated in children with *muscular dystrophy* by M-mode echography by Ahmad *et al.* (1978). They found little or no evidence of myocardial impairment in 13 children and adolescents with the Duchenne variety of dystrophy. However, considerable impairment of LV function sometimes does occur, and the LV posterior wall appears particularly involved (Fig. L-5), which is in accord with previous electrocardiographic and pathologic studies. In a larger and more recent series of 36 patients, all but 2 had some abnormality

of LV size or function (Danilowicz *et al.*, 1980).

Friedrich's ataxia. Earlier reports had suggested that IHSS was the type of cardiomyopathy typical of this disease, but a recent study of seven patients (St. John Sutton *et al.*, 1980) revealed that the rule was a symmetrically hypertrophied LV with normal to small cavity. Septal motion was grossly normal. More subtle indices of contractility, such as peak rates of LV wall thickening and diastolic thinning, were impaired in some cases.

Left ventricular hypertrophy, mild LV dilatation, and impaired LV performance are often seen in patients with *acromegaly* and may be secondary to hypertension or coronary disease, to which acromegalics have a predilection (Martins *et al.*, 1977). However, 3 of 16 patients in Martins' series had mild concentric LV hypertrophy that could be attributed to acromegaly itself in the absence of other causes. These three patients had had the endocrinopathy for over 13 years; other patients with acromegaly of shorter duration showed no echographic abnormalities.

M-mode echocardiography has been employed to assess LV function in patients suffering from *sickle cell anemia* (Rees *et al.*, 1978). Although all asymptomatic children had normal LV function, diminished LV performance was detected in some who complained of dyspnea or failure on moderate effort. Val-Meijas *et al.* (1979) found abnormal low ejection fractions in sickle cell disease only in older patients (over 23 years) and postulated a deleterious effect of repeated crises on the myocardium. However, Gerry *et al.* (1976) found no evidence of LV dysfunction on echocardiography in a series of adults with sickle cell anemia. This also has been my experience, even in patients with symptoms apparently referable to the heart.

Mir (1978) did M-mode echograms in 38 patients with acute *leukemia or lymphoma* before chemotherapy and found that approximately half of them had impaired LV function as manifested in low LV internal dimension systolic shortening fractions and increased LV end-systolic dimension. Serial echocardiography confirmed the deleterious effect on LV myocardium of the cytotoxic drug daunorubicin in some of these patients.

Doxorubicin toxicity. In a prospective study

of children given doxorubicin (Adriamycin) for malignancies, abnormal LV function as reflected in decrease of shortening fraction occurred in 43 per cent but irreversible cardiac failure in only 4 per cent. There was marked individual variation in response; the total dose and age of patient were not obviously related to myocardial deterioration (Biencaniello et al., 1980).

Collagen diseases. Echocardiograms showing cardiomyopathy of the dilated or congestive type have been described in polymyositis by Henderson et al. (1980). Scleroderma can cause cardiomyopathy of either the dilated or the infiltrative restrictive type (Eggebrecht and Kleiger, 1977; Gottdiener et al., 1979).

Chronic renal failure. The incidence or even existence of myocardial disease secondary to uremia is controversal. Dilated cardiomyopathy does occur in patients on long-term hemodialysis (D'Cruz et al., 1978).

Drueke et al. (1980) found that LV function improved after parathyroidectomy. Cohen et al. (1979), on the other hand, found that the indices of LV contractility remained normal in seven young patients (average age, 24 years) on long-term hemodialysis.

A practical point worth noting by echocardiographers is that LV volumes (systolic, diastolic, and stroke volume) are significantly larger just before dialysis than just after it (Vaziri and Prakash, 1979) because of the fluid retention and expanded blood volume prior to dialysis.

RESTRICTIVE CARDIOMYOPATHY

This category of myocardial disease, much rarer than the dilated and hypertrophic varieties, does not denote a single clinicopathologic entity. It embraces several different conditions of varied etiology, pathology, and pathophysiology. Consequently, the echocardiographic features are also diverse; unfortunately, they are also rather nonspecific and not as distinctive as the ultrasound features of dilated (congestive) and hypertrophic types of cardiomyopathy.

Cardiac amyloidosis (Fig. L-10) is a variety of restrictive cardiomyopathy that may be suspected when the echocardiogram reveals symmetrically thickened LV posterior wall and ventricular septum, normal or slightly increased LV internal dimension, and normal or mildly impaired contractile function as reflected in LV internal dimension systolic shortening fraction (Child et al., 1976, 1979; Borer et al., 1977; Chiaramida et al., 1980; Siqueira-Filhos et al., 1981; Carroll et al., 1982; St. John Sutton et al., 1982). The presence of a small to moderate pericardial effusion, left atrial enlargement, and diminished systolic thickening of septum and LV wall strengthens the diagnosis. Siqueira-Filhos et al. (1981) pointed out that whereas the LV thickening is commonly concentric, it is sometimes asymmetric, the septal thickness being 1.3 times or more the LV posterior wall thickness. These authors reported that 2-D echography contributed further diagnostic information: thickened papillary muscles, thickened valve leaflets, thickened RV walls, and a characteristic "granular sparkling" of the thickened LV walls that the authors consider almost pathognomonic.

Most of the above findings are not present in constrictive pericarditis, the main clinical and hemodynamic differential diagnosis of amyloid and other restrictive cardiomyopathies. Thus echocardiography is of great diagnostic help in this situation. However, the *echographic* picture of the amyloid heart is not unlike that of hypertrophic cardiomyopathy in several respects. Septal and LV wall thickening without LV dilatation, associated with symptoms of congestive failure, is common to both. A sparkling or hyperrefractile appearance of the septum, especially the basal portion, may be seen in hypertrophic cardiomyopathy, but this peculiar echographic texture is said to be more diffuse in cardiac amyloidosis (Siqueira-Filhos et al., 1981). SAM and midsystolic aortic valve nearclosure of course are indicative of the hypertrophic rather than restrictive type of cardiomyopathy, and atrial arrhythmias strengthen the diagnostic suspicion. High ECG voltage suggestive of LV hypertrophy is conspicuous by its absence in cardiac amyloidosis. On the other hand, thick-walled, small-chambered left ventricles due to hypertension or hypertrophic cardiomyopathy have real LV myocardial hypertrophy and so exhibit high QRS voltage on the ECG (Carroll et al., 1982).

Infiltration of the myocardium by other pathologic elements, as in hemochromatosis

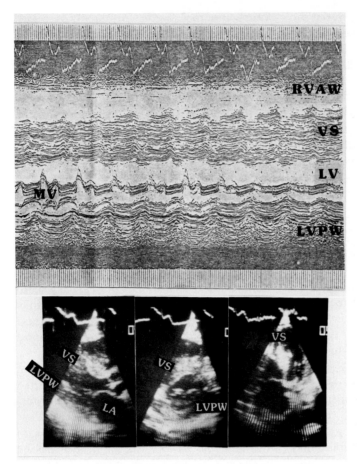

Fig. L-10. *Upper.* M-mode echogram of a 73-year-old man with congestive failure who had extensive cardiac amyloid cardiomyopathy at autopsy. The ventricular septum is abnormally thick, more so than the LV posterior wall. The LV chamber size is low normal. The septum and LV wall appear hypokinetic.

Lower. 2-D echogram of the same patient in the long-axis view (*left*), short-axis view (*center*) and apical 4-chamber view (*right*). The septum appears abnormally thick. An unduly small LA chamber was an atypical feature of this case.

(Cutler *et al.*, 1980), sarcoidosis (Kinney *et al.*, 1980), and neoplastic infiltration (Kubac *et al.*, 1980), and so forth, can lead to cardiac failure and somewhat similar echocardiographic features. Cabin *et al.* (1981) recently described an instance of massive lymphomatous infiltration of the heart; the patient presented in congestive failure and echography showed marked concentric "hypertrophy" simulating hypertrophic cardiomyopathy.

A different variety of restrictive cardiomyopathy includes entities such as Loeffler's endocardial fibrosis and thrombosis associated with hypereosinophilia, and endomyocardial fibrosis of the type commonly seen in Africa. Occasional instances of the syndrome do occur in Western countries (Chew *et al.*, 1977). The main pathologic feature is impressive endocardial fibrotic scarring and often thrombus deposition in either or both ventricles, resulting in partial obliteration and impaired contraction of the affected chamber.

Echocardiographic findings in the African type in the Ivory Coast (Dienot *et al.*, 1980) and in a series studied in England (Chew *et al.*, 1977) include paradoxic systolic motion of the ventricular septum, increased systolic thickening of the septum, prominent septal "dip" (brief sharp posterior motion) in early diastole, dilatation of the RV outflow tract (anterior to the aortic root) but not of the RV body, tricuspid valve thickening, steep mitral EF slope (more than 200 mm/sec), and normal LV size.

Hall *et al.* (1977) reported a patient with hypereosinophilic syndrome in whom serial M-mode echocardiograms one year apart demonstrated progressive decrease in RV dimension and increase in RV wall thickness. At autopsy, marked endocardial fibrous thickening was noted in both ventricles, with superimposed mural thrombi and partial obliteration of the RV cavity. Unfortunately, these features are mostly nonspecific and inconsistent (Benotti *et al.*, 1980); they may serve to support a clinical suspicion of restrictive cardiomyopathy, but do not present the echocardiographer with a clear-cut diagnostic echographic appearance as with hypertrophic or dilated cardiomyopathy.

REFERENCES

CONGESTIVE (DILATED) CARDIOMYOPATHY

Abbasi, A. S.; Chahine, R. A.; MacAlpine, R. N.; et al.: Ultrasound in the diagnosis of primary congestive cardiomyopathy. Chest, 63:937, 1973.

Burch, G. E.; Giles, T. D.; and Martinez, E.: Echocardiographic detection of abnormal motion of the interventricular septum in ischemic cardiomyopathy. Am. J. Med., 57:293, 1974.

Chandaratna, P. A. N., and Aronow, W. S.: Mitral valve ring in normal versus dilated left ventricle: Cross-sectional echocardiographic study. Chest, 79:151, 1981.

Corya, B. E.; Feigenbaum, H.; Rasmussen, S.; et al.: Echocardiographic features of congestive cardiomyopathy compared with normal subjects and patients with coronary artery disease. Circulation, 49:1153, 1974.

D'Cruz, I. A.; Lalmalani, G. G.; and Vaidya, P. V.: Cardiac failure and infarction ECG pattern in a chronic alcoholic. Arch. Intern. Med., 140:391, 1980.

D'Cruz, I. A.; Lalmalani, G. G.; Sambasivan, C. C.; et al.: The superiority of mitral E point–ventricular septum separation to other echocardiographic indicators of left ventricular performance. Clin. Cardiol., 2:140, 1979.

DeMaria, A. N.; Bommer, W.; Lee, G.; et al.: Value and limitations of two-dimensional echocardiography in assessment of cardiomyopathy. Am. J. Cardiol., 46:1224, 1980.

Ghafour, A. S., and Gutgesell, H. P.: Echocardiographic evaluation of left ventricular function in children with congestive cardiomyopathy. Am. J. Cardiol., 44:1332, 1979.

Isner, J. M.; Virmani, R.; Itscoitz, S. B.; et al.: Left and right ventricular myocardial infarction in idiopathic dilated cardiomyopathy. Am. Heart J., 99:235, 1980.

Kotler, M. N.; Guss, S.; and Reichek, N. M.: Echocardiography and compound B ultrasonography in congestive cardiomyopathy. J.C.U., 1:258, 1973.

Kramer, N. E.; Rathod, R.; Chawla, K. K.; et al.: Echocardiographic diagnosis of left ventricular mural thrombi occurring in cardiomyopathy. Am. Heart J., 96:381, 1978.

Levisman, J. A.: Echocardiographic diagnosis of mitral regurgitation and congestive cardiomyopathy. Am. Heart J., 93:33, 1977.

Massie, B. M.; Schiller, M. B.; Ratshin, R. A.; et al.: Mitral-septal separation: A new echocardiographic index of left ventricular function. Am. J. Cardiol., 39:1008, 1977.

Mintz, G. S.; Kotler, M. N.; Segal, B. L.; et al.: Echocardiographic features of cardiomyopathy. Cardiovasc. Clin., 9:123, 1978.

Morganroth, J., and Chen, C. C.: Noninvasive diagnosis of the cardiomyopathies. Med. Clin. North Am., 64:33, 1980.

Packer, M.; Meller, J.; Medina, N.; et al.: Importance of left ventricular chamber size in determining the response of hydralazine in severe chronic heart failure. N. Engl. J. Med., 303:250, 1980.

Pollick, C.; Pittman, M.; Filly, K.; et. al.: Mitral and aortic valve orifice area in normal subjects and in patients with congestive cardiomyopathy. Am. J. Cardiol., 49:1191, 1982.

Roberts, W. C., and Ferran, V. J.: Pathological anatomy of the cardiomyopathies. Hum. Pathol., 6:287, 1975.

SPECIFIC FORMS OF MYOCARDIAL DISEASE

Rheumatic Myocarditis

Lewis, B. S.; Geft, I. L.; Milo, S.; et al.: Echocardiography and valve replacement in the critically ill patients with acute rheumatic carditis. Ann. Thorac. Surg., 27:529, 1979.

Shieken, R. M., and Kerber, R. E.: Echocardiographic abnormalities in acute rheumatic fever. Am. J. Cardiol., 38:458, 1976.

Chagas' Disease

Aquatella, H.; Schiller, N. B.; Pnigbo, J. J.; et al.: M-mode and two-dimensional echocardiography in chronic Chagas' heart disease. A clinical pathological study. Circulation, 62:787, 1980.

Alcoholism

Akanas, A.; Udoshi, M.; and Sadjadi, S. A.: The heart in chronic alcoholism: A noninvasive study. Am. Heart J., 99:9, 1980.

Mathews, E. C.; Gardin, J.; Henry, W. L.; et al.: Echocardiographic abnormalities in chronic alcoholics with and without overt congestive heart failure. Am. J. Cardiol., 47:570, 1981.

Muscular Dystrophy

Ahmad, M.; Sanderson, J. E.; Dubowitz, V.; et al.: Echocardiographic assessment of left ventricular function in Duchenne's muscular dystrophy. Br. Heart J., 40:734, 1978.

Danilowicz, D.; Rutkowski, M.; Myung, D.; et al.: Echocardiography in Duchenne muscular dystrophy. Muscle Nerve, 3:298, 1980.

Goldberg, S. J.; Feldman, L.; Reinecke, C.; et al.: Echocardiographic determination of contraction and relaxation measurements of the left ventricular wall in normal subjects and patients with muscular dystrophy. Circulation, 62:1061, 1980.

Friedrich's Ataxia

St. John Sutton, M. G.; Olukotun, A. Y.; Tajik, A. J.; et al.: Left ventricular function in Friedrich's ataxia. An echocardiographic study. Br. Heart J., 44:309, 1980.

Acromegaly

Martins, J. B.; Kerber, R. F.; Sherman, B. M.; et al.: Cardiac size and function in acromegaly. Circulation, 56:863, 1977.

Savage, D. D.; Henry, W. L.; Eastman, R. C.; et al.: Echocardiographic assessment of cardiac anatomy and function in acromegalic patients. Am. J. Med., 67:823, 1979.

Sickle Cell Anemia

Gerry, J. L.; Baird, M. S.; and Fortuin, N. G.: Evaluation of left ventricular function in patients with sickle cell anemia. Am. J. Med., 60:968, 1976.

Rees, A. N.; Stefadouros, M. A.; and Strong, W. B.: Left ventricular performance in children with homozygous sickle cell anemia. Br. Heart J., 40:690, 1978.

Val-Meijas, J.; Lee, W. K.; Weisse, A. B.; et al.: Left ventricular performance during and after sickle cell crisis. Am. Heart J., 97:585, 1979.

Leukemia and Lymphoma

Mir, M. A.: Evidence for non-infiltrative cardiomyopathy in acute leukemia and lymphoma. A clinical and echocardiographic study. *Br. Heart J.,* **40:**725, 1978.

Doxorubicin Toxicity

Biencaniello, T.; Meyer, R. A.; Wong, K. Y.; *et al.:* Doxorubicin cardiotoxicity in children. *J. Pediatr.,* **97:**45, 1980.

Collagen Diseases

Eggebrecht, R. F., and Kleiger, R. E.: Echocardiographic patterns in scleroderma. *Chest,* **71:**47, 1977.

Gottdiener, J. S.; Montsopoulos, H. M.; and Gecker, J. L.: Echocardiographic identification of cardiac abnormality in scleroderma and related disorders. *Am. J. Med.,* **66:**391, 1979.

Henderson, A.; Cumming, W. J.; Williams, D. O.; *et al.:* Cardiac complications of polymyositis. *J. Neurosci.,* **47:**425, 1980.

Chronic Renal Failure

Cohen, M. V.; Diaz, P.; and Scheur, J.: Echocardiographic assessment of left ventricular function in patients with chronic uremia. *Clin. Nephrol.,* **12:**156, 1979.

D'Cruz, I. A.; Bhatt, G. R.; Cohen, H. C.; and Glick, G.: Echocardiographic diagnosis of cardiac involvement in chronic renal failure. *Arch. Intern. Med.,* **138:**720, 1978.

Drueke, T.; Fauchet, M.; Fleury, J.; *et al.:* Effect of parathyroidectomy in left ventricular function in hemodialysis patients. *Lancet,* **1:**112, 1980.

Vaziri, N. D., and Prakash, R.: Echocardiographic evaluation of the effect of hemodialysis on cardiac size and function in patients with end-stage renal disease. *Am. J. Med. Sci.,* **278:**201, 1979.

Sarcoidosis

Kinney, E. L.; Jackson, G. L.; Reeves, W. C.; *et al.:* Thallium-scan myocardial defects and echocardiography abnormalities in patients with sarcoidosis without clinical cardiac dysfunction. *Am. J. Med.,* **68:**497, 1980.

RESTRICTIVE (INFILTRATIVE) CARDIOMYOPATHY

Benotti, J. R.; Grossman, W.; and Cohn, P. F.: Clinical profile of restrictive cardiomyopathy. *Circulation,* **61:**1206, 1980.

Borer, J. S.; Henry, W. L.; and Epstein, S. E.: Echocardiographic observations in patients with systemic infiltrative disease involving the heart. *Am. J. Cardiol.,* **39:**184, 1977.

Cabin, H. S.; Costello, R. M.; Vasudevan, G.; *et al.:* Cardiac lymphoma mimicking hypertrophic cardiomyopathy. *Am. Heart J.,* **102:**466, 1981.

Carroll, J. D.; Gaasch, W. H.; and McAdam, P. W. J.: Amyloid cardiomyopathy: Characterization by a distinctive voltage-mass relation. *Am. J. Cardiol.,* **49:**9, 1982.

Chew, C. Y. C.; Ziady, G. M.; Raphael, M. J.; *et al.:* Primary restrictive cardiomyopathy: Non-tropical endomyocardial fibrosis and hypereosinophilic heart disease. *Br. Heart J.,* **39:**399, 1977.

Chiaramida, S. A.; Goldman, M. A.; Zema, M. J.; *et al.:* Real-time cross-sectional echocardiographic diagnosis of infiltrative cardiomyopathy due to amyloid. *J.C.U.,* **8:**58, 1980.

Child, J. S.; Krivokapich, J.; and Abbasi, A. S.: Increased right ventricular wall thickness on echocardiography in amyloid infiltrative cardiomyopathy. *Am. J. Cardiol.,* **44:**1391, 1979.

Child, J. S.; Levisman, J. A.; Abbasi, A. S.; *et al.:* Echocardiographic manifestations of infiltrative cardiomyopathy: A report of seven cases due to amyloid. *Chest,* **70:**726, 1976.

Cutler, D. J.; Isner, J. M.; Bracey, A. W.; *et al.:* Hemachromatosis heart disease: An unemphasized cause of potentially reversible restrictive cardiomyopathy. *Am. J. Med.,* **69:**923, 1980.

Dienot, B.; Ekra, A.; and Bertrand, E.: L'échocardiographie du 23 cas de fibroses endomyocardiques constrictives droites ou bilatérales. *Arch. Mal. Coeur,* **72:**1101, 1980.

Hall, S. W.; Theologides, A.; and From, A. H. L.: Hypereosinophilic syndrome with biventricular involvement. *Circulation,* **55:**217, 1977.

Kubac, G.; Doris, I.; Oudro, M.; *et al.:* Malignant granular cell myoblastoma with metastatic cardiac involvement. *Am. Heart J.,* **100:**227, 1980.

St. John Sutton, M. G.; Reichek, N.; Kastor, J. A.; *et al.:* Computerized M-mode echocardiographic analysis of left ventricular dysfunction in cardiac amyloid. *Circulation,* **66:**790, 1982.

Siqueira-Filhos, A. G.; Cunha, C. L. P.; Tajik, A. J.; *et al.:* M-mode and two-dimensional echocardiographic features in cardiac amyloidosis. *Circulation,* **63:**188, 1981.

M

Prosthetic Valves

The value and limitations of echocardiography in the assessment of patients with prosthetic valves are often not clearly understood by many cardiologists and internists. A wide variety of valve prostheses has been used over the last 15 years, although many of them enjoyed only a transient popularity and were in vogue only in certain centers. As a rule, the surgeons at any particular center usually have a few favorite models that they use exclusively. Therefore, no echocardiographer can become familiar with the appearances and malfunctions of all different types of valves. One should aim at becoming well acquainted with the prosthetic valves used locally, but welcome the opportunity to study patients with other models implanted at some other institution or during an earlier era.

The following is a brief discussion of the diagnostic role of M-mode and 2-D echocardiography with regard to prosthetic valves:

The presence and type of valve prosthesis are usually known to the clinician and echocardiographer from the information provided by the patient or the medical record. However, it is not uncommon for this data to be unavailable from either source for various reasons. In such circumstances, echocardiography may not enable one to diagnose the exact model but can usually ascertain to which of the following categories it belongs (Mehlman, 1981):

a. Ball-cage type, such as the Starr-Edwards (Figs. M-1 to M-4) and Braunwald-Cutter valves,

b. Disk-cage, such as the Beall and Kay-Shiley valves,

c. Tilting disk, such as the Bjork-Shiley (Figs. M-5 to M-10) and Lillehei-Kaster valves,

d. Double tilting disk, such as the St. Jude valve (Hidajat *et al.*, 1980; DePace *et al.*, 1981; Tri *et al.*, 1981; Feldman *et al.*, 1982),

e. Bioprosthetic, such as the Edwards and Hancock heterograft valves (Figs. M-11 to M-13).

MECHANICAL PROSTHETIC VALVES

Precise identification of the type of valve model is possible by careful observation of the chest x-ray (Mehlman and Resnekov, 1978).

1. All mechanical valves consist of a fixed part (sewing ring and cage or struts) and a moving component (ball or disk). In the ball-cage and disk-cage types (categories **a** and **b** above), motion of the ball or disk is parallel to motion of the sewing ring and to the "long axis" of the valve. This is not true of the tilting disk types, in which the direction of disk tilt may or may not be in the direction of the ultrasound beam, depending on how such asymmetric valves have been implanted. Ball or disk motion takes place abruptly at the onset and cessation of systole (Figs. M-1 to M-3), and the echocardiographer's efforts are directed to recording this opening and closing motion. Movement toward the transducer is recorded on the echogram as "anterior" motion and away from the transducer as "posterior" motion. The slope of such motion can be measured on the tracing and indicates the velocity of motion.

2. Ball or disk motion may be recorded when the valve is viewed from the usual (left parasternal) site. However, the amplitude of the motion is appreciated best if the ultrasound beam is parallel to the direction of motion. For this reason, apical scanning is sometimes used for recording mitral mechanical valves and the right

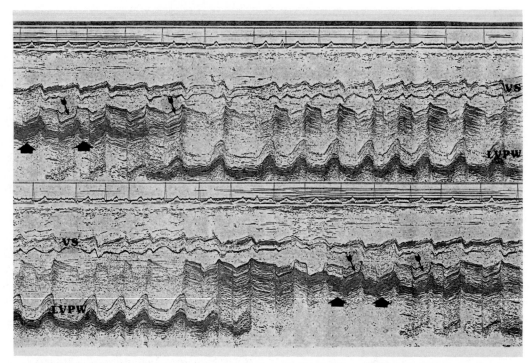

Fig. M-1. M-mode echocardiogram showing a scan from LA to LV in the upper panel and a scan from LV to LA in the lower panel, in a patient with a Starr-Edwards mitral valve. The prosthetic ball (*thin arrows*) can be seen to move anteriorly in diastole and posteriorly in systole. Dense echoes in and around the sewing ring region (*broad arrows*) are apparent posterior to the anterior ball echoes; these echoes could possibly simulate an LV thrombus or an LA myxoma (*right, upper panel*).

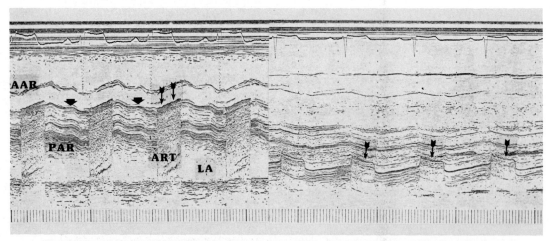

Fig. M-2. M-mode echocardiogram of a patient with a Starr-Edwards prosthetic valve in the aortic position. The left panel shows the aortic root, viewed from the left parasternal region. The linear echoes running parallel to the anterior and posterior aortic root echoes arise from the struts of the prosthetic valve (*broad arrows*). The ball is visible only during systole, its appearance and disappearance being equally abrupt (*thin arrows*). The apparent extension of its echoes into the LA is artefactual (ART). In the right panel the prosthetic valve has been visualized by the right supraclavicular approach. The superior surface of the prosthetic ball appears as a sharp linear echo that moves abruptly toward the transducer early in systole and away from it an end-systole (*thin arrows*).

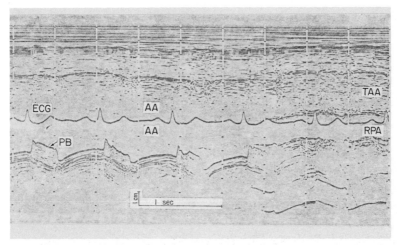

Fig. M-3. M-mode echocardiogram obtained by the right supraclavicular approach. In the left of the figure, the superior surface of the ball of a Starr-Edwards valve can be seen moving anteriorly in systole. The transducer was then directed more leftward, bringing the transverse aortic arch and right pulmonary artery into view.

supraclavicular approach (Figs. M-1 and M-2) for viewing similar aortic valves.

3. Abnormally *decreased* motion of a prosthetic ball (Fig. M-4) or disk could be due to formation of thrombus or vegetations in the valve area or, alternatively, to swelling or crack-

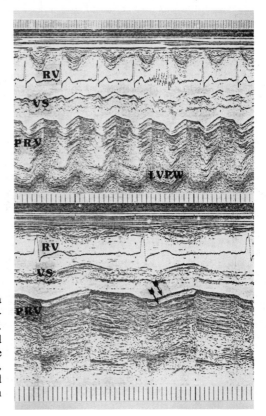

Fig. M-4. Segments from the M-mode echogram of a patient in congestive heart failure who had had Starr-Edwards mitral ball-valve replacement 8 years previously. Both panels show the prosthetic valve, but paper speed is faster and the scale expanded in the lower panel. The amplitude of ball motion is abnormally small (*arrows, lower panel*), attributable to fibrosis and thrombus around the valve, which also explains the wide dense echoes in the prosthetic valve area.

ing of the ball. Theoretically, echocardiography could be used to diagnose such clinically important complications; in practice, this is difficult because (a) motion of the ball or disk recorded on the echogram is not an absolute value, but only the vector or component of such motion

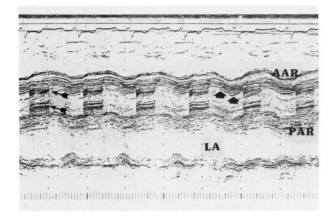

Fig. M-5. M-mode echocardiogram of a patient with a prosthetic aortic valve of the disk type. Echoes arising from the disk appear as a pair of dense parallel bandlike echoes within the aortic root, during systole (*thin arrows*). The strut of the valve is a dense echo parallel to the aortic root (*broad arrows*).

projected on the beam axis, which can vary with anatomic variation in cardiac position and alignment, scanning site, beam angulation, and so forth; (b) part of the motion recorded is not of the ball with reference to the sewing ring, but of the valve ring itself, which in turn results from ventricular contraction and relaxation. For these reasons, pathologically diminished ball or disk motion can be diagnosed with certainty only if the abnormality is extreme. Rarely, the ball or disk may actually fail to open in some beats or do so after a significant delay (as compared to other beats). Abnormal decrease in valve motion is appreciated better if serial echograms are available for comparison. At one time, it was routine in some centers to obtain periodic echograms for this purpose in all patients after valve replacement, but this is seldom done now because the yield of abnormal findings is too small to justify the expense and effort.

The Bjork-Shiley valve (Figs. M-5 to M-10), a popular tilting-disk valve, has received considerable attention from echocardiographers (Douglas and Williams, 1974; Ben-Ziv et al., 1974; Chandaratna et al., 1976; Srivastava et al., 1976; Bernal-Ramirez and Phillips, 1977; Chun et al., 1979; Copans et al., 1980; Griffiths et al., 1980). Normal motion of the disk, as measured on the M-mode echogram, is 10 to 18 mm (Chandaratna et al., 1976). M-mode abnormalities associated with the Bjork-Shiley valve include: (a) slow and rounded opening and closure contours (Fig. M-8) suggest thrombosis in the valve (Bernal-Ramirez and Phillips, 1977); (b) a characteristic "hump" in early diastole, accompanied by vigorous posterior septal

motion in systole, suggests a paravalvular leak (Bernal-Ramirez and Phillips, 1977; Chun et al., 1979).

4. *Artefacts.* Since the metallic and other constituents of mechanical valves are very strong reflectors of ultrasound, patients with prosthetic valves exhibit dense echoes that may artefactually extend beyond the expected site and appear in neighboring cardiac chambers. Thus prosthetic mitral or aortic valve echoes may appear in the atrial area on the tracing. Another potential source of fallacy is mistaking dense valvar or paravalvar echoes for thrombi (Fig. M-6), vegetations, mitral annulus calcification, or even a stenotic mitral valve. Since ultrasound passes through silastic material at a slower velocity than through blood and myocardium, the silastic ball of a Starr-Edwards valve, much in use about a decade ago, appears much larger on the echogram than it really is, so that the ball echo may even extend beyond the left ventricular posterior wall echo.

5. In spite of the potentially confusing effect of dense echoes arising from prosthetic valve components, it is sometimes possible for an experienced echographer to suspect valvar thrombi when the intravalvar echoes exceed, in extent and density, what is usual or expected for that valve (Lewis et al., 1983), especially if ball or disk motion seems impaired (Fig. M-9). Two-D echography is superior to the M-mode technique for this purpose (Mehlman and Talano, 1982).

6. Another useful role of 2-D echography is in those instances of bacterial endocarditis (on a prosthetic valve) wherein the vegetations are mobile and exhibit oscillating or undulating

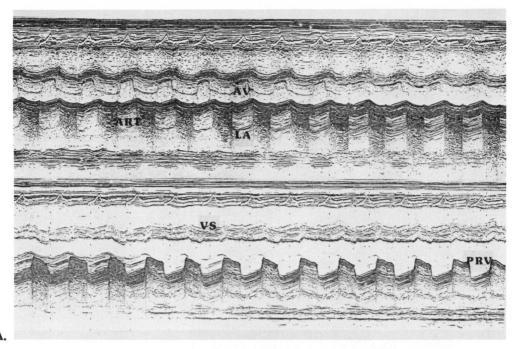

A.

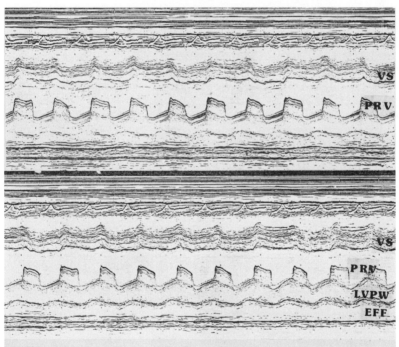

B.

Fig. M-6. M-mode echograms of a patient with a Bjork-Shiley tilting-disk valve in the mitral position.

Fig. M-6. *A.* The upper panel shows the aortic root and LA. A dense abnormal echo, apparently within the LA chamber, is visible in diastole; this is due to the disk of the prosthetic valve. Other dense echoes, arising from the sewing ring, appear behind the posterior aortic root in the right half of the figure as the transducer is slightly angled toward the LV. The lower panel shows motion of the prosthetic disk in the LV. In the right half of the figure it bears some resemblance to a stenotic mitral valve.

Fig. M-6. *B.* The same patient, with a Bjork-Shiley disk mitral valve: the resemblance to a stenotic mitral valve is more marked here.

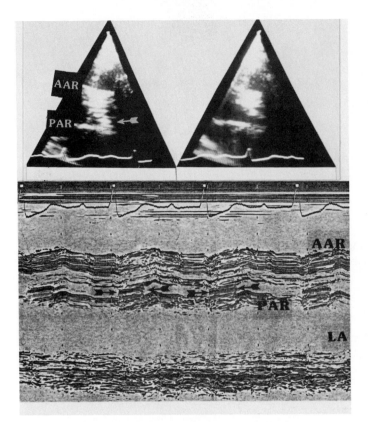

Fig. M-7. 2-D echogram (*upper*) in systole (*left*) and diastole (*right*), in a patient with a disk-type prosthetic aortic valve. The lower panel is from the M-mode echogram of the same patient and shows the aortic root. In both M-mode and 2-D echograms, the prosthetic valve produces dense echoes within the anterior part of the aorta, while the disk appears in the posterior part only during systole (*arrows*).

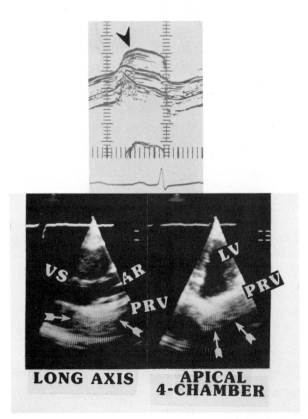

Fig. M-8. M-mode echogram of a 29-year-old woman with a partly clotted and partly fibrotic Bjork-Shiley mitral valve, which was shown to be stenotic on cardiac catheterization. Note the rounded outline of disk motion (*arrowhead*) on the M-mode tracing. The 2-D echogram in the long-axis view (*left*) and apical 4-chamber view (*right*) reveals excessive dense echoes (*arrows*) in the prosthetic area.

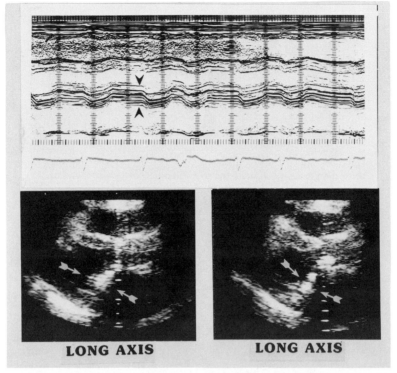

Fig. M-9. Echocardiogram of a 60-year-old woman with proven thrombosis of a Bjork-Shiley mitral valve. In the M-mode echogram (*above*) the prosthetic valve (*arrow heads*) appears unduly full of dense echoes, and no disk motion is evident. In the 2-D echogram (*below*), in the long-axis view, the dense echoes in the valve area (*arrows*) represent thrombi.

motion. Such appearances are diagnostically valuable because nonmobile vegetations produce echoes that are indistinguishable from those originating in prosthetic structures or surrounding fibrosis.

7. Phonocardiography has proven useful in conjunction with M-mode echography in detecting impaired ball or disk motion (Brodie *et al.,* 1976; Waggoner *et al.,* 1980; Mintz *et al.,* 1982), usually caused by local thrombus formation. Valve opening or closing is normally accompanied by sharp, loud clicking sounds as the ball or disk strikes against the fixed cage or struts. In patients with mitral prostheses, the aortic valve closing–to–mitral valve opening interval is increased (delayed mitral opening) if the prosthetic valve is "stuck" due to thrombus formation. In patients with prosthetic aortic valves, an increase in Q-to-aortic opening interval, and mitral closure–to–aortic opening interval, similarly suggests valve sticking (Berndt *et al.,* 1976; Cunha *et al.,* 1980; Griffiths *et al.,* 1980). Echophonocardiographic abnormalities were detected in as many as 71 per cent

of patients with prosthetic valve malfunction in the large Mayo Clinic series (Cunha *et al.,* 1980).

8. Echocardiographic findings with regard to structures other than the prosthetic valve itself may be helpful in diagnosing valve malfunction; thus (a) an unduly hyperdynamic LV, reflected in high systolic fractional shortening of the LV internal dimension and absence of abnormal septal motion, suggests LV diastolic overload caused by a paravalvar leak; (b) definite diastolic flutter of the mitral valve and perhaps left margin of the ventricular septum signifies aortic regurgitation.

9. Dehiscence of a prosthetic valve over part of its circumferential attachment is a frequent complication of postoperative endocarditis. Abnormal rocking motion of the prosthesis can produce abnormal echoes in the vicinity of aortic root echoes or in the LV outflow tract (Salem *et al.,* 1979; Schapira *et al.,* 1979; Cunha *et al.,* 1980; Strasberg *et al.,* 1980). This abnormality is even better demonstrated on 2-D echography.

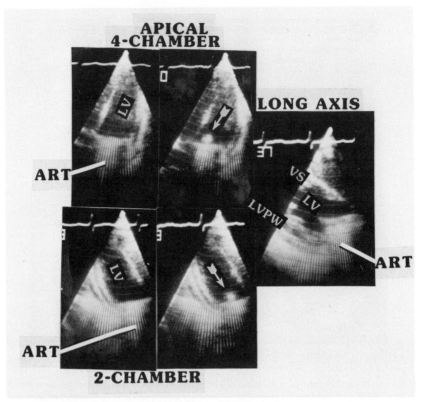

Fig. M-10. 2-D echogram in a patient with a mitral Bjork-Shiley prosthetic valve. Artefactual (ART) echo masses, due to reverberations from the prosthetic valve, appear larger in systole than in diastole (*left frames*). The disk can be seen in diastole (*arrows*). The reverberatory artefacts, apparently occupying the LA, should not be mistaken for a thrombus.

10. Echocardiographic visualization of an extruded disk of a Beall valve, lying loose and moving randomly in the LV, has been reported (Chen *et al.,* 1982).

11. If the mitral chordae have not been removed at the time of valve replacement, echoes from the loose or "floating" chordae can produce bizarre echographic appearances that may perplex the unwary (Gallego *et al.,* 1982).

BIOPROSTHETIC VALVES

(Bloch *et al.,* 1976, 1977; Horowitz *et al.,* 1976; Chandaratna and San Pedro, 1978; Harston *et al.,* 1978; Brown *et al.,* 1978; Schapira *et al.,* 1979; Alam *et al.,* 1979; Alam and Goldstein, 1980; Strasberg *et al.,* 1980; Perry *et al.,* 1981).

Bioprosthetic (porcine) valves resemble the mechanical valves echocardiographically in the sense that the sewing ring and stents produce dense echoes that tend to spread artefactually into neighboring areas because of the beam-width effect. These dense echoes may also obscure motion of the valve leaflets. Leaflet motion is appreciated better on 2-D than on M-mode echography (Fig. M-11); in normal valves the leaflets appear thin and delicate with brisk motion. The following echographic abnormalities of the leaflets have been described:

1. Dense, thickened (more than 3 mm thick) leaflet echoes with diminished motion suggest sclerosis or calcification.

2. Mitral regurgitation may manifest with systolic flutter (Alam *et al.,* 1979) and usually is caused by a leaflet tear. Systolic flutter does not occur with normal valves.

3. A flail leaflet tends to protrude into the left atrium in systole, as viewed on 2-D echography.

4. Vegetations of endocarditis may be recognized as dense nodules attached to the leaflets on the 2-D echogram (Fig. M-12); they may

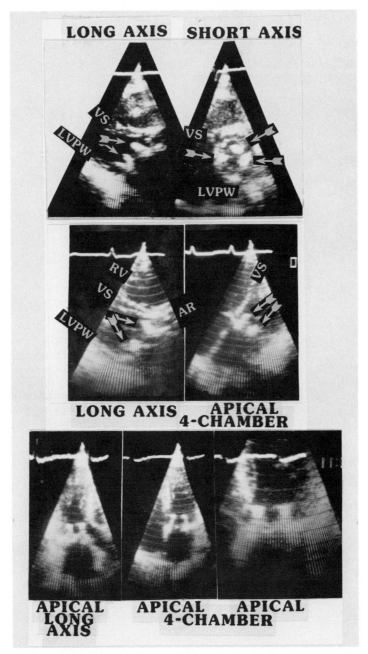

Fig. M-11. *Upper.* 2-D echocardiogram of a patient with prosthetic (porcine) mitral and aortic valves. The projecting stents (*arrows*) are clear in the long-axis view (*left*) as they protrude into the LV cavity. In the short-axis view (*right*), the stents (*arrows*) are visible around the mitral orifice within the LV.

    Center. 2-D echocardiogram of a patient with prosthetic (porcine) mitral and aortic valves, in the long-axis view (*right*). The posterior stent of the mitral valve could resemble posterior submitral (mitral annulus) calcification. However, the characteristic contour of the anterior stent in both views, typical of the prosthetic heterograft valve, provides a ready clue to the correct diagnosis (apart from the history of valve replacement). The arrows indicate the stents of the prosthetic mitral valve.

    Lower. 2-D echogram of a patient with a porcine prosthetic mitral valve. The first frame is in the apical long-axis view; the second frame is in the apical 4-chamber view; the third is an expanded apical 4-chamber view of the prosthetic valve. Its stents are easily recognizable. In real-time viewing, the leaflets of the prosthetic valve can be seen to move briskly between the stents.

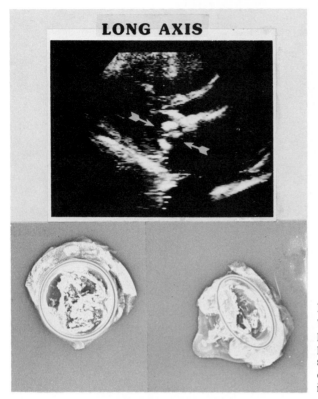

LONG AXIS

Fig. M-12. 2-D echogram of a 19-year-old woman who had had porcine mitral valve replacement 3 years previously. At autopsy the prosthetic valve was calcified and clotted, as seen in the xenoradiograph. The arrows indicate the valvar pathology on the 2-D echogram in the long-axis view.

be difficult or impossible to differentiate from mere sclerotic changes, especially in valves of long standing.

5. Thrombi may manifest as dense echoes within the stents, but separate from the leaflet echoes (Bloch *et al.*, 1976b).

6. Diastolic flutter of the leaflets of a mitral prosthesis occurs when aortic regurgitation

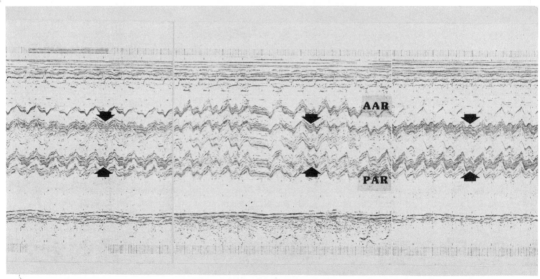

Fig. M-13. M-mode echocardiogram of a prosthetic porcine aortic valve. The stents of the prosthetic valve can be seen well within the aortic root (*broad arrows*). The anterior and posterior aortic roots thus appear to have a double outline. The leaflets show motion like that of a normal aortic valve (*left*).

Fig. M-14. 2-D echogram, in the apical view, of a child with a porcine mitral valve (PPV). A paravalvar aneurysm or pocket (*arrow*) appears in diastole (*left frame*). It expands in systole (*center frame*). In a different view (*right frame*), approaching the apical long-axis view, a space appears posterior to the prosthetic valve (*arrow*). The space represents a posterior pocket. The presence of these paravalvar pockets, or aneurysms, was confirmed by angiocardiography, and could have been due to the prosthesis having been sewn not to the mitral annulus but to the atrial wall above annulus level.

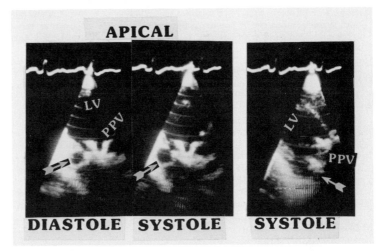

coexists. However, the flutter is more prominent on the posterior leaflet, whereas with native mitral valves flutter is always greater on the anterior leaflet.

7. I have seen an instance of a paravalvar aneurysm or pocket (Fig. M-14) possibly caused by a mitral bioprosthesis being sewed on too high, i.e., not to the mitral annulus but to the left atrial wall above it.

Bioprosthetic valves in the aortic position appear echocardiographically very much like native aortic valves, except that the stents are responsible for a duplication of the anterior and posterior aortic root echoes (Fig. M-13).

REFERENCES

Alam, M.; Madrazo, A. C.; Magilligan, D. J.; *et al.:* M-mode and two-dimensional echocardiographic features of porcine valve dysfunction. *Am. J. Cardiol.,* **43:**502, 1979.

Alam, M., and Goldstein, S.: Echocardiographic features of a stenotic porcine aortic valve. *Am. Heart J.,* **100:**517, 1980.

Ben-Ziv, J.; Hildner, F. J.; Chandaratna, P. A.; *et al.:* Thrombosis on Bjork-Shiley aortic valve prosthesis: Clinical, arteriographic, echocardiographic and therapeutic observations in seven cases. *Am. J. Cardiol.,* **34:**538, 1974.

Bernal-Ramirez, J. A., and Phillips, J. H.: Echocardiographic study of malfunction of the Bjork-Shiley prosthetic heart valve in the mitral position. *Am. J. Cardiol.,* **40:**449, 1977.

Berndt, T. B.; Goodman, D. J.; and Popp, R. L.: Echocardiographic and phonocardiographic confirmation of suspected caged mitral valve malfunction. Chest, **70:**221, 1976.

Bloch, W. N.; Felner, J. M.; Wickliffe, C.; *et al.:* Echocardiogram of the porcine aortic bioprosthesis in the mitral position. *Am. J. Cardiol.,* **38:**293, 1976a.

Bloch, W. N.; Felner, J. M.; Wickliffe, C.; *et al.:* Echocardiographic diagnosis of thrombus on a heterograft aortic valve in the mitral position. *Chest,* **70:**339, 1976b.

Bloch, W. N.; Felner, J. M.; Schlant, R. C.; *et al.:* The echocardiogram of the porcine aortic bioprosthesis in the aortic position. *Chest,* **72:**640, 1977.

Brodie, B. R.; Grossman, W.; McLaurin, L.; *et al.:* Diagnosis of prosthetic mitral valve malfunction with combined echo-phonocardiography. *Circulation,* **53:**93, 1976.

Brown, J. W.; Dunn, J. M.; and Spooner, E.: Late spontaneous disruption of a porcine xenograft mitral valve. *J. Thorac. Cardiovasc. Surg.,* **75:**606, 1978.

Chandaratna, P. A. N.; Lopez, J. M.; Hildner, F. J.; *et al.:* Diagnosis of Bjork-Shiley aortic valve dysfunction by echocardiography. *Am. Heart J.,* **91:**318, 1976.

Chandaratna, P. A. N., and San Pedro, S. B.: Echocardiographic features of the normal and malfunctioning porcine xenograft valve. *Am. Heart J.,* **95:**548, 1978.

Chen, C. C.; Morganroth, J.; and Pauletto, F. J.: Embolized disc from a Beall mitral valve prosthesis. *Chest,* **81:**108, 1982.

Chun, P. K. C.; Rajfer, S. I.; Donohue, D. J.; *et al.:* Bjork-Shiley mitral valvular dehiscence. *Am. Heart J.,* **99:**230, 1979.

Copans, H.; Lakier, J. B.; Kinsley, R. H.; *et al.:* Thrombosed Bjork-Shiley mitral prostheses. *Circulation,* **61:**169, 1980.

Cunha, C. L. P.; Giuliani, E. R.; Callahan, J. A.; *et al.:* Echocardiographic findings in patients with prosthetic heart valve malfunction. *Mayo Clin. Proc.,* **55:**231, 1980.

DePace, N. L.; Kotler, M. N.; Mintz, G. S.; *et al.:* Echocardiographic and phonocardiographic assessment of the St. Jude cardiac valve prosthesis. *Chest,* **80:**272, 1981.

Douglas, J. E., and Williams, G. D.: Echocardiographic evaluation of the Bjork-Shiley prosthetic valve. *Circulation,* **50:**52, 1974.

Feldman, H. J.; Gray, R. J.; Chaux, A.; *et al.:* Noninvasive in vivo and in vitro study of the St. Jude mitral valve prosthesis. *Am. J. Cardiol.,* **40:**1101, 1982.

Gallego, F. G.; Oliver, J. M.; and Sotillo, J. F.: Echocardiographic detection of free mitral chordae tendineae after mitral valve replacement. *Cor Vasa,* **1:**273, 1982.

Griffiths, B. E.; Charles, R.; and Coulshed, N.: Echophonocardiography in diagnosis of mitral paravalvular regurgitation with Bjork-Shiley prosthetic valve. *Br. Heart J.,* **43:**325, 1980.

Harston, W. E.; Robertson, R. M.; Friesinger, G. C.: Echocardiographic evaluation of porcine heterograft valves in the mitral and aortic positions. *Am. Heart J.,* **96**:448, 1978.

Hidajat, H. C.; Gottwik, M. G.; Thormann, J.; *et al.:* Echocardiographic identification and analysis of function of the St. Jude medical heart valve prosthesis. *Eur. J. Cardiol.,* **12**:167, 1980.

Horowitz, M. S.; Tecklenberg, P. L.; Goodman, D. J.; *et al.:* Echocardiographic evaluation of the stent mounted aortic bioprosthetic valve in the mitral position. *Circulation,* **54**:91, 1976.

Lewis, B. S.; Agathengelou, N. E.; DosSantos, L. A.; *et al.:* Real-time 2-dimensional echocardiographic visualization of thrombus on a Bjork-Shiley mitral valve prosthesis. *Am. J. Cardiol.,* **51**:908, 1983.

Mehlman, D. J.: Ultrasonic visualization of prosthetic heart valves. *Semin. Ultrasound.,* **2**:134, 1981.

Mehlman, D. J., and Resnekov, L.: A guide to radiographic identification of prosthetic heart valves. *Circulation,* **57**:613, 1978.

Mehlman, D. J., and Talano, J. V.: Detection of atrioventricular disc valve malfunction by two-dimensional echocardiography. *Am. Heart. J.,* **104**:1378, 1982.

Mintz, G. S.; Carlson, E. B.; and Kotler, M. N.: Comparison of noninvasive techniques in evaluation of the nontissue cardiac valve prosthesis. *Am. J. Cardiol.,* **49**:39, 1982.

Perry, L. W.; Midgley, F. M.; Galioto, F. M.; *et al.:* Two-dimensional echocardiographic evaluation of mitral bioprosthetic function in children. *Am. Heart. J.,* **102**:1022, 1981.

Salem, B. I.; Pechacek, L. W.; and Leachman, R. D.: Major dehiscence of a prosthetic aortic valve. Detection by echocardiography. *Chest,* **75**:513, 1979.

Schapira, J. N.; Martin, R. P.; and Fowles, R. E.: Two-dimensional echocardiographic assessment of patients with bioprosthetic valves. *Am. J. Cardiol.,* **43**:510, 1979.

Srivastava, T. N.; Hussain, M.; Gray, L. A.; *et al.:* Echocardiographic diagnosis of a stuck Bjork-Shiley aortic valve prosthesis. *Chest,* **70**:94, 1976.

Strasberg, B.; Kanakis, C.; Eckner, F.; *et al.:* Echocardiographic demonstration of porcine mitral valve vegetation and dehiscence. *Eur. J. Cardiol.,* **12**:41, 1980.

Tri, T. B.; Schatz, R. A.; Watson, T. D.; *et al.:* Echocardiographic evaluation of the St. Jude medical prosthetic valve. *Chest,* **80**:278, 1981.

Waggoner, A. D.; Quinones, M. A.; Young, J. B.; *et al.:* Echophonocardiography evaluation of obstruction of prosthetic mitral valve. *Chest,* **78**:60, 1980.

N

Pericardial Disease

PERICARDIAL EFFUSIONS OF SMALL AND MODERATE SIZES

The principle of the ultrasound diagnosis of pericardial effusion is simple. It is that fluid transmits rather than reflects ultrasound (thus the cardiac chambers, always full of blood, appear echo free on the echocardiogram). An accumulation of pericardial fluid between the left ventricular posterior wall and the posterior parietal pericardium, therefore, manifests on the echocardiogram as a clear space between the echo of the left ventricular posterior wall and that of the parietal pericardium. Normally, in the absence of any effusion, the left ventricular epicardial and the pericardial echoes show no separation, the epicardium-pericardium interface being represented by a single strong echo or two linear parallel echoes very close (1 or 2 mm) to each other. Similarly, fluid in the anterior pericardial space between the right ventricular anterior wall and anterior parietal pericardium shows as an anterior echo-free space.

In practical terms, the echocardiographer's task therefore consists of recording adequately, with best possible definition: (1) the endocardium and epicardium of the ventricular wall, (2) the parietal pericardium, and (3) the echo-free region itself (Fig. N-1).

Technical aspects of visualizing the left ventricular posterior wall and the characteristics of endocardial and epicardial motion have been well described in detail (Feigenbaum et al., 1965, 1966; Feigenbaum, 1970; Moss and Bruhn, 1966; Goldberg et al., 1967; Pate et al., 1967; Rothman et al., 1967; Klein and Segal, 1968; Abbasi et al., 1973; Tajik, 1977). Of the two, the epicardial echo is stronger and easier to record. The endocardial echo can be distinguished from it, as well as from other lin-

ear echoes in the vicinity (posterior mitral chordae tendineae and posterior mitral leaflet), by its characteristic contour and the fact that it exhibits faster anterior motion during systole than these other neighboring echoes. The left ventricular endocardial and epicardial echoes can be further identified because, on close examination with suitable gain-setting, the space between them shows a typical "myocardial" pattern of fine linear echoes in diastole altering to a fine mottling or stippling during systole and, to a lesser degree, during atrial contraction and the phase of early rapid ventricular filling (D'Cruz et al., 1976).

The pericardial echo is usually the strongest one in the whole echocardiographic field. Electronic ingenuity has devised gray scale, switched gain, and other means of enhancing the prominence of the pericardial echo, so that recent commercially available echocardiographic equipment enables even a novice to locate the pericardial echo with ease.

Another way of identifying the pericardial echo is by progressively decreasing the gain. The endocardial echo, the weakest, is the first to disappear, leaving the epicardial and pericardial echoes visible; next to vanish is the epicardial echo, so that the sole remaining one is that of the pericardium (Fig. N-2, lower panel). Although this general rule is usually true, it often happens in subacute or chronic pericarditis with effusion that the epicardium is thickened and sclerotic. The left ventricular epicardial echo in such patients is as dense and prominent as the pericardial echo; decreasing the gain does not eliminate the epicardial before the pericardial echo.

Yet another means of confirming the identity of the pericardial and left ventricular posterior

PERICARDIAL EFFUSIONS ECHO PATTERNS

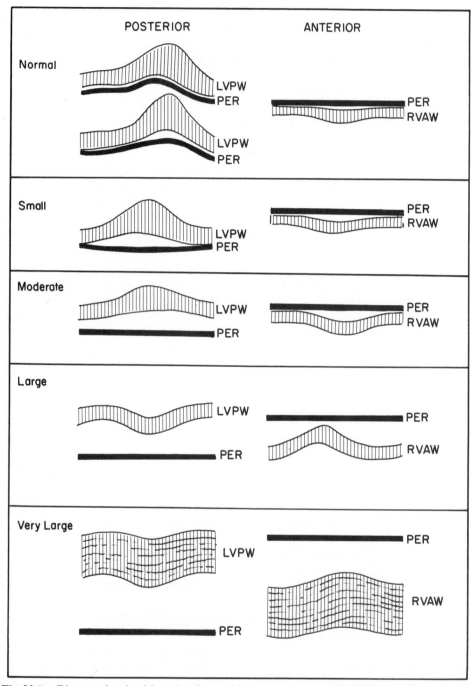

Fig. N-1. Diagram showing M-mode echographic patterns in pericardial effusions. The posterior pericardial space is depicted on the left; the anterior pericardial space, on the right. As the size of the effusion increases, from small to very large, the width of the echo-free space increases, and ventricular wall motion abnormally increases due to enhanced cardiac mobility.

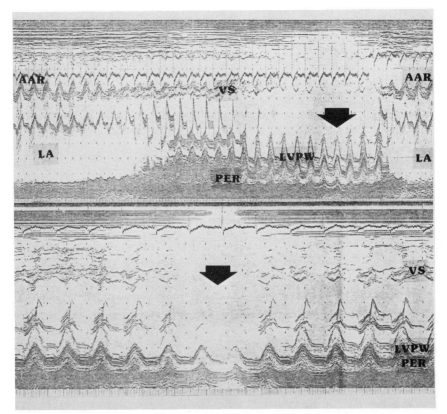

Fig. N-2. M-mode echocardiogram of a patient who had had mitral valvotomy one week earlier. The upper panel depicts a scan from LA to LV, and then back to LA, at a paper speed of 10 mm/sec. In the lower panel, showing the LV, the paper speed was 25 mm/sec. In both panels, a small space can be seen between LV posterior wall and pericardium; it contains small stippled or short linear echoes. When the damping is increased (*arrows*) this space appears echo free. Such echocardiographic appearances are very common during the first week or two after any cardiac operation, and represent a small accumulation of pericardial exudate undergoing organization.

wall echoes is to record continuous scans from left ventricle to left atrium. In patients with pericardial effusion, the width of the echo-free pericardial space attenuates behind the atrioventricular junction and terminates behind the left atrium. The left ventricular posterior wall becomes continuous with the left atrial posterior wall, while the pericardial echo posterior to the left ventricle continues just behind the left atrial posterior wall and contiguous to it, perhaps fusing with it (Fig. N-2, upper panel).

This maneuver, a very useful one in routine echocardiography, was formerly thought to be a foolproof method for diagnosing the presence of a pericardial effusion. However, there are two exceptions which need to be kept in mind:

1. Although pericardial effusions usually do not extend into the space behind the left atrium (the oblique pericardial sinus), occasionally they may do so. First described by Lemire *et al.* (1976), such a finding is nearly always seen only with large pericardial effusions.

2. It is often taught that scanning from left ventricle to left atrium demonstrates narrowing and obliteration of the retroventricular echo-free space in pericardial effusion, but not in pleural effusion, because pleural effusions extend posterior to the left atrium. Nevertheless, the left atrial posterior surface is mostly related to posterior mediastinal structures; the left atrium is really medial as well as anterior to the pleural cavity. A sweep from left ventricle medially and upward to the left atrium in a patient with a pleural effusion often demonstrates a "disappearance" of the effusion at about the moment that the left atrium comes into view. Thus the narrowing and ending of an echo-free space as a scan moves from left

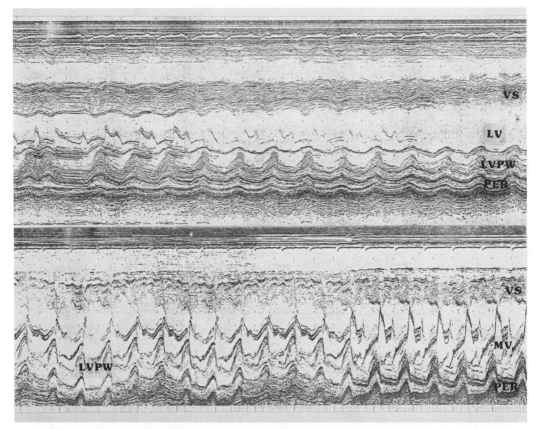

Fig. N-3.   M-mode echocardiogram of a patient with a small pericardial effusion. A separation between LV posterior wall and thickened pericardium, suggestive of pericardial fluid, is visible at mitral valve level (*left*) but is not as evident at chordae level (*right*).

M-mode echocardiogram of a patient with a small pericardial effusion. A small pericardial space, between LV posterior wall and pericardium, can be seen best in the right third of the figure. However, the pericardial echo is not flat but instead follows the motion of the LV posterior wall. This is attributable to intrapericardial adhesions, which are in fact evident in the center of the figure.

ventricle to left atrium is not necessarily a reliable means of distinguishing a pericardial from a pleural effusion.

It was not until Horowitz *et al.* (1974) published their study, systematically correlating the echographic patterns of ventricular wall–pericardial separation with the quantity of fluid directly suctioned off from the pericardial sac at thoracotomy, that a scientific basis was established for roughly quantifying pericardial effusions in routine clinical practice. This series consisted of 43 patients who underwent cardiac or thoracic surgery for various indications; by measuring the entire fluid content of the pericardial sac, a more reliable estimation of the volume of the effusion was possible than by paracentesis which, of course, cannot achieve a complete removal of the pericardial contents.

The basic concepts and guidelines laid down by Horowitz *et al.* have been widely accepted and applied.

Thus it is commonly acknowledged that a small echo-free space between the parietal pericardium and the left ventricular posterior wall in systole, but not in diastole, signifies a small pericardial effusion (Fig. N-3, upper panel; Fig. N-4). When the separation between epicardium and parietal pericardium exists throughout the cardiac cycle, the effusion is believed to be of moderate size (Figs. N-5 and N-6).

Horowitz *et al.* (1974) noted that when a patient showed the classic pattern of epicardial-pericardial separation throughout the cardiac cycle, the visualization of "a large anterior echo-free space made a moderately large pericardial effusion likely." They noted that "in

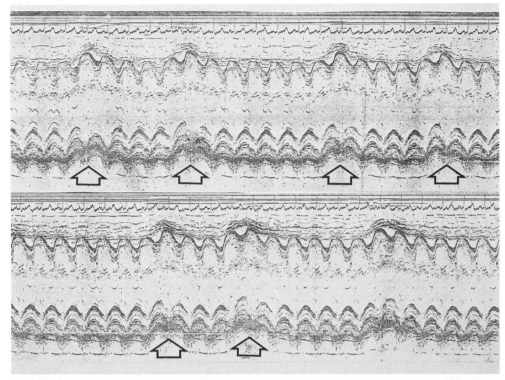

Fig. N-4. Segments from the M-mode echocardiogram of a patient with a small pericardial effusion (subcostal approach). A small echo-free space anterior as well as posterior to the heart is seen in systole only. The posterior pericardial space is more apparent in the upper panel; the anterior pericardial space, in the lower panel. Note that, in the subcostal view, the heart moves toward the transducer during inspiration (*arrows*).

the absence of this diagnostic posterior echo-free space, an anterior echo-free space had no diagnostic significance as it was found in 11 patients with less than 16 ml of pericardial fluid." Possible alternative explanations for an echo-free space anterior to the right ventricular anterior wall include epicardial fat, retrosternal connective tissue, the thymus, retrosternal goiter, and various anterior mediastinal masses.

With the patient in a supine position, an echo-free space does not usually appear between right ventricular anterior wall and anterior pericardium until about 1 cm epicardial-pericardial separation has appeared posteriorly. Anterior effusions often widen if the patient sits up. Another situation associated with an anterior echo-free space as wide, or wider than, the posterior pericardial space is that of patients who have had recent cardiac surgery, or who have had a pericardial window created surgically for recurrent or refractory pericardial effusion (usually cases of chronic renal failure).

In actual practice, the echographic diagnosis of small pericardial effusions is not as easy as the preceding paragraphs may imply. In children, adolescents, or adults who for some reason exhibit hyperdynamic cardiac contraction, a slight separation between left ventricular wall and pericardium may occur during vigorous systole. This pattern resembles that in patients with minimal or small effusion inasmuch as a small echo-free space can be visualized in systole but not in diastole. Differentiation between these two possible interpretations is facilitated by attention to the following points:

1. If the parietal pericardial echo remains "flat" throughout the cardiac cycle (i.e., does not exhibit an anterior systolic motion similar to that of the left ventricular posterior wall epicardial echo), the diagnosis of a small pericardial effusion is favored. The pericardial fluid is presumed to act as a buffer, insulating or dissociating the parietal pericardium from ventricular wall motion. On the other hand, if the pericardium moves anteriorly during systole, closely following epicardial motion, this echo-

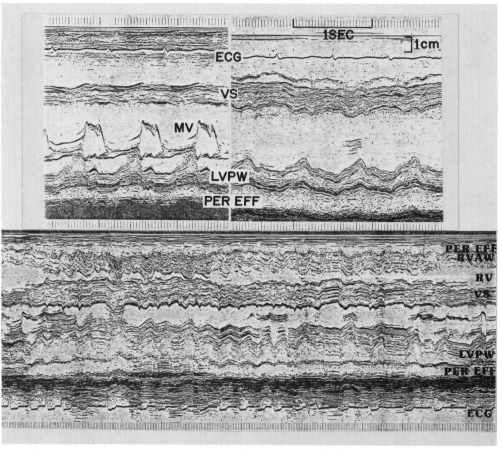

Fig. N-5. *Upper.* M-mode echocardiogram showing a posterior pericardial effusion of moderate size. A somewhat unusual pattern of LV posterior wall motion in early diastole to middiastole is visible at mitral valve level (*left*) but not at mid-LV level (*right*). The mechanism of such minor alterations in LV mobility is uncertain, but may be related to the presence of pericardial fluid.

Lower. M-mode echocardiogram of a patient with a pericardial effusion of moderate size. The LV is concentrically hypertrophied. Note the RV dimension varies from normal to almost zero at different levels of the scan: an abnormally small RV dimension has been considered by some to be an important sign of cardiac tamponade. This patient had no tamponade.

graphic pattern is likely to be a normal variant.

2. If the epicardial-pericardial separation occurs not only in systole but also in much of diastole, such that the diastolic contact between the two is very brief, a pericardial effusion is probably present. On the other hand, a slight separation of only 2 or 3 mm between epicardium and pericardium that is limited to ventricular systole is likely to be within the normal range.

It must be added that the various diagnostic patterns described above are not infallable criteria, because the same patient can exhibit different patterns with only minor changes in transducer direction (Fig. N-7).

3. Frequently, more pericardial fluid collects at and near the cardiac apex than near the basal left ventricle. Thus only a slight epicardial-pericardial separation may be visualized at mitral valve level (small effusion pattern), which broadens to a more complete separation (moderate effusion pattern) of 1 cm or more at mid- or apical left ventricular level. The ventricle therefore should be scanned as extensively as possible from base to apex in patients with suspected pericardial effusions.

4. An apparent echo-free space between epicardium and pericardium, which remains of constant width during both systole and diastole, suggests the presence of thickened adherent

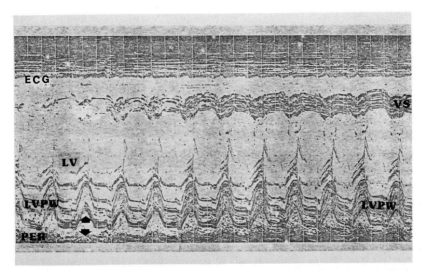

Fig. N-6. M-mode echogram of a patient with a small to moderate pericardial effusion. At a suitable degree of damping (*left of figure*), the posterior pericardial space, representing fluid, is evident. With lesser damping (*right of figure*), the space posterior to the LV posterior wall is not echo free, so that the presence of a pericardial effusion is not clearly demonstrated.

pericardium rather than pericardial effusion. Horowitz *et al.* (1974) noted this pattern in two of their patients who had pericardial thickening but no pericardial effusion at surgery. Feigenbaum (1981) has also commented on this pattern as indicative of pericardial thickening.

5. When the transducer is directed to the posteromedial wall of the left ventricle, the ventricular wall systolic excursion may increase markedly with distortion of the normal endocardial and epicardial contour (Fig. N-7). A triangular echo-free space posterior to the ventricular wall in such a tracing is an artefact and does not signify pericardial fluid. A small shift in transducer direction always succeeds in visualizing the ventricular epicardium and endocardium in proper contour, with no epicardial-pericardial separation. The echo-free peri-

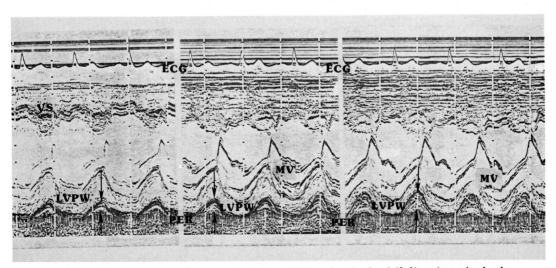

Fig. N-7. M-mode echocardiogram, showing the LV at chordae level (*left*) and at mitral valve level (*middle and right*). In the left and middle panels a very small space is demonstrated in systole between the epicardial and the pericardial echoes, which may not exceed normal. In the right panel an apparently larger systolic space opens up, suggesting a small pericardial effusion. It is an artefact caused by too medial an angulation of the transducer. Note that the LV wall appears distorted in this panel for the same reason.

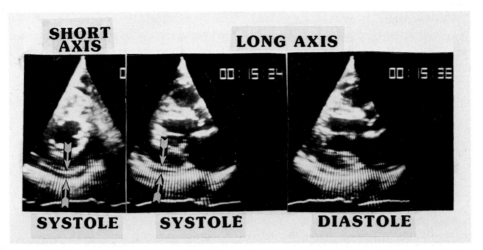

Fig. N-8. 2-D echogram of a patient with a small pericardial effusion. A narrow echo-free space is present between the LV and pericardium posteriorly (*arrows*) in systole (*left and center*) but is barely detectable in diastole (*right*).

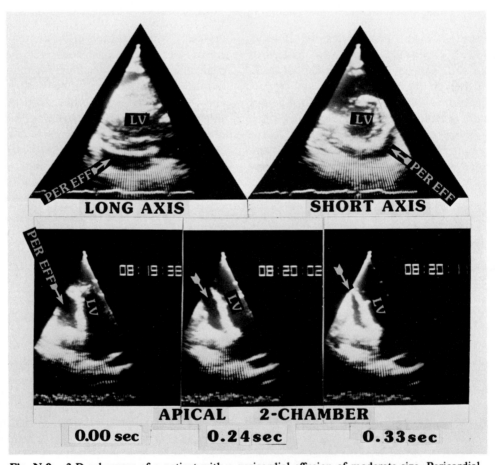

Fig. N-9. 2-D echogram of a patient with a pericardial effusion of moderate size. Pericardial fluid posterior to the LV is seen as an echo-free space in the long-axis view (*upper left*), short-axis view (*upper right*), and apical 2-chamber view (*lower 3 frames*). The latter show a striking fluctuation in width of the posterior pericardial space during different phases of the same cardiac cycle.

cardial space, widening in systole, can be seen well on 2-D echography (Figs. N-8 and N-9).

Practical difficulties or pitfalls in the technique and interpretation of M-mode echocardiography with regard to pericardial effusions have been discussed by several investigators (Jacobs *et al.,* 1978; Walinsky, 1978; D'Cruz *et al.,* 1977; Horowitz *et al.,* 1979). Others have examined the correlation between clinical and echocardiographic findings in patients with pericardial disease (Berger *et al.,* 1978; Markiewicz *et al.,* 1980).

LARGE PERICARDIAL EFFUSIONS
(Figs. N-10 to N-18)

As may be expected, large pericardial effusions exhibit larger widths of echo-free space anterior and posterior to the heart than are seen in effusions of small to moderate size. In addition, certain other echographic features are noted,

most of which are due to increased mobility of the heart within a voluminous fluid-filled space (Feigenbaum *et al.,* 1966; Nanda *et al.,* 1976).

In large pericardial effusions, a wide space of up to 4 cm or even more is visualized, anterior as well as posterior to the heart, which often broadens as the left ventricle is scanned from base to apex (Figs. N-10 and N-11). Although the width of the posterior echo-free space usually exceeds that of the anterior echo-free space, exceptions to this are not uncommon.

Common to most large pericardial effusions is an abnormal oscillatory or pendulous motion of the heart as a whole. In the absence of excessive pericardial fluid, the restraining effect of the pericardium, pleura, and surrounding structures prevents an undue range of ventricular motion, which comprises not only an anteroposterior component but also a rotatory component

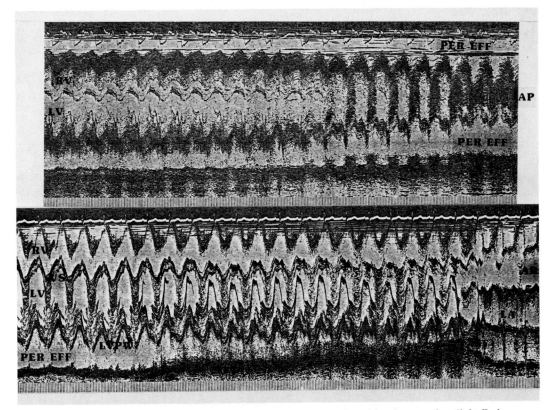

Fig. N-10. M-mode scan from base to apex of LV in a patient with a large pericardial effusion. The pericardial fluid is more abundant around the apex. Note also, in the lower panel, abnormal posterior systolic motion of the LV posterior wall, due to swinging ventricular motion. The mitral valve partakes of this systolic posterior motion, which is sometimes referred to as pseudoprolapse.

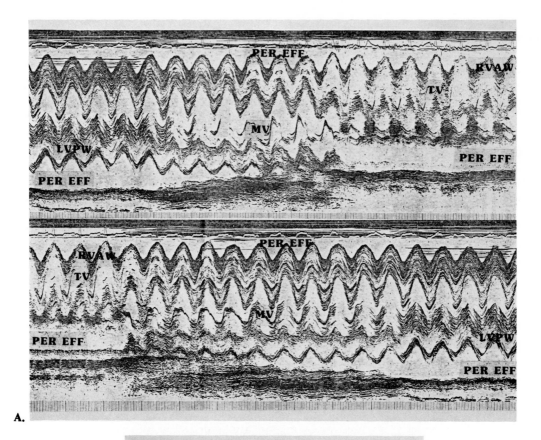

A.

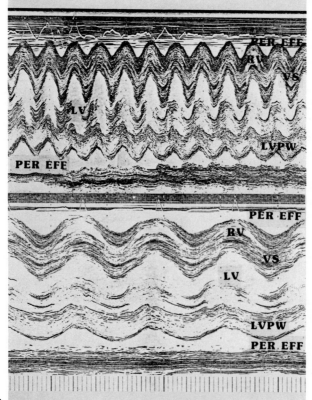

B.

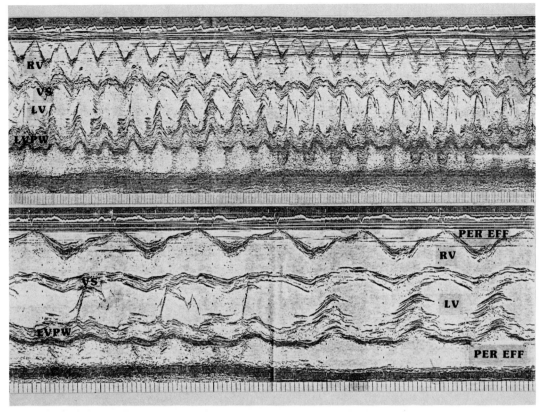

Fig. N-12. M-mode echocardiogram, showing the LV at different levels, of a patient with a large pericardial effusion. The ventricles display abnormal mobility, resulting in abnormal patterns of LV posterior wall motion, which varies at different LV levels. The anterior motion of the LV posterior wall appears normal until it is examined with reference to the ECG and motion of the RV wall and septum, when it is evident that the anterior LV wall motion occurs in diastole.

around the ventricular long axis. In large effusions, on the other hand, the heart is allowed free play to float and bounce from side to side within the fluid with every beat. Whereas the base of the heart is anchored to the mediastinum in the region of the great vessels, venae cavae, and pulmonary veins, the ventricles lie suspended and untrammeled in a lake of pericardial fluid. Every ventricular contraction, therefore, results in an exaggerated range of mobility; the ultrasound transducer records that component of the motion which occurs along the axis of the beam (more or less in the anteroposterior direction).

Enhanced cardiac mobility of mild degree may consist merely of a "flattening" of left ventricular posterior wall configuration, the normal anterior systolic excursion being blunted or ab-

Fig. N-11. *A.* M-mode echocardiogram of a patient with a large pericardial effusion and cardiac tamponade. The ventricles exhibit a swinging motion, so that the RV anterior wall, ventricular septum, and LV posterior wall all move posteriorly in systole and anteriorly in diastole. The RV appears unduly narrow, a finding suggestive of tamponade.

Fig. N-11. *B.* The upper panel depicts a scan from the LV at papillary muscle level to the LV at basal level and then rightward to the RV and RA. The anterior pericardial width shows little change during the scan. The posterior pericardial space tapers at mitral level and then widens again behind the RA. In the lower panel, a scan has been made in the reverse direction, from the right heart to the base and then toward the apex of the LV. Ventricular swinging and an abnormally small RV dimension are evident, as in *A.*

LEFT VENTRICULAR POSTERIOR WALL MOTION PATTERNS
IN PERICARDIAL EFFUSIONS

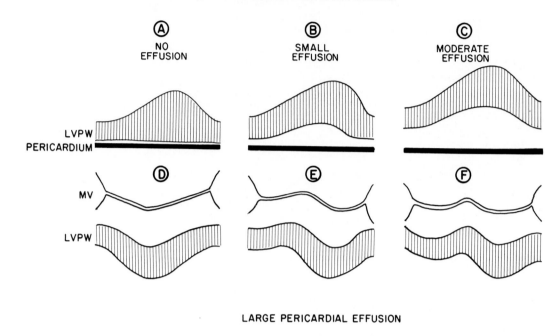

Fig. N-13.   Diagram showing patterns of LV posterior wall motion in normal (*A*), small (*B*), and moderate (*C*), pericardial effusions. Motion is anterior during systole in *B* and *C*. In large pericardial effusions (*C, D, E*), the LV posterior wall moves abnormally in systole: posterior motion may begin in early (*D*) or in midsystole (*E, F*).

sent. A somewhat greater extent of abnormal mobility results in so-called congruous motion of the anterior and posterior borders of the heart. Whereas normally the right ventricular anterior wall and the left ventricular posterior wall move toward each other in systole and away from each other in early diastole, in large pericardial effusions the echoes of these two structures may appear to move in the same direction (i.e., parallel) during the whole cardiac cycle (Figs. N-12 and N-13). Different LV posterior wall motion patterns may be observed simultaneously at different LV levels (Fig. N-12).

"PSEUDOMITRAL PROLAPSE"
(Figs. N-10, N-12, N-13)

Echoes of various cardiac structures such as the ventricular septum and mitral valve partake of the exaggerated motion of the heart as a whole, sometimes producing an apparent abnormality akin to that seen in various disease states. Thus, "pseudoparadoxic" septal motion has been described, also pseudomitral prolapse (Nanda *et al.,* 1976; Levisman and Abbasi, 1976; Lemire *et al.,* 1976; Owens *et al.,* 1976; Vignola *et al.,* 1976). The latter term refers to a posterior motion of the mitral valve in systole associated with a corresponding posterior systolic motion of the whole heart (including the adjacent left ventricular posterior wall) in patients with large pericardial effusions (Fig. N-13). After drainage of the effusion, such abnormal mitral and ventricular wall motion promptly disappears. Vignola *et al.* (1976) have noted that the contour of such pseudomitral prolapse on the echogram depended on the heart rate. The pseudoprolapse appeared in early or late systole if the heart rate exceeded 120/min, and a holosystolic pseudoprolapse if the rate was below 120/min. In practice, it is unlikely that pseudoprolapse would ever be mistaken for true prolapse by an experienced echocardiographer because it is difficult to overlook the presence of a large pericardial effusion and

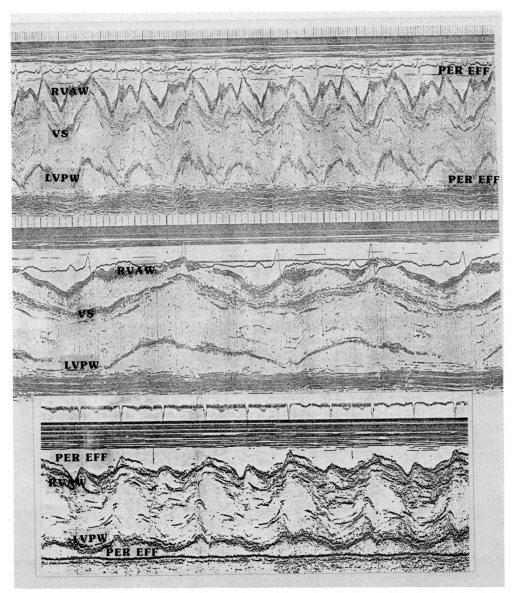

Fig. N-14. *Upper and Center.* M-mode echocardiogram in a woman with a large pericardial effusion secondary to breast carcinoma. The ECG shows alternation of contour. Cardiac position and motion also alternate from beat to beat. The lower panel is taken at much faster paper speed.

Lower. M-mode echocardiogram of a patient with a large pericardial effusion causing cardiac tamponade. The heart exhibits a swinging motion. Alternation in cardiac position and motion is evident from beat to beat. ECG alternans was also noted, but is not very obvious in the lead recorded in this tracing.

the concomitant abnormal mobility of the left ventricular posterior wall.

Nanda, Gramiak, and Gross (1976) analyzed the echocardiograms of 34 patients with large pericardial effusions; 22 (65 per cent) of these demonstrated apparent systolic motion abnormalities of one or more valves, all of which

were observed to disappear after marked decrease or removal of the effusion had taken place in those cases in whom serial echograms were available. Systolic anterior motion (SAM) of the anterior mitral leaflet, resembling that of idiopathic hypertrophic subaortic stenosis, was seen in four cases; mitral prolapse patterns

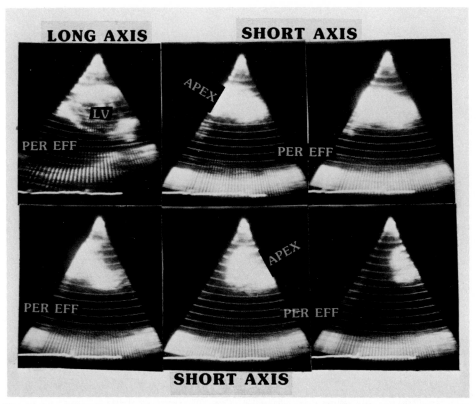

Fig. N-15. 2-D echogram of a young woman with cholesterol pericarditis. Calibration marks are 1 cm apart. The left upper frame, in the long-axis view, shows a very large pericardial effusion, with the bulk of fluid posterior to the ventricles. In all the other frames, the cardiac apex is visualized in short-axis view as a dense echo within a large echo-free expanse of pericardial fluid. Swinging motion of the ventricles is partly responsible for variable position and contour of the apex in the different frames.

in five cases; and tricuspid prolapse patterns in four. Midsystolic notching or "premature" closure motion of the aortic or pulmonic valve was noted in a few instances. Nanda *et al.* offer possible explanations for the occurrence of these "pseudo-SAM" or pseudoprolapse echo patterns in patients with large pericardial effusions:

1. Excessive rocking or rotatory motion of the heart adds vectors that are superimposed on normal patterns of valve motion.

2. "Swinging" of the heart produces alterations in the deceleration and acceleration of the mass of blood contained within the heart chambers, which in turn could well affect valve motion.

THE "SWINGING HEART"

In its most extreme form, excessive pendulous motion of the heart within a very large pericardial effusion gives rise to a characteristic ap-

pearance referred to as the swinging heart. A considerable width of anterior and posterior echo-free space is visualized, between which the echoes arising from the heart itself exhibit oscillations or irregular sine-wavelike undulations of large amplitude (Figs. N-10 to N-12, N-14, N-17). The anterior and posterior borders of the heart are defined sharply, while the intervening area shows a near-homogenous appearance in which individual cardiac structures cannot be distinguished easily. At times, the right ventricular anterior wall produces a sharp, dense echo, but only indistinct, feeble echoes are recorded from the rest of the heart.

Abnormal cardiac mobility, including swinging of the heart in large pericardial effusions, was first described by Feigenbaum *et al.* (1966). Subsequently, Gabor *et al.* (1971) reported one patient, and Usher and Popp (1972) two patients, all of whom had a swinging heart on echocardiography and electrical alternans on

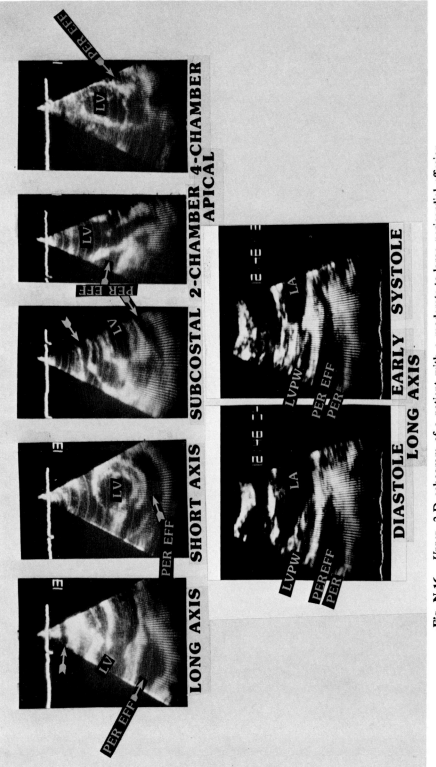

Fig. N-16. *Upper.* 2-D echogram of a patient with a moderate-to-large pericardial effusion, in 5 different views: parasternal long- and short-axis views, subcostal view, and apical 2-chamber (long-axis) and 4-chamber views. Posterior pericardial fluid is demonstrated in the first four frames; posterolateral fluid, in the last frame. A small anterior effusion can be detected in the first three frames.

Lower. 2-D echogram, in the long-axis view, in another patient with a large pericardial effusion. The pericardial effusion is seen as an echo-free space posterior to the LV posterior wall, which does not extend behind the LA in diastole (*left*) but does so in early systole (*right*).

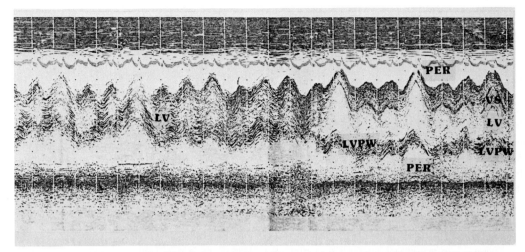

Fig. N-17. M-mode echogram in a patient with a very large pericardial effusion (1.7 liters removed). A typical "swinging heart" appearance presented. With the ultrasound beam passing through the heart near its apex (*left*) the cardiac width appears narrow and individual structures cannot be identified. As the scan continues to the base of the heart, the cardiac width increases (*right*) and some cardiac structures can be distinguished.

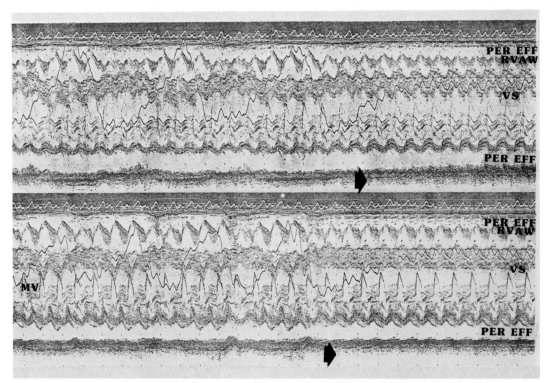

Fig. N-18. M-mode echographic tracing in a patient with a large pericardial effusion and mild tamponade. The LV is visualized at chordae level in the upper panel and at mitral valve level in the lower panel. The respiratory excursions are recorded so that the trace moves upward during inspiration and downward during expiration. Inspiratory RV enlargement is accompanied by decrease in LV size; during expiration the opposite occurs. When the patient held his breath (*arrows*) the respiratory fluctuations in ventricular dimensions were no longer apparent.

electrocardiography, an association that had been noted earlier by Feigenbaum.

Electrical alternans is seen in only a minority of patients with large pericardial effusions. Several authors have noted that almost invariably cardiac tamponade is present. Its interest to echocardiographers lies in the fact that echocardiography provides a good explanation for the mechanism of QRS alternation. These patients have excessive pendulous cardiac motion within large effusions, the so-called swinging heart appearance (Fig. N-14). Cardiac position is found to alternate from beat to beat in the echocardiogram; in every alternate beat, the heart seems more anterior than in the intervening beats. Another way of describing the phenomenon is to state that the cycle of cardiac motion is half that of the heart rate; having "flipped" into an abnormal position after one beat, the heart returns to its original position only after the impetus of the next beat, after which the cycle repeats itself every two beats. Alternation of motion from beat to beat can be demonstrated even on the left atrial posterior wall echo (Sotolongo and Horton, 1981).

Electrical alternans in association with pericardial effusions is most often encountered in malignant effusions, less commonly with tuberculous or uremic effusions. The heart rate is an important determining factor; it has been thought that tachycardia is necessary, although in one case of Usher and Popp (1972) the rate was 90/min.

TRANSDUCER DIRECTION AND THE SWINGING HEART

It is not generally recognized that patients with large pericardial effusions may exhibit a classic swinging heart appearance in some scans, whereas in other scans at the same examination an appearance suggestive of a moderate or even small effusion is obtained. The swinging heart appears as a narrow, undulating band of indistinct echoes, with a large expanse of echo-free space anterior and posterior to it. Such an appearance is visualized when the transducer is directed caudally, either in a sagittal plane or in a downward and rightward inclination. On the other hand, with a cephalad or less caudad transducer direction, the posterior echo-free space decreases markedly in width, while the

cardiac diameter (right ventricular anterior wall to left ventricular posterior wall) increases, the anterior echo-free space remaining the same.

It is suggested (D'Cruz et al., 1977) that when a swinging heart appearance is detected on the oscilloscope screen, the transducer beam should be directed more cephalad toward the base of the heart, when it may result in diminution in the swinging motion and better visualization of individual cardiac structures. Conversely, in patients who apparently have only a moderate-sized pericardial effusion, aiming the transducer beam downward, or downward and medially, may surprisingly reveal a swinging heart appearance, suggesting that the effusion is probably larger than it seemed at first.

PERICARDIAL FLUID BEHIND THE LEFT ATRIUM

Until 1976, it was believed that pericardial fluid did not accumulate behind the left atrium. The disappearance of an echo-free space between left ventricular posterior wall and pericardium during a scan from left ventricle to left atrium was thought to confirm the presence of a pericardial effusion. On the other hand, the detection of an echo-free space behind both left atrium and left ventricle was considered diagnostic of pleural effusion.

However, the Mayo Clinic group (Lemire et al., 1976) described five patients with large pericardial effusions in whom pericardial fluid was shown to extend posterior to the left atrium. This pericardial pocket, communicating with the main pericardial cavity, is known to anatomists as the oblique sinus, and its continuity with the main body of pericardial fluid is readily demonstrated in scans from left ventricle to left atrium or vice versa.

Tajik (1978) subsequently reported that the Mayo Clinic series of such patients had increased to 11. All his patients had large pericardial effusions and some degree of swinging heart phenomenon. Tajik drew attention to the large amplitude of the left atrial posterior wall motion; fluid from the main pericardial cavity thus is allowed to ebb and flow into the oblique sinus with every beat. This peculiar echographic configuration of the left atrial posterior wall motion not only serves to differentiate such retroatrial pericardial fluid from a pleural effusion behind the left atrium, but also helps in alerting the echocardiographer to the probability that the pericardial effusion is of large size.

The abnormal oscillatory left atrial posterior wall motion in such patients may be so similar to a like motion of the left ventricular posterior wall that the distinction between atrial and ventricular walls may be difficult to make on contour alone, even in a continuous scan from ventricle to atrium or vice versa.

Tajik (1978) noted that in 3 of his 11 patients it was possible to visualize fluid behind the left atrium at one site but not at others (slightly altering the transducer direction). The explanation for this finding is that the entire left atrial posterior wall is not covered by pericardium; there are sites of pericardial reflection near the entry of the pulmonary veins where no pericardial fluid is seen.

Two-Dimensional Echocardiography

The sensitivity of 2-D echography may not exceed that of the M-mode technique for detecting pericardial fluid anterior and posterior to the heart. However, 2-D echography (Figs. N-8, N-9, N-15, N-16, N-22, N-35, N-42, N-43) has further advantages (Martin et al., 1978; D'Cruz, 1982, 1983): (1) it can demonstrate the distribution of fluid within the pericardial sac and detect loculated effusions, (2) swinging cardiac motion is better presented, (3) certain echographic signs of tamponade are better visualized (see below), and (4) it is most helpful in selecting the safest and most effective site for paracentesis.

PERICARDIAL EFFUSION WITH TAMPONADE

In clinical practice, the diagnosis of cardiac tamponade in patients with pericardial effusions is made at the bedside on the basis of physical signs such as engorged neck veins, hepatomegaly, hypotension, and a paradoxic pulse. However, under certain circumstances, such as obesity, recent chest trauma or surgery, and associated heart or lung disease, the physical signs of tamponade are difficult to elicit or interpret. It is in this type of predicament that the

echocardiographic signs of tamponade may be of value to the clinician in assessing the course or prognosis and determining the management of patients with known or suspected pericardial effusions. In addition, one occasionally sees several patients with intrathoracic spread of lung or breast malignancy in whom the presence of a large pericardial effusion with tamponade was first revealed by echocardiography, their symptoms having previously been attributed to pleural, pulmonary, or mediastinal involvement.

Until a few years ago, it was believed that although cardiac ultrasound was the best means of diagnosing pericardial effusions, it was incapable of detecting tamponade. However, over the period 1975 to 1977, several descriptions appeared of echocardiographic abnormalities associated with cardiac tamponade that promptly disappeared when the cardiac compression was relieved. These echographic signs include:

1. Respiratory phasic changes in ventricular dimension (Fig. N-18). During inspiration, the RV undergoes a striking increase in dimension while the LV dimension shows a reciprocal (though less dramatic) decrease in dimension (D'Cruz et al., 1975). During inspiration in normal individuals, the LVID undergoes a small decrease (average, about 3 mm) as compared to the LVID during expiration (Brenner and Waugh, 1978). In patients with moderate to large pericardial effusions *without* cardiac tamponade, the respiratory variations in LV and RV remain small (Fig. N-19).

Simultaneously with inspiratory increase in RV and decrease in LV sizes, the anterior mitral diastolic excursion decreases and the EF slope may become flatter. These echocardiographic signs of cardiac tamponade were confirmed by Cosio et al. (1977), Sakamoto et al. (1977), and Settle et al. (1977). The latter two groups of authors also described marked inspiratory decrease in duration of aortic valve opening. The inspiratory decrease in LV size, in diastolic opening of the mitral valve and its EF slope, and in aortic valve ejection period is in accord with the inspiratory decrease of pulse volume and pulse pressure (well known to clinicians, for a century, as the paradoxic pulse) and the inspiratory decrease in LV stroke volume demonstrated by hemodynamic and radionuclide

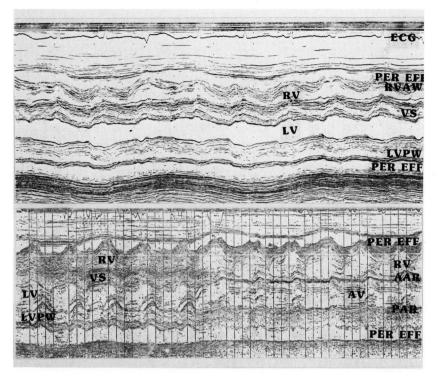

Fig. N-19. *Upper.* M-mode echocardiogram (subcostal approach) of a patient with a moderate pericardial effusion. During inspiration the heart moves toward the transducer, and the RV enlarges. The LV shows little reciprocal change in dimension, perhaps because it is hypertrophied; the ventricular septum may resist displacement toward the left ventricle in diastole.

Lower. M-mode echocardiogram (subcostal approach) in a patient with a moderate to large pericardial effusion. A scan has been made from LV to aortic root, and posterior pericardial fluid is visible posterior to both.

studies (Ruskin *et al.,* 1973; Yeh, 1978) in the setting of cardiac tamponade.

Apart from the respiratory fluctuations, the mitral EF slope tends to be lower during tamponade than it was before tamponade developed or after tamponade is relieved (D'Cruz *et al.,* 1975; Vignola *et al.,* 1976).

Settle *et al.* (1977) made the important observation that the marked respiratory phasic changes in RV and LV dimensions, so conspicuous in patients with large pericardial effusions with tamponade, were not found in 20 patients with large effusions who did *not* have tamponade and paradoxic pulse. This suggests that phasic changes in ventricular dimension and mitral motion in patients with tamponade are real and not artefactual due to the ultrasound beam transecting different segments of the ventricles and mitral valve in inspiration than in expiration. On the other hand, Schiller and Botvinick (1977) reported phasic changes in ventricular dimensions and mitral diastolic motion

in patients with large pericardial effusions but no tamponade. The apparent contradictory nature of their data can perhaps be explained by the fact that their criteria for diagnosis of tamponade were more stringent (hypotension below 100 mmHg systolic).

2. Schiller and Botvinick (1977) described right ventricular narrowing or "compression" in a series of patients with cardiac tamponade. It is presumed that the high intrapericardial pressure in tamponade compresses the thinner-walled RV to a greater extent than the much thicker-walled LV. RV dimension was measured at the level of the mitral chordae tendineae at end-diastole and end-expiration, with the patient in the left oblique position. These authors found that the RV dimension thus measured was 4 ± 2 mm in their patients with tamponade, whereas it was 24 ± 5 mm in normal subjects. The upper normal limit for their patients with tamponade was of the order of 7 to 9 mm. Schiller and Botvinick also found

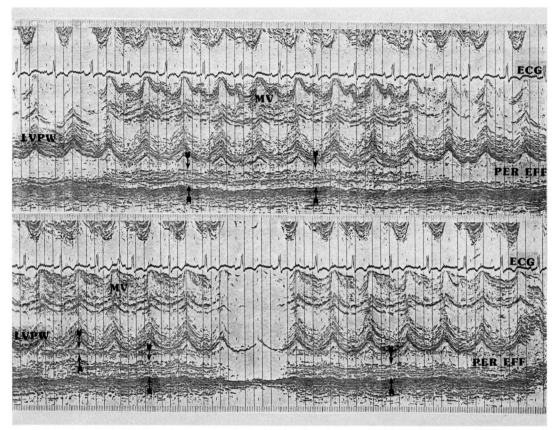

Fig. N-20. M-mode echocardiogram of a patient with chronic renal failure and a moderate pericardial effusion. A layer of solid material about 1 cm thick, presumably fibrin, is apparent contiguous to the parietal pericardium (*arrows*). A thinner layer is visible adjacent to the epicardium, in the lower panel (*arrows, left*). Increased damping (*center of lower panel*) suppresses echoes from LV posterior wall and fibrin, but the strong pericardial echo persists.

that the dimension of the RV outflow tract (distance between anterior aortic root and RV anterior wall) was smaller (29 ± 3 mm) in the patients with tamponade than in normal subjects (43 ± 6 mm), and that such RV outflow tract compression tended to occur in the most severe cases of tamponade.

RV narrowing, as defined by Schiller and Botvinick, is not incompatible with the phasic respiratory changes in ventricular dimension in cardiac tamponade described by D'Cruz et al. (1975). Schiller noted inspiratory increase and expiratory decrease in RV dimension in his patients with tamponade; in fact, the RV narrowing, so extreme at end-expiration, was often absent at end-inspiration.

However, the RV, unlike the LV, is not a chamber of simple and symmetric shape. It is of irregular width, broader in the region of its inflow and outflow areas than in its mid- and apical portions. Moreover, the true RV dimension is sometimes difficult to ascertain because of trabeculae and parts of the tricuspid apparatus traversing the RV chamber. The proper elicitation of Schiller's sign (RV narrowing in tamponade) requires careful attention to recording technique: "RV end-diastolic dimensions could be artificially reduced in those patients with large effusion and accentuated in those with tamponade by sweeping near the apex, by moving the transducer laterally from the sternal edge, or by using a low intercostal space" (Schiller and Botvinick, 1977).

Two-dimensional echocardiographic visualization of RV narrowing was observed by Schiller and Botvinick (1977). I have also encountered this finding, but have been impressed even more by dramatic respiratory fluctuations in RV dimension, well visualized on long-axis, short-axis, as well as apical views.

3. Vignola *et al.* (1976) described an unusual early systolic notch on the RV anterior wall echo in four patients with cardiac tamponade, which was not present in 15 of 16 other patients with moderate to large pericardial effusions but no tamponade, and which disappeared with relief of tamponade. Vignola noted that this notch occurred 0.04 ± 0.01 sec after onset of the QRS complex and pointed out that it coincided with the isovolumic phase of ventricular contraction. However, neither he nor others have a satisfactory explanation of why the RV anterior wall motion should exhibit this abnormality only in patients with tamponade. The sensitivity and specificity of the sign in a large series of patients are unknown.

4. "Collapse" or sharp posterior "dip" of the RV anterior wall in early diastole, just after mitral valve opening, has recently been described as a valuable sign of tamponade (Armstrong *et al.,* 1982; Engel *et al.,* 1982).

5. Indentation or buckling inward of the RA wall in the 2-D apical four-chamber view, just after P wave inscription, has been reported by Miller *et al.* (1982) as a reliable sign of tamponade.

Echocardiographic Appearances Simulating Those of Tamponade

Prominent respiratory fluctuations in ventricular dimensions and mitral valve diastolic motion have been reported in association with pulmonary embolization (Winer *et al.,* 1977), chronic obstructive pulmonary disease (Kronzon *et al.,* 1980; Settle *et al.,* 1980), bronchial asthma (Jardin *et al.,* 1982), and compression of the heart and superior mediastinum by a large thymoma (Canedo *et al.,* 1977). Such phasic changes thus are not entirely specific for cardiac tamponade; rather, their diagnostic value lies in signifying the presence or absence of tamponade in patients with known pericardial effusions, especially if previous tracings are available for comparison.

The diagnostic potential of marked respiratory fluctuations in RV and LV dimensions, and in mitral diastolic motion, in fact may be compared to the paradoxic pulse, which has proved a useful and dependable sign of cardiac tamponade in patients with known or suspected pericardial effusions for almost a century. In fact, phasic respiratory changes in LV dimension and mitral valve excursion correlate very consistently with the presence of a paradoxic pulse, whether the cause is cardiac tamponade or chronic lung disease (Kronzon *et al.,* 1981). The paradoxic pulse, too, is nonspecific in the sense that it can occur with respiratory airway obstruction, constrictive pericarditis, and so forth; yet it has not been abandoned by clinicians. Like it, the echocardiographic signs of tamponade have a useful role in clinical cardiology, provided their limitations and diagnostic significance are understood properly.

Atypical Features of Tamponade in Certain Special Situations

Pulsus paradoxus and phasic respiratory variations in ventricular dimension were absent in five patients with atrial septal defect in spite of the fact that they had large pericardial effusions and tamponade. This was attributed to equilibration of pressure across the atrial septal defect (Winer and Kronzon, 1979).

The clinical picture of tamponade need not always be accompanied by a large pericardial effusion compressing the ventricles from all sides. A loculated yet big pericardial effusion related to only one aspect of the cardiac surface (Jones *et al.,* 1977; Friedman *et al.,* 1979; Dunlap *et al.,* 1982) on occasion can cause the syndrome of tamponade. Kronzon *et al.* (1983) reported three instances of cardiac tamponade following cardiac surgery, due to loculated pericardial effusion or hematoma compressing the right atrium, diagnosed by 2-D echography in the apical 4-chamber view. When tamponade occurs in patients with hypertrophic cardiomyopathy, it may provoke abnormal systolic mitral motion (SAM), which subsides as the tamponade resolves (Schulman *et al.,* 1981).

INTRAPERICARDIAL ECHOES

In most pericardial effusions, the space between visceral and parietal pericardium is echo free. Exceptions to this rule include:

1. Amorphous ill-defined echoes, commonly seen in the subacute or healing phase of acute pericarditis of various etiologies. Such echoes are commonplace immediately after cardiac surgery and probably represent organizing ex-

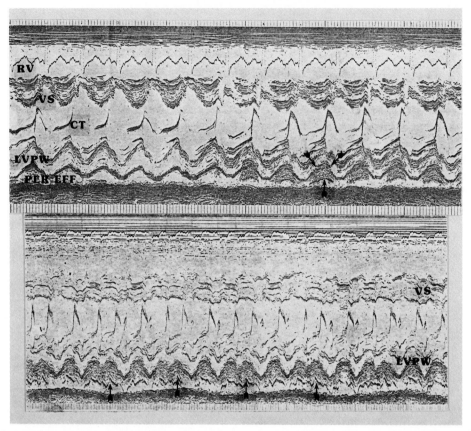

Fig. N-21. M-mode echocardiograms in two patients with pericarditis showing evidence of fibrin adherent to the LV posterior wall. Small to moderate posterior pericardial effusions were present in both. In the upper panel, a dense layer of fibrin is evident on the epicardial surface of the LV posterior wall. In both panels a linear undulating echo can be discerned (*arrows*), which probably represents a small fibrinous tag or adhesion fluttering within the pericardial fluid.

udate. In some cases, they fill the whole posterior pericardial space; in others, they gather near the atrioventricular junction behind the basal LV.

2. Sometimes a well-defined layer of low echo density appears adherent or at least contiguous to the posterior parietal pericardium (Fig. N-20). In other cases, small echoes appear like tags attached to the ventricular wall and move with it (Fig. N-21). Slight changes in transducer direction can cause them to appear or disappear from view. Such tags or shaggy attachments are seen even better on 2-D echo; they move along with the ventricular wall, and close observation may show that they undulate in the pericardial fluid as it is agitated by ventricular motion. Such echoes probably arise from fibrin adherent to the visceral or parietal pericardium, producing the bread-and-butter

appearance well known to pathologists as typical of acute fibrinous pericarditis. In my experience, echo evidence of such fibrinous tags, strands, or layers within the pericardial sac is particularly common in patients with chronic renal failure on long-term dialysis (D'Cruz *et al.*, 1978).

3. Recently, Martin *et al.* (1980) have called attention to bandlike intrapericardial echoes seen on 2-D echocardiography, bridging the echo-free pericardial space between visceral and parietal pericardium (Fig. N-22). In some of their patients, such pericardial adhesions appeared to divide the pericardial space into separate compartments, i.e., the pericardial effusion was loculated. Such adhesions or loculation also may be evident on M-mode echography (Figs. N-23 and N-24).

The combination of a pericardial effusion and

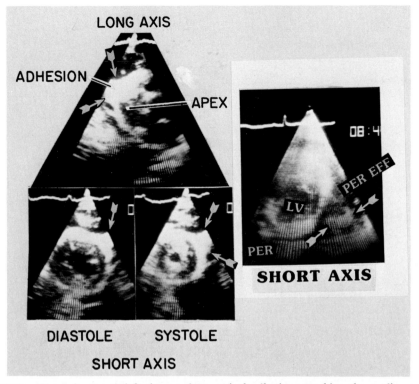

Fig. N-22. The 3 frames at left show a dense apical adhesion attaching the cardiac apex to the parietal pericardium. The left upper frame is in the long-axis view; the 2 lower frames, in the short-axis view.

The right frame is a 2-D echogram, in the short-axis view, of a patient with a large pericardial effusion secondary to malignant involvement of the pericardium by an anaplastic mediastinal neoplasm. At autopsy a few days later the pericardial sac contained much fibrin. The intrapericardial echoes probably arise from fibrin. However, true intrapericardial metastases can present similarly (Chandaratna, P.A.N., and Aronow, W.S.: Detection of pericardial metastases by cross-sectional echocardiography. *Circulation*, **63**:197, 1981).

pleural effusion (with the pericardial-pleural interface separating the two effusions extending as a conspicuous band across the echo-free space) could conceivably be mistaken for an intrapericardial adhesion between visceral and parietal pericardium. There are two features that help in differentiating the two situations:

a. Intrapericardial bands tend to show an undulatory motion when viewed in real time, whereas the pericardial-pleural membrane is stationary.

b. Pericardial adhesions tend to be radially aligned, especially in the short-axis view, i.e., they extend from ventricular wall to parietal pericardium, whereas the pleural-pericardial echo is tangential to the ventricular wall.

4. An intrapericardial thrombus, following pericardiocentesis, has been visualized by 2-D echography (Shuster and Nanda, 1982).

PERICARDIAL THICKENING (FIBROSIS, SCLEROSIS, CALCIFICATION) (Figs. N-25 to N-30)

Although the ultrasound diagnosis of pericardial effusions was established in 1965 (Feigenbaum *et al.*), it was not until a decade later that abnormal appearances of the pericardial membrane itself received attention in the echocardiographic literature. M-mode tracings depicting thickened pericardium were briefly described and illustrated by Feigenbaum (1976) and mentioned by Horowitz *et al.* (1974). Liedtke *et al.* (1976) reported a case of pneumococcal pericarditis in which echocardiography indicated a pericardial effusion of moderate size but no fluid could be aspirated, and at surgery the pericardium was thickened and contained inpissated exudate but no fluid.

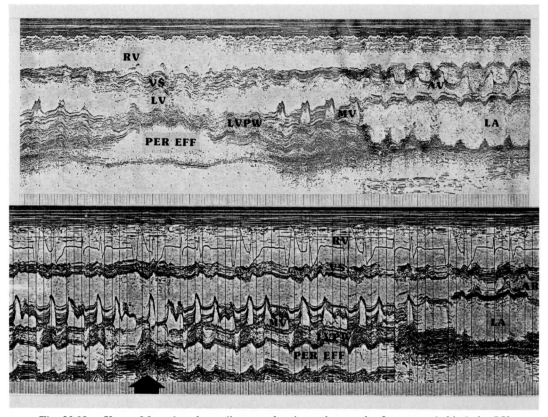

Fig. N-23.   *Upper.* M-mode echocardiogram showing a large echo-free space behind the LV near its apex but little or no separation between pericardium and LV posterior wall at basal (mitral valve) level. The pericardial effusion appears to be localized in the retrocardiac area near the apex. No fluid can be seen anteriorly.

Lower. M-mode echocardiogram of a patient with a loculated posterior pericardial effusion. A scan has been made from LV to LA, and at one site (*arrow*) an adhesion appears to tether the parietal pericardium to the LV posterior wall. This might account for the fact that the pericardial echo is not flat, but instead moves parallel to the LV posterior wall. The absence of any pericardial effusion anteriorly is attributable to anterior pericardial adhesions.

An important paper (Allen *et al.*, 1977) documenting the evolution of ultrasound appearances as blood clotted experimentally within the pericardial sac in dogs and during the transformation from pericardial effusion to constrictive pericarditis in two patients emphasized the value of serial echocardiography in pericardial disease. Chandaratna and Imaizumi (1978) reported thickening of the pericardium in eight patients proven at surgery or autopsy; in four, the pericardium and contiguous pleura were sharply outlined by the pericardial effusion anterior to them and the pleural effusion posteriorly, so that the thickness of the pericardiopleural membrane could be measured easily.

More recently, a variety of M-mode echographic patterns has been shown to be associated with anatomically proven thick pericardium. Thus Schnittger *et al.* (1978) described as many as seven different patterns encountered in a series of 167 patients, in 49 of whom pericardial thickening was confirmed by direct inspection at surgery or autopsy. Horowitz *et al.* (1979) studied a smaller series of 11 patients with similarly documented evidence of thick pericardium and concluded that the echographic patterns conformed to three clinicopathologic types: (1) chronically fibrosed and thickened pericardium without associated pericardial exudate; (2) effusive-contrictive or subacute wet pericarditis; and (3) subacute dry pericarditis. Both papers marked an important echographic advance, inasmuch as they validated certain M-mode appearances that echo-

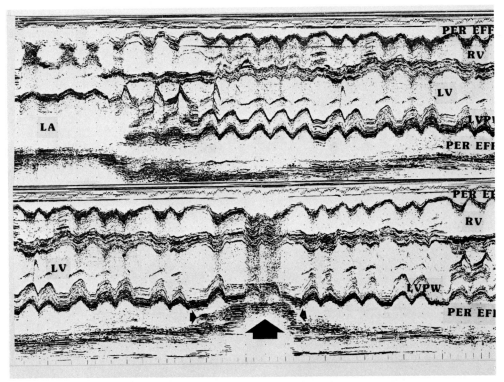

Fig. N-24. M-mode echocardiographic scans in a patient with a large pericardial effusion. A wide echo-free posterior pericardial space is visible in the upper panel, and also in the lower panel except at one site (*center*) where intrapericardial adhesions tether the LV to the parietal pericardium. This might account for the absence of abnormal swinging motion of the heart commonly seen in large pericardial effusions.

cardiographers had suspected were indicative of pericardial thickening. However, the echocardiographer's lot was perhaps made no easier because now he was required to memorize a multitude of diverse patterns and cope with different systems of classification and terminology.

If clinical or hemodynamic findings of pericardial constriction were found exclusively or predominantly in patients with certain M-mode patterns and not in others, the pains taken to learn the characteristics of each would perhaps have been justified. But both Schnittger *et al.* (1978) and Horowitz *et al.* (1979) found that constrictive pericarditis had no particular association with any individual pattern or patterns.

I have found the following approach to pericardial thickening (including fibrotic, sclerotic, or calcific change) useful and simple in routine practice:

1. In the *presence* of pericardial effusion, the epicardium (visceral pericardium) (Fig. N-26) or the parietal pericardium or both are thickened and sclerotic. The thickened membrane is easily visualized as a dense layer of variable thickness: in the case of the epicardium, it is of course adherent to the LV posterior wall and moves with it; the parietal pericardium, on the other hand, remains more or less flat and may appear as a single thick layer or a stratified aggregation of multiple linear parallel echoes.

2. In the *absence* of obvious pericardial fluid separating the visceral and parietal pericardium, thickened pericardium can manifest as any of the following patterns. Although morphologically distinct, there is little clinical or functional significance specifically attached to any of these patterns:

a. A definite *single layer,* a few millimeters thick, which may appear clear (echo free) or may contain small punctate or stippled echoes. This narrow space easily could be mistaken for a small pericardial effusion, from which it can be distinguished by the observation that it is of constant width during all phases of the cardiac cycle; a pericardial effusion, on the other

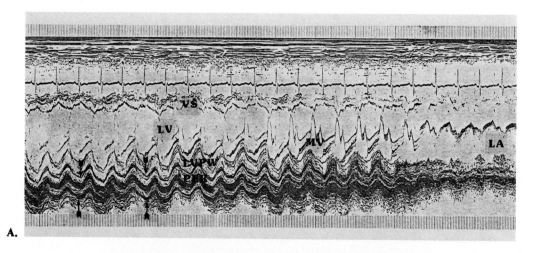

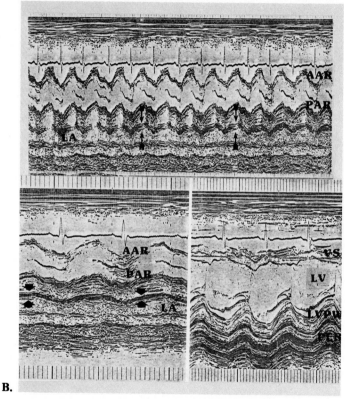

Fig. N-25. *A.* M-mode echocardiogram of a patient with considerable thickening of the posterior pericardium, which manifests as dense stratified echoes posterior to the LV posterior wall (*arrows*). Motion of the thickened pericardium is parallel to that of the LV posterior wall epicardium, presumably due to the fact that the former is adherent to the latter.

Fig. N-25. *B.* M-mode echocardiogram of a patient with considerable thickening of the pericardium (*right lower panel*). A dense linear echo can be noted posterior and parallel to the posterior aortic root in the upper and left lower panels (*arrows*), which may represent pericardial thickening in the region of the transverse sinus (a recess of the pericardial space posterior to the ascending aorta).

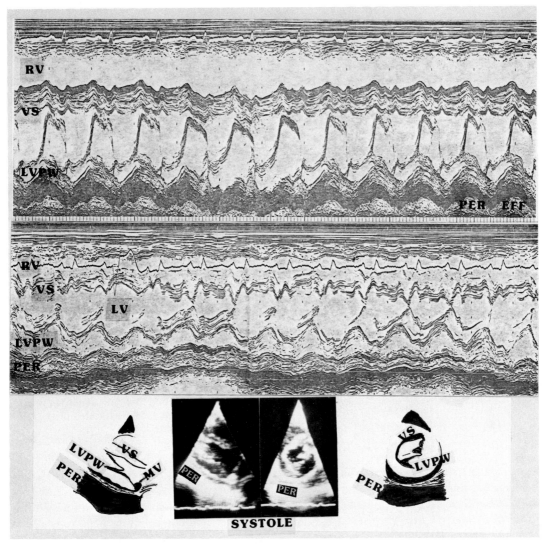

Fig. N-26. *Upper.* M-mode echogram, showing a small pericardial effusion posteriorly, of a man with acute pericarditis.

Center. M-mode echogram 2 months later shows no effusion but pericardial thickening is evident.

Lower. 2-D echogram, also 2 months after the uppermost scan, in long- and short-axis views, shows pericardial thickening.

hand, is associated with systolic widening of the pericardial space.

b. *Stratified* pericardial echoes (Fig. N-25) appearing on the tracing as multiple parallel linear echoes moving parallel to the LV posterior wall, to which both visceral and parietal layers of pericardium are closely adherent. Calcification eventually may occur within or between these pericardial strata, in which case they appear markedly dense and persist after the LV posterior wall and all other cardiac

structures have been fully suppressed by turning down the gain or increasing the reject.

c. The identities of the visceral and parietal pericardium distinctly recognizable and separated by a space varying from a few millimeters to 2 cm or more in width. This "pericardial" space is not echo free but is filled with amorphous irregular or mottled echoes (Fig. N-26), which are at least as dense as the endocardial and myocardial echoes of the LV posterior wall. The parietal pericardium does not

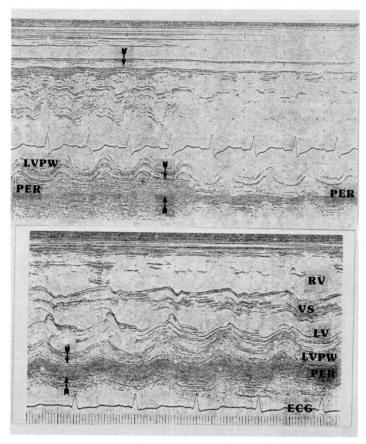

Fig. N-27. M-mode echograms from two proven cases of constrictive pericarditis; constriction developed within a few weeks of the effusive phase in one patient (*upper*), and within a few months of the effusive phase in the other (*lower*). In the upper panel, the damping has been increased in the right half, suppressing the LV posterior wall echo, but not the pericardial echo. Note the thickened pericardium (*arrows*) in both panels. Systolic septal motion is abnormal in both, but better delineated in the lower panel.

move parallel to the LV posterior wall, although it may show some slight anterior motion in systole. The echo appearances thus are very like those of a moderate-size pericardial effusion, except that the space between LV wall and parietal pericardium is not echo free but full of smudgy, irregular echoes. Such a pattern is the rule during the days or weeks following cardiac surgery and also very common in the subacute or recovery stage of acute pericarditis, whatever the etiology. It probably represents organization of inflammatory pericardial exudate and corresponds to type 6 of Schnittger *et al.* (1978). Interestingly, a similar pattern was obtained experimentally with freshly clotted blood in the pericardial sac (Allen *et al.,* 1977). Schnittger *et al.* (1978) found that in some patients with this echo morphology pericardial fluid is present, mixed with aggregations of fibrinous or coagulated exudate; in others, no fluid is found within the pericardial sac, the organization of exudate having proceeded completely to fibrosis. If serial echocardiograms are done in pa-

tients with this pattern, the amorphous, mottled or smudgy echoes eventually disappear, the posterior pericardial space narrows, and a thickened pericardium as in **a** or **b** above is all that persists.

Exceptionally, in pyogenic pericarditis, an accelerated transformation from pericardial exudate to dense fibrosis occurs within a few weeks, concomitant with the development of pericardial constriction (Fig. N-27). Echocardiographically, a dense echogenic "halo" is evident between, and distinct from, the thickened visceral and parietal pericardial echoes (Woolf and Gewitz, 1982).

An important practical maneuver in establishing pericardial sclerosis is to increase the damping control so that the myocardial echoes (LV wall and septum) are suppressed. The dense echoes of thickened pericardium persist (Figs. N-28 and N-29).

Pericardial calcification manifests as very thick and extremely dense pericardial echoes (Fig. N-29). In some such cases, infiltration of

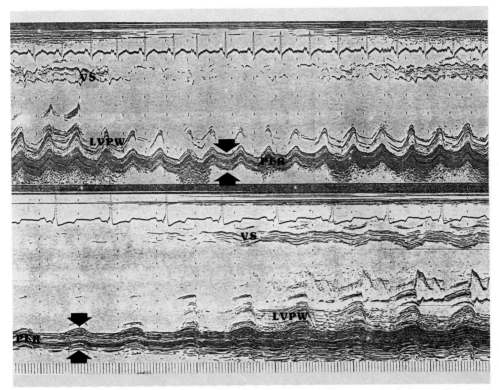

Fig. N-28. M-mode echocardiograms of two patients with pericardial thickening. In both cases, the thickened sclerotic pericardium is of about the thickness of the LV posterior wall. When the damping is increased (*middle, upper panel; left, lower panel*), the LV wall endocardial echo is suppressed, so that the thick pericardium (*arrows*) could possibly be mistaken for the LV posterior wall.

calcification in the LV wall can be suspected if unduly dense echoes extend into the LV wall echo (D'Cruz *et al.,* 1978).

CONSTRICTIVE PERICARDITIS

Although several echocardiographic abnormalities have been described in patients with constrictive pericarditis, none of them is present in every case and none is entirely specific. Hence, cardiac ultrasound is not as reliable in the diagnosis of pericardial constriction as it is in the detection of pericardial effusions; the echocardiogram is at best suggestive rather than conclusive of constriction, and the probability becomes stronger if two or more of the various abnormalities are present. Moreover, the physical signs compatible with pericardial constriction have to be taken into consideration; it would be rash to diagnose constrictive pericarditis on the echogram alone if the patient exhibits no evidence at all of raised venous pressure.

On the other hand, if the clinical presentation is that of congestive heart failure of uncertain cause, echocardiography can be of real help if it reveals abnormal findings that turn the clinician's suspicions toward the possibility of pericardial constriction, which might otherwise have been overlooked or misdiagnosed as cardiomyopathy.

M-mode findings include one or more of the following in various combinations:

1. *Pericardial thickening* has been discussed above. Hemodynamic evidence of pericardial constriction is obtained in only a minority of patients with one of the M-mode patterns of pericardial fibrosis or calcification (24 of 167 in Schnittger *et al.'s* series, 1978). Conversely, few echocardiographers would venture to suggest the diagnosis of pericardial constriction in the *absence* of pericardial thickening.

2. Abnormal systolic motion of the ventricular septum (Fig. N-27) is a common abnormality. Pool *et al.* (1975) found it in all of their

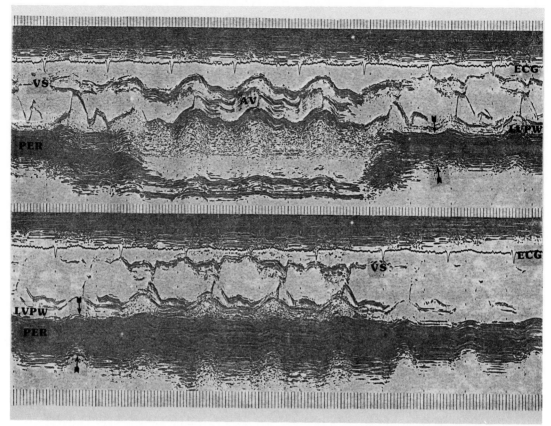

Fig. N-29. M-mode echogram of a patient with pericardial constriction in whom the pericardium was heavily calcified (detected by radiography and at surgery). In the upper panel a scan has been made from LV to LA (which is dilated) and then back to LV. In the lower panel, damping has been increased in the left and right ends of the figure to suppress myocardial echoes, but the dense pericardial echoes largely persist.

five patients with pericardial constriction; Gibson *et al.* (1976) in eight of their ten patients. However, others (Schnittger *et al.*, 1978; Candell-Riera *et al.*, 1978; Voelkel *et al.*, 1978) report a lower incidence, even if "abnormal septal motion" is taken to include not only frankly paradoxic septal motion (type A) but also "akinetic" or so-called type B motion and "hypokinetic" septal motion (posterior systolic motion less than 3 mm).

Although it may move toward the transducer rather than away from it (as it normally should), the ventricular septum usually undergoes normal systolic thickening, in this respect resembling the paradoxic septal motion of atrial septal defect. The brief, rapid, early systolic posterior motion (that precedes the paradoxic motion) of left bundle branch block does not occur in constrictive pericarditis, nor does the lack of systolic thickening typical of septal infarction

or cardiomyopathy. There is no completely satisfactory explanation for why the ventricular septum moves paradoxically in systole in patients with constrictive pericarditis. The failure in most cases for septal systolic motion to normalize after surgical removal of constricting pericardium is likewise a mystery.

In conclusion, it may be stated that abnormal septal motion in a patient with obvious pericardial thickening suggests the possibility of pericardial constriction if no other cause for septal abnormality (for instance, recent open-heart surgery or left bundle branch block) is evident. On the other hand, normal systolic septal motion does not exclude constrictive pericarditis.

3. Candell-Riera *et al.* (1978) from Barcelona, Spain, focused their attention on diastolic rather than systolic motion of the ventricular septum. They found that seven of their eight patients with constrictive pericarditis showed

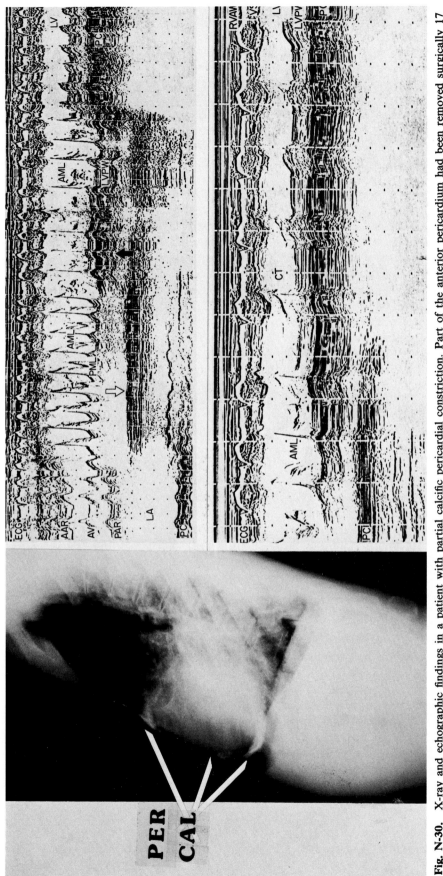

Fig. N-30. X-ray and echographic findings in a patient with partial calcific pericardial constriction. Part of the anterior pericardium had been removed surgically 17 years earlier. Cardiac catheterization at the time of these scans showed classic hemodynamic signs of constriction.

Lateral chest radiograph (*left*) shows anterior and inferior pericardial calcification (PER CAL). M-mode echocardiographic scans are shown on the right. In the upper panel the scan moves from aortic root–left atrium to the atrioventricular junction and then the left ventricle. Calcification is apparent in the LA wall (*open arrow*), as well as in the LV wall (*solid arrow*). The LV is more dilated at basal level (*center of figure*) than toward the apex (*right of figure*). The latter region is shown in the lower panel, at a faster paper speed. Note the flat LV posterior wall diastolic motion (absence of LV expansion after mitral LV filling).

(Reproduced from D'Cruz, I. A., et al.: Echocardiographic diagnosis of partial pericardial constriction of the left ventricle. *Radiology* **127**:755, 1978, with permission of the publishers.)

a peculiar early diastolic motion abnormality on the M-mode tracing "consisting of a sudden anterior displacement followed by a brisk posterior rebound." The onset of the anterior component of this motion coincided with the pericardial knock sound. If the specificity and sensitivity of this unusual echographic septal configuration are confirmed by other observers, this "Spanish notch" (as it is known to echocardiographers) may prove a useful indicator of pericardial constriction. The fact that the abnormal early diastolic septal motion disappeared in six of Candell-Riera's seven patients following surgical relief of the constriction tends to confirm that the abnormality of septal motion is related to the abnormal hemodynamic events in the LV (rapid mitral LV filling immediately after mitral valve opening, abruptly followed by resistance to further filling and rise in LV pressure). Tei et al. (1983) found another type of "notch": a brief anterior septal motion that occurs during and just after the P wave on the ECG, a consistent finding in constrictive pericarditis but not in restrictive cardiomyopathy.

4. "Flat" diastolic motion of the LV posterior wall was well described and illustrated by Feigenbaum (1976). Normally, the LV posterior wall endocardial echo exhibits a rapid posterior motion in early diastole and then a gentle posterior drift through the remainder of diastole. This mid to late diastolic filling of the LV is associated with a small but appreciable gradual increase in LV dimension, the transition from rapid early LV filling to slow filling being marked by a rather sharp angulation of the LV posterior wall endocardium.

In patients with constrictive pericarditis, the unyielding, thick pericardium limits any further LV expansion after the initial rapid filling. Consequently, the LV posterior wall contour appears flat and parallel to that of the ventricular septum and chest wall on the M-mode echogram.

This echocardiographic sign has been further refined or quantified by Voelkel et al. (1978), who measured the distance from the "crystal artefact" (i.e., the transducer face) to the LV posterior wall endocardium at (a) the end of early rapid diastolic filling and (b) the end of diastole. Normally, the latter measurement exceeds the former by 1.5 to 4 mm, the LV posterior wall having moved further away from the transducer to this extent as the LV gradually filled. In 11 of their 12 patients with constrictive pericarditis, flat LV posterior wall contour manifested as a negligible (less than 1 mm) difference between the early and late diastolic measurements.

5. A steep EF (or EFo) slope of the anterior mitral leaflet was demonstrated by Feigenbaum (1976) in a patient with constrictive pericarditis, and others have subsequently confirmed its incidence in some cases of this disease. However, it is present only in a minority (2 of 14 patients of Schnittger et al., 1978) of instances and is such a nonspecific sign that it is of little diagnostic value.

6. In a patient with pericardial thickening, the *absence* of LV dilatation, of LV hypertrophy, and of poor LV function (as estimated echocardiographically by diminished LVID systolic fractional shortening and increased mitral E point–septal separation) in conjunction with the clinical picture of unexplained congestive heart failure.

7. Premature pulmonary valve opening (Wann et al., 1977; Tanaka et al., 1979) has been reported, but its incidence in constrictive pericarditis remains uncertain. Tanaka et al. (1979) showed that the pulmonic valve "A" wave is much deeper and wider than normal; their hemodynamic studies suggested that the pulmonic valve opened during atrial contraction. The presence of a pericardial effusion on echocardiography does not exclude the diagnosis of hemodynamically significant constrictive pericarditis if the parietal pericardium is thickened and other findings suggesting possible constriction have been detected. This variety of pericarditis—"effusive-constrictive"—is, in fact, not uncommon and formed a substantial proportion of the series of Horowitz et al. (1979) and that of Schnittger et al. (1978).

Since most of the echocardiographic features of constrictive pericarditis are nonspecific, it is not surprising that the differential diagnosis of this entity includes a wide variety of cardiac conditions:

1. Pericardial thickening without constriction is far more common than constrictive pericarditis, as mentioned above. Even very thick pericardium is compatible with the absence of constriction if other echocardiographic and clinical signs of constriction are lacking.

2. The clinical presentation of a large pericardial effusion with cardiac tamponade is not very different from that of constrictive pericarditis, but their echocardiographic appearances are very dissimilar. However, it must be kept in mind that hemodynamically important constriction frequently complicates effusive-constrictive pericarditis. It is also possible for thickened pericardium to be mistaken for a small pericardial effusion, but cardiac tamponade usually does not complicate small effusions, with the exception of traumatic hemopericardium.

3. Other causes of paradoxic septal motion (such as, for example, anteroseptal infarction, atrial septal defect, left bundle branch block, and recent open-heart surgery) can be distinguished to some extent on the basis of other echographic findings: thus a large right ventricle suggests atrial septal defect or tricuspid regurgitation; an initial brief posterior component of septal motion would be typical of left bundle branch block.

Constrictive pericarditis has been reported as a complication of coronary artery bypass surgery (Cohen and Greenberg, 1979; Kutcher et al., 1982). However, some pericardial thickening and abnormal septal systolic motion are the rule after coronary surgery, and one should be wary of making the diagnosis of pericardial constriction unless good additional evidence points in the same direction.

2-D echographic studies in constrictive pericarditis (Lewis, 1982; D'Cruz et al., 1982) revealed the following diagnostic features: (1) a striking disparity between small ventricular and dilated atrial chambers; (2) a dense, rigid, thick pericardial shell that abruptly limits ventricular filling in early diastole; (3) dilated inferior vena cava and hepatic veins; and (4) bulging of the atrial and ventricular septa toward the left side during inspiration.

Partial constriction of the LV, resulting from incomplete surgical removal of constricting pericardium, can present with unusual and even bizarre echocardiographic appearances (D'Cruz et al., 1977). In one such case, the apical and near-apical LV appeared small with flat, parallel diastolic motion of the LV posterior wall and ventricular septum, whereas the unconstricted basal LV at mitral valve level was of much larger width. Penetration of the LV myocardial wall, and even the left atrial wall, by pericardial calcification was apparent on the echocardiogram and confirmed at surgery.

Absence of the pericardium (either following pericardiectomy or congenital) is associated with apparent RV dilatation and abnormal systolic septal motion (Payvardi and Kerber, 1976). Nicholisi et al. (1982) confirmed these M-mode findings, and showed by 2-D echography that they were due to abnormal intrathoracic position and systolic motion of the untrammeled heart rather than to real change in cardiac structure during contraction.

ECHOCARDIOGRAPHIC APPEARANCES SIMULATING ANTERIOR PERICARDIAL EFFUSION (Figs. N-31 and N-32)

Normally, the RV anterior wall echo and the chest wall echo are contiguous. In fact, a sharp line of demarcation between the two may be difficult to demonstrate.

An anterior pericardial effusion is the most common cause of separation between the chest wall and RV; this separation by an echo-free space varies from a few millimeters, in systole only, to a large width of several centimeters. The presence of anterior pericardial fluid permits a greater amplitude of posterior systolic excursion of the RV anterior wall than would occur normally.

When an echo-free space anterior to the heart is associated with an echo-free space posterior to the heart, the diagnosis of pericardial effusion may be presumed unless proved otherwise. (The other possibilities include pericardial thickening and tumor encasement of the heart by malignant tissue.)

When an echo-free space anterior to the RV anterior wall is *not* accompanied by an echo-free space posterior to the LV posterior wall, an anterior pericardial effusion cannot be presumed. Other possible causes of such an anterior echo-free space between chest wall and RV anterior wall include the following:

1. Pericardial fat is probably a common

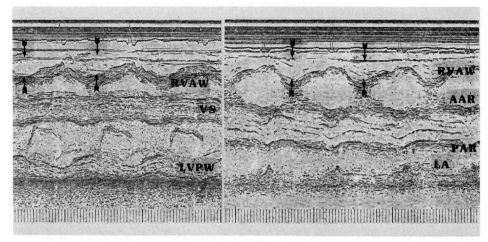

Fig. N-31. M-mode echocardiogram at mitral valve level (*left*) and aortic valve level (*right*) showing an echo-free space anterior to the RV. On 2-D echography this space was well defined and localized. The patient had had a sternal marrow puncture the previous day; the anterior echo-free space was presumed to be a retrosternal hematoma, not a pericardial effusion.

cause. Nanda and Gramiak (1978) have stated that an anterior echo-free space up to 15 mm wide caused by pericardial fat has been proven at surgery. They remarked that such a space narrows as an LV scan moves toward the apex, whereas echo-free spaces caused by pericardial fluid tend to be broader near the LV apex than near its base. Recent studies correlating echographic and CT scan findings demonstrate that pericardial fat is a common cause of echo-free space, anterior as well as posterior to the heart (Wada *et al.*, 1982; Isner *et al.*, 1983).

2. Immediately after cardiac surgery, the pericardial sac is often left widely open; blood clots or exudates accumulate in the anterior mediastium and it is very common to record an echo-free space of 1 cm or more between chest wall and the right ventricle.

3. Extracardiac anterior mediastinal masses are rare, but a variety of such anterior space–occupying lesions have been reported: pericardial cyst (Felner *et al.*, 1975; Hynes *et al.*, 1983), diaphragmatic hernia through the foramen of Morgagni (Popp and Harrison, 1974), lymphoma (Case Records, MGH, 1976), thymoma (Canedo *et al.*, 1977), malignant metastases in the anterior chest wall or anterior mediastinal space (Chandaratna *et al.*, 1978), pericardial infiltration by malignant metastases (Come *et al.*, 1981). Figure N-31 demonstrates a retrosternal hematoma resulting from a sternal puncture procedure for investigation of ane-

mia. In the case of cystic masses, the space anterior to the RV anterior wall may be truly echo free (Figure N-32), but if the mass consists of solid tumor tissue, this space may contain stratified multilinear echoes as in the patient of Canedo *et al.* (1977); i.e., it does not seem echo free unless the gain is turned down considerably.

Exceptionally, an extracardiac mediastinal mass may be so large that it displaces the heart as a whole from its usual location. Ultrasound scanning from the conventional left parasternal site may then reveal, instead of expected cardiac structures, a clear echo-free space, as in the instance of a giant mediastinal cyst (Koch *et al.*, 1977) and that of a large cystic thymoma (Schloss *et al.*, 1975). In both of these cases, the large mediastinal mass compressed the heart to such an extent that a clinical and hemodynamic picture simulating cardiac tamponade or constrictive pericarditis was produced. A somewhat similar presentation was reported in the patient of Canedo *et al.* (1977) with a large superior mediastinal thymoma, and in Case No. 4 of Chandaratna *et al.* (1978) with a large cystic intrapericardial hematoma in a patient on anticoagulant therapy; in both, a large space intervened anteriorly between RV anterior wall and chest wall.

The combination of a large echo-free space anterior to the heart, engorged neck veins, and raised diastolic pressures in the right heart

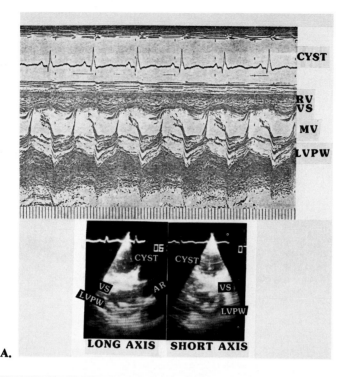

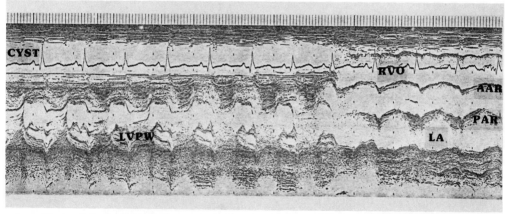

Fig. N-32. *A.* M-mode echogram recorded from the second left intercostal space, with the transducer directed posteriorly, inferiorly, and to the right. The patient was a 10-year-old girl who presented with a pulsatile swelling at the upper left sternal border. At surgery a cystic chondroma was removed; the tumor had the size, shape, and rigidity of a Ping-Pong ball and it overlay and deformed the right ventricle. The cyst manifests as an echo-free space immediately under the chest wall, in the M-mode echogram as well as the 2-D echogram (*below*). The RV chamber has been compressed at this site. The echo-free space representing the cyst could easily be mistaken for the RV chamber or for an anterior pericardial effusion.

Fig. N-32. *B.* An M-mode scan has been made from LV to aortic root level. The cyst compresses the RV anterior to the LV, but not the RV outflow (RVO) region anterior to the aortic root.

EXTRACARDIAC SPACES: DIFFERENT ECHOGRAPHIC PATTERNS

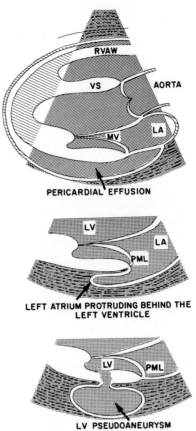

Fig. N-33. Diagram showing typical 2-D echographic contours of a pericardial effusion and of other structures or conditions that could simulate it by presenting as an echo-free space posterior or anterior to the heart.

chambers and pulmonary artery wedge could conceivably lead to the erroneous diagnosis of pericardial effusion with tamponade and attempts at paracentesis. Cardiac tamponade due to a large pericardial effusion can be excluded by noting (1) the absence of a wide echo-free pericardial space *posterior* to the heart, and (2) the absence of a swinging oscillatory cardiac motion, a usual (although not necessarily invariable) accompaniment of pericardial effusions large enough to produce tamponade.

Two-dimensional echocardiography is helpful inasmuch as it confirms these two distinguishing features, and in the case of an anterior mediastinal mass would delineate not only the presence but also the shape of the mass, demonstrating perhaps a distortion of the right ventricular contour due to encroachment or com-

pression by the tumor (Nishimura *et al.,* 1982).

An unusual instance of a hydatid cyst imbedded in the LV apical region (Oliver *et al.,* 1982) and of an LV pseudoaneurysm anterior to the LV in the subcostal view (Kessler *et al.,* 1982) could possibly have simulated loculated pericardial effusions, inasmuch as a large anterior abnormal echo-free space was demonstrated by 2-D echography.

Inadequate technique or interpretation, especially in inexperienced hands, can produce the illusion of an echo-free anterior space where, in fact, no such space exists:

1. If the ventricular septum is mistaken for RV anterior wall, the RV chamber could be mistaken for an anterior pericardial effusion. This could happen possibly if the left septal border appears as a bandlike echo rather than

EXTRACARDIAC SPACES : DIFFERENT ECHOGRAPHIC PATTERNS

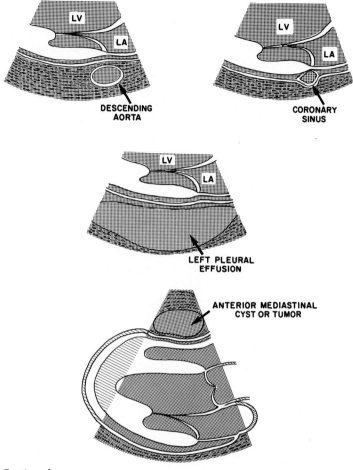

Fig. N-33.   *Continued*

a thin linear echo, in which case the right septal border may be mistaken for the RV anterior wall.

2. If a catheter or pacemaker wire in the RV chamber is mistaken for the RV anterior wall, the space between it and the true RV anterior wall echo could be taken, in error, for an anterior pericardial effusion.

ECHOCARDIOGRAPHIC APPEARANCES SIMULATING POSTERIOR PERICARDIAL EFFUSION (Fig. N-33)

NORMAL ANATOMIC STRUCTURES

The *coronary sinus,* the descending thoracic *aorta,* and the left lower *pulmonary vein* may all appear as small echo-free spaces behind the heart, usually not more than 1 or 2 cm wide. Should the coronary sinus be dilated (because a persistent left superior vena cava or anomalous pulmonary veins drain into it), or should the descending aorta be dilated (by atherosclerotic or syphilitic disease), the echo-free space may be even larger.

The chief diagnostic feature of the echo-free space, in the case of each of these structures, is that it is localized to the region just posterior to the junction of the left atrium and left ventricle, i.e., the basal LV at mitral valve level but not the mid-LV at chordae level. Therefore, scanning from the echo-free space toward the LV apex causes it to disappear, whereas in pericardial effusion the echo-free space caused by pericardial fluid is usually wider near the apex than it is near the base of the LV.

Two-D echocardiography is very helpful in identifying these structures and differentiating them from pericardial and pleural effusions. In the long-axis view, the coronary sinus appears as a small, round space in very close proximity to the atrioventricular junction. The descending aorta is also represented by a roundish, echofree space that is rather larger than that of the coronary sinus and on a slightly more posterior plane (Figs. N-34 and N-35).

Although the base of the posterior *papillary muscle* merges with the LV posterior wall and appears on the M-mode echocardiogram as an abrupt thickening of the latter structure to twice its thickness elsewhere, the apex or projecting dome of the papillary muscle may appear as a conspicuous bandlike echo anterior to the LV posterior wall. An inexperienced echocardiographer could mistake the papillary muscle echo for the LV posterior wall, in which case the actual LV posterior wall may be labeled a posterior pericardial effusion, especially if the gain or reject setting is such as to suppress the ven-

tricular wall intramural echoes. The correct identification of papillary muscle and LV posterior wall echoes becomes evident if the LV is scanned from apex to base or vice versa; the papillary muscle echoes become continuous with chordae tendineae and then mitral cusp echoes. Likewise, the LV posterior wall echo is recognized by its typical endocardial motion and intramural echographic pattern.

Mitral annulus calcification, located in the plane between mitral valve and LV posterior wall, appears in the M-mode echogram as a dense band that may be mistaken for the LV posterior wall, particularly if the gain or reject setting has been turned down to suppress echoes arising from LV myocardium (Hirschfeld and Emilson, 1975). The thickness of the LV posterior wall behind the annulus calcification could then be mistaken for a moderate-size pericardial effusion. The true diagnosis is made by noting that (1) scanning upward and medially to the left atrium usually causes the mitral annulus calcification echo to end abruptly (Fig. B-14), whereas the LV posterior wall echo becomes continuous with the left atrial posterior wall

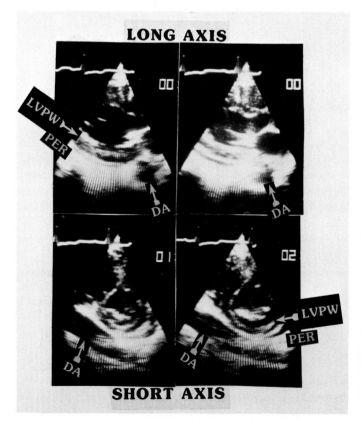

LONG AXIS

SHORT AXIS

Fig. N-34. 2-D echogram of a patient with chronic renal failure and thickened pericardium. The descending aorta (DA) appears as a small echofree space within the dense pericardial echo, posterior to the left atrioventricular junction, in the long-axis view (*upper*). In the short-axis view (*lower*) the descending aorta is visualized in approximately its long axis as an elongated echo-free space with nearly parallel borders, posterior to the LV. This characteristic retrocardiac space should not be mistaken for a pericardial or pleural effusion, which are also retrocardiac but of different contour.

SHORT AXIS

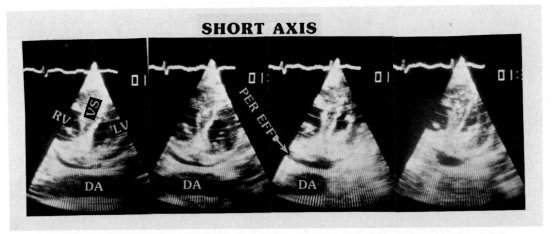

Fig. N-35. 2-D echogram in a plane near to the short axis showing the relationship of the right and left ventricles to the descending aorta (DA). A small pericardial effusion facilitates demarcation of the ventricular wall from the pericardium. The descending aorta produces an echo-free space with parallel borders, which is lost to view with slight change in transducer direction (*third and fourth frames*). These characteristics distinguish it from pleural effusions.

echo; (2) appropriate increase of the gain settings displays the LV posterior wall and other structures adjacent to the mitral annulus calcification.

Two-D echocardiography reveals mitral annulus calcification as a conspicuous round or oval blob in the long-axis view and a crescentic bar in the short-axis view, between the mitral leaflets and LV posterior wall. The 2-D appearances of a posterior pericardial effusion are entirely different.

Reverberations of the pericardial echo or LV posterior wall echoes are often recorded on the M-mode tracing several centimeters posterior to the true pericardial or ventricular wall echo. If the reverberatory echoes are mistakenly labeled pericardial echoes, the space between them and the true epicardial-pericardial echo could be misdiagnosed as a large pericardial effusion. Reverberations can be identified easily by their contours running parallel to the true or original echoes anterior to them, and echocardiographers soon learn by experience to recognize them by their morphology for what they are.

Tumor encasement of the heart is rare but a possibility that must be kept in mind in any patient who apparently has a pericardial effusion of moderate size and who is known to have or have had a malignant neoplasm. Since the malignant tissue surrounds the ventricles anteriorly as well as posteriorly, the echocardio-

graphic resemblance to a pericardial effusion can be very close, but any attempt at paracentesis is unsuccessful because the pericardial space is occupied by solid tissue. Documented examples of this type include the patient of Foote *et al.* (1977), a 46-year-old man with pericardial spread of lung carcinoma and cardiac catheterization findings simulating constrictive pericarditis; the 16-year-old patient of Lin *et al.* (1978) with a primary tumor (angiosarcoma) of the pericardium; and three patients described by Come *et al.* (1981).

That *left atrial enlargement* exceptionally may extend behind the LV posterior wall at its base, simulating a pericardial effusion in the M-mode tracing, was shown by Ratshin *et al.* (1974). Careful scanning from left atrium to left ventricle, or vice versa, demonstrates that the space behind the LV is continuous with the left atrial chamber (Fig. N-36). The abnormal space does not extend as far as the mid-LV level, nor does it continue behind the left atrial posterior wall. Two-D echocardiography reveals the prolongation of the left atrium as it lies behind the basal LV (Reeves *et al.*, 1981).

Extension of a *pancreatic pseudocyst* into the posterior mediastinum can present as a large echo-free space posterior to the LV (Shah and Schwartz, 1980). Compression of the LV at basal (mitral valve) level by the large cystic mass produced a striking distortion of the normal echographic morphology of this region

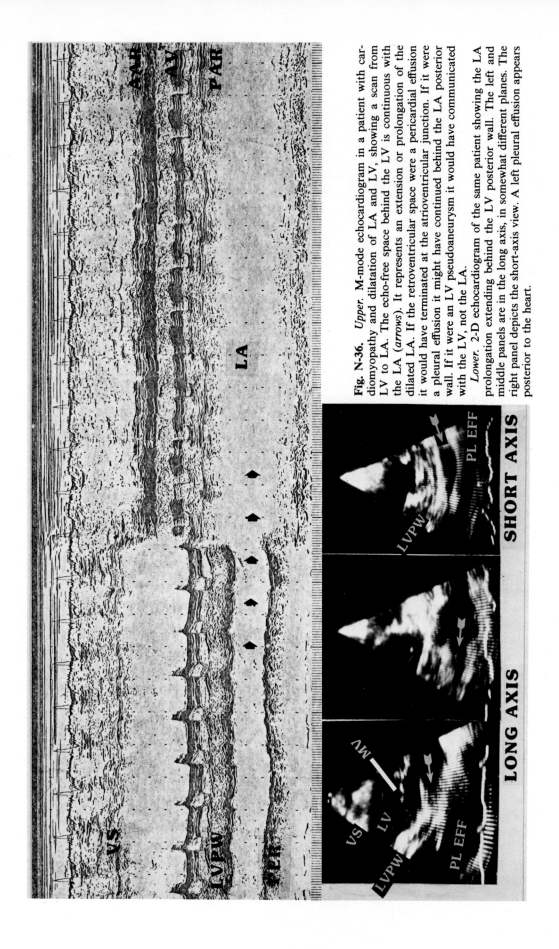

Fig. N-36. *Upper.* M-mode echocardiogram in a patient with cardiomyopathy and dilatation of LA and LV, showing a scan from LV to LA. The echo-free space behind the LV is continuous with the LA (*arrows*). It represents an extension or prolongation of the dilated LA. If the retroventricular space were a pericardial effusion it would have terminated at the atrioventricular junction. If it were a pleural effusion it might have continued behind the LA posterior wall. If it were an LV pseudoaneurysm it would have communicated with the LV, not the LA.

Lower. 2-D echocardiogram of the same patient showing the LA prolongation extending behind the LV posterior wall. The left and middle panels are in the long axis, in somewhat different planes. The right panel depicts the short-axis view. A left pleural effusion appears posterior to the heart.

such that the pericardium, LV posterior wall, and posterior mitral leaflet seemed to merge into one dense echo, which moved anteriorly in diastole and posteriorly in systole, i.e., parallel to and just behind the anterior mitral leaflet echo. Drainage of the pancreatic pseudocyst caused the large retrocardiac space to disappear and the LV posterior wall pattern to return to normal.

A large *aneurysm-fistula involving the proximal circumflex coronary artery* and coronary sinus mimicked a posterior pericardial effusion because it caused an echo-free space behind the basal LV (Come *et al.,* 1981).

PLEURAL EFFUSION (FIGS. N-37 TO N-43)

A left pleural effusion is probably the most common and important differential diagnosis of a large posterior pericardial effusion. In both conditions, a wide echo-free space is evident posterior to the heart. The following features help in distinguishing between them:

1. When an M-mode scan is made from LV to left atrium, the echo-free space behind the LV posterior wall continues behind the left atrial posterior wall in pleural effusions, whereas in pericardial effusions the echo-free space tapers and then ends at the atrioventricular junction so that no space is seen behind the left atrial posterior wall. There are two important exceptions to this rule that weaken its value as a diagnostic criterion:

a. Scanning from left ventricle to left atrium in patients with a left pleural effusion may result in the echo-free space disappearing from view as the ultrasound beam sweeps medially to bring the left atrium in view. The reason for this is that the left atrial chamber is related posterolaterally to the pleura, but posteromedially to posterior mediastinal structures such as the esophagus, descending aorta, and anterior spinal muscles. An echo-free space therefore would appear behind the left atrial posterior wall when the ultrasound beam transects the left atrium laterally, but not when it passes through the medial "mediastinal" part.

b. In patients with large pericardial effusions, fluid sometimes may be visualized immediately posterior to the left atrial posterior wall; this small echo-free space can be shown to be continuous with the larger echo-free space behind the LV posterior wall. This is possible because there normally exists a potential space (a pericardial recess named the oblique sinus) behind the left atrium that communicates with the main pericardial cavity. Fluid does not accumulate here in echocardiographically obvious quantity in small to moderate pericardial effusions, but it does so in large effusions with large "swinging" cardiac oscillations, in which case the left atrial posterior wall exhibits a vigorous motion of large amplitude synchronous with heart rate. This typical left atrial posterior wall pattern of motion is helpful in identifying the retroatrial space as pericardial, because in the case of pleural fluid behind the left atrium the left atrial posterior wall retains its normal flattish contour.

2. When the patient is turned to the left lateral position, pleural fluid gravitates away from behind the heart to the most dependent part of the pleural cavity. The echo-free retrocardiac space therefore becomes narrow or disappears. On the other hand, an echo-free space behind the left ventricle caused by pericardial fluid will show little change in the left lateral position.

3. With the patient supine, pleural fluid tends to gravitate posteriorly, so that an ultrasound transducer positioned at the left posterior axillary line will record an echo-free space under the chest wall in patients with pleural effusions. No echo-free space would be obtained at this location in the case of pericardial effusions, because the pericardial sac is separated from this part of the chest wall by a considerable volume of lung tissue.

4. The 2-D appearances of large pericardial effusions are different from those of pleural effusions. Whereas the echo-free pericardial space tends to surround the ventricles on all sides, as demonstrated in long-axis, short-axis, apical, and (if possible) subcostal views, the pleural space is situated posterior and perhaps posterolateral to the heart. Large swinging or pendulous oscillations of the heart, easily appreciated on 2-D echocardiography, are the rule in large pericardial effusions but do not occur with pleural effusions.

5. Recently, Haaz *et al.* (1980) and Lewandowski *et al.* (1981) have described how identification of the descending aorta echo on 2-D

[*Text continued on page 425.*]

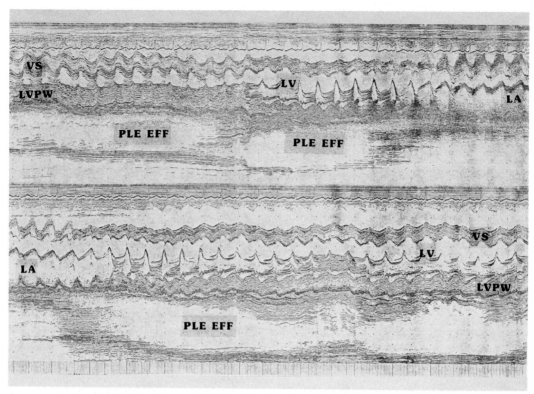

A.

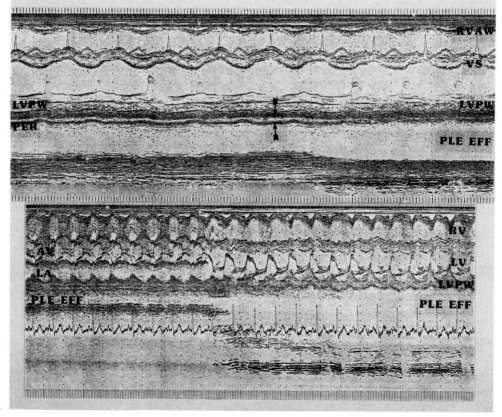

B.

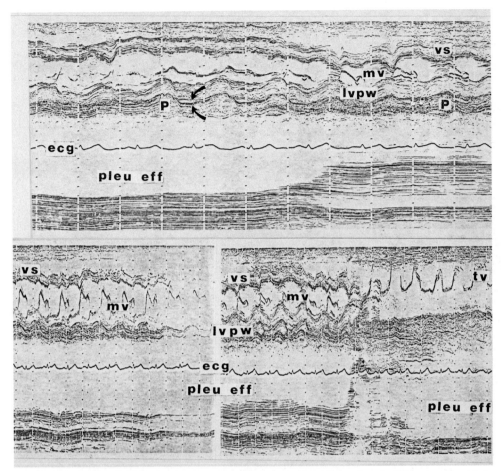

Fig. N-38. *Upper.* M-mode echocardiogram showing a large left pleural effusion, represented by a very wide echo-free space posterior to the heart. A separation between LV posterior wall and pericardium can be seen (*arrows*), thus identifying the large echo-free space behind it as a pleural rather than pericardial effusion.

Lower. M-mode echocardiogram of the same patient showing the left pleural effusion behind the LV (*left*). In the right panel, a rightward scan has been made from the LV to the tricuspid valve and right atrium. With the transducer beam sharply angled into the right hemithorax, a large echo-free space behind the heart is visible in this location also, suggesting a right pleural effusion. X-rays of the chest revealed large bilateral pleural effusions.

Fig. N-37. *A.* (*Opposite*) M-mode echogram of a patient with a left pleural effusion. The upper panel is a scan from LV (at papillary muscle level) to LA; the lower panel is a scan in the reverse direction, from LA to LV at mitral and then chordae level. A very narrow pericardial space, better recognized in the lower panel, permits identification of the large echo-free space as pleural fluid. The pleural effusion does not extend behind the LA in this case. Pleural adhesion or thickening is evident.

Fig. N-37. *B.* (*Opposite*) M-mode echograms in two patients with left pleural effusions.

Upper. M-mode echogram of a patient with inferior wall myocardial infarction. The ventricular septum moves well, in contrast to the akinetic LV posterior wall. A small pericardial effusion (*arrows*) permits identification of the posterior parietal pericardium. The wide echo-free space posterior to it can thus be identified as a pleural effusion.

Lower. M-mode echogram showing a scan from LA to LV. A large pleural effusion is visible behind the LV; it also extends behind the LA. (Alternatively this narrow space could be the descending aorta.)

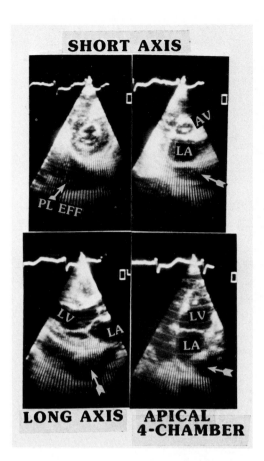

SHORT AXIS

LONG AXIS **APICAL 4-CHAMBER**

Fig. N-39. 2-D echogram of a patient with a left pleural effusion (*arrows*). In the short-axis view it appears behind the LA (*upper right*) and also behind the LV (*upper left*). In the latter it does not have the crescentic shape associated with pericardial effusions. In the parasternal long-axis view (*lower left*) the posterior echo-free space can be seen posterior to the LV, as well as the LA. In the apical 4-chamber view, the pleural effusion is visualized as a broad, somewhat triangular space posterolateral to the LA.

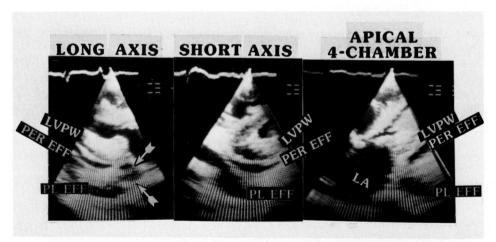

Fig. N-40. 2-D echogram of a patient with a small pericardial effusion and also a small pleural effusion. Thickened pleura separates the two effusions, as seen in the long-axis view (*left*), short-axis view (*center*) and apical 4-chamber view (*right*). The descending aorta (*left, arrows*) lies in a plane posterior to that of the pericardial effusion, but anterior to that of the pleural effusion. The LV shows considerable concentric hypertrophy, with very thick walls and a narrow LV chamber.

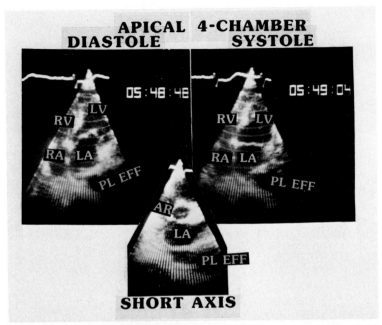

Fig. N-41. 2-D echogram of a patient with a left pleural effusion (PL EFF), which manifests as an echo-free space posterolateral to the LA in the apical 4-chamber view (*upper*). It can also be seen posterior to the LA in the short-axis view (*lower*). The contour of this pleural space is different from the narrow slitlike space sometimes seen posterior to the LA in pericardial effusions.

echocardiography can help in differentiating pleural from posterior pericardial effusions. In the 2-D long-axis view, the descending thoracic aorta appears as a small, circular, echo-free area posterior to the atrioventricular groove; in the short-axis view, it is a small, circular or oval space behind the LV posterior wall. Pericardial effusions manifest as an echo-free space between the LV posterior wall and aorta. A left pleural effusion appears as an echo-free space posterior to the descending aorta. In other words, the descending aorta serves as a marker of the pericardial-pleural interface.

COMBINED PERICARDIAL AND PLEURAL EFFUSIONS (Figs. N-42 and N-43)

It is not uncommon for pericardial and left pleural effusions to coexist in the same patient as, for example, in chronic renal failure; systemic lupus; intrathoracic spread of bronchogenic, breast, or other malignancies; congestive heart failure; and so forth. Concomitant effusions in both serous cavities, although difficult

to diagnose with certainty on the chest x-ray, are a boon to the echocardiographer because recognition of the pericardial space and the pleural space behind it is rendered easier. The contiguous parietal pericardium and pleura may appear on the M-mode echogram as a linear or bandlike echo suspended between an anterior echo-free space (pericardial effusion) and a posterior echo-free space (pleural effusion).

Even when the pericardial effusion is quite small, it serves the useful purpose of separating the pericardial echo from the subjacent LV posterior wall, enabling the echocardiographer to identify reliably the pericardium and the space behind it as a pleural effusion.

On 2-D echocardiography also, the membrane produced by the juxtaposed parietal pericardium and pleura forms a conspicuous demarcation between the pericardial space immediately behind the LV and the pleural space posterior to that in short-axis as well as long-axis views. If the descending thoracic aorta can be identified as a small, oval or round space, it will be seen to be situated in the place between pleural and pericardial effusions.

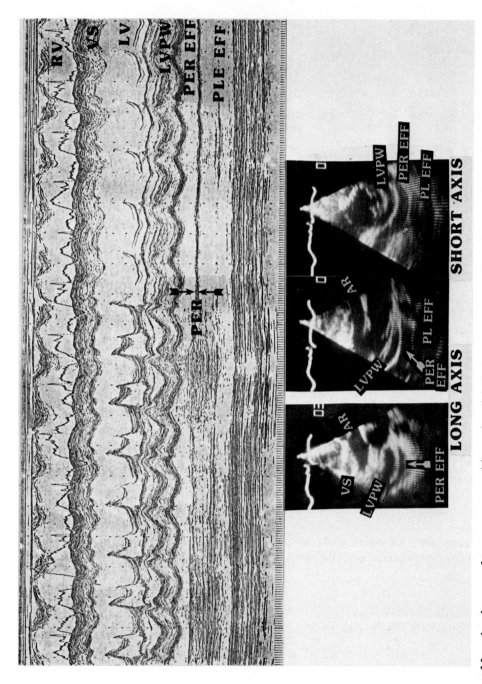

Fig. N-42. *Upper.* M-mode echogram of a young woman with a pericardial effusion of moderate size, as well as a left pleural effusion. The pleural effusion is not obvious at mitral valve level (*left*) but appears as a clear echo-free space at chordae level (*right*). A thin, well-defined linear echo marks the pericardial-pleural interface separating the two effusions (*arrows*).

Lower. 2-D echogram of same patient. In the first frame (long axis) only the pericardial effusion is evident. In the second frame (long axis in a slightly different plane), both the pericardial and pleural effusions are apparent. The third frame (short axis) also demonstrates the pleural effusion posterior to the pericardial effusion, separated from it by a thin linear echo (pericardial-pleural interface).

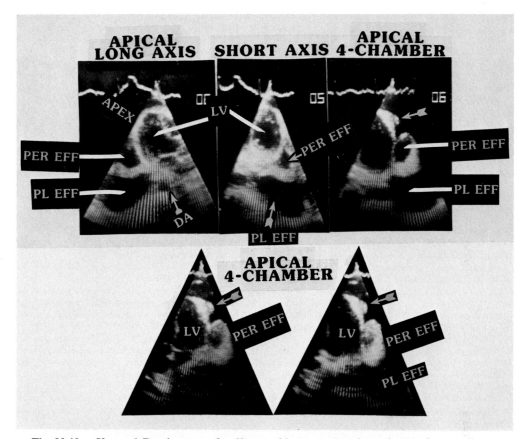

Fig. N-43. *Upper.* 2-D echogram of a 60-year-old man under chemotherapy for a malignant lymphoma A. A pleural effusion is demonstrated, as is an unusual loculated pericardial effusion restricted to the posterolateral LV wall at mid-LV level. In addition, a small nodule on the LV surface near its apex (*arrow in right frame*), the nature of which is uncertain, is visible.
Lower. 4-chamber apical view showing the small nodule and loculated pericardial effusion.

REFERENCES

PERICARDIAL EFFUSIONS

Abbasi, A. S.; Ellis, N.; and Flynn, J. U.: Echocardiographic M-scan technique in the diagnosis of pericardial effusion. *J.C.U.*, **1**:300, 1973.

Berger, M.; Bobak, L.; Jelveh, M.; *et al.:* Pericardial effusion diagnosed by echocardiography: Clinical and electrocardiographic findings in 171 patients. *Chest,* **74**:183, 1978.

D'Cruz, I.; Hirsch, L.; Prabhu, R.; *et al.:* Intramural myocardial echographic patterns during the cardiac cycle. *Circulation,* **54,** Suppl. II:84, 1976 (Abstr.).

D'Cruz, I.; Prabhu, R.; Cohen, H. C.; *et al.:* Potential pitfalls in quantification of pericardial effusions by echocardiography. *Br. Heart J.,* **39**:529, 1977.

D'Cruz, I.A.: Pericardial effusion and pericardial disease. In *Cardiac Ultrasound Workbook,* ed. J. V. Talano. Grune & Stratton, New York, 1982.

D'Cruz, I. A.: Pericardial disease. In *Textbook on Two-Dimensional Echocardiography,* eds. J. V. Talano and J. M. Gardin. Grune & Stratton, New York, 1983.

Feigenbaum, H.: Echocardiographic diagnosis of pericardial effusion. *Am. J. Cardiol.,* **26**:475, 1970.

Feigenbaum, H.; Waldhausen, J. A.; and Hyde, L. P.: Ultrasound diagnosis of pericardial effusion. *JAMA,* **191**:107, 1965.

Feigenbaum, H.; Zaky, A.; and Grabhorn, L.: Cardiac motion in patients with pericardial effusion: A study using ultrasound cardiography. *Circulation,* **34**:611, 1966.

Friedman, M. J.; Sahn, D. J.; and Haber, K.: Two-dimensional echocardiography and B-mode ultrasonography for the diagnosis of loculated pericardial effusion. *Circulation,* **60**:1644, 1979.

Gabor, G. E.; Winsberg, F.; and Bloom, H. S.: Electrical and mechanical alternation in pericardial effusion. *Chest,* **59**:341, 1971.

Goldberg, B. B.; Ostrum, B. J.; and Isard, J. J.: Ultrasonic determination of pericardial effusion. *JAMA,* **202**:103, 1967.

Greene, D. A.; Kleid, J. J.; and Naidu, S.: Unusual echocardiographic manifestation of pericardial effusion. *Am. J. Cardiol.,* **39**:112, 1977.

Hochberg, M. S.; Merrill, W. H.; Gruber, M.; *et al.:* Delayed cardiac tamponade associated with prophylactic anticoagulation in patients undergoing coronary bypass grafting: Early diagnosis with two-dimensional echocardiography. *J. Thorac. Cardiovasc. Surg.,* **75**:777, 1978.

Horowitz, M. S.; Schultz, C. S.; Stinson, E. B.; *et al.:* Sensitivity and specificity of echocardiographic diagnosis of pericardial effusion. *Circulation,* **50**:239, 1974.

Horowitz, M. S.; Rossen, R.; and Harrison, D. C.: Echocardiographic diagnosis of pericardial disease. *Am. Heart J.,* **97:**420, 1979.

Jacobs, W. R.; Talano, J. V.; and Loeb, H. S.: Echocardiographic interpretation of pericardial effusion. *Arch. Intern. Med.,* **138:**622, 1978.

Kleid, J. J., and Segal, B. L.: Pericardial effusion diagnosed by reflected ultrasound. *Am. J. Cardiol.,* **22:**57, 1968.

Krueger, S. K.; Zucker, R. P.; Dzindzio, B. S.; *et al.:* Swinging heart syndrome with predominant anterior pericardial effusion. *J.C.U.,* **4:**113, 1976.

Lemire, F.; Tajik, A. J.; Giuliani, E. R.; *et al.:* Further echocardiographic observations in pericardial effusion. *Mayo Clin. Proc.,* **51:**13, 1976.

Levisman, J. A.; and Abbasi, A. S.: Abnormal motion of the mitral valve with pericardial effusion: Pseudo-prolapse of the mitral valve. *Am. Heart J.,* **91:**18, 1976.

Markiewicz, W.; Brik, A.; Brook, G.; *et al.:* Pericardial rub in pericardial effusion: Lack of correlation with amount of fluid. *Chest,* **77:**643, 1980.

Martin, R. P.; Rakowski, H.; French, J.; and Popp, R. L.: Localization of pericardial effusion with wide angle phased array echocardiography. *Am. J. Cardiol.,* **42:**904, 1978.

Matsuo, H.; Matsumoto, M.; Hamanaka, Y.; *et al.:* Rotational excursion of heart in massive pericardial effusion studied by phased-array echocardiography. *Br. Heart J.,* **41:**513, 1979.

Moss, A., and Bruhn, F.: The echocardiogram: An ultrasound technic for the detection of pericardial effusion. *N. Engl. J. Med.,* **274:**380, 1966.

Nanda, N. C.; Gramiak, R.; and Gross, G. M.: Echocardiography of cardiac valves in pericardial effusion. *Circulation,* **59:**500, 1976.

Owens, J. S.; Kotler, M. N.; Segal, B. L.; *et al.:* Pseudoprolapse of the mitral valve in a patient with pericardial effusion. *Chest,* **69:**214, 1976.

Pate, J. W.; Gardner, H. C.; and Norman, R. S.: Diagnosis of pericardial effusion by echocardiography. *Ann. Surg.,* **165:**826, 1967.

Rothman, J.; Chase, N. E.; Kricheff, I.; *et al.:* Ultrasonic diagnosis of pericardial effusion. *Circulation,* **35:**358, 1967.

Sotolongo, R. P., and Horton, J. D.: Total electrical alternans in pericardial tamponade. *Am. Heart J.,* **101:**853, 1981.

Tajik, A. J.: Echocardiography in pericardial effusion. *Am. J. Med.,* **63:**29, 1977.

Tajik, A. J.: Echocardiographic evaluation of pericardial disease. *Prog. Cardiovasc. Dis.,* **21:**133, 1978.

Usher, B. W., and Popp, R. L.: Electrical alternans. Mechanism in pericardial effusion. *Am. Heart J.,* **83:**459, 1972.

Walinsky, P.: Pitfalls in the diagnosis of pericardial effusion. *Cardiovasc. Clin.,* **9:**111, 1978.

PERICARDIAL EFFUSION WITH TAMPONADE

Armstrong, W. F.; Schilt, R. F.; Helper, D. J.; *et al.:* Diastolic collapse of the right ventricle with cardiac tamponade. An echocardiographic study. *Circulation,* **65:**1491, 1982.

Baum, V. C.; Tanoff, H.; and Hoffman, J. I. E.: Pulsus paradoxus in a patient with tricuspid atresia and hypoplastic right heart. *Circulation,* **62:**651, 1980.

Brenner, J. L., and Waugh, R. A.: Effect of phasic respiration on left ventricular dimension and performance in a normal population. An echocardiographic study. *Circulation,* **57:**122, 1978.

Bulkey, B. H.; Humphries, J. O. N.; and Hutchins, G. M.: Purulent pericarditis with asymmetric cardiac tamponade: A cause of death months after coronary artery bypass surgery. *Am. Heart J.,* **93:**776, 1977.

Cosio, F.; Martinez, J. P.; Serrano, C. M.; *et al.:* Abnormal septal motion in cardiac tamponade with pulsus paradoxus. Echocardiographic and hemodynamic observations. *Chest,* **71:**787, 1977.

D'Cruz, I. A.; Cohen, H. C.; Prabhu, R.; and Glick, G.: Diagnosis of cardiac tamponade by echocardiography: Changes in mitral valve motion and ventricular dimensions, with special reference to paradoxical pulse. *Circulation,* **52:**460, 1975.

Dunlap, T. E.; Sorkin, R. P.; Mori, K. W.; *et al.:* Massive organized intrapericardial hematoma mimicking constrictive pericarditis. *Am. Heart J.,* **104:**1373, 1982.

Engel, P. J.; Hon, H.; Fowler, N. O.; *et al.:* Echocardiographic study of right ventricular wall motion in cardiac tamponade. *Am. J. Cardiol.,* **50:**1018, 1982.

Friedman, M. J.; Sahn, D. J.; and Haber, K.: Two-dimensional echocardiography and B-mode ultrasonography for the diagnosis of loculated pericardial effusion. *Circulation,* **60:**1644, 1979.

Gillam, L. D.; Guyer, D. E.; Stewart, W. J.; *et al.:* A comparison of right atrial and right ventricular inversion as echocardiographic markers of cardiac tamponade. *J.A.C.C.,* **1:**738, 1983 (Abstr.).

Hochberg, M. S.; Merrill, W. H.; Grumer, M.; *et al.:* Delayed cardiac tamponade associated with prophylactic anticoagulation in patients undergoing coronary bypass grafting: Early diagnosis with two-dimensional echocardiography. *J. Thorac. Cardiovasc. Surg.,* **75:**777, 1978.

Ieri, A., and Zipoli, A.: Abnormal diastolic motion of interventricular septum during inspiratory phase. Echocardiographic study. *Br. Heart J.,* **43:**702, 1980.

Jardin, F.; Farcot, J. C.; Boisante, L.; *et al.:* Mechanism of paradoxical pulse in bronchial asthma. *Circulation,* **66:**887, 1982.

Jones, M. R.; Vine, D. L.; Attas, M.; *et al.:* Late isolated left ventricular tamponade. Clinical, hemodynamic and echocardiographic manifestations of a previously unreported postoperative complication. *J. Thorac. Cardiovasc. Surg.,* **77:**142, 1977.

Kronzon, I.; Winer, H. E.; Weiss, E. C.; *et al.:* Echocardiographic observations of paradoxic pulse without pericardial disease. *Chest,* **78:**474, 1980.

Kronzon, I.; Winer, H.; Weiss, E.; *et al.:* Echocardiography in paradoxical pulse. *Chest,* **80:**376, 1981 (Abstr.).

Kronzon, I.; Cohen, M. L.; and Winer, H. E.: Cardiac tamponade by loculated pericardial hematoma. *J.A.C.C.,* **1:**913, 1983.

Lerman, B. B.; Talano, J. V.; Meyers, S. N.; *et al.:* Reciprocal changes in ventricular dimensions related to respiration. *Arch. Intern. Med.,* **140:**685, 1980.

Martins, J. B., and Kerber, R. E.: Can cardiac tamponade be diagnosed by echocardiography? Experimental studies. *Circulation,* **60:**737, 1979.

Miller, S. W.; Feldman, L.; Palacios, I.; *et al.:* Compression of the superior vena cava and right atrium in cardiac tamponade. *Am. J. Cardiol.,* **50:**1287, 1982.

Orzan, F.; Guttin, J.; and Dear, W. E.: Atypical late cardiac tamponade after mitral valve replacement: Case presentation with hemodynamic and echocardiographic observations. *Cathet. Cardiovasc. Diagn.,* **3:**297, 1977.

Ravindranathan, M. P.; Lipat, G.; and Sanders, M.: Unusual echocardiographic findings in pericardial tamponade. *Am. Heart J.,* **98:**225, 1979.

Rinkenberger, R. L.; Polumbo, R. A.; Bolton, M. R.; *et*

al.: Mechanism of electrical alternans in patients with pericardial effusion. *Cathet. Cardiovasc. Diagn.,* 4:63, 1978.

Ruskin, J.; Bache, J. R.; Remberg, J. C.; *et al.:* Pressure-flow studies in man: Effect of respiration on left ventricular stroke volume. *Circulation,* 48:79, 1973.

Sakamoto, T.; Tei, C.; Hayashi, T.; Ishiyasu, H.; *et al.:* Echocardiogram in pulsus paradoxus: Respiration dependent cyclic changes in mitral and aortic valve motion: A case report. *Jpn. Heart J.,* 18:883, 1977.

Sbarboro, J. A., and Brooks, H. L.: Pericardial effusion and electrical alternans: Echocardiographic assessment. *Postgrad. Med.,* 63:105, 1978.

Schiller, N. B., and Botvinick, E. H.: Right ventricular compression as a sign of cardiac tamponade: An analysis of echocardiographic ventricular dimensions and their clinical implications. *Circulation,* 56:774, 1977.

Shindler, D. M.; Reddy, K.; Shindler, O.; *et al.:* Failure of the aortic valve to open during inspiration in cardiac tamponade. *Chest,* 82:797, 1982.

Schulman, P.; Come, P. C.; Isaacs, R.; *et al.:* Left ventricular outflow obstruction induced by tamponade in hypertrophic cardiomyopathy. *Chest,* 80:110, 1981.

Settle, H. P.; Adolph, R. J.; Fowler, N. O.; *et al.:* Echocardiographic study of cardiac tamponade. *Circulation,* 56:951, 1977.

Settle, H. P.; Engle, P. J.; and Fowler, N. O.: Echocardiographic study of the paradoxical arterial pulse in chronic obstructive lung disease. *Circulation,* 62:1297, 1980.

Vignola, P. A.; Pohost, G. M.; Curfman, G. D.; *et al.:* Correlation of echocardiographic and clinical findings in patients with pericardial effusion. *Am. J. Cardiol.,* 37:701, 1976.

Winer, H. E., and Kronzon, I.: Absence of paradoxical pulse in patients with cardiac tamponade and atrial septal defects. *Am. J. Cardiol.,* 44:378, 1979.

Winer, H.; Kronzon, I.; and Glassman, E.: Echocardiographic findings in severe paradoxical pulse due to pulmonary embolization. *Am. J. Cardiol.,* 40:808, 1977.

Yeh, E. L.: Varying ejection fractions of both ventricles in paradoxical pulses. *Chest,* 74:687, 1978.

ABNORMAL INTRAPERICARDIAL ECHOES

Chandaratna, P. A., and Aronow, W. S.: Detection of pericardial metastases by cross-section echocardiography. *Circulation,* 63:197, 1981.

Chiaramida, S. A.; Goldman, M. A.; Zema, M. J.; *et al.:* Echocardiographic identification of intrapericardial fibrous strands in acute pericarditis with pericardial effusion. *Chest,* 77:85, 1980.

D'Cruz, I. A.; Bhatt, G. S.; Cohen, H. L.; *et al.:* Echocardiographic detection of cardiac involvement in patients with chronic renal failure. *Arch. Intern. Med.,* 138:720, 1978.

Friedman, M. J.; Sahn, D. J.; and Haber, K.: Two-dimensional echocardiography and B-mode ultrasonography for the diagnosis of loculated pericardial effusion. *Circulation,* 60:1644, 1979.

Martin, R. P.; Bowden, R.; Filly, K.; *et al.:* Intrapericardial abnormalities in patients with pericardial effusion. Findings by two-dimensional echocardiography. *Circulation,* 61:578, 1980.

Schuster, A. H., and Nanda, N. C.: Pericardiocentesis induced intrapericardial thrombus: Detection by two-dimensional echocardiography. *Am. Heart J.,* 104:308, 1982.

PERICARDIAL THICKENING AND CONSTRICTION

Allen, J. W.; Harrison, E. C.; Camp, J. C.; *et al.:* The role of serial echocardiography in the evaluation and differential diagnosis of pericardial disease. *Am. Heart J.,* 93:560, 1977.

Candell-Riera, J.; Garcia del Castillo, H.; Permanyermizalda, G.; *et al.:* Echocardiographic features of the interventricular septum in chronic constrictive pericarditis. *Circulation,* 57:1154, 1978.

Chandaratna, P. A. N., and Imaizumi, T.: Echocardiographic diagnosis of thickened pericardium. *Cardiovasc. Med.,* Dec., 1978, p. 1279.

Cohen, M. V.; and Greenberg, M. A.: Constrictive pericarditis: Early and late complication of cardiac surgery. *Am. J. Cardiol.,* 43:657, 1979.

D'Cruz, I. A.; Levinsky, R.; Anagnostopoulos, C.; *et al.:* Echocardiographic diagnosis of partial pericardial constriction of the left ventricle. *Radiology,* 127:755, 1978.

Feigenbaum, H.: *Echocardiography,* 2nd ed. Lea & Febiger, Philadelphia, 1976.

Gibson, T. C.; Grossman, W.; McLaurin, L. P.; *et al.:* An echocardiographic study of the interventricular septum in constrictive pericarditis. *Br. Heart J.,* 38:738, 1976.

Hancock, E. W.: Subacute effusive-constrictive pericarditis. *Circulation,* 43:183, 1971.

Horowitz, M. S.; Rossen, R.; and Harrison, D. C.: Echocardiographic diagnosis of pericardial disease. *Am. Heart J.,* 97:420, 1979.

Kutcher, M. A.; King, S. B.; Alimurung, B. N.; *et al.:* Constrictive pericarditis as a complication of cardiac surgery. *Am. J. Cardiol.,* 50:742, 1982.

Lewis, B. S.: Real time two-dimensional echocardiography in constrictive pericarditis. *Am. J. Cardiol.,* 49:1789, 1982.

Lewis, J. R.; Parker, J. O.; and Burggraf, G. W.: Echocardiography: Pericardial thickening and constrictive pericarditis. *Am. J. Cardiol.,* 42:383, 1978.

Liedtke, A. J.; DeJoseph, R. L.; and Zelis, R.: Echocardiographic observations in inflammatory pericarditis. *Ann. Intern. Med.,* 84:873, 1976.

Pool, P. E.; Seagren, S. C.; Abbasi, A. S.; Charuzi, Y.; and Kraus, R.: Echocardiographic manifestations of constrictive pericarditis. Abnormal septal motion. *Chest,* 68:684, 1975.

Schnittger, I.; Bowden, R. E.; Abrams, J.; *et al.:* Echocardiography: Pericardial thickening and constrictive pericarditis. *Am. J. Cardiol.,* 42:388, 1978.

Schwartz, D. J.; Thanavaro, S.; Keliger, R. E.; *et al.:* Epicardial pacemaker complicated by cardiac tamponade and constrictive pericarditis. *Chest,* 76:226, 1979.

Tanaka, L.; Nichimoto, M.; Takeuchi, K.; *et al.:* Presystolic pulmonary valve opening in constrictive pericarditis. *Jpn. Heart J.,* 20:419, 1979.

Tei, C.; Child, J. S.; Tanaka, H.; *et al.:* Atrial systolic notch on the interventricular septal echogram: An echocardiographic sign of constrictive pericarditis. *J.A.C.C.,* 1:907, 1983.

Voelkel, A. G.; Pietro, D. A.; Folland, E. D.; *et al.:* Echocardiographic features of constrictive pericarditis. *Circulation,* 58:871, 1978.

Wann, L. S.; Weyman, A. E.; Dillon, J. C.; *et al.:* Premature pulmonary valve opening. *Circulation,* 55:128, 1977.

Woolf, P. R., and Gewitz, M. H.: Echocardiographic indications for pericardectomy in purulent pericarditis. *Am. J. Cardiol.,* 49:1041, 1982 (Abstr.).

Absent Pericardium

Nicolisi, G. L.; Borgioni, L.; Alberti, E.; et al.: M-mode and two-dimensional echocardiography in congenital absence of the pericardium. Chest, 81:610, 1982.

Payvandi, M. N., and Kerber, R. E.: Echocardiography in congenital and acquired absence of the pericardium. Circulation, 53:86, 1976.

ECHOCARDIOGRAPHIC APPEARANCES
SIMULATING ANTERIOR PERICARDIAL
EFFUSION

Pericardial or Mediastinal Cysts; Pseudoaneurysms

Felner, J. M.; Fleming, W. H.; and Franch, R. H.: Echocardiographic identification of a pericardial cyst. Chest, 68:386, 1975.

Friday, R. O.: Paracardiac cyst: Diagnosis by ultrasound and puncture. Letter to the Editor. JAMA, 226:82, 1973.

Hynes, J. K.; Tajik, A. J.; Osborn, M. G.; et al.: Two-dimensional echocardiographic diagnosis of pericardial cyst. Prof. Mayo Clin., 58:60, 1983.

Koch, P. C.; Kronzon, I.; Winer, H. E.; et al.: Displacement of the heart by a giant mediastinal cyst. Am. J. Cardiol., 40:445, 1977.

Levy, R.; Rozanski, A.; Charuzi, Y.; et al.: Complementary roles of two-dimensional echocardiography and radionuclide ventriculography in ventricular aneurysm. Am. Heart J., 102:1066, 1981.

Oliver, J. M.; Benito, L. P.; Ferrufino, O.; et al.: Cardiac hydatid cyst diagnosed by two-dimensional echocardiography. Am. Heart J., 104:164, 1982.

Schloss, M.; Kronzon, I.; Geller, P. M.; et al.: Cystic thymoma simulating constrictive pericarditis: The role of echocardiography in the differential diagnosis. J. Thorac. Cardiovasc. Surg., 70:143, 1975.

Anterior Mediastinal Tumor

Canedo, M. I.; Otken, L.; and Stefadouros, M. A.: Echocardiographic features of cardiac compression by a thymoma simulating cardiac tamponade and obstruction of the superior vena cava. Br. Heart J., 39:1038, 1977.

Case Records of Massachusetts General Hospital: Case 50–1976: Hodgkin's mass in anterior mediastinum. N. Engl. J. Med., 295:1367, 1976.

Chandaratna, P. A. N.; Littman, B. B.; Serafini, A.; et al.: Echocardiographic evaluation of extracardiac masses. Br. Heart J., 40:741, 1978.

Gottdiener, J. S.; and Maron, B. J.: Posterior cardiac displacement by anterior mediastinal tumor. Chest, 77:784, 1980.

Nishimura, T.; Kondo, M.; Miyazaki, S.; et al.: Two-dimensional echocardiographic findings of cardiovascular involvement by invasive thymoma. Chest, 81:752, 1982.

Panella, J. S.; Paige, M. L.; Victor, T. A.; et al.: Angiosarcoma of the heart. Diagnosis by echocardiography. Chest, 76:221, 1979.

Epicardial Fat

Gramiak, R., and Nanda, N. C.: Clinical Echocardiography. C. V. Mosby, St. Louis, 1978, p. 276.

Isner, J. M.; Carter, B. C.; Roberts, W. C.; et al.: Subepicardial adipose tissue producing echocardiographic appearance of pericardial effusion. Documentation by computed tomography and necropsy. Am. J. Cardiol., 51:656, 1983.

Wada, T.; Honda, M.; and Matsuyama, S.: What do extra echo spaces on echocardiography represent? A correlated study with computed tomography. Am. J. Cardiol., 45:1020, 1982 (Abstr.).

Diaphragmatic Hernia (Foramen of Morgagni)

Popp, R. L., and Harrison, D. C.: Echocardiography. In: Weissler, A. M. (ed.): Noninvasive Cardiology. Grune & Stratton, New York, 1974, pp. 149–226.

ECHOCARDIOGRAPHIC APPEARANCES
SIMULATING POSTERIOR PERICARDIAL
EFFUSION

Pleural Effusion

Feigenbaum, H.: Echocardiography, 3rd ed. Lea & Febiger, Philadelphia, 1981, pp. 485–489.

Haaz, W. S.; Mintz, G. S.; Kotler, M. N.; et al.: Two-dimensional echocardiographic recognition of the descending thoracic aorta: Value in differentiating pericardial from pleural effusions. Am. J. Cardiol., 46:739, 1980.

Lewandowski, B. J.; Jaffe, N. M.; and Winsberg, F.: Relationship between the pericardial and pleural spaces in cross-sectional imaging. J.C.U., 9:271, 1981.

Mitral Annulus Calcification

Hirschfeld, D. S., and Emilson, B. B.: Echocardiogram in calcified mitral annulus. Am. J. Cardiol., 36:354, 1975.

Left Atrial Enlargement

Ratshin, R. A.; Smith, M.; and Hood, W. P.: Possible false-positive diagnosis of pericardial effusion by echocardiography in presence of large left atrium. Chest, 65:112, 1974.

Reeves, W. C.; Ciotola, T.; Babb, J. D.; et al.: Prolapsed left atrium behind the left ventricular posterior wall: Two-dimensional echocardiographic and angiographic features. Am. J. Cardiol., 47:708, 1981.

Coronary Sinus

Cohen, B. E.; Winer, H. E.; and Kronzon, I.: Echocardiographic findings in patients with left superior vena cava and dilated coronary sinus. Am. J. Cardiol., 44:158, 1979.

Hibi, N.; Fukui, Y.; Nishimura, K.; et al.: Cross-sectional echocardiographic study on persistent left superior vena cava. Am. Heart J., 100:69, 1980.

Orsmond, G. S.; Ruttenberg, H. D.; Bessinger, F. B.; et al.: Echocardiographic features of total anomalous pulmonary venous connection to the coronary sinus. Am. J. Cardiol., 41:597, 1978.

Snider, A. R.; Ports, T. A.; and Silverman, N. H.: Venous anomalies of the coronary sinus: Detection by M-mode, two-dimensional and contrast echocardiography. Circulation, 60:721, 1979.

Pancreatic Pseudocyst

Shah, A., and Schwartz, H.: Echocardiographic features of cardiac compression by mediastinal pancreatic pseudocyst. Chest, 77:440, 1980.

Tumor Compressing Left Atrium

Yoshikawa, J.; Sabah, I.; Yanagihara, Y.; et al.: Cross-sectional echocardiographic diagnosis of large left atrial tumor and extracardiac tumor compression the left atrium: Limitation of M-mode echocardiography in distinguishing the two lesions. Am. J. Cardiol., 42:853, 1978.

Subvalvular LV Aneurysm

Hickey, A. J., and Braye, S.: Annular subvalvular left ventricular aneurysm mimicking a pericardial effusion on echocardiogram. Aust. N.Z. J. Med., 9:251, 1979.

Coronary Arteriovenous Aneurysm

Come, P. C.; Riley, M. F.; and Fortuin, N. J.: Echocardiographic mimicry of pericardial effusion. *Am. J. Cardiol.,* **47:**365, 1981.

Pericardial Tumors

Come, P. C.; Riley, M. F.; and Fortuin, N. J.: Echocardiographic mimicry of pericardial effusion. *Am. J. Cardiol.,* **47:**365, 1981.

Foote, W. C.; Jefferson, C. M.; and Price, H. L.: False-positive echocardiographic diagnosis of pericardial effusion. Result of tumor encasement of the heart simulating constrictive pericarditis. *Chest,* **71:**546, 1977.

Lin, T. K.; Stech, J. M.; and Eckert, W. G.: Pericardial angiosarcoma simulating pericardial effusion by echocardiography. *Chest,* **73:**881, 1978.

Millman, A.; Meller, J.; Motro, M.; *et al.:* Pericardial tumor or fibrosis mimicking pericardial effusion by echocardiography. *Ann. Intern. Med.,* **86:**434, 1977.

PERICARDIAL INVOLVEMENT IN SPECIFIC DISEASES

Chronic Renal Failure

D'Cruz, I. A.; Bhatt, G. R.; Cohen, H. C.; *et al.:* Echocardiographic detection of cardiac involvement in patients with chronic renal failure. *Arch. Intern. Med.,* **138:**720, 1978.

Goldstein, D. H.; Nagar, C.; Srivastava, N.; *et al.:* Clinically silent pericardial effusions in patients on long-term hemodialysis. *Chest,* **72:**744, 1977.

Kleiman, J. H.; Motta, J.; Jordan, E.; *et al.:* Pericardial effusions in patients with end-stage renal disease. *Br. Heart J.,* **40:**190, 1978.

Luft, F. C.; Gilman, J. K.; and Weyman, A. E.: Pericarditis in the patient with uremia. Clinical and echocardiographic evaluation. *Nephron,* **25:**160, 1980.

Winney, R. J.; Wright, N.; Sumerling, M. D.; *et al.:* Echocardiography in uremic pericarditis with effusion. *Nephron,* **18:**209, 1977.

Yoshida, K.; Shina, A.; Asano, Y.; *et al.:* Uremic pericardial effusion: Detection and evaluation of uremic pericardial effusion by echocardiography. *Clin. Nephrol.,* **13:**260, 1980.

Collagen Diseases

Collins, R. L.; Turner, R. A.; Nomeir, A. M.; *et al.:* Cardiopulmonary manifestations of systemic lupus erythematosus. *J. Rheumatol.,* **5:**279, 1978.

Elkayam, U.; Weiss, S.; and Laniado, S.: Pericardial effusion and mitral valve involvement in systemic lupus erythematosus. Echocardiographic study. *Ann. Rheum. Dis.,* **36:**349, 1977.

Nomeir, A. M.; Turner, R. A.; and Watts, L. E.: Cardiac involvement in rheumatoid arthritis. *Arthritis Rheum.,* **22:**561, 1979.

Weiss, S.; Zyskind, A.; Rosenthal, T.; *et al.:* Cardiac involvement in progressive systemic sclerosis—an echocardiographic study. *Z. Rheumatol.,* **39:**190, 1980.

Cardiac Failure

Kessler, K. M.; Rodriguez, D.; Rahim, A.; *et al.:* Echocardiographic observations regarding pericardial effusions associated with cardiac disease. *Chest,* **78:**736, 1980.

Postcardiac Surgery

Clapp, S. K.; Garson, A.; Gutgesell, H. P.; *et al.:* Postoperative pericardial effusion and its relation to post pericardiotomy syndrome. *Pediatrics,* **66:**585, 1980.

Righetti, A.; Crawford, M. H.; O'Rourke, R. A.; *et al.:* Echocardiographic and roentgenographic determination of left ventricular size after coronary arterial bypass graft surgery. *Chest,* **72:**455, 1977.

Postradiation Malignant Lymphoma

Markiewicz, W.; Glatstein, E.; London, E. J.; *et al.:* Echocardiographic detection of pericardial effusion and pericardial thickening in malignant lymphoma. *Radiology,* **123:**161, 1977.

Hypothyroidism

Hardisty, C. A.; Naik, D. R.; and Munro, D. S.: Pericardial effusion in hypothyroidism. *Clin. Endocrinol. (Oxf.),* **13:**349, 1980.

Pregnancy

Haiat, R.; Halphen, C.; Clement, F.; *et al.:* Silent pericardial effusion in late pregnancy. *Chest,* **74:**717, 1981.

O

Bacterial Endocarditis—General Remarks

Since the description of the M-mode appearances of valvular vegetations by Dillon et al. (1973) and Spangler et al. (1973), this application of echocardiography has aroused great interest among internists and cardiologists. Subsequently, the M-mode features of vegetations were described in fuller detail (Wann et al., 1976; Roy et al., 1976; Andy et al., 1977). The screening of patients presenting with unexplained fever or cerebrovascular accidents for possible vegetations on the heart valves constitutes a large proportion of the patient load in most echocardiographic laboratories.

The 2-D characteristics of bacterial endocarditis were reported by Gilbert et al. (1977), and recently the echocardiographic literature has been enriched by a spate of papers from several leading centers (Mintz et al., 1979; Wann et al., 1979; Stewart et al., 1980; Strom et al., 1980; Martin et al., 1980; Davis et al., 1980; Talano and Mehlman, 1981; Come et al., 1982). These authors have attempted to answer the following practical clinical questions:

1. With what frequency are valvular vegetations detected by echocardiography? What is the incidence of false negatives?

2. How does the diagnostic ability of the M-mode technique compare with that of 2-D echography?

3. Are there any echocardiographic characteristics that can serve as predictors for prognosis and therefore in deciding the necessity for valve replacement?

4. Can serial echocardiograms provide reliable information about the cause of bacterial endocarditis? What is the "natural history" of the echographic appearances of vegetations?

The answers to these queries are contained in the following general conclusions:

1. Evidence of vegetations or valve destruction, or both, was detected in three quarters or more of all patients with definite endocarditis (Wann et al., 1979; Martin et al., 1980), but others (Mintz et al., 1979) reported a sensitivity in the 50 per cent range.

2. Martin et al. (1980) found 2-D echocardiography much superior to the M-mode technique in making a definite diagnosis of vegetations, but others (Mintz et al., 1979; Wann et al., 1979) reported that M-mode and 2-D echography could detect valvular vegetations with almost equal frequency. However, Mintz et al. (1979) found that 2-D echography was far superior to the M-mode technique in visualizing complications of endocarditis such as flail aortic, mitral, or tricuspid leaflets, aortic root abscess, and sinus of Valsalva aneurysms. Stafford et al. (1979) pointed out that the size and shape of vegetations were appreciated better by 2-D echography, whereas the density of the echoes (quality of echo reflection) showed up better in M-mode echocardiograms.

Martin et al. (1980) distinguished between vegetations recognizable as definite "masses" and others with abnormal but nonspecific morphology, not specifically recognizable as a mass lesion. They found that the mass type of lesion was specific for vegetations, since 15 patients without endocarditis (but initially referred for clinically suspected intracardiac infection) did not show such appearances. Two-D echography could identify mass lesions diagnostic of vegetations in about four fifths of patients proven to have endocarditis; nonspecific changes were noted in the remaining cases. On the other hand, M-mode echocardiography identified specific mass lesions of vegetations in only about one seventh of patients and nonspecific valve changes in another one third. These authors thus found 2-D echocardiography considerably superior to the M-mode technique in the diagnosis of bacterial endocarditis. In particular, the 2-D technique is very useful in detecting tricuspid and prosthetic valve vegetations. By M-mode echocardiography, good visualization of the tricuspid valve is difficult to achieve unless the RV is dilated; prosthetic valve echoes are usually so dense and pervasive that the identification of abnormal echoes due to vegetations within them is impossible on the M-mode tracing.

3. Patients suffering from bacterial endocarditis who exhibit vegetations on echocardiography tend to have more severe disease in the sense that they have a higher incidence of embolism, congestive heart failure, and the necessity for valve surgery (Wann *et al.,* 1976; Stewart *et al.,* 1980). However, it is now generally agreed that patients who show vegetations and do not undergo surgery are *not* doomed. The demonstration of a flail aortic or mitral leaflet, by M-mode or 2-D echography, is usually associated with severe regurgitation, often with rapidly worsening left heart failure, and surgical therapy sooner or later. The M-mode finding of premature mitral valve closure in a patient with aortic valve endocarditis indicates very severe aortic regurgitation and necessitates early valve replacement. The size of vegetations has no bearing on prognosis. According to some, and in the experience of Talano and Mehlman (1981), vegetations that are large (over 5 mm) or pedunculated carry a higher risk of embolization and death.

4. Serial echocardiography, in some cases over many months, in patients who made a clinical recovery with antibiotic therapy (Stafford *et al.,* 1979; Stewart *et al.,* 1980) brought to light the somewhat surprising finding that abnormal echoes representing the vegetation on the valves persist long beyond bacteriologic cure and even indefinitely in the majority of cases. They may decrease in size in some instances and also become more dense, presumably because the vegetations and the valves affected heal by dense scarring and perhaps calcification. Should such a patient subsequently come under suspicion for new bacterial endocarditis, the residual abnormalities of the old, healed vegetations can easily confuse the echocardiographer and make the diagnosis of new vegetations difficult or impossible. Such predicaments are not rare among drug addicts and patients in chronic renal failure on dialysis.

5. Echocardiography can be of great diagnostic value in culture-negative bacterial endocarditis. In a series of 11 such instances, 5 of whom had infected native valves and 6 prosthetic valves, Rubenson *et al.* (1981) showed that vegetations were detectable in 8. Moreover, complications such as paravalvar abscess and valve dehiscence, revealed by echography in some cases, were of crucial interest to the cardiac surgeon.

Certain practical echocardiographic details, applicable to patients with suspected bacterial endocarditis, are worth mentioning:

1. Setting the gain too high will exaggerate the size of the vegetation and may cause it to coalesce indistinctly with neighboring structures. Too low a gain setting may suppress small vegetations (Berger *et al.,* 1980). Suspicious echoes should be recorded in as many views as possible, and later viewed carefully in slow motion as well as real time.

2. The echocardiographic examination itself is best performed by the experienced physician-echocardiographer, who is fully aware of the clinical findings and can concentrate his attention on specific areas under suspicion so as to obtain the maximum diagnostic information. Far-reaching decisions regarding surgical intervention or prolonged high-dose antibiotic therapy may well depend on the echocardiographic verdict.

Talano and Mehlman (1981) recently have analyzed the cumulative data from 12 echocardiographic-clinical correlative studies (including their own); 7 of these were restricted to the M-mode technique, whereas 5 utilized 2-D echography. Of the total 425 patients reported, 257 (60 per cent) had vegetation-positive endocarditis and 168 (40 per cent) vegetation-negative endocarditis. It became strikingly obvious that the presence of vegetations in a patient with bacterial endocarditis worsened the prognosis in several ways: the mortality was higher (14 versus 4 per cent); valve replacement therapy was required much more often (53 versus 7 per cent); congestive heart failure was twice as common (57 versus 24 per cent); and embolization was many times as frequent (33 versus 4 per cent).

In their own series of 32 patients studied by both M-mode and 2-D techniques, Talano and Mehlman found that the diagnostic sensitivity of echocardiography was 88 per cent and the specificity (in patients presenting as suspected bacterial endocarditis) was 96 per cent.

In conclusion, the optimal diagnostic use of echocardiography in bacterial endocarditis depends not only on skillful recording and reliable interpretation of the echocardiogram itself, but also on (1) proper awareness of the sensitivity and specificity of the technique in identifying vegetations, (2) significance of associated echographic appearances suggesting hemodynamic deterioration, abscess extension, or flail valve motion, and (3) basing management decisions not on the echogram alone, but on the entire clinical picture.

REFERENCES

Andy, J. J.; Sheikh, M. U.; Ali, N.; et al.: Echocardiographic observations in opiate addicts with active infective endocarditis. Am. J. Cardiol., 40:17, 1977.

Berger, M.; Delfin, L. A.; Jelveh, M.; et al.: Two-dimensional echocardiographic findings in right-sided infective endocarditis. Circulation, 61:855, 1980.

Come, P. C.; Isaacs, R. E.; and Riley, M. F.: Diagnostic accurracy of M-mode echocardiography in active infective endocarditis and prognostic implications of ultrasound-detectable vegetations. Am. Heart J., 103:839, 1982.

Davis, R. S.; Strom, J. A.; Frishman, W.; et al.: The demonstration of vegetations by echocardiography in bacterial endocarditis. Am. J. Med., 69:57, 1980.

Dillon, J. C.; Feigenbaum, H.; and Konecke, L. L.: Echocardiographic manifestations of valvular vegetations. Am. Heart J., 86:698, 1973.

Gilbert, B. W.; Haney, R. S.; Crawford, F.; et al.: Two-dimensional echocardiographic assessment of vegetative endocarditis. Circulation, 55:346, 1977.

Martin, R. P.; Meltzer, R. S.; Chia, B. L.; et al.: Clinical utility of two-dimensional echocardiography in infective endocarditis. Am. J. Cardiol., 46:379, 1980.

Mintz, G. S.; Kotler, M. N.; Segal, B. L.; et al.: Comparison of two-dimensional and M-mode echocardiography in the evaluation of patients with infective endocarditis. Am. J. Cardiol., 43:738, 1979.

Roy, P.; Tajik, A. J.; Guiliani, E. R.; et al.: Spectrum of echocardiographic findings in bacterial endocarditis. N. Engl. J. Med., 295:135, 1976.

Rubenson, D. S.; Tucker, C. R.; Stinson, E. B.; et al.: The use of echocardiography in diagnosing culture-negative endocarditis. Circulation, 64:641, 1981.

Spangler, R. D.; Johnson, M. J.; Holmes, H. J.; et al.: Echocardiographic demonstration of bacterial vegetations in active infective endocarditis. J.C.U., 1:126, 1973.

Stafford, A.; Wann, L. S.; Dillon, J. C.; et al.: Serial echocardiographic appearance of healing bacterial vegetations. Am. J. Cardiol., 44:754, 1979.

Stewart, J. A.; Silimperi, D.; Harris, P.; et al.: Echocardiographic documentation of vegetative lesions in infective endocarditis: Clinical implications. Circulation, 61:374, 1980.

Strom, J.; Becker, R.; Davis, R.; et al.: Echocardiographic and surgical correlations in bacterial endocarditis. Circulation, 62:1164, 1980.

Talano, J. V., and Mehlman, D. J.: Two-dimensional echocardiography in infective endocarditis. Semin. Ultrasound, 2:149, 1981.

Wann, L. S.; Dillon, J. C.; Weyman, A. E.; et al.: Echocardiography in bacterial endocarditis. N. Engl. J. Med., 295:135, 1976.

Wann, L. S.; Hollain, C. C.; Dillon, J. C.; et al.: Comparison of M-mode and cross-sectional echocardiography in infective endocarditis. Circulation, 60:728, 1979.

Index